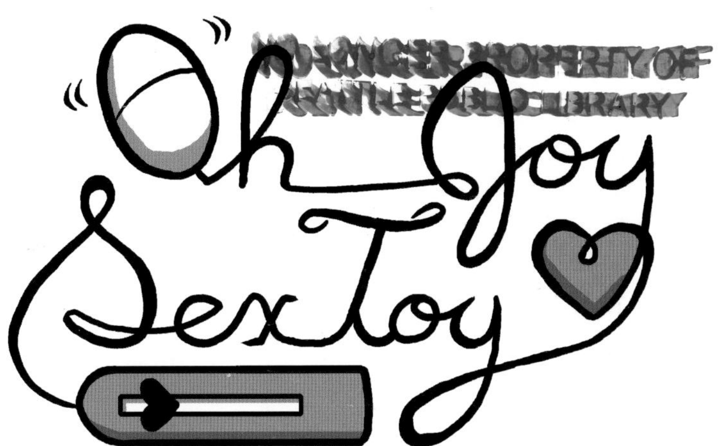
Oh Joy
Sex Toy

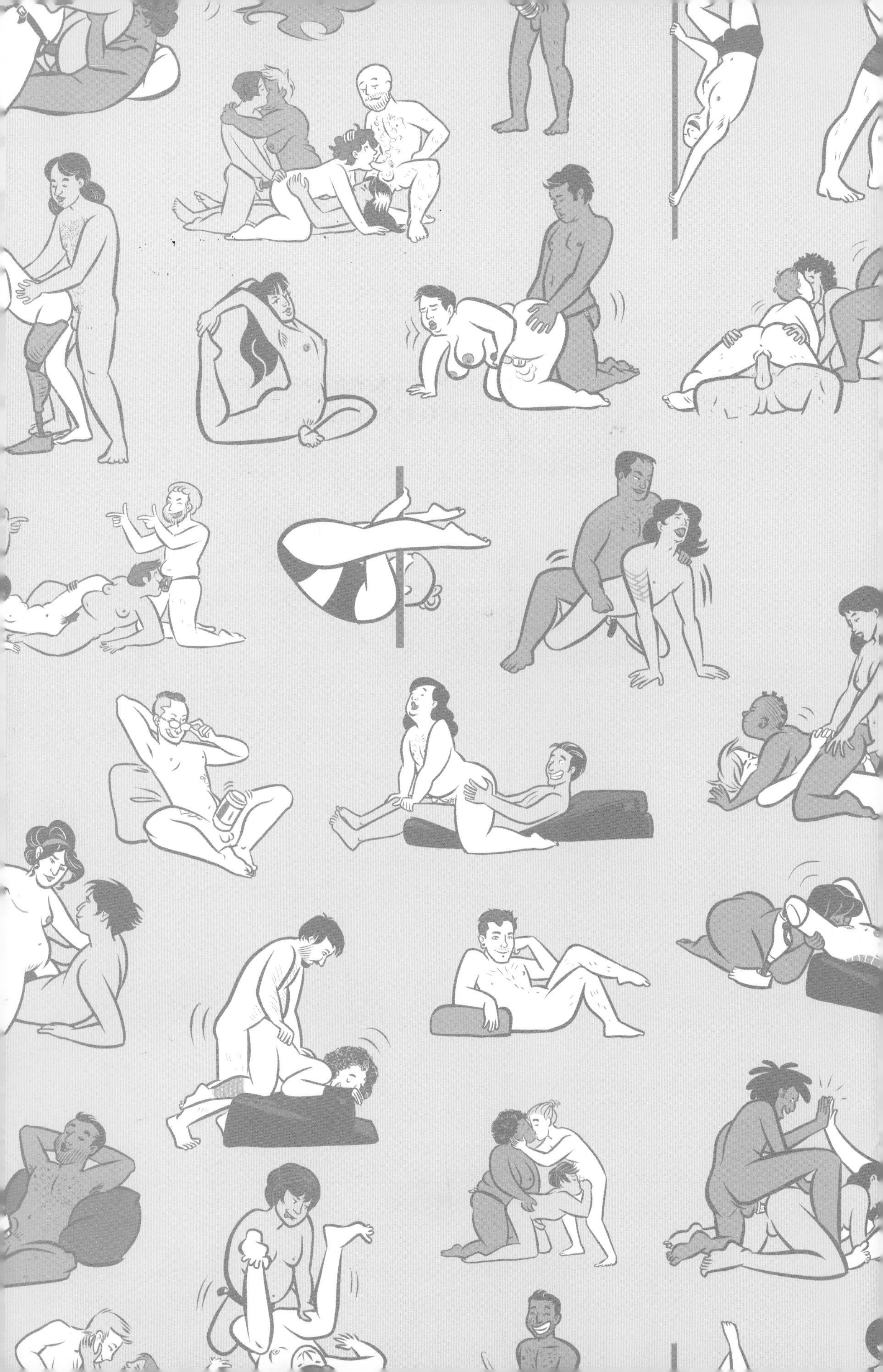

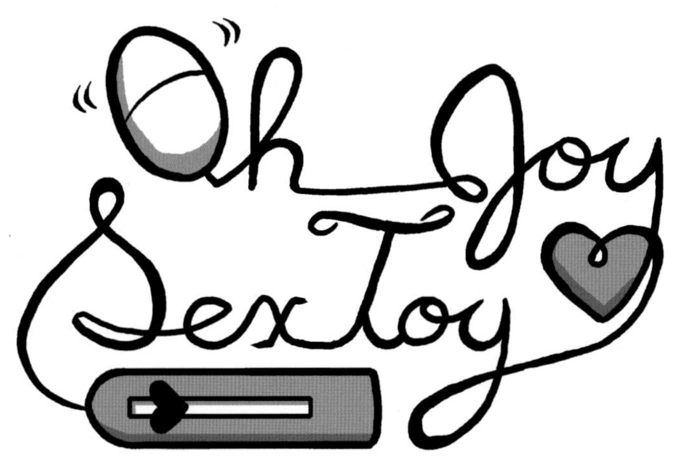

created by

ERIKA MOEN

&

MATTHEW NOLAN

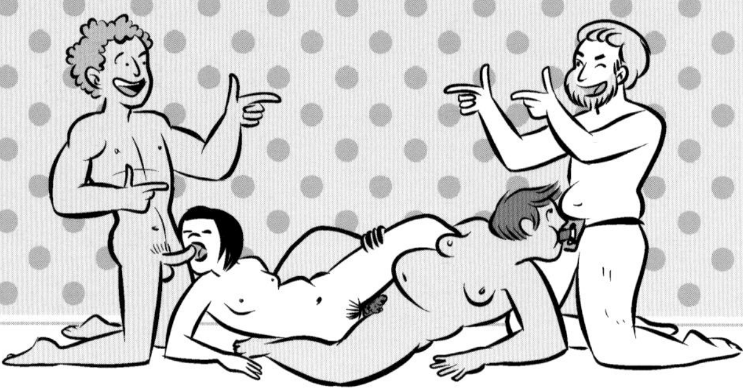

Collection Design
Matthew Nolan and Allyson Haller

Published by Erika Moen Comics & Illustration, LLC
Persiscope Studio
333 SW 5th Ave, Suite 500
Portland, OR 97204

First edition: November 2015
ISBN 978-0-9823437-9-1

OhJoySexToy.com

Table of Contents

Introduction

ERIKA MOEN AND MATTHEW NOLAN JUST GET IT.

It's still mighty rare in the worlds we live in, to find sex information for those of any age, that is complete and holistic, fun without being flippant, sexy without being smug. Where even sound factual information about parts of sex thought to be un-sexy by a lot of people (like infections and contraception or economics) still has a giant jet stream of pleasure and joy running through it all.

But Erika Moen and Matthew Nolan get it. And Oh Joy Sex Toy gives it.

Sex toy reviews are at the core of what you'll find here. In these you'll find a straightforward detailed and enjoyable approach that makes even a lackluster review feel like it was worth your while. I suspect there have been a few times, in fact, where the making or the reading of the comic was a lot more fun than the toy itself.

But you'll also find information on lubricants, contraceptive methods, STIs, safer sex tools and other sexual health issues. It covers negotiating sex within relationships, starter guides for sexual activities like oral or anal sex (starring the anal safety snails, who I really wish were the kind I found in my garden), advice on how to navigate everything from online personals to strip club etiquette and restraint to consent. There are things for everyone to learn in all of this, even for those of us who have been working as sex geeks for a very long time.

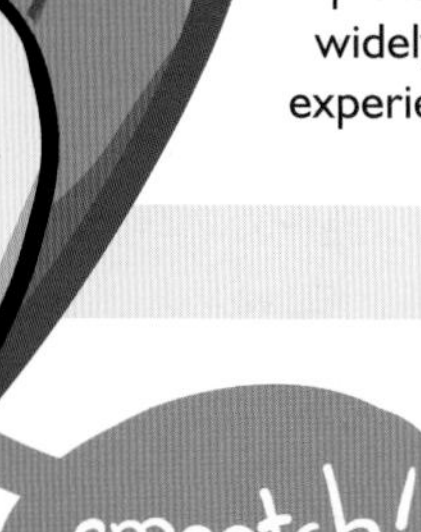

Erika and Matthew do something else I deeply appreciate: they pull together people from different areas of sexuality work, rather than keeping everyone in the segregated boxes we all too often stay shut in. Putting porn actors and actresses together with sex toy purveyors, illustrators with sex and relationships educators, neurosex geeks with swingers. They give you the benefit of the big picture from an awful lot of perspectives, meshed together from a group that rarely find opportunities that allow this kind of creative and intellectual union.

There's something special that seems to happen when sexuality information is centered around sex toys: it effortlessly encourages sex as a way for people to bring play back into their lives (though hopefully, it never left). Then you add Erika and Matthew's wit and whimsy, wonderful illustration style and the radically fantastic guests to that built-in center of play and pleasure. If more sex ed was like this, everyone would be a sex geek. If more sex ed was like this, I truly believe everyone would be having exceptional sexual lives they felt better about.

Did you know that some people — quite a lot of people really — still don't get that sex is primarily about play and pleasure? It's bonkers, I know, but it's true. What kind of play and pleasure we're talking about obviously varies widely from person to person, experience to experience. But when we get all the way down

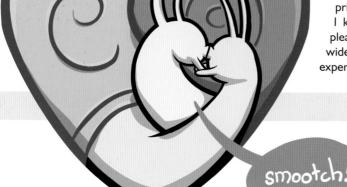

to the real nitty-gritty, sex is ultimately about the pleasure found in play. Whether we include others in our sexual lives or not, it's about being creative, spontaneous, curious to explore and enjoy our senses, our bodies, our hearts and our minds and — including the wondrous weirdness of them all — being free.

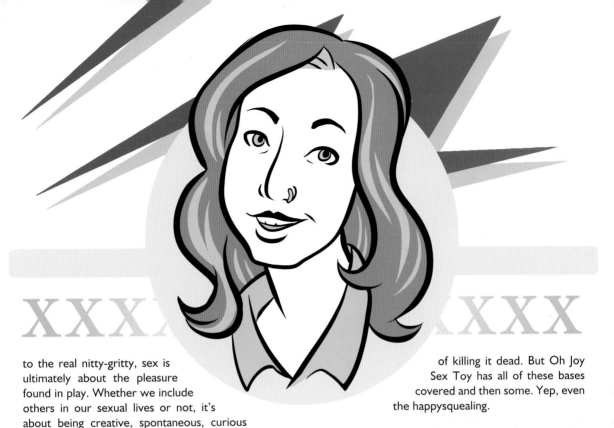

Play, pleasure and discussing sex and what can happen within it seriously aren't mutually exclusive. A lot of people really don't get that part, and that's mighty sad, because that truly is where all of the richest and most interesting of what sex can offer us is usually found.

I'm often asked for sex information resources for those who are older than the teens and emerging adults we serve at Scarleteen. Sadly, while there's a lot of information and sexuality content for adults out there, there's not a whole lot I feel very excited about. There's very little I feel wiggle-in-your-chair-happysqueal about and little where I find all the pieces I think of as essential in place. The facts are factual, the scope wide and holistic, the information truly inclusive as well as sound and supportive, and the approach accessible and — imagine! — also enjoyable and fun. It's in support of your sexybuzz-on instead of killing it dead. But Oh Joy Sex Toy has all of these bases covered and then some. Yep, even the happysquealing.

It's one of those rare projects in this field that has all the right pistons firing when it comes to sex, sexuality information and education. It's designed for an incredibly wide range of ages and ways of being a sexual active person with a sexuality. It brings something new, fresh and unexpected to the table that is both delightful and so needed.

Erika Moen and Matthew Nolan get it. And now you have what they get so well, right here in your greedy little hands.

Enjoy it. Keep hot liquids at a safe distance while reading and don't read it on the bus if you don't want to have to fight the compulsion to show everyone on board what you're laughing at so hard. Then go play already, for crying out loud. Play is truly a serious business, it's one of the biggest parts of what makes them joyful. We need it in our lives, most certainly including our sexual lives.

- Heather Corinna
Founder of Scarlateen.com

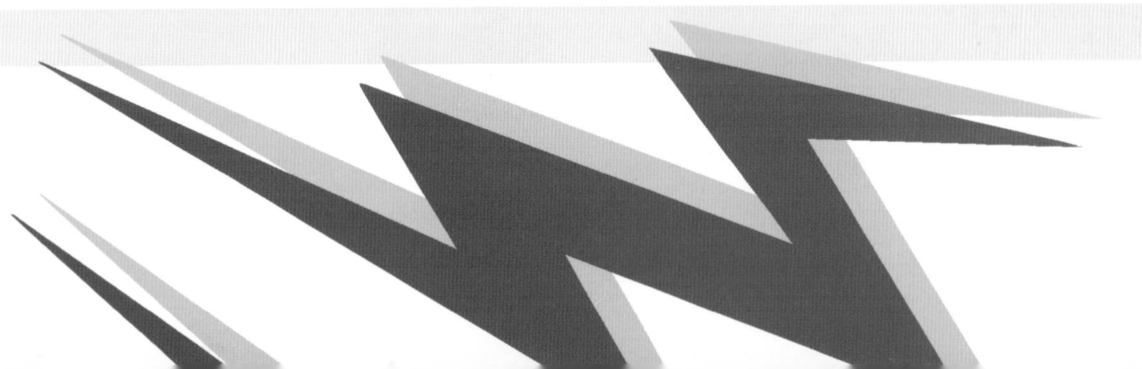

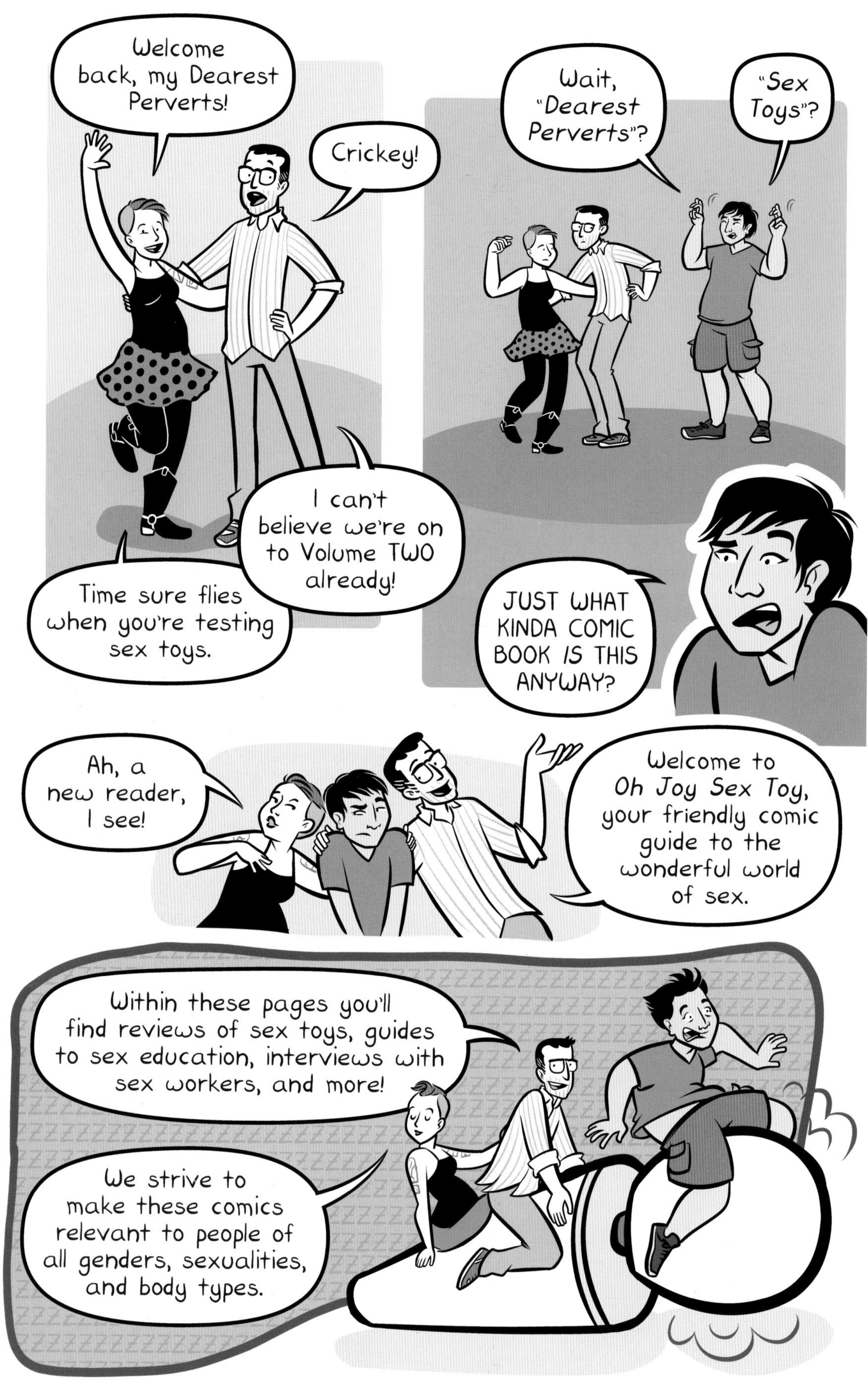
Welcome back, my Dearest Perverts!
Crickey!
Wait, "Dearest Perverts"?
"Sex Toys"?
I can't believe we're on to Volume TWO already!
Time sure flies when you're testing sex toys.
JUST WHAT KINDA COMIC BOOK IS THIS ANYWAY?
Ah, a new reader, I see!
Welcome to Oh Joy Sex Toy, your friendly comic guide to the wonderful world of sex.
Within these pages you'll find reviews of sex toys, guides to sex education, interviews with sex workers, and more!
We strive to make these comics relevant to people of all genders, sexualities, and body types.

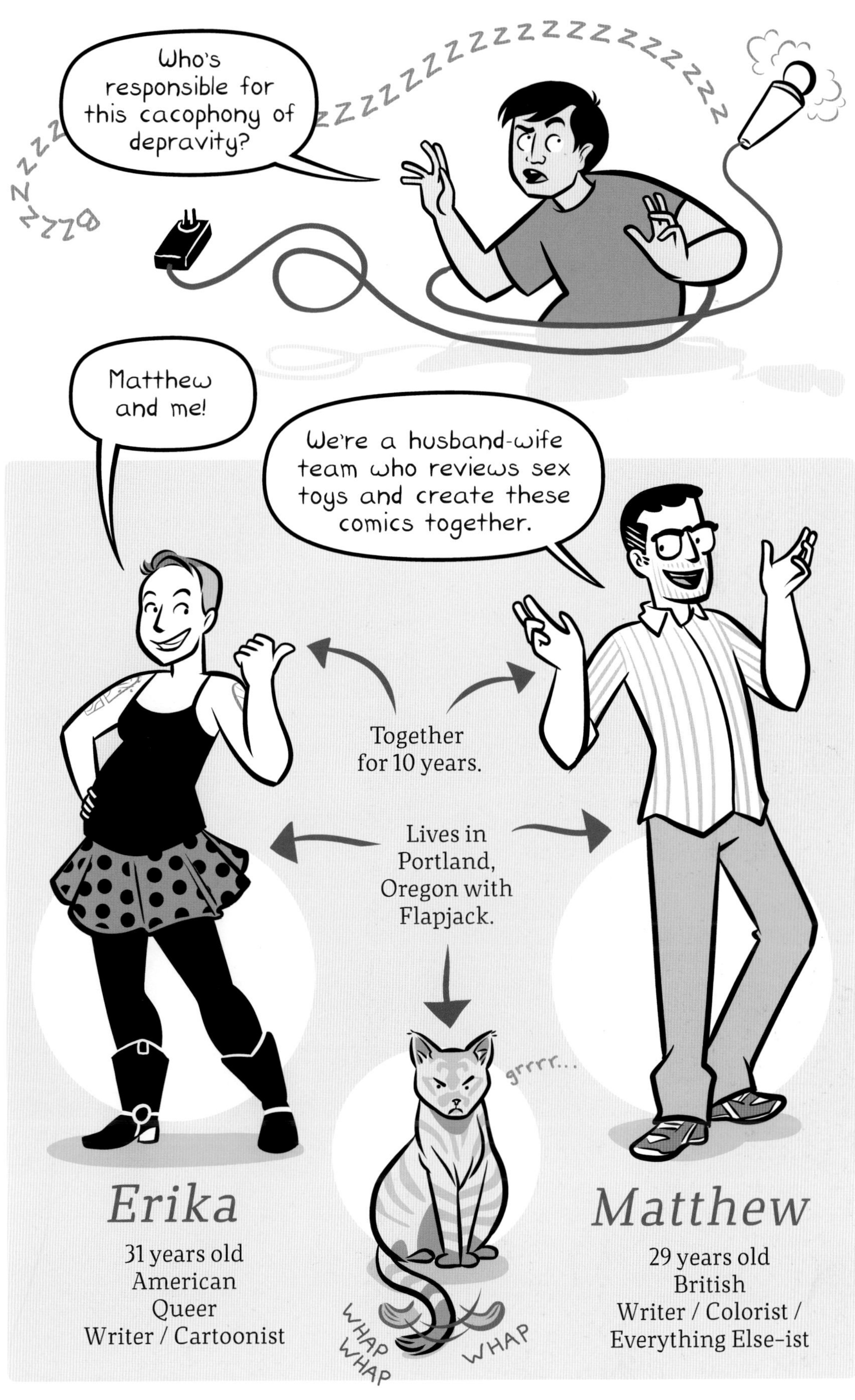
BZZZZZZZZZZZZZZZZZZZZZZZZZZZZZZZ
Who's responsible for this cacophony of depravity?
Matthew and me!
We're a husband-wife team who reviews sex toys and create these comics together.
Together for 10 years.
Lives in Portland, Oregon with Flapjack.
grrrr...
Erika
31 years old
American
Queer
Writer / Cartoonist
WHAP WHAP
WHAP
Matthew
29 years old
British
Writer / Colorist / Everything Else-ist

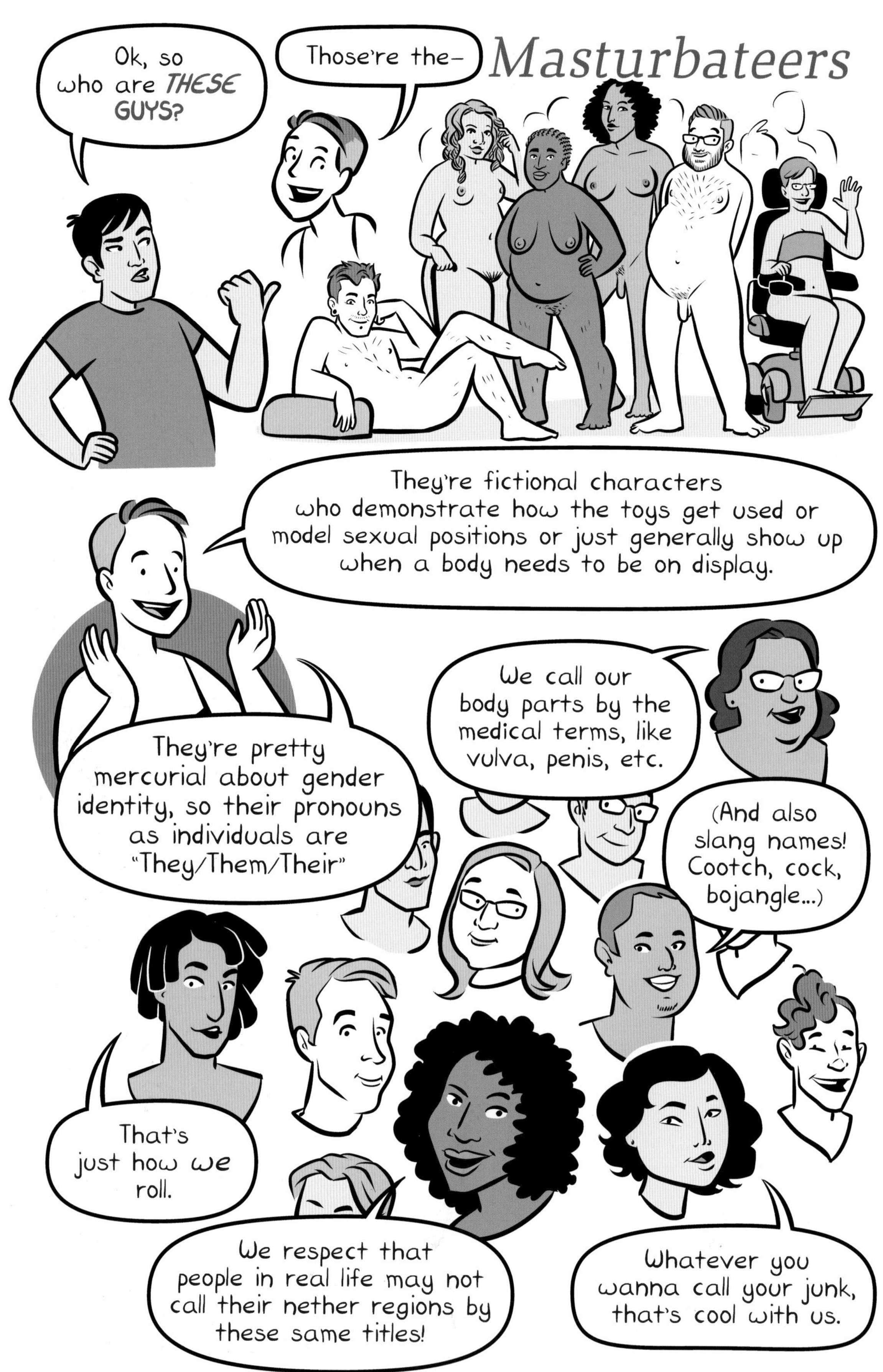
Ok, so who are THESE GUYS?
Those're the–
Masturbateers
They're fictional characters who demonstrate how the toys get used or model sexual positions or just generally show up when a body needs to be on display.
They're pretty mercurial about gender identity, so their pronouns as individuals are "They/Them/Their"
We call our body parts by the medical terms, like vulva, penis, etc.
(And also slang names! Cootch, cock, bojangle...)
That's just how we roll.
We respect that people in real life may not call their nether regions by these same titles!
Whatever you wanna call your junk, that's cool with us.

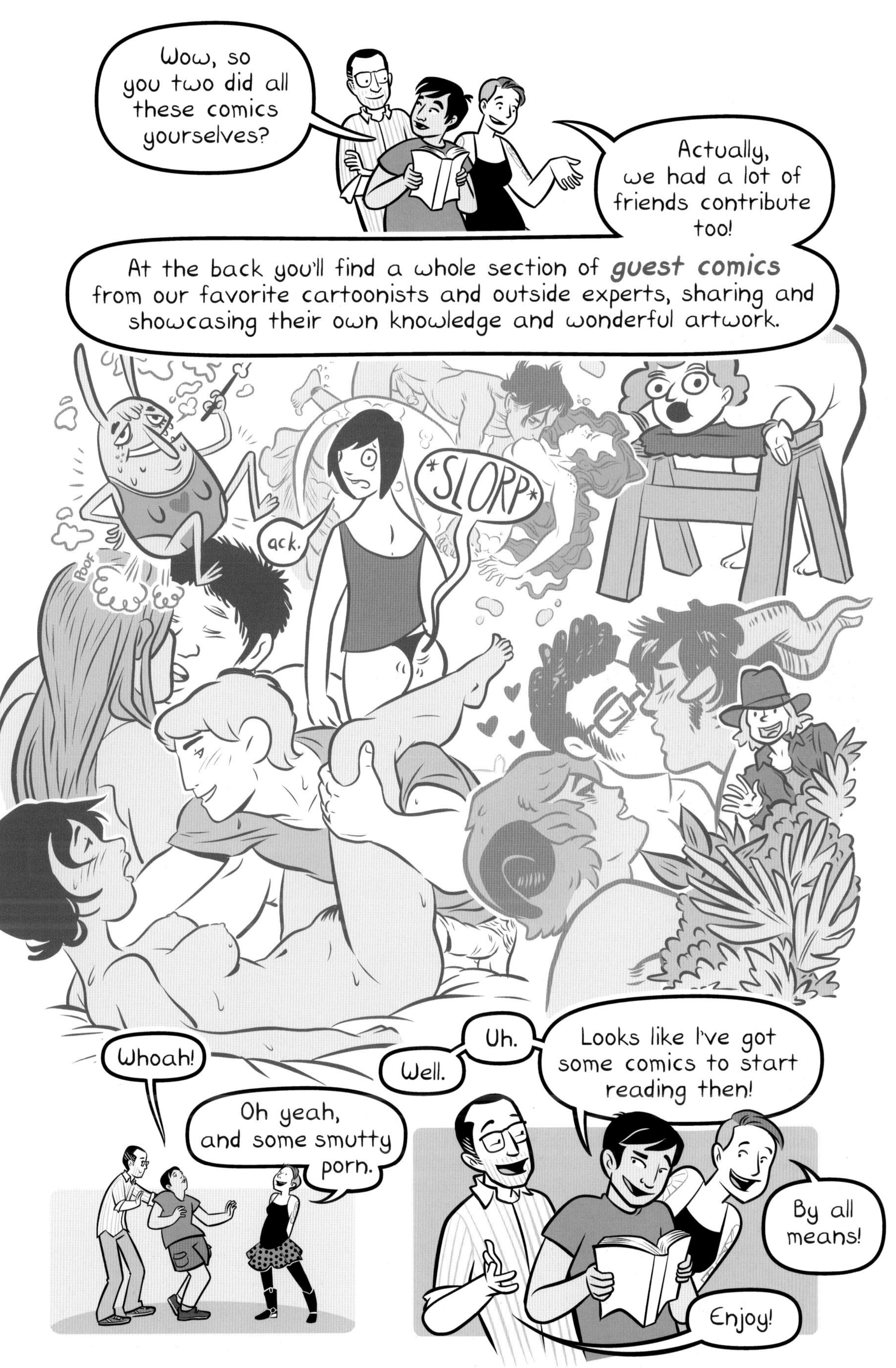
Wow, so you two did all these comics yourselves?
Actually, we had a lot of friends contribute too!
At the back you'll find a whole section of ***guest comics*** from our favorite cartoonists and outside experts, sharing and showcasing their own knowledge and wonderful artwork.
ack.
SLORP
POOF
Whoah!
Oh yeah, and some smutty porn.
Uh.
Well.
Looks like I've got some comics to start reading then!
By all means!
Enjoy!

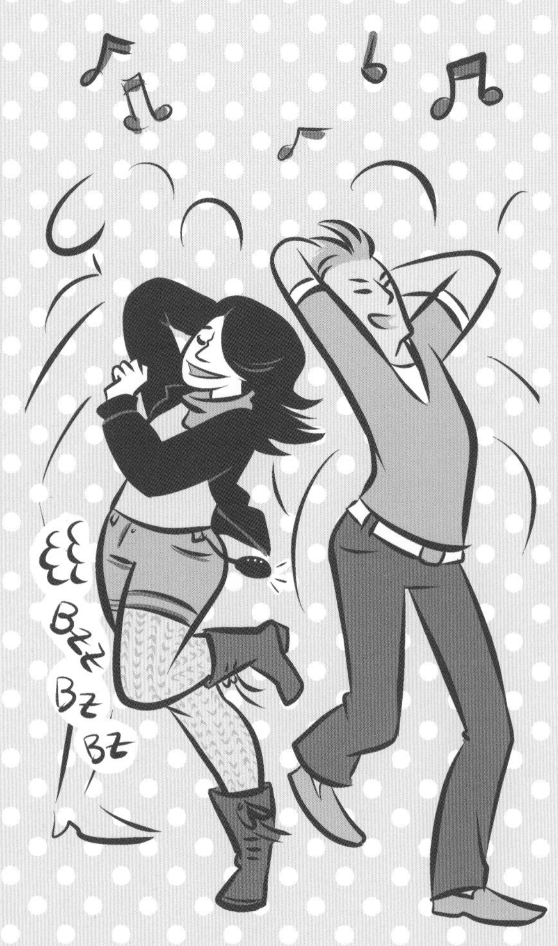
Bzzz
Bz
Bz

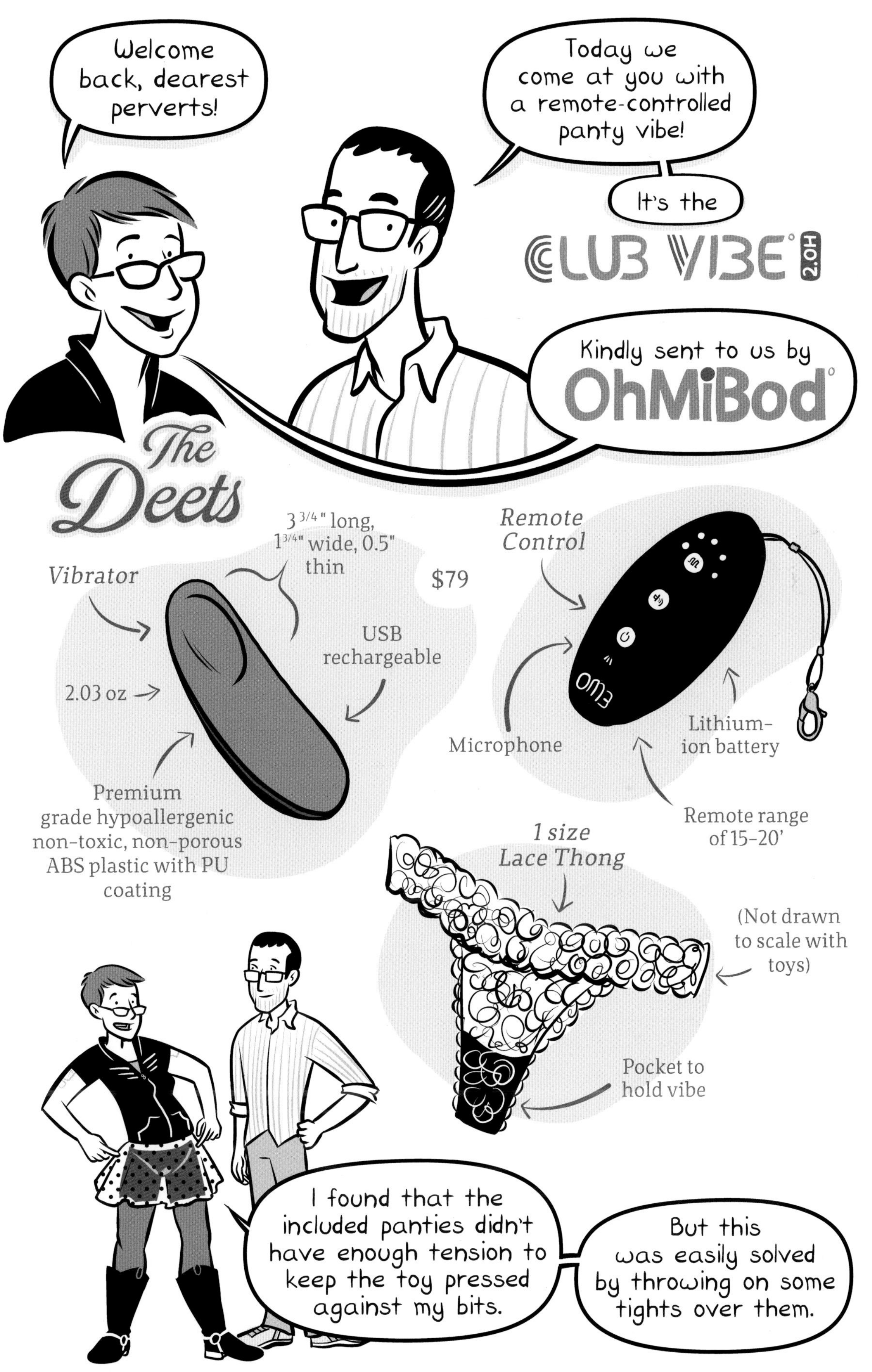

Welcome back, dearest perverts!
Today we come at you with a remote-controlled panty vibe!
It's the
CLUB VIBE 2.OH
Kindly sent to us by
OhMiBod
The Deets
Vibrator
3 3/4" long, 1 3/4" wide, 0.5" thin
$79
USB rechargeable
2.03 oz
Premium grade hypoallergenic non-toxic, non-porous ABS plastic with PU coating
Remote Control
Microphone
Lithium-ion battery
Remote range of 15-20'
1 size Lace Thong
(Not drawn to scale with toys)
Pocket to hold vibe
I found that the included panties didn't have enough tension to keep the toy pressed against my bits.
But this was easily solved by throwing on some tights over them.

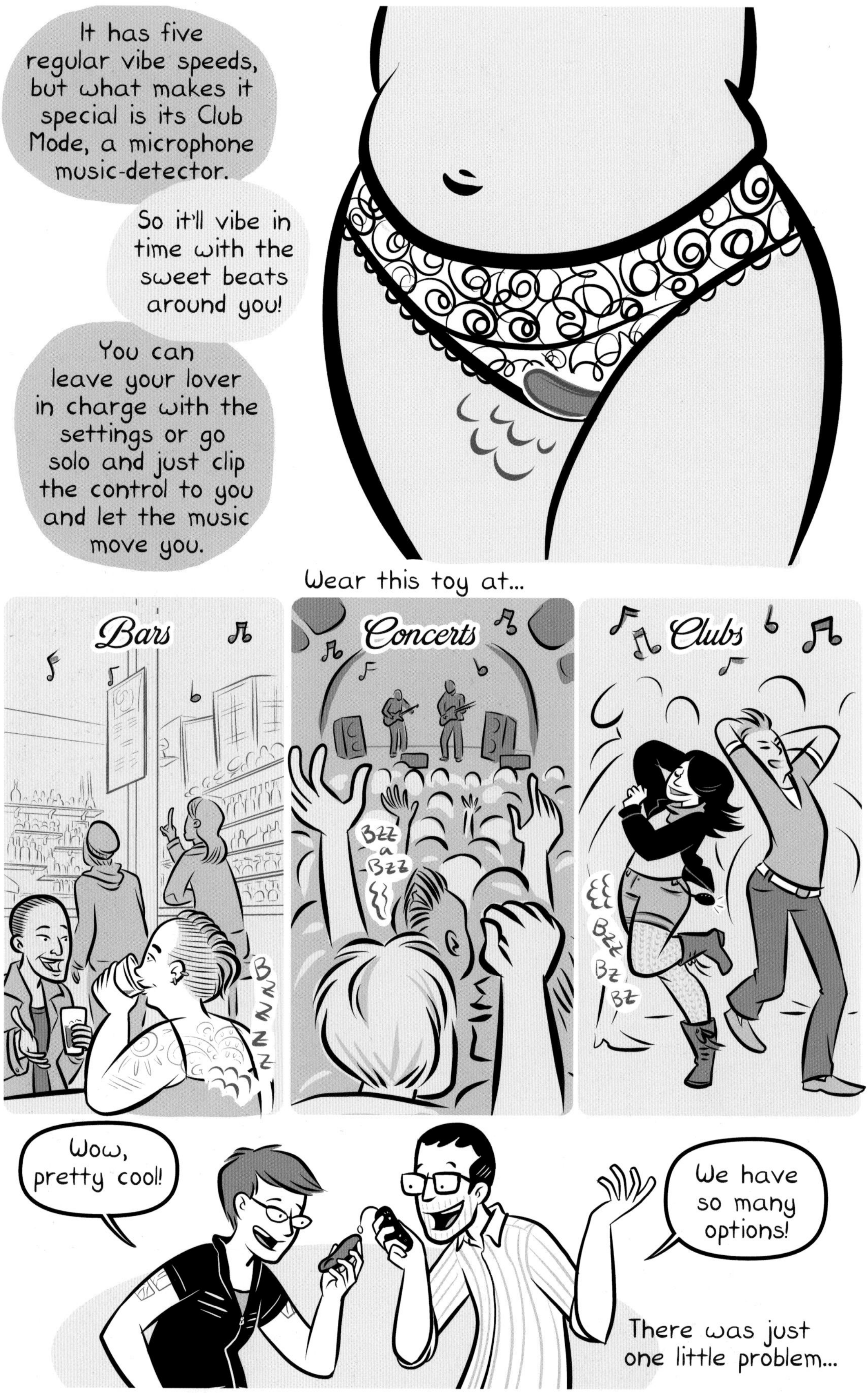

It has five regular vibe speeds, but what makes it special is its Club Mode, a microphone music-detector.

So it'll vibe in time with the sweet beats around you!

You can leave your lover in charge with the settings or go solo and just clip the control to you and let the music move you.

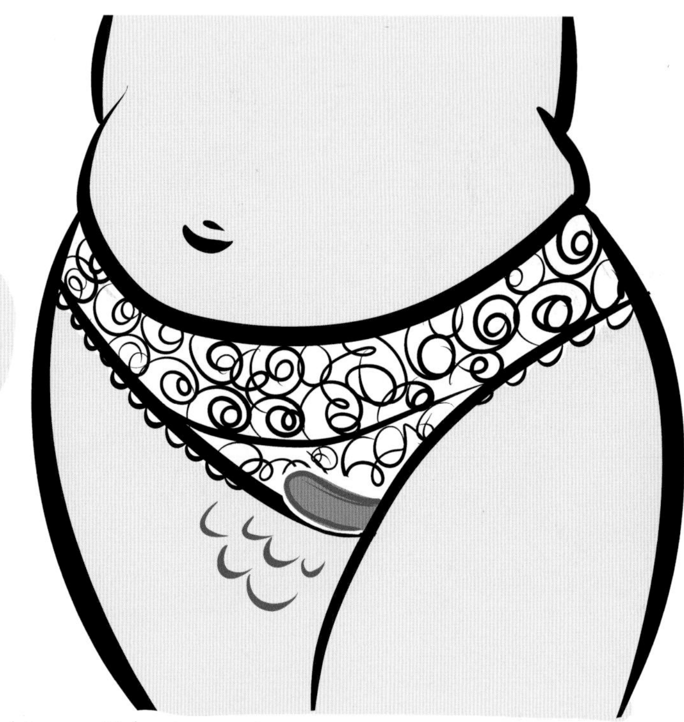

Wear this toy at...

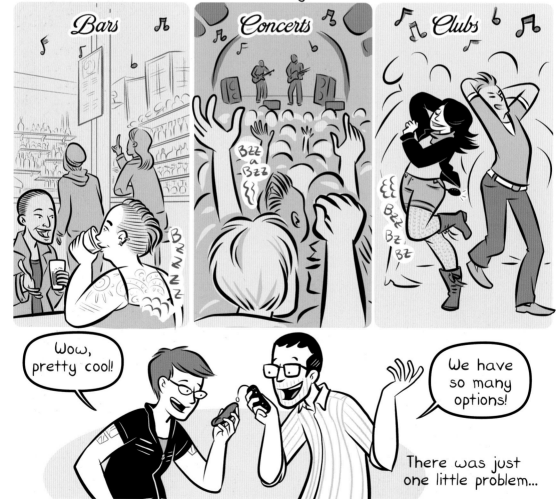

There was just one little problem...

How we feel about:

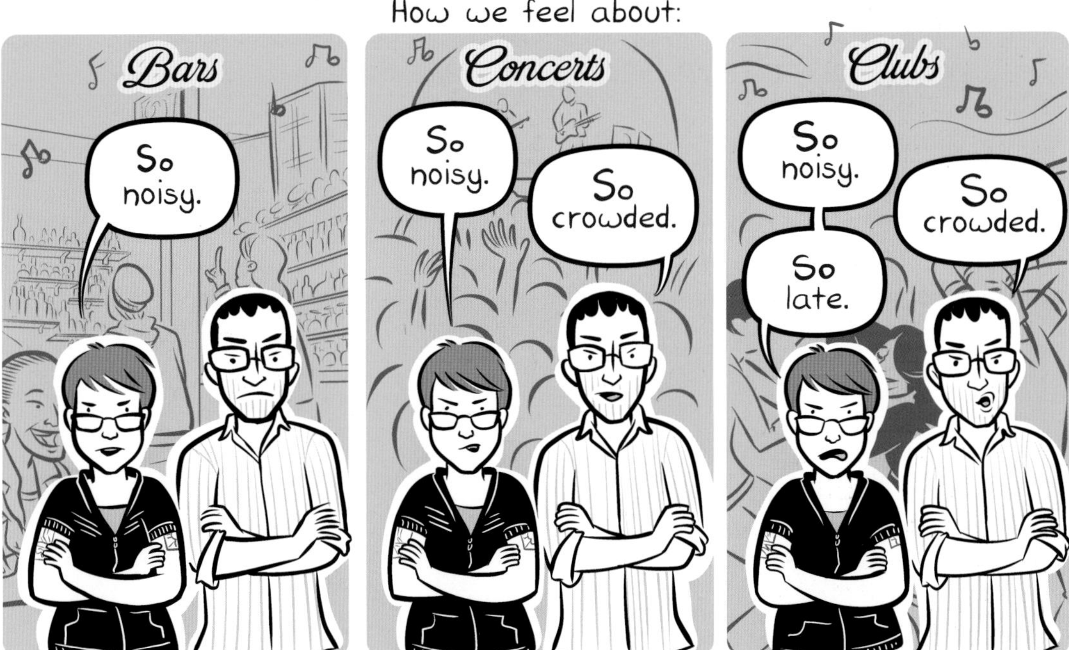

Bars
So noisy.
Concerts
So noisy.
So crowded.
Clubs
So noisy.
So late.
So crowded.

We're kind of the most boring couple on the face of the earth.

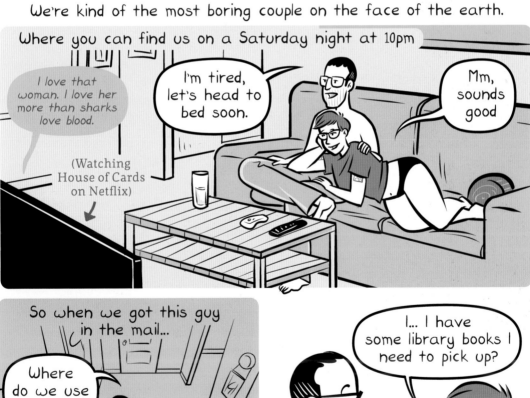

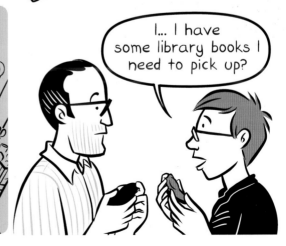

Where you can find us on a Saturday night at 10pm

I love that woman. I love her more than sharks love blood.

I'm tired, let's head to bed soon.

Mm, sounds good

(Watching House of Cards on Netflix)

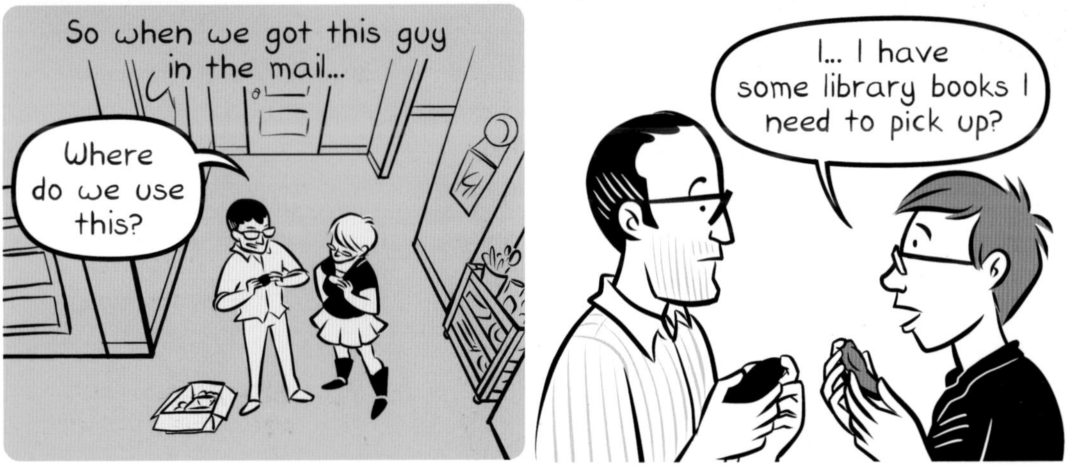

So when we got this guy in the mail...

Where do we use this?

I... I have some library books I need to pick up?

This vibe is definitely quiet and would be completely undetectable to others in a noisy venue...

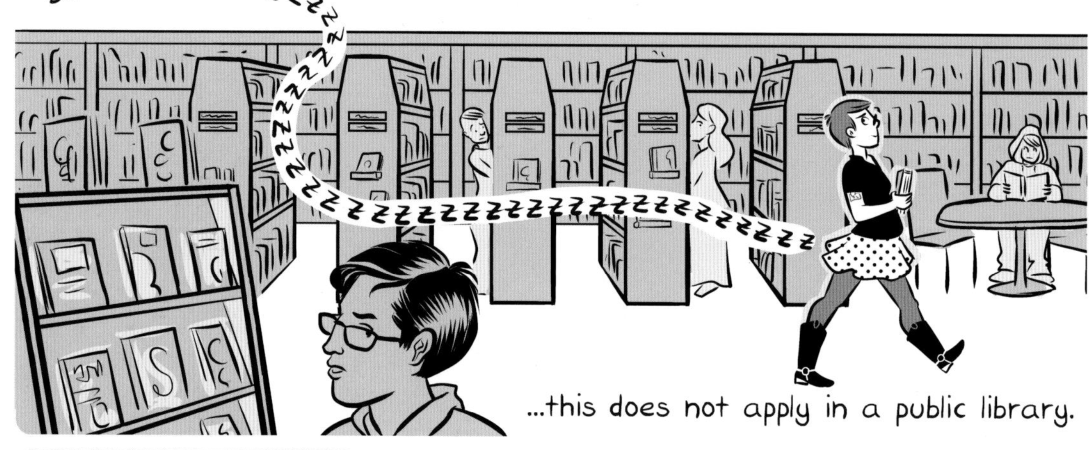

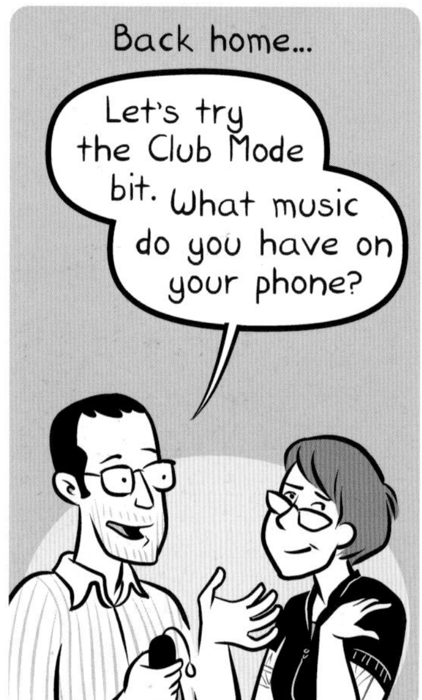

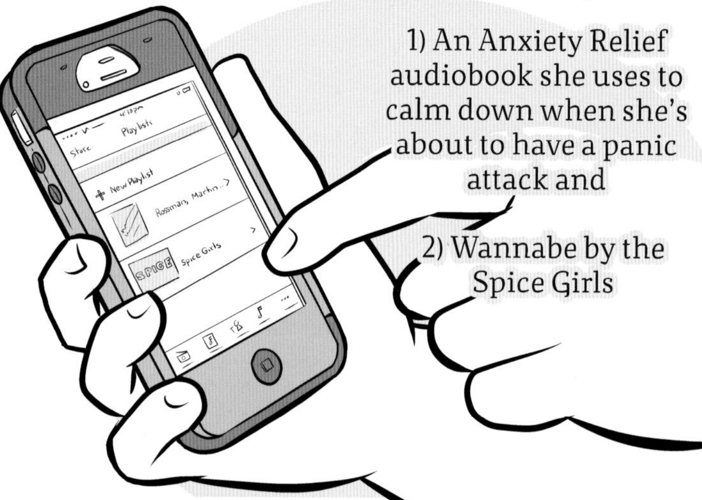

...this does not apply in a public library.

Back home...
Let's try the Club Mode bit. What music do you have on your phone?

FUN FACT:
Erika only has two audio files on her phone.
1) An Anxiety Relief audiobook she uses to calm down when she's about to have a panic attack and
2) Wannabe by the Spice Girls
Playlists
New Playlist
Spice Girls

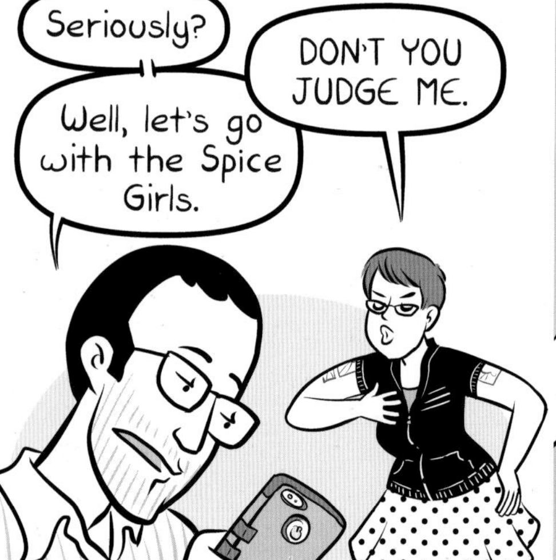

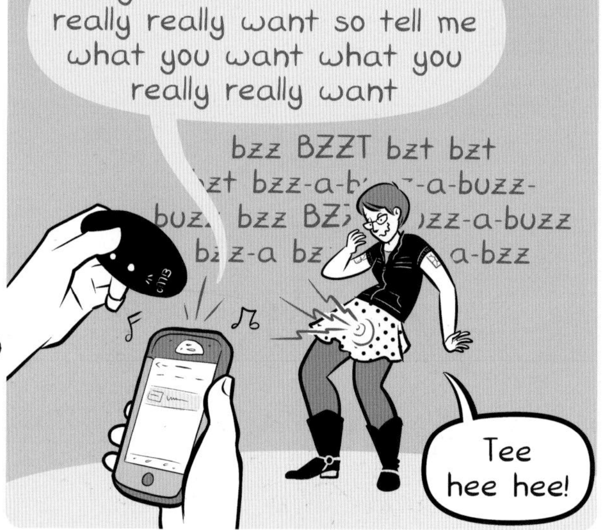

DON'T YOU JUDGE ME.

I tell you what I want what I really really want so tell me what you want what you really really want
bzz BZZT bzt bzt

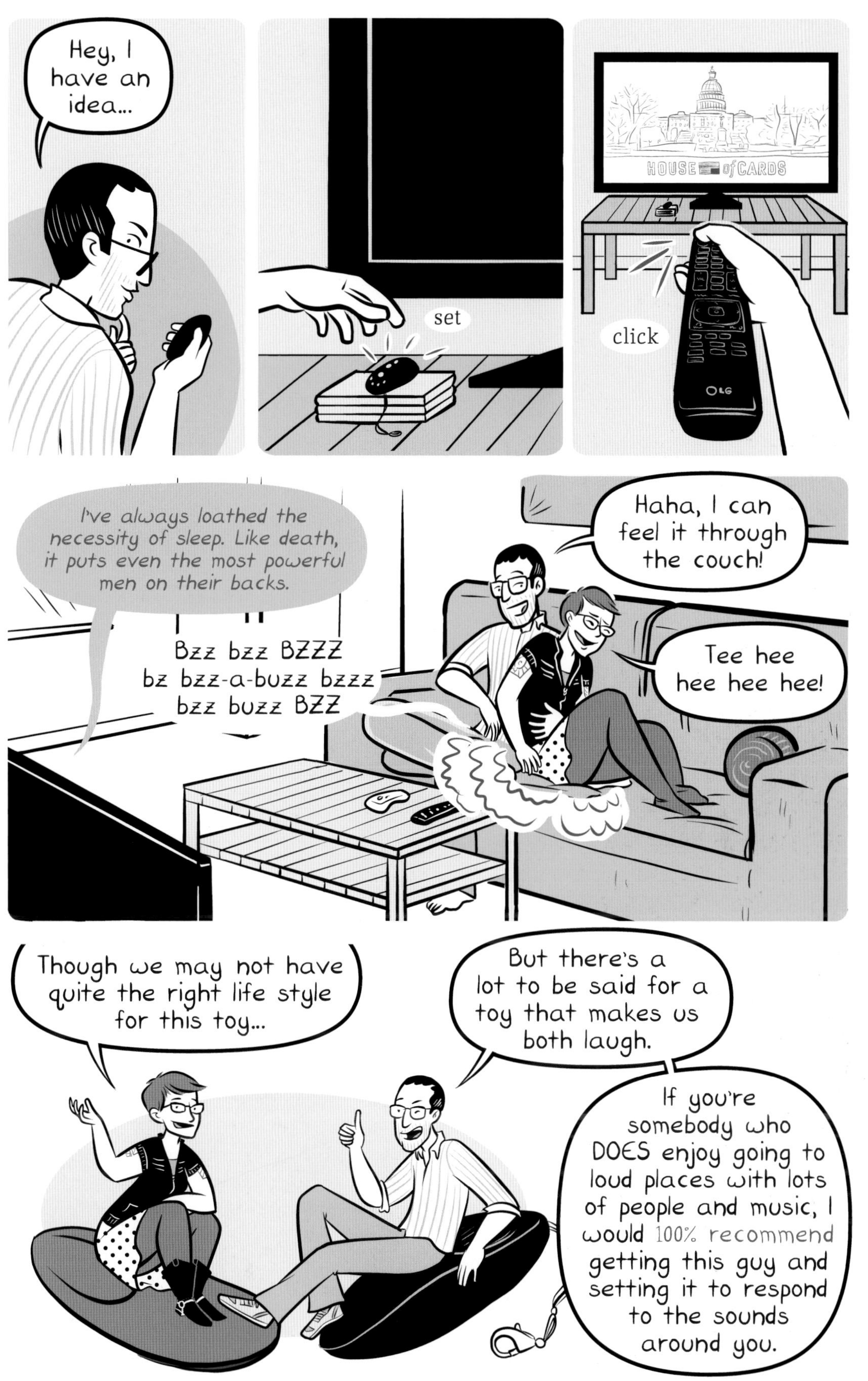
Hey, I have an idea...
set
HOUSE of CARDS
click
I've always loathed the necessity of sleep. Like death, it puts even the most powerful men on their backs.
Haha, I can feel it through the couch!
Tee hee hee hee hee!
Bzz bzz BZZZ
bz bzz-a-buzz bzzz
bzz buzz BZZ
Though we may not have quite the right life style for this toy...
But there's a lot to be said for a toy that makes us both laugh.
If you're somebody who DOES enjoy going to loud places with lots of people and music, I would 100% recommend getting this guy and setting it to respond to the sounds around you.

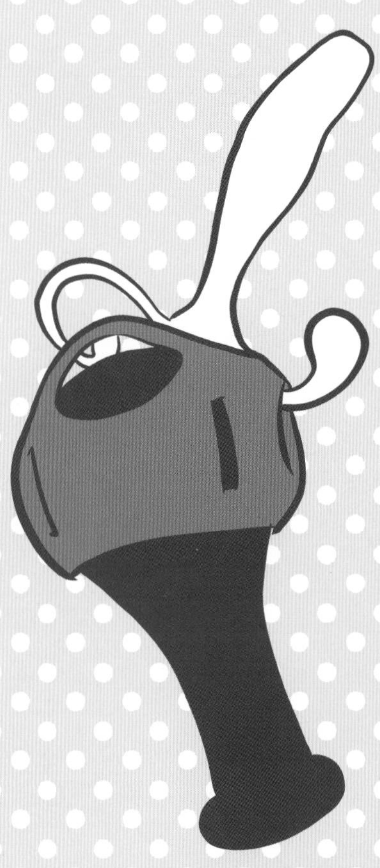

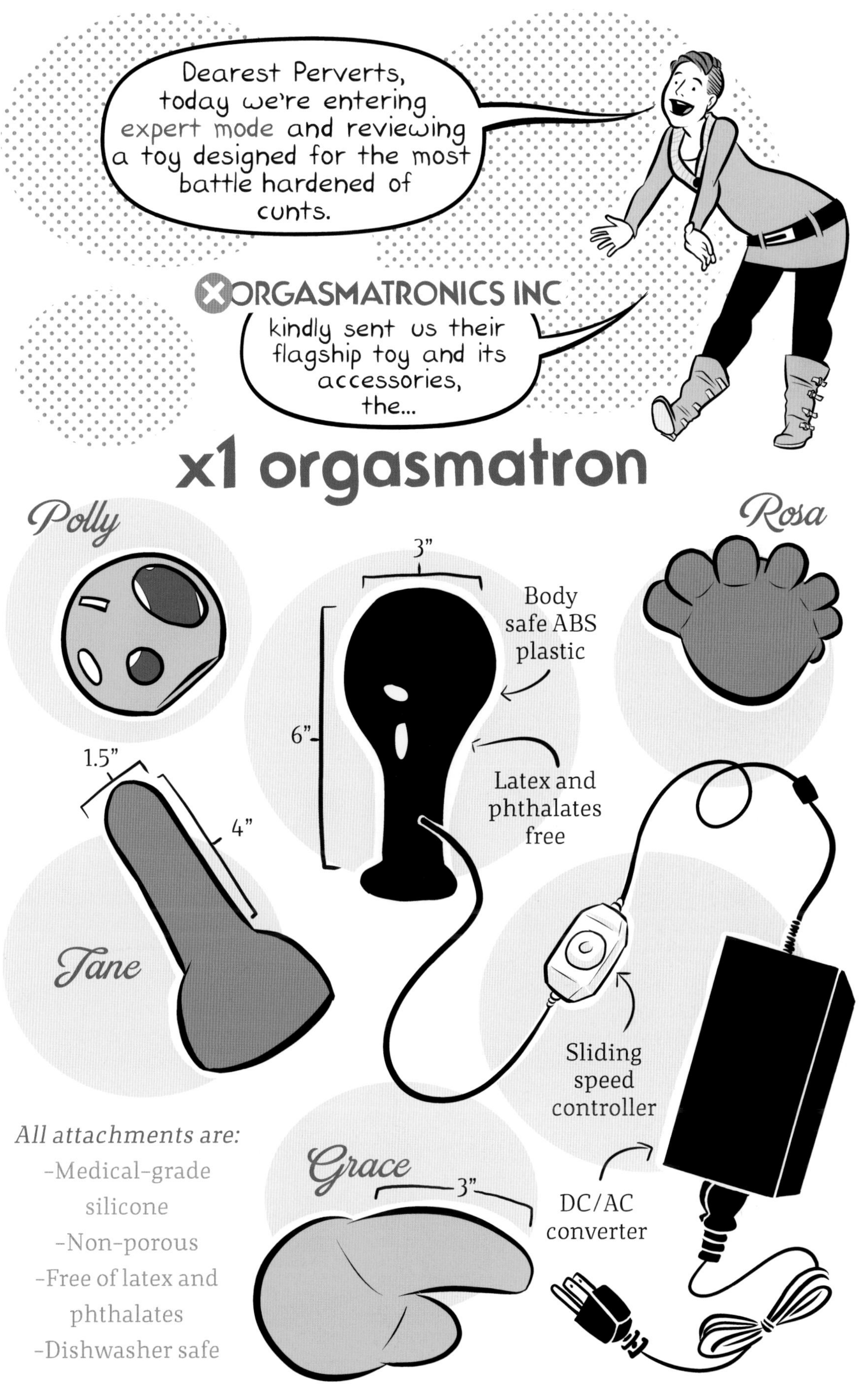
Dearest Perverts, today we're entering expert mode and reviewing a toy designed for the most battle hardened of cunts.
ORGASMATRONICS INC
kindly sent us their flagship toy and its accessories, the...
x1 orgasmatron
Polly
Rosa
3"
6"
Body safe ABS plastic
Latex and phthalates free
1.5"
4"
Jane
Sliding speed controller
All attachments are:
-Medical-grade silicone
-Non-porous
-Free of latex and phthalates
-Dishwasher safe
Grace
3"
DC/AC converter

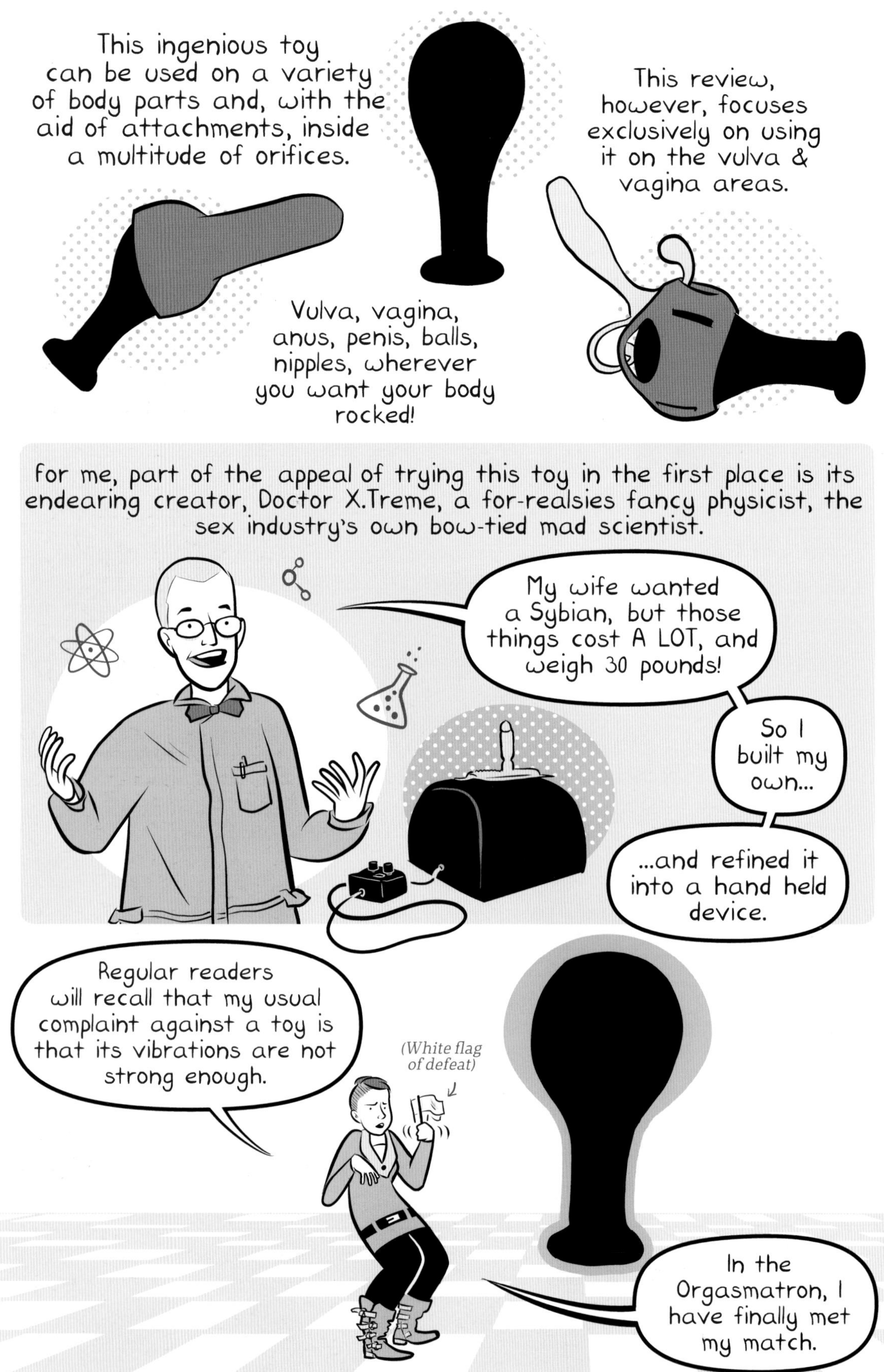
This ingenious toy can be used on a variety of body parts and, with the aid of attachments, inside a multitude of orifices.
Vulva, vagina, anus, penis, balls, nipples, wherever you want your body rocked!
This review, however, focuses exclusively on using it on the vulva & vagina areas.
For me, part of the appeal of trying this toy in the first place is its endearing creator, Doctor X.Treme, a for-realsies fancy physicist, the sex industry's own bow-tied mad scientist.
My wife wanted a Sybian, but those things cost A LOT, and weigh 30 pounds!
So I built my own...
...and refined it into a hand held device.
Regular readers will recall that my usual complaint against a toy is that its vibrations are not strong enough.
(White flag of defeat)
In the Orgasmatron, I have finally met my match.

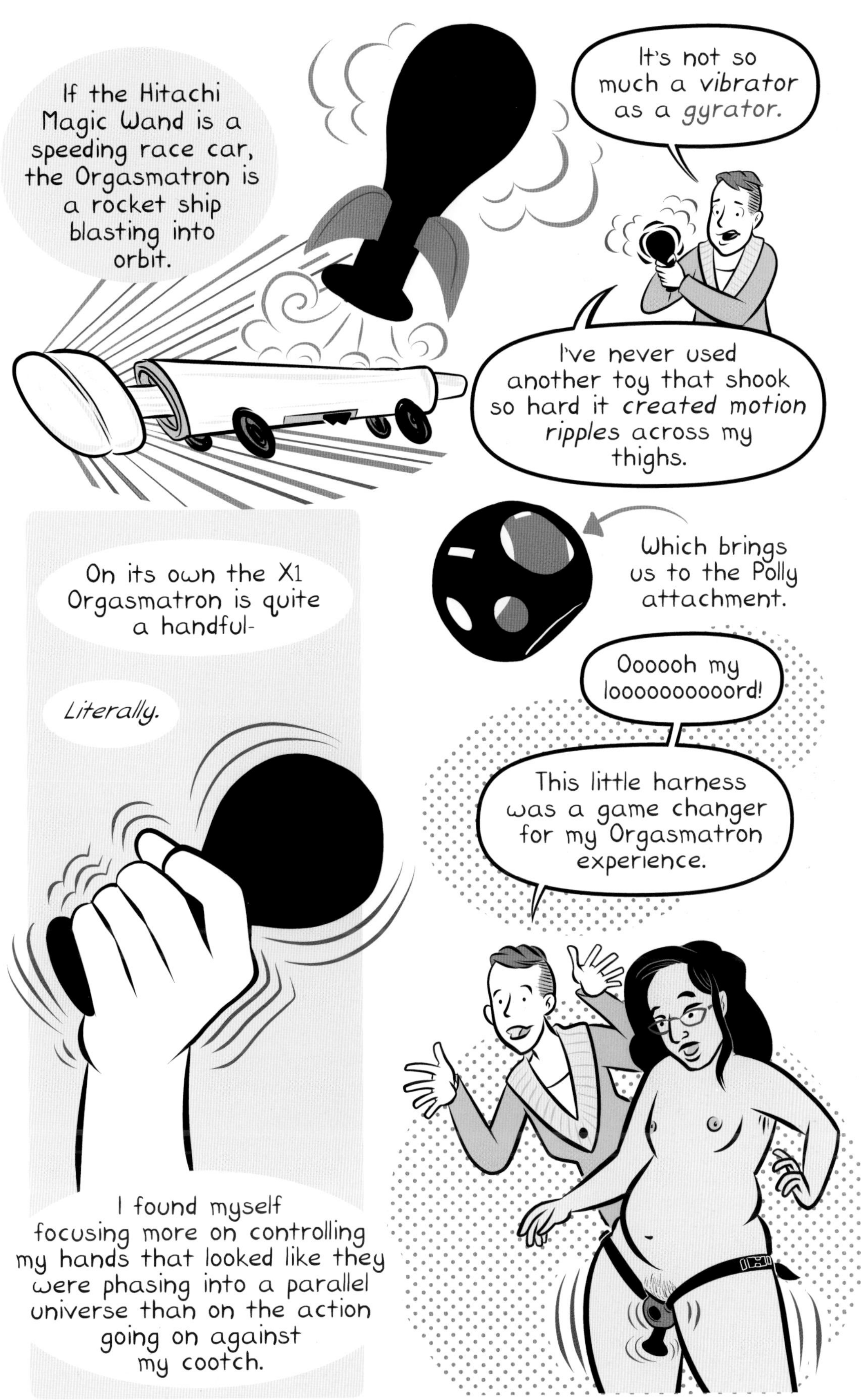
If the Hitachi Magic Wand is a speeding race car, the Orgasmatron is a rocket ship blasting into orbit.
It's not so much a *vibrator* as a *gyrator.*
I've never used another toy that shook so hard it *created motion ripples* across my thighs.
On its own the X1 Orgasmatron is quite a handful-
Literally.
I found myself focusing more on controlling my hands that looked like they were phasing into a parallel universe than on the action going on against my cootch.
Which brings us to the Polly attachment.
Oooooh my looooooooooord!
This little harness was a game changer for my Orgasmatron experience.

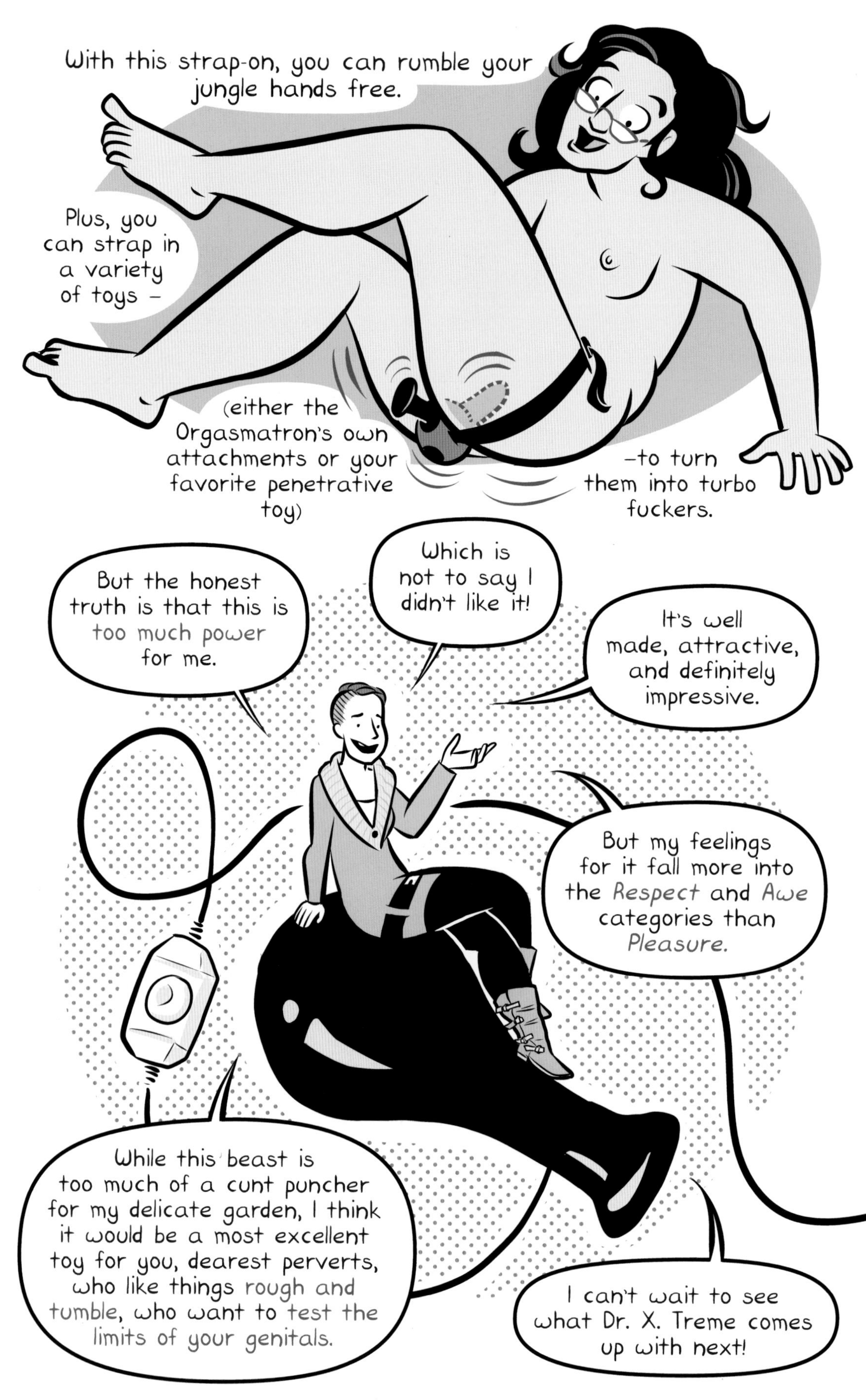
With this strap-on, you can rumble your jungle hands free.
Plus, you can strap in a variety of toys –
(either the Orgasmatron's own attachments or your favorite penetrative toy)
–to turn them into turbo fuckers.
But the honest truth is that this is too much power for me.
Which is not to say I didn't like it!
It's well made, attractive, and definitely impressive.
But my feelings for it fall more into the Respect and Awe categories than Pleasure.
While this beast is too much of a cunt puncher for my delicate garden, I think it would be a most excellent toy for you, dearest perverts, who like things rough and tumble, who want to test the limits of your genitals.
I can't wait to see what Dr. X. Treme comes up with next!

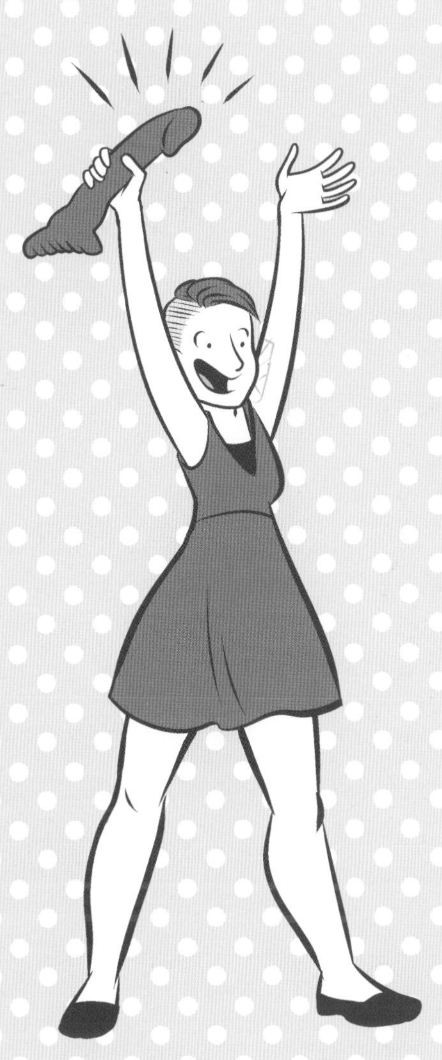

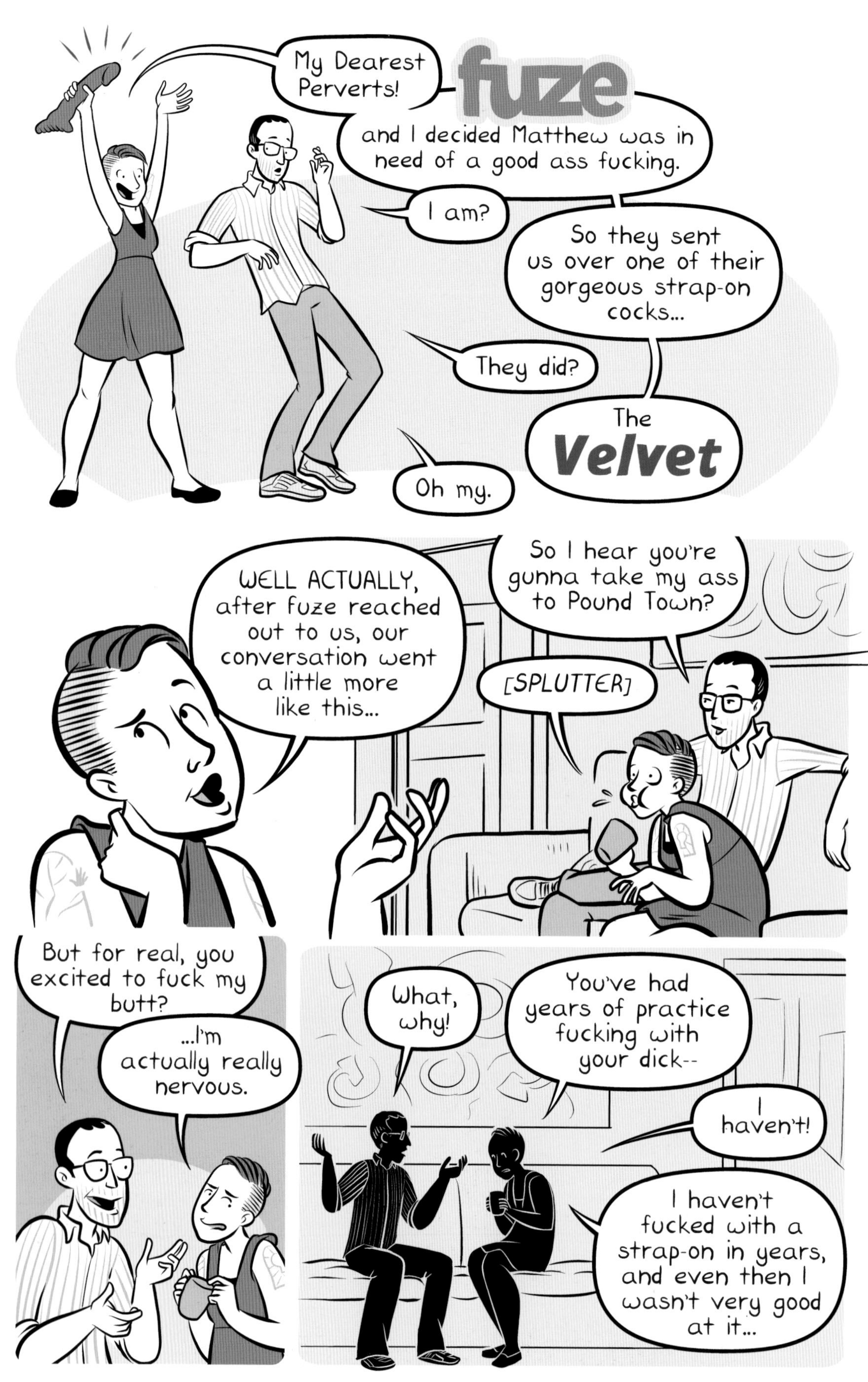
My Dearest Perverts!
fuze
and I decided Matthew was in need of a good ass fucking.
I am?
So they sent us over one of their gorgeous strap-on cocks...
They did?
The Velvet
Oh my.
WELL ACTUALLY, after fuze reached out to us, our conversation went a little more like this...
So I hear you're gunna take my ass to Pound Town?
[SPLUTTER]
But for real, you excited to fuck my butt?
...I'm actually really nervous.
What, why!
You've had years of practice fucking with your dick--
I haven't!
I haven't fucked with a strap-on in years, and even then I wasn't very good at it...

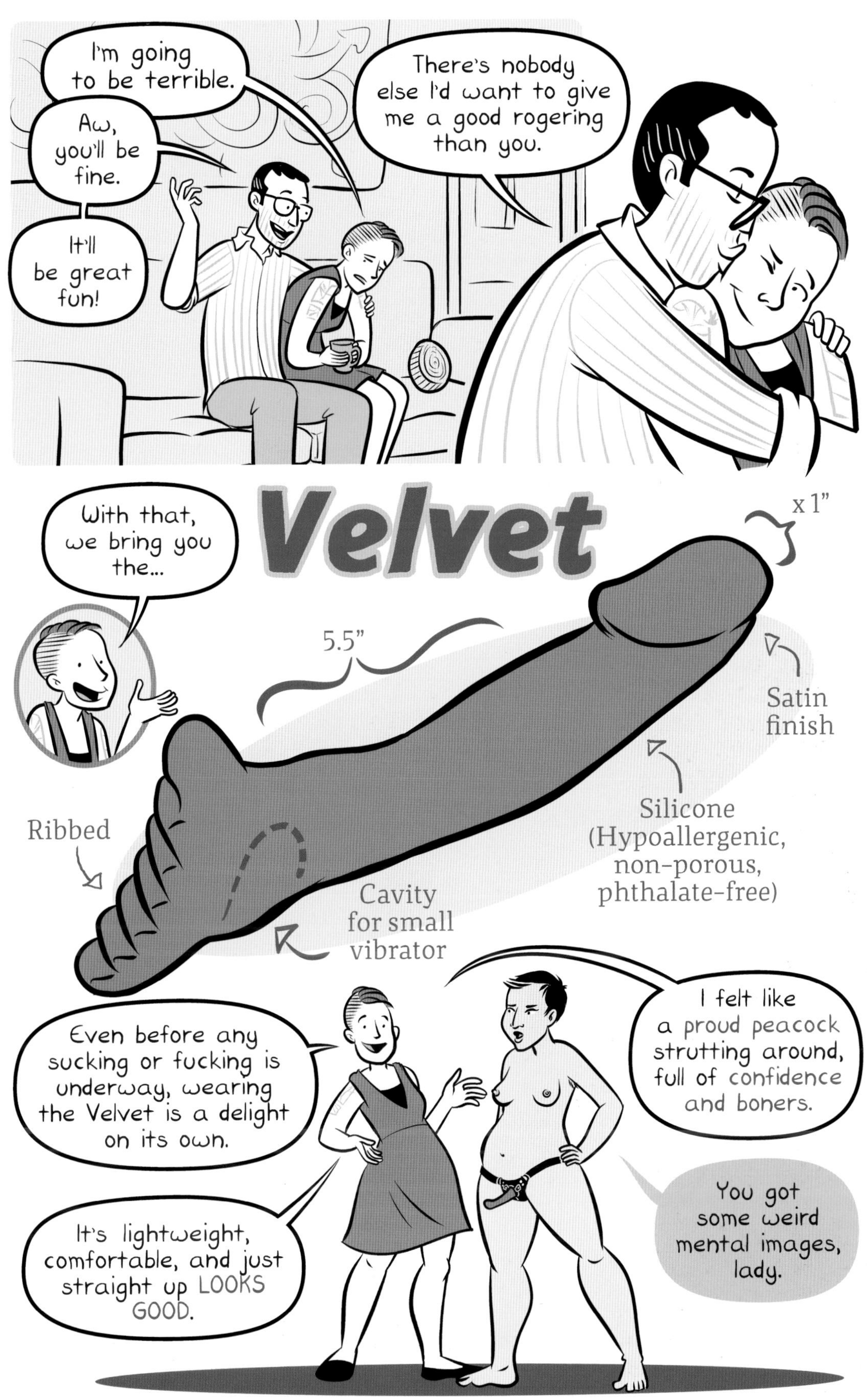
I'm going to be terrible.
Aw, you'll be fine.
It'll be great fun!
There's nobody else I'd want to give me a good rogering than you.
With that, we bring you the...
Velvet
x 1"
5.5"
Satin finish
Silicone (Hypoallergenic, non-porous, phthalate-free)
Ribbed
Cavity for small vibrator
Even before any sucking or fucking is underway, wearing the Velvet is a delight on its own.
I felt like a proud peacock strutting around, full of confidence and boners.
It's lightweight, comfortable, and just straight up LOOKS GOOD.
You got some weird mental images, lady.

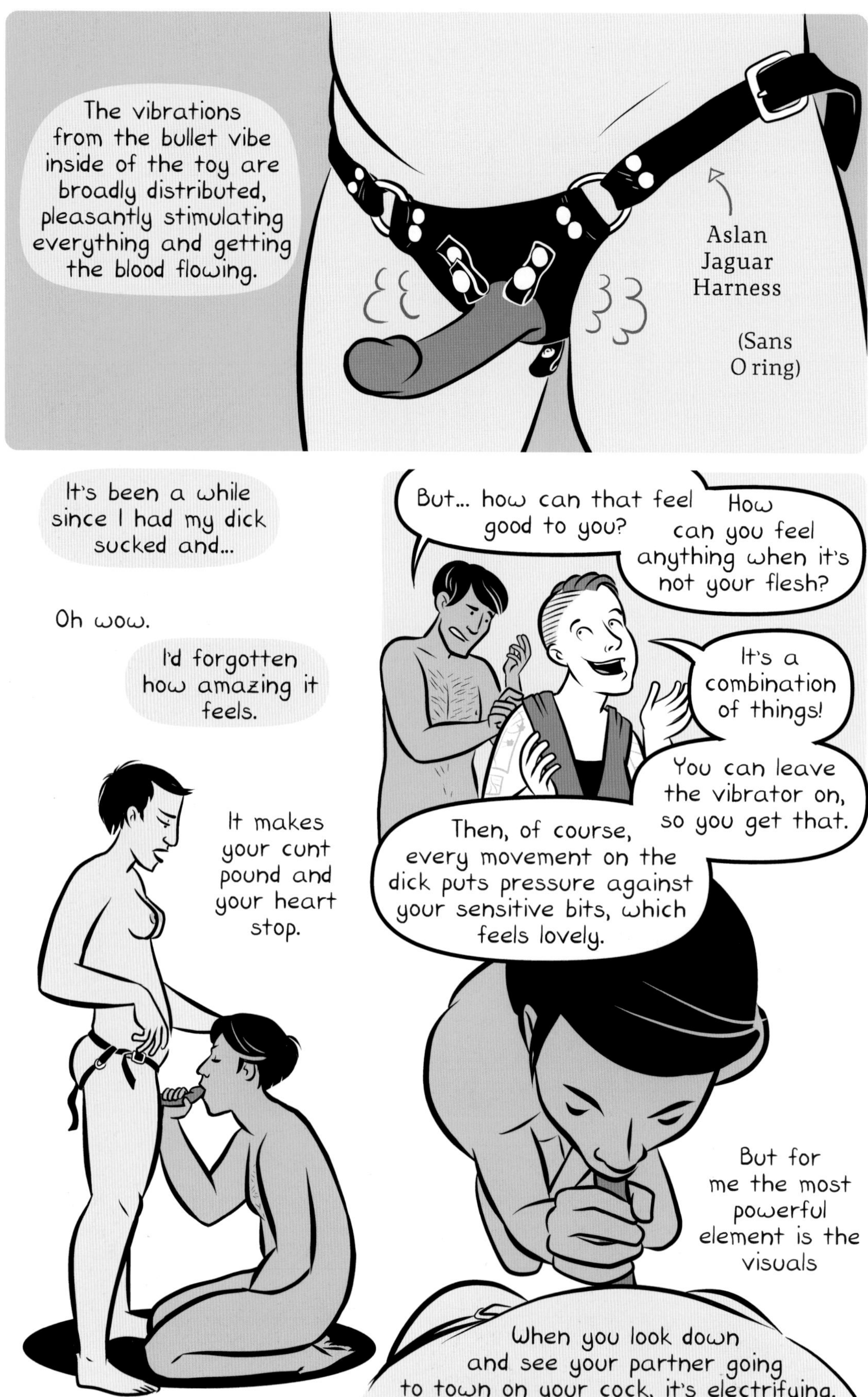
The vibrations from the bullet vibe inside of the toy are broadly distributed, pleasantly stimulating everything and getting the blood flowing.
Aslan Jaguar Harness
(Sans O ring)
It's been a while since I had my dick sucked and...
Oh wow.
I'd forgotten how amazing it feels.
It makes your cunt pound and your heart stop.
But... how can that feel good to you?
How can you feel anything when it's not your flesh?
It's a combination of things!
You can leave the vibrator on, so you get that.
Then, of course, every movement on the dick puts pressure against your sensitive bits, which feels lovely.
But for me the most powerful element is the visuals
When you look down and see your partner going to town on your cock, it's electrifying.

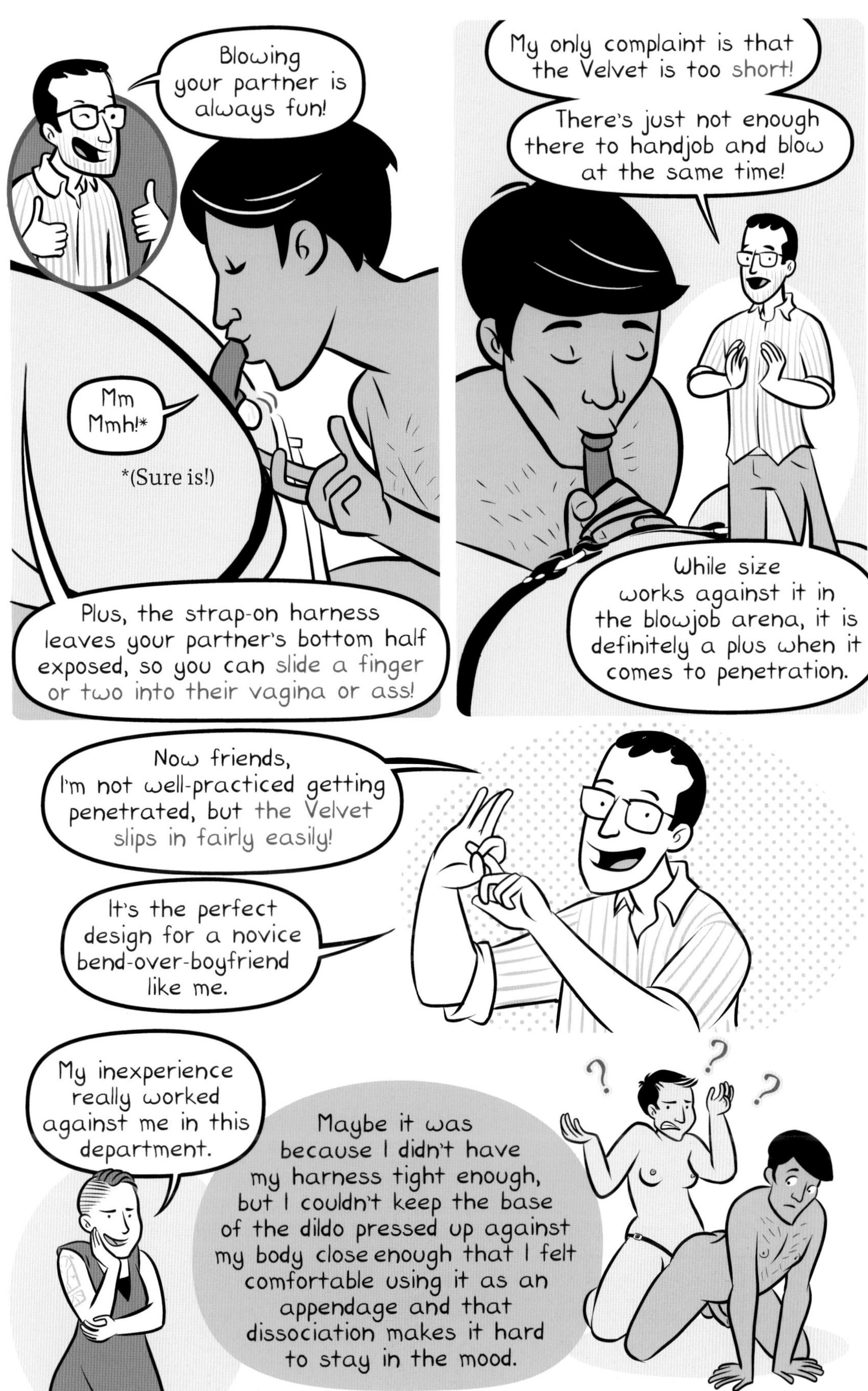
Blowing your partner is always fun!
Mm Mmh!*
*(Sure is!)
Plus, the strap-on harness leaves your partner's bottom half exposed, so you can slide a finger or two into their vagina or ass!
My only complaint is that the Velvet is too short!
There's just not enough there to handjob and blow at the same time!
While size works against it in the blowjob arena, it is definitely a plus when it comes to penetration.
Now friends, I'm not well-practiced getting penetrated, but the Velvet slips in fairly easily!
It's the perfect design for a novice bend-over-boyfriend like me.
My inexperience really worked against me in this department.
Maybe it was because I didn't have my harness tight enough, but I couldn't keep the base of the dildo pressed up against my body close enough that I felt comfortable using it as an appendage and that dissociation makes it hard to stay in the mood.
? ? ?

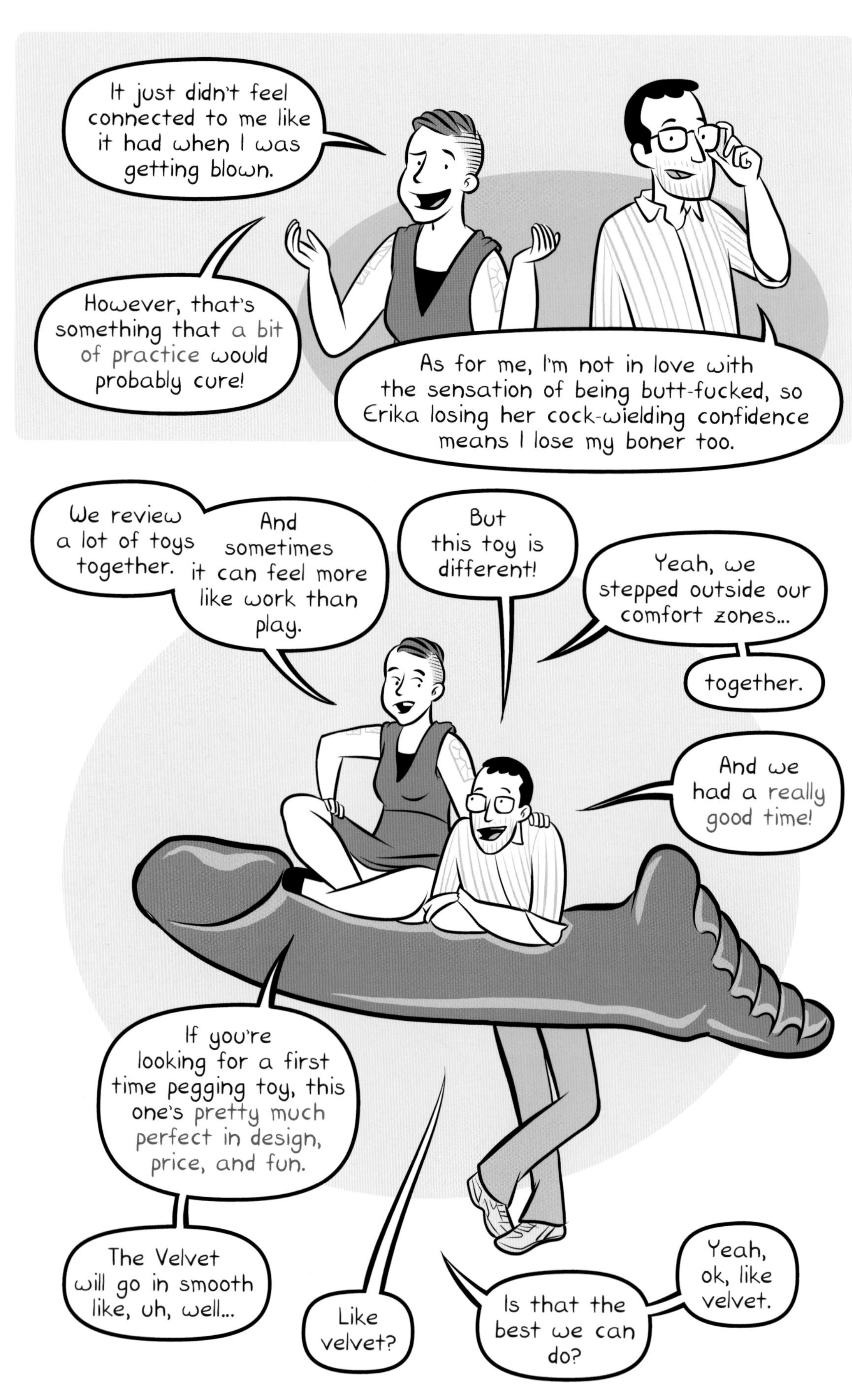
It just didn't feel connected to me like it had when I was getting blown.
However, that's something that a bit of practice would probably cure!
As for me, I'm not in love with the sensation of being butt-fucked, so Erika losing her cock-wielding confidence means I lose my boner too.
We review a lot of toys together.
And sometimes it can feel more like work than play.
But this toy is different!
Yeah, we stepped outside our comfort zones...
together.
And we had a really good time!
If you're looking for a first time pegging toy, this one's pretty much perfect in design, price, and fun.
The Velvet will go in smooth like, uh, well...
Like velvet?
Is that the best we can do?
Yeah, ok, like velvet.

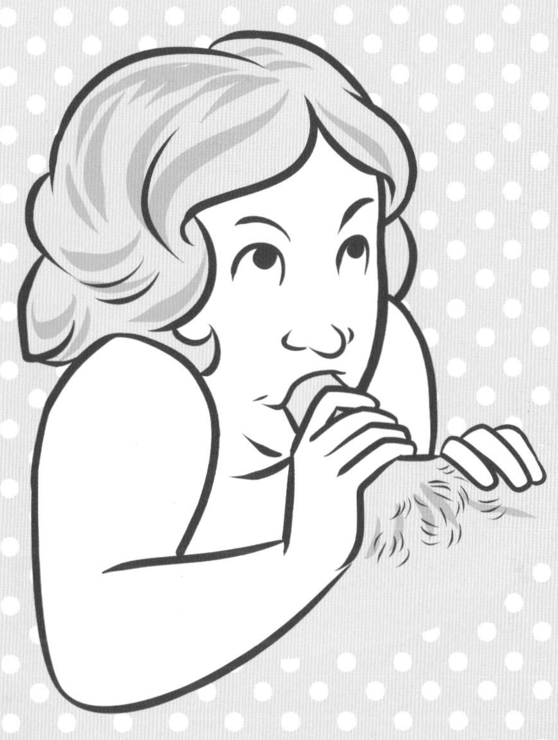

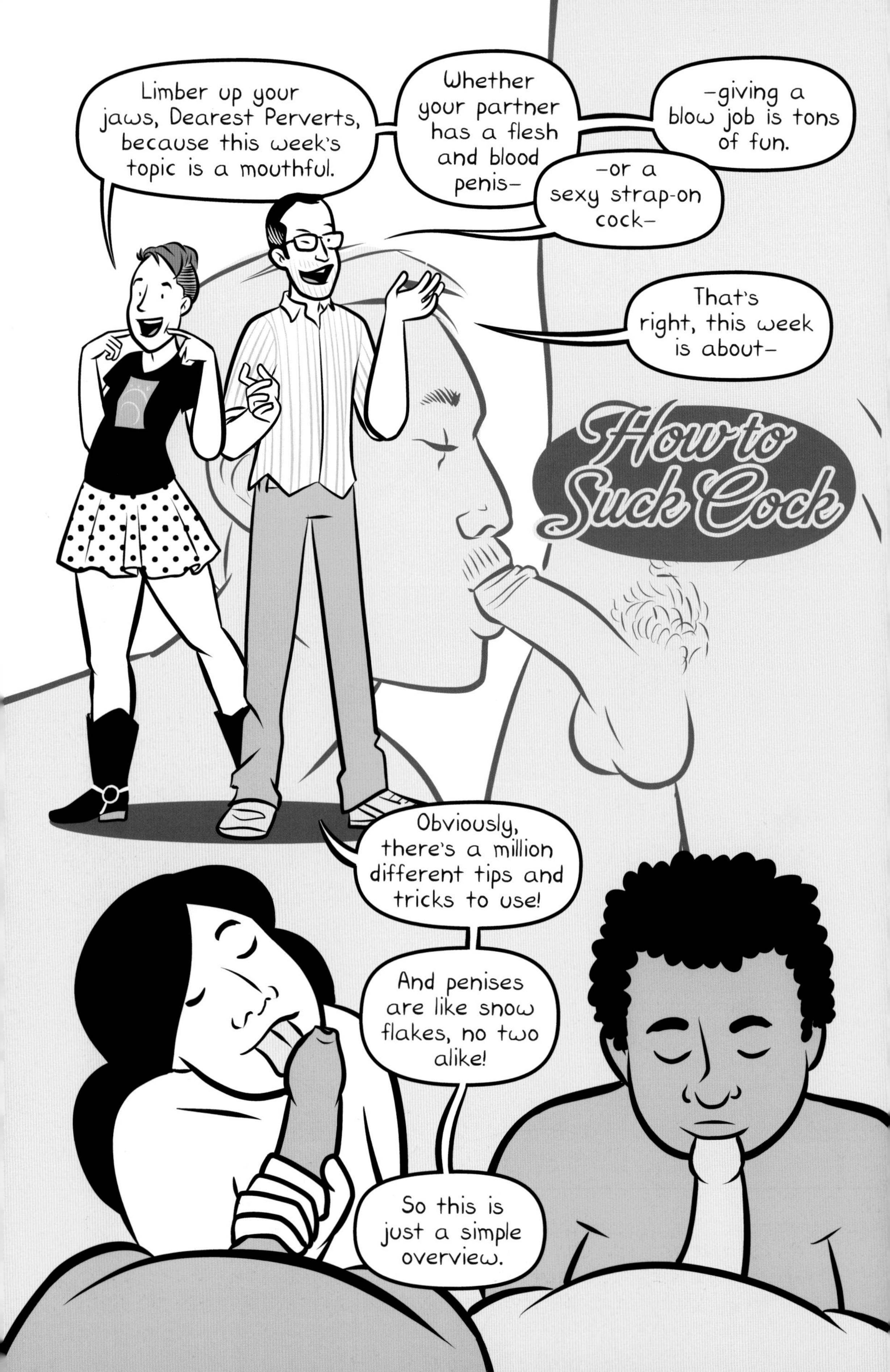
Limber up your jaws, Dearest Perverts, because this week's topic is a mouthful.
Whether your partner has a flesh and blood penis–
–or a sexy strap-on cock–
–giving a blow job is tons of fun.
That's right, this week is about–
How to Suck Cock
Obviously, there's a million different tips and tricks to use!
And penises are like snow flakes, no two alike!
So this is just a simple overview.

Meet the Penis

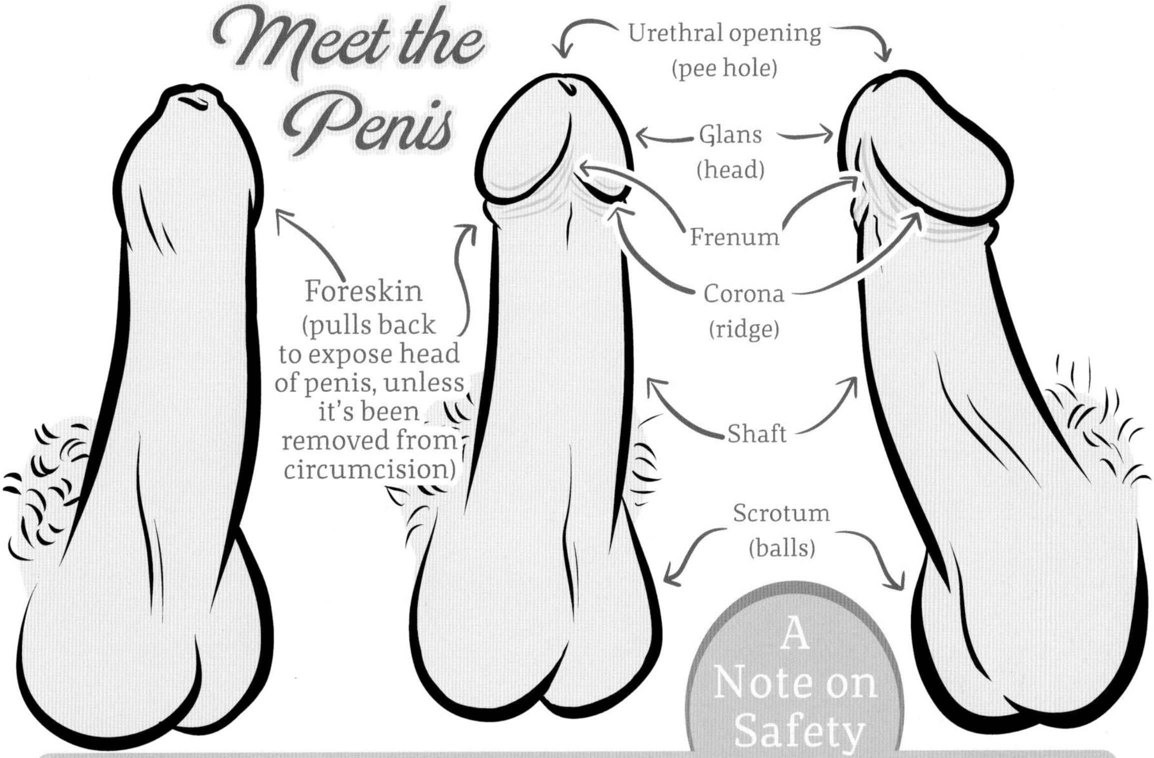

Urethral opening (pee hole)

Glans (head)

Frenum

Corona (ridge)

Foreskin (pulls back to expose head of penis, unless it's been removed from circumcision)

Shaft

Scrotum (balls)

A Note on Safety

STIs can be transmitted between saliva and semen, so to prevent spreading anything infectious between partners, put a condom on the penis before it goes in anyone's mouth.

Communicate

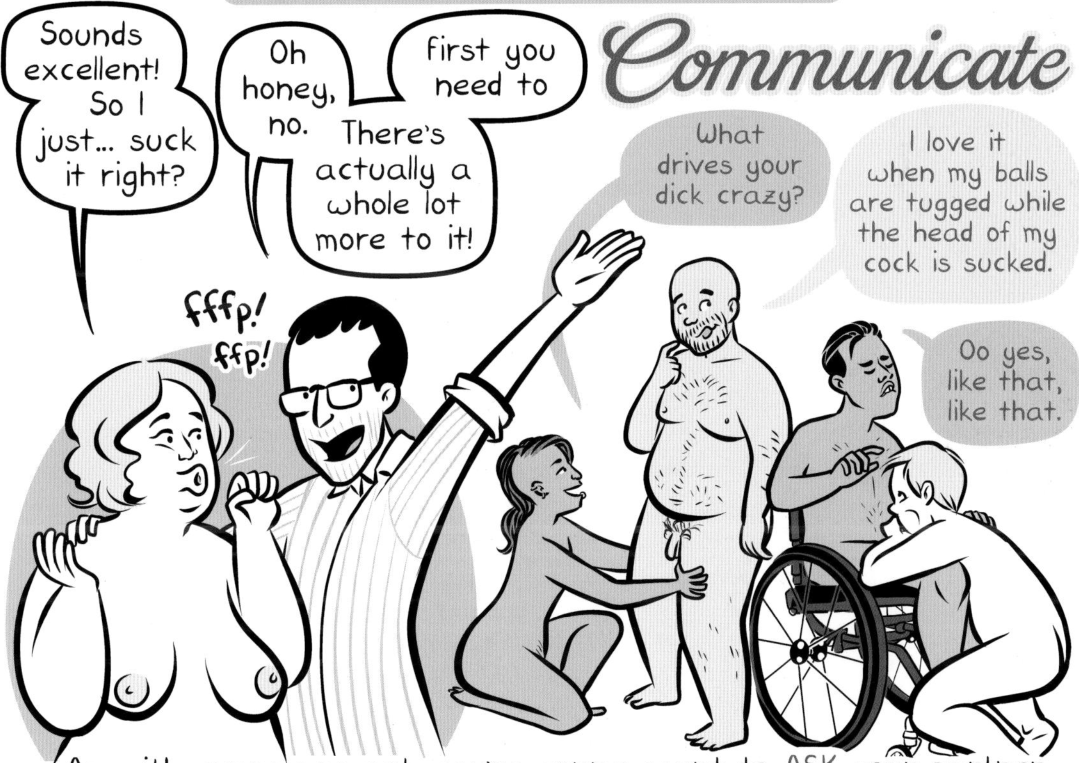
Sounds excellent! So I just... suck it right?
Oh honey, no.
first you need to
There's actually a whole lot more to it!
fffp! ffp!
What drives your dick crazy?
I love it when my balls are tugged while the head of my cock is sucked.
Oo yes, like that, like that.

As with every sex act, you're gonna want to ASK your partner what they like, TELL your partner what you want, give the giver positive reinforcement when they're doing something you do like.

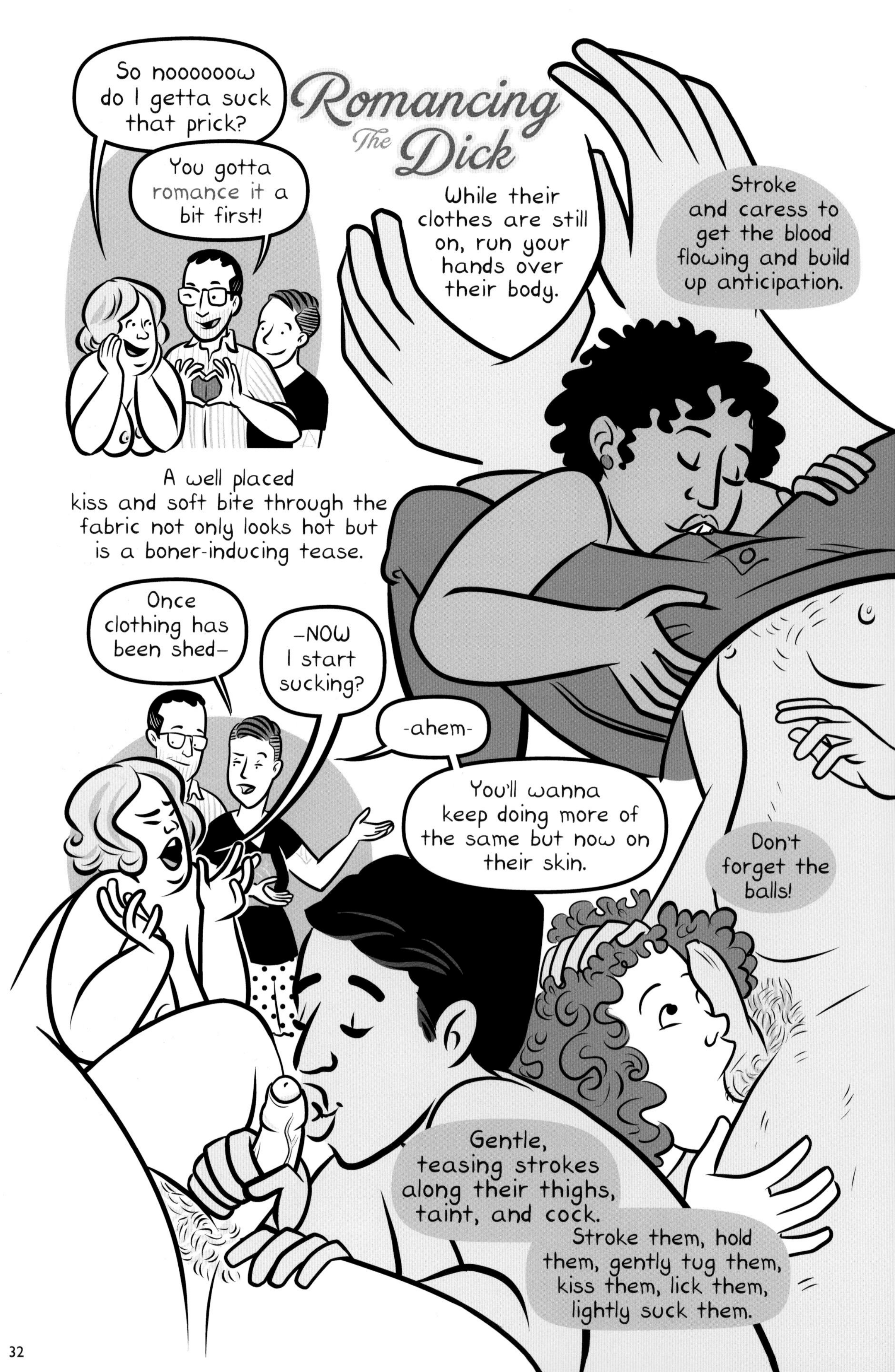
Romancing The Dick
So noooooow do I getta suck that prick?
You gotta romance it a bit first!
While their clothes are still on, run your hands over their body.
Stroke and caress to get the blood flowing and build up anticipation.
A well placed kiss and soft bite through the fabric not only looks hot but is a boner-inducing tease.
Once clothing has been shed–
–NOW I start sucking?
-ahem-
You'll wanna keep doing more of the same but now on their skin.
Don't forget the balls!
Gentle, teasing strokes along their thighs, taint, and cock.
Stroke them, hold them, gently tug them, kiss them, lick them, lightly suck them.

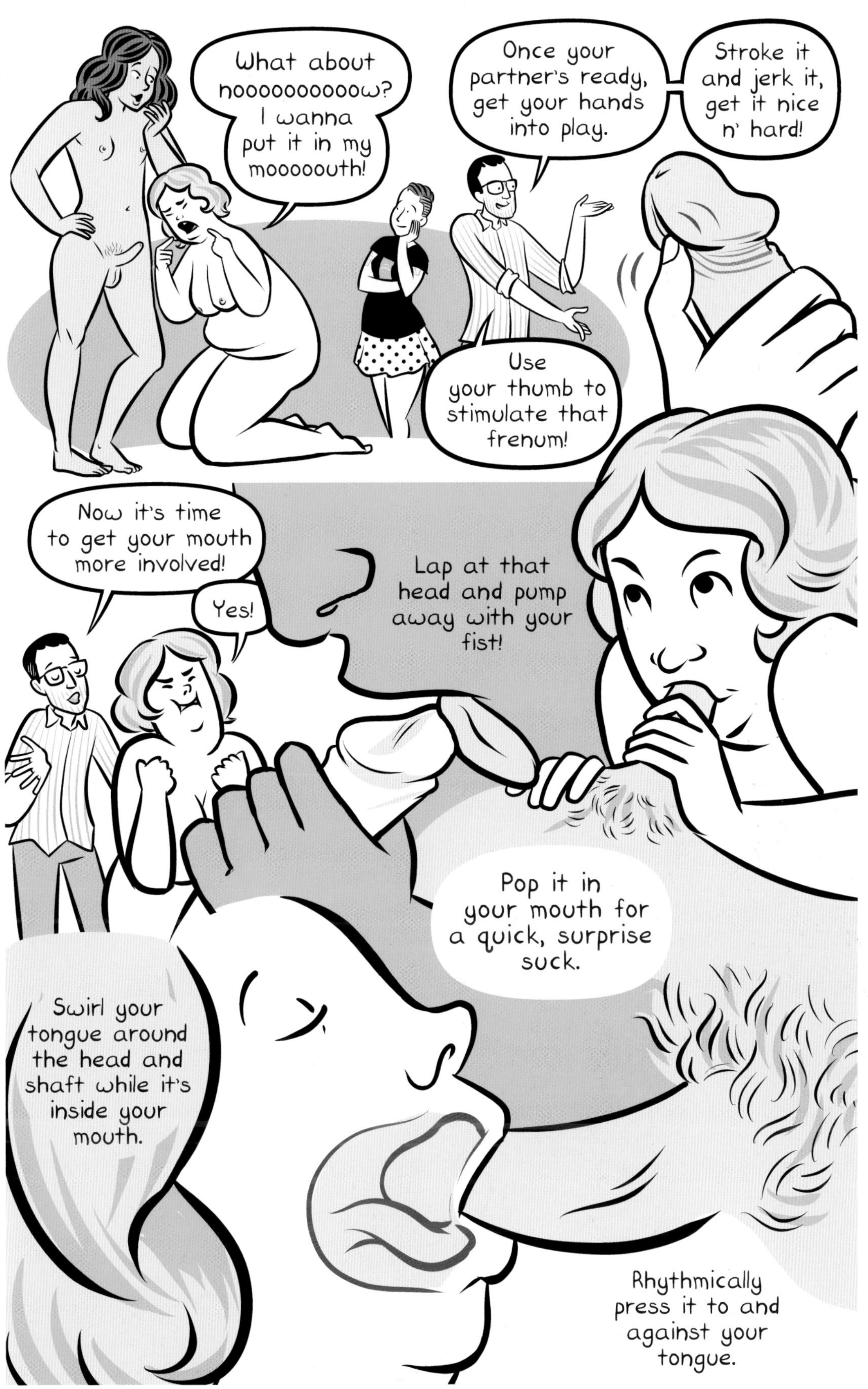
What about noooooooooow? I wanna put it in my mooooouth!
Once your partner's ready, get your hands into play.
Stroke it and jerk it, get it nice n' hard!
Use your thumb to stimulate that frenum!
Now it's time to get your mouth more involved!
Yes!
Lap at that head and pump away with your fist!
Pop it in your mouth for a quick, surprise suck.
Swirl your tongue around the head and shaft while it's inside your mouth.
Rhythmically press it to and against your tongue.

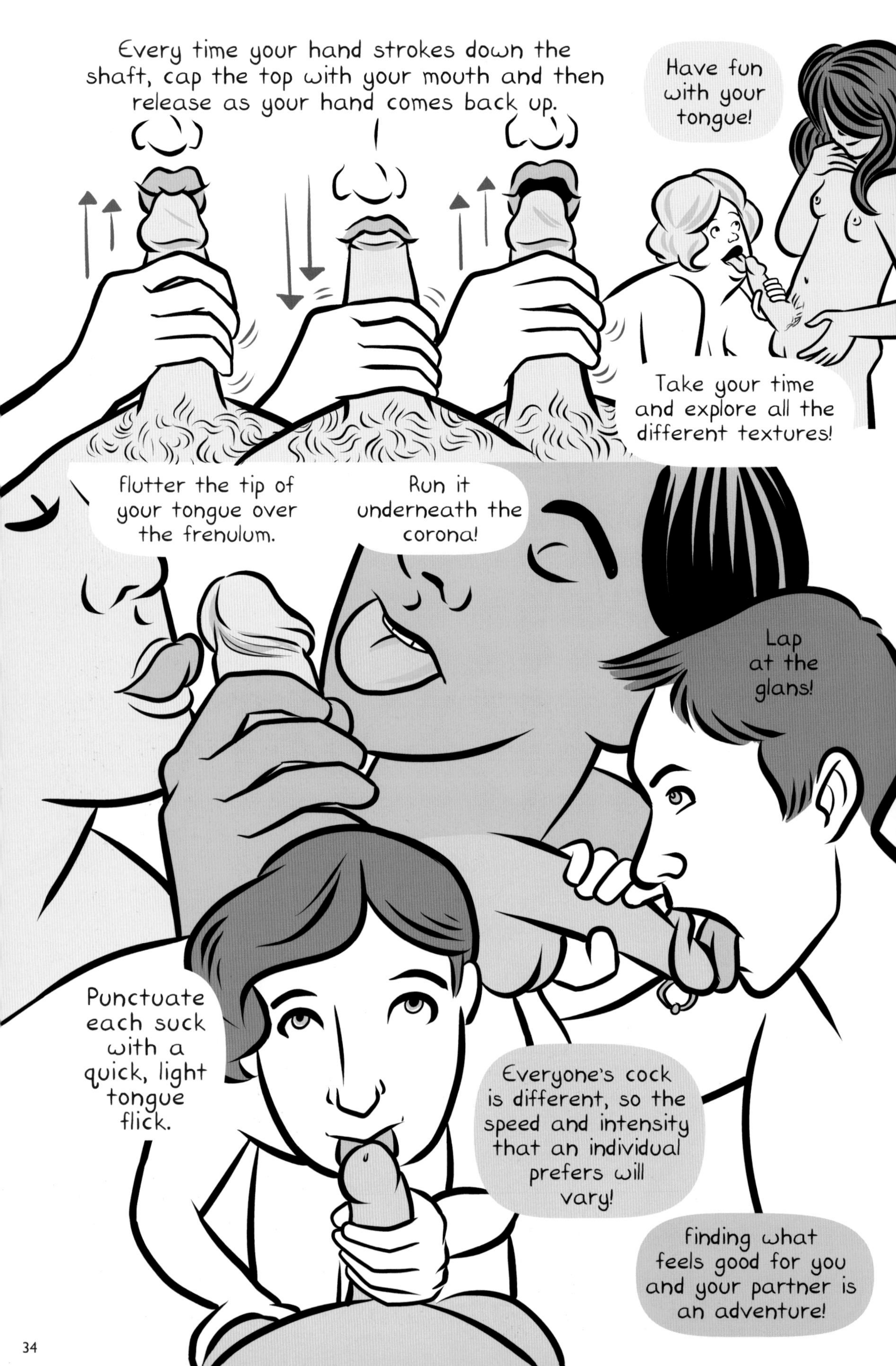
Every time your hand strokes down the shaft, cap the top with your mouth and then release as your hand comes back up.
Have fun with your tongue!
Take your time and explore all the different textures!
flutter the tip of your tongue over the frenulum.
Run it underneath the corona!
Lap at the glans!
Punctuate each suck with a quick, light tongue flick.
Everyone's cock is different, so the speed and intensity that an individual prefers will vary!
finding what feels good for you and your partner is an adventure!

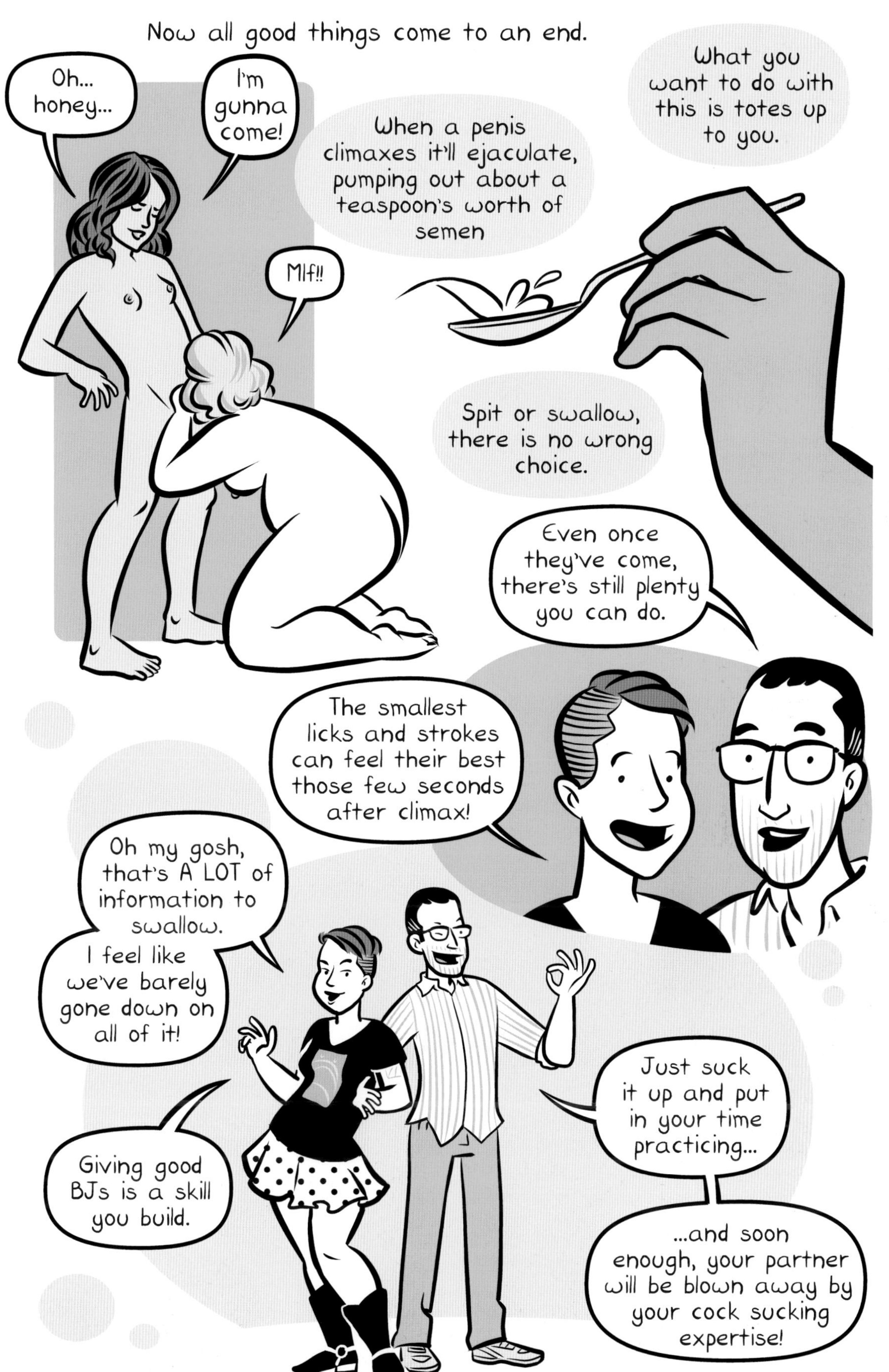
Now all good things come to an end.
Oh... honey...
I'm gunna come!
Mlf!!
When a penis climaxes it'll ejaculate, pumping out about a teaspoon's worth of semen
What you want to do with this is totes up to you.
Spit or swallow, there is no wrong choice.
Even once they've come, there's still plenty you can do.
The smallest licks and strokes can feel their best those few seconds after climax!
Oh my gosh, that's A LOT of information to swallow.
I feel like we've barely gone down on all of it!
Giving good BJs is a skill you build.
Just suck it up and put in your time practicing...
...and soon enough, your partner will be blown away by your cock sucking expertise!

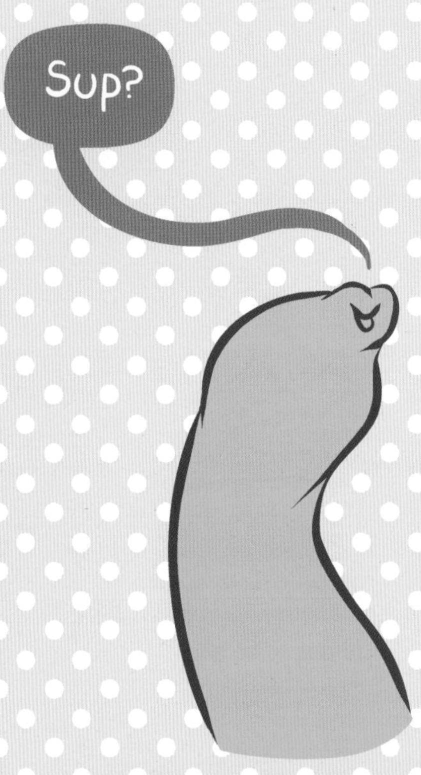
Sup?

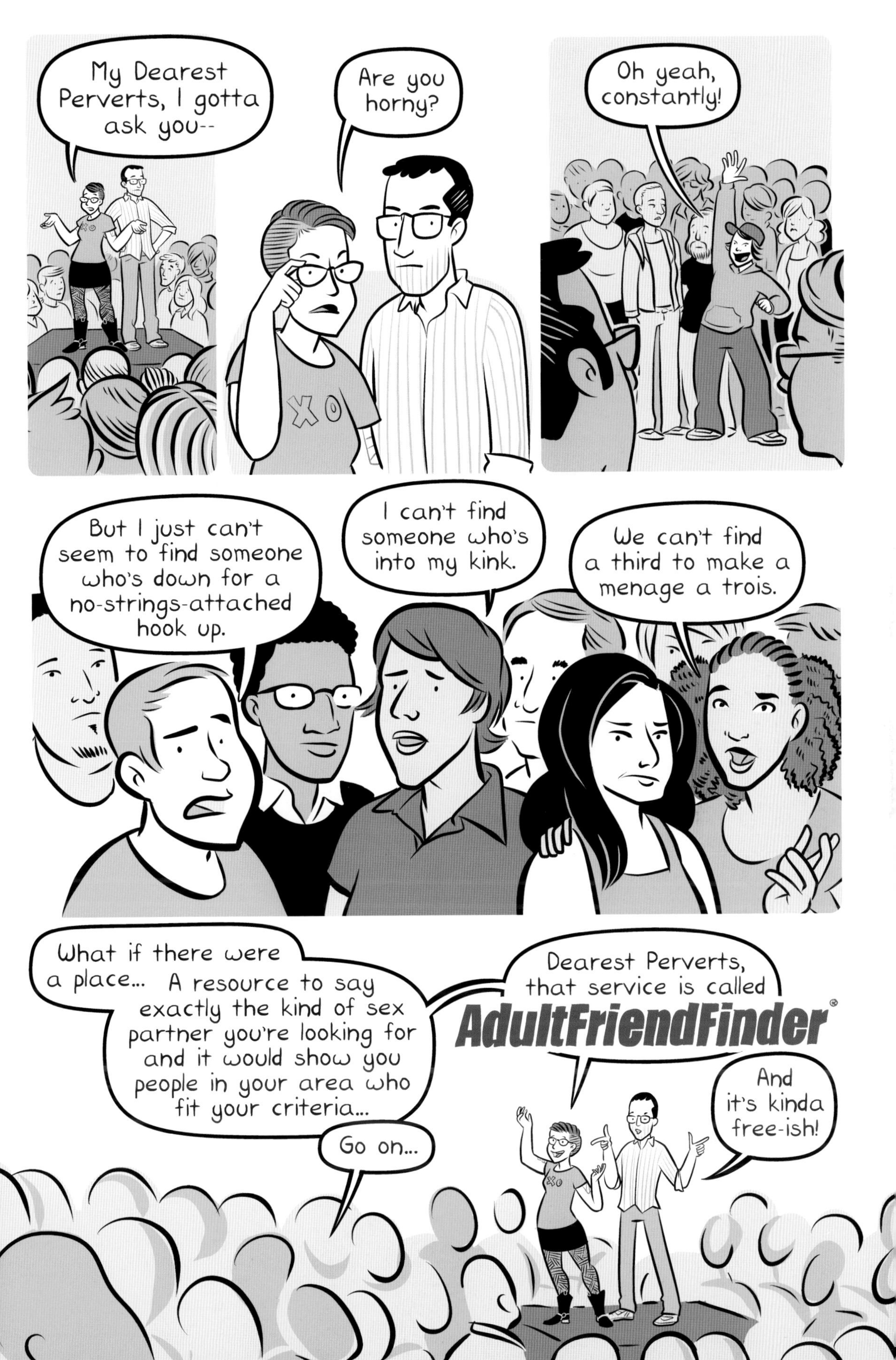
My Dearest Perverts, I gotta ask you--
Are you horny?
Oh yeah, constantly!
But I just can't seem to find someone who's down for a no-strings-attached hook up.
I can't find someone who's into my kink.
We can't find a third to make a menage a trois.
What if there were a place... A resource to say exactly the kind of sex partner you're looking for and it would show you people in your area who fit your criteria...
Go on...
Dearest Perverts, that service is called AdultFriendFinder®
And it's kinda free-ish!

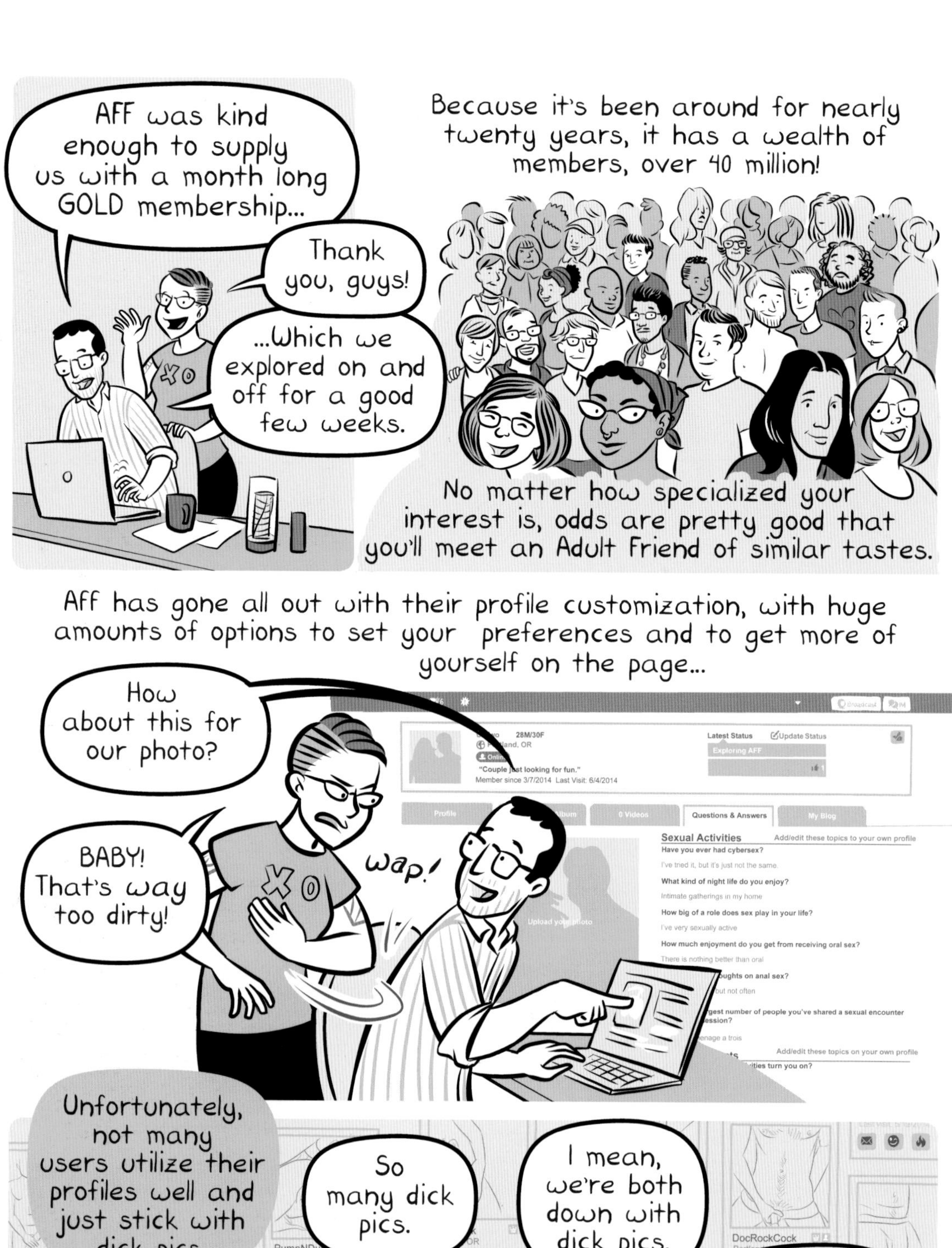
AFF was kind enough to supply us with a month long GOLD membership...
Thank you, guys!
...Which we explored on and off for a good few weeks.
Because it's been around for nearly twenty years, it has a wealth of members, over 40 million!
No matter how specialized your interest is, odds are pretty good that you'll meet an Adult Friend of similar tastes.
AFF has gone all out with their profile customization, with huge amounts of options to set your preferences and to get more of yourself on the page...
How about this for our photo?
BABY! That's way too dirty!
wap!
Sexual Activities
Questions & Answers
Unfortunately, not many users utilize their profiles well and just stick with dick pics.
So many dick pics.
I mean, we're both down with dick pics.
Oh man...
But c'mon, everything in moderation!
Maybe if AFF limited the amount of cock shots you could upload...?
PumpNDu
GirthBrooks
CooterLootr
DocRockCock
nodramaplz

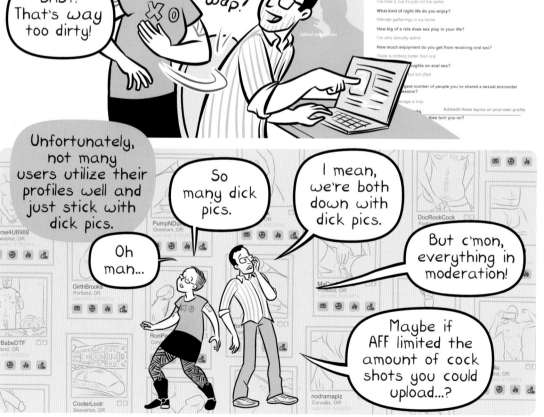

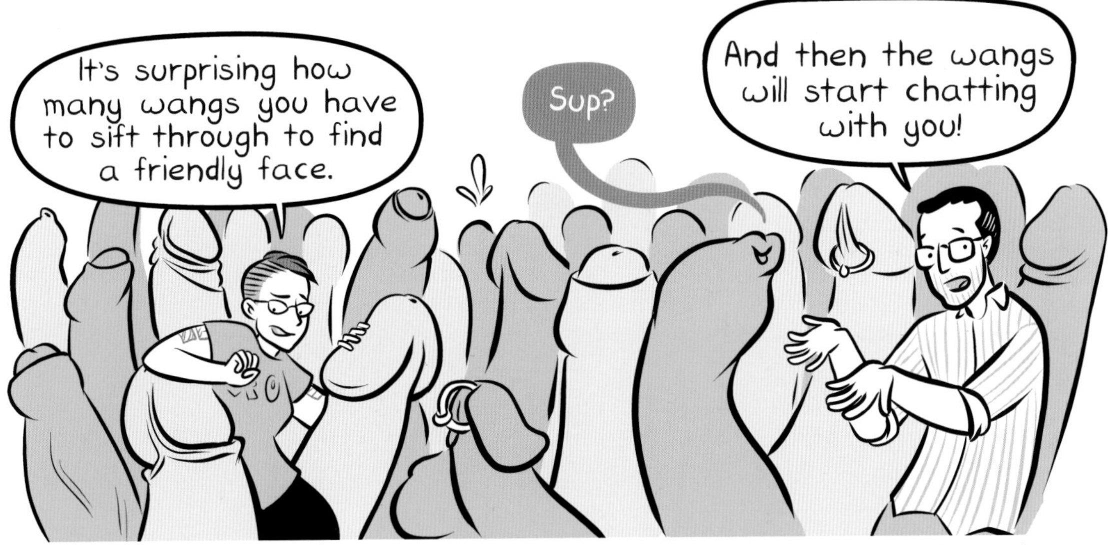

We were honestly surprised at how much people just wanted to chat.

If you can weed out the fake and 'whack off' accounts run by seemingly illiterate 16 year olds, you can manage to get some rewarding flirty conversations with your friendly local perverts.

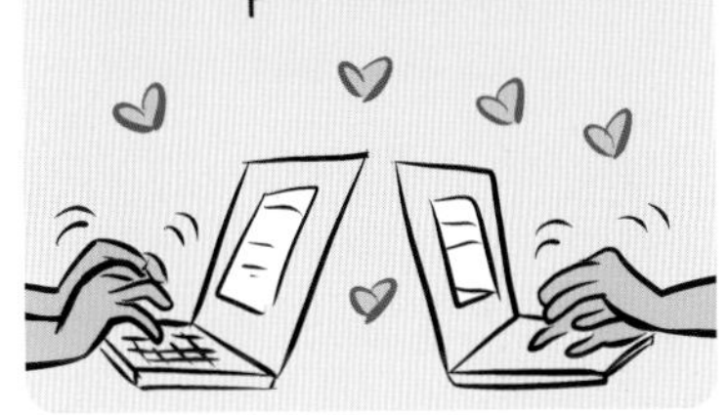

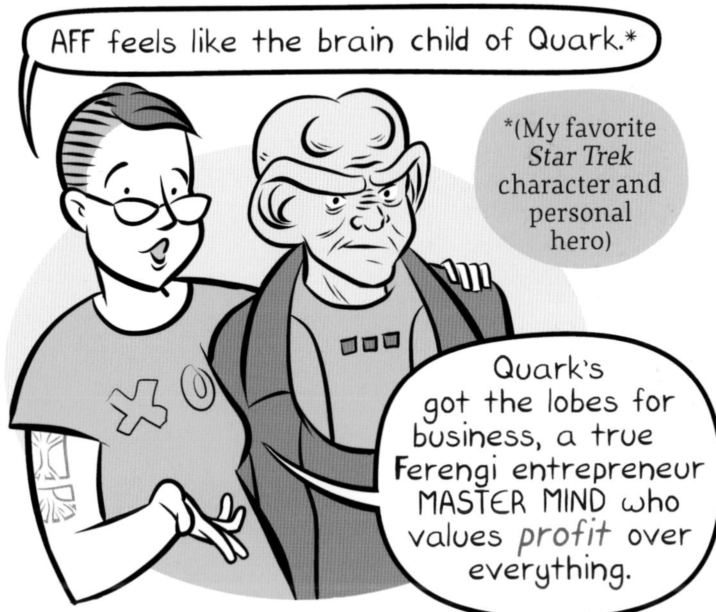

AFF feels like the brain child of Quark.*
*(My favorite *Star Trek* character and personal hero)
Quark's got the lobes for business, a true Ferengi entrepreneur MASTER MIND who values *profit* over everything.

Ferengi society operates on an aggressively capitalist model.

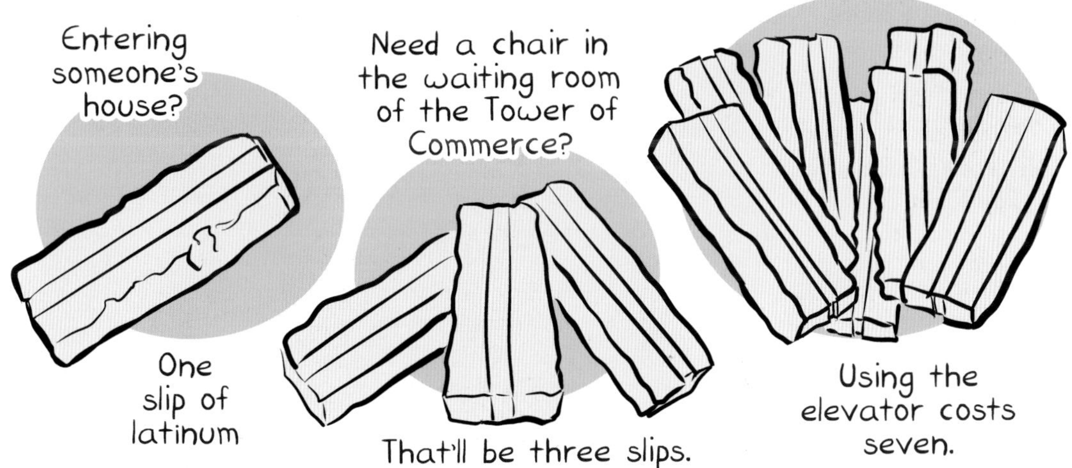

Entering someone's house?
One slip of latinum
Need a chair in the waiting room of the Tower of Commerce?
That'll be three slips.
Using the elevator costs seven.

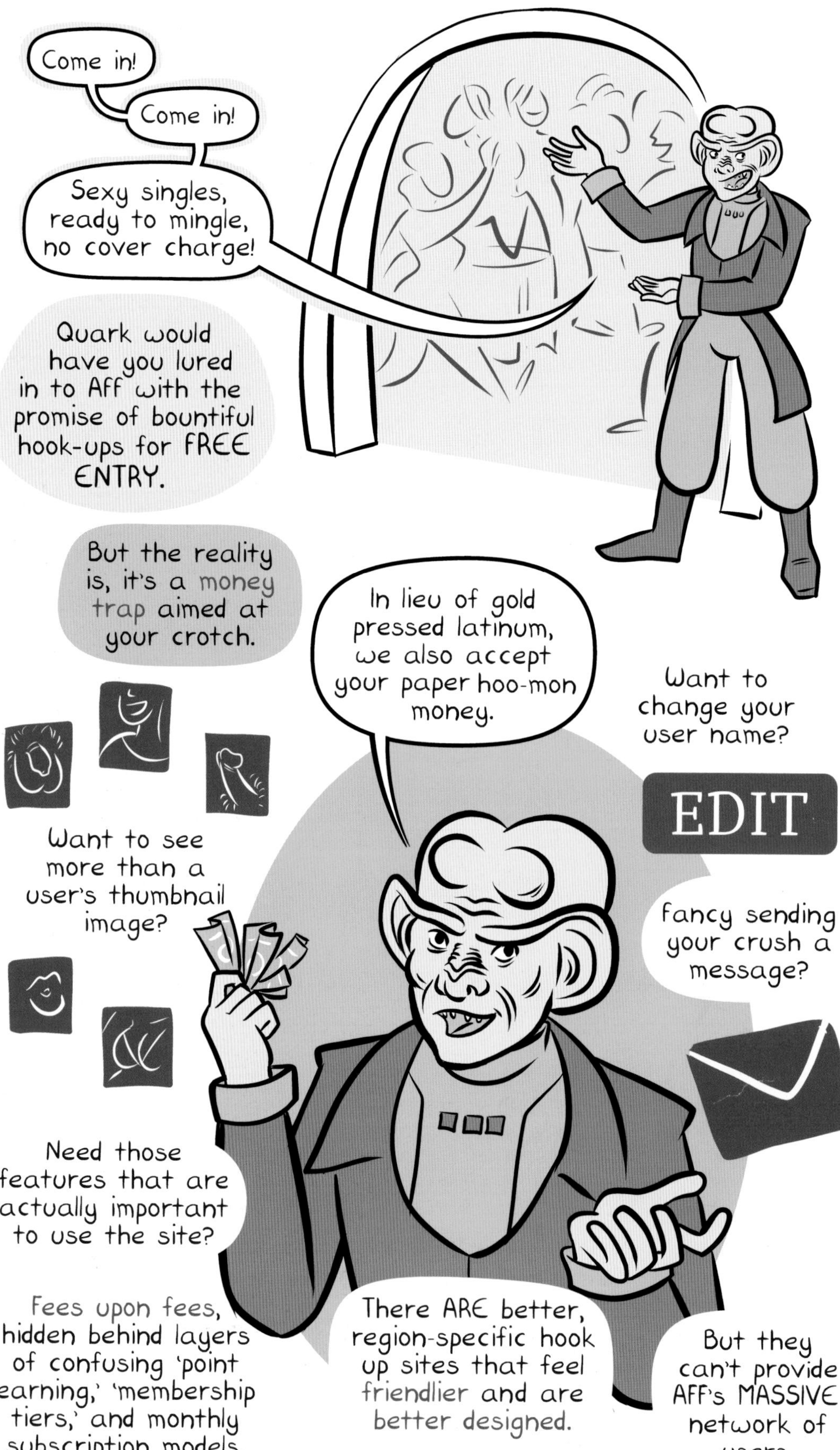
Come in!
Come in!
Sexy singles, ready to mingle, no cover charge!
Quark would have you lured in to Aff with the promise of bountiful hook-ups for FREE ENTRY.
But the reality is, it's a money trap aimed at your crotch.
In lieu of gold pressed latinum, we also accept your paper hoo-mon money.
Want to change your user name?
EDIT
Want to see more than a user's thumbnail image?
fancy sending your crush a message?
Need those features that are actually important to use the site?
Fees upon fees, hidden behind layers of confusing 'point earning,' 'membership tiers,' and monthly subscription models.
There ARE better, region-specific hook up sites that feel friendlier and are better designed.
But they can't provide AFF's MASSIVE network of users.

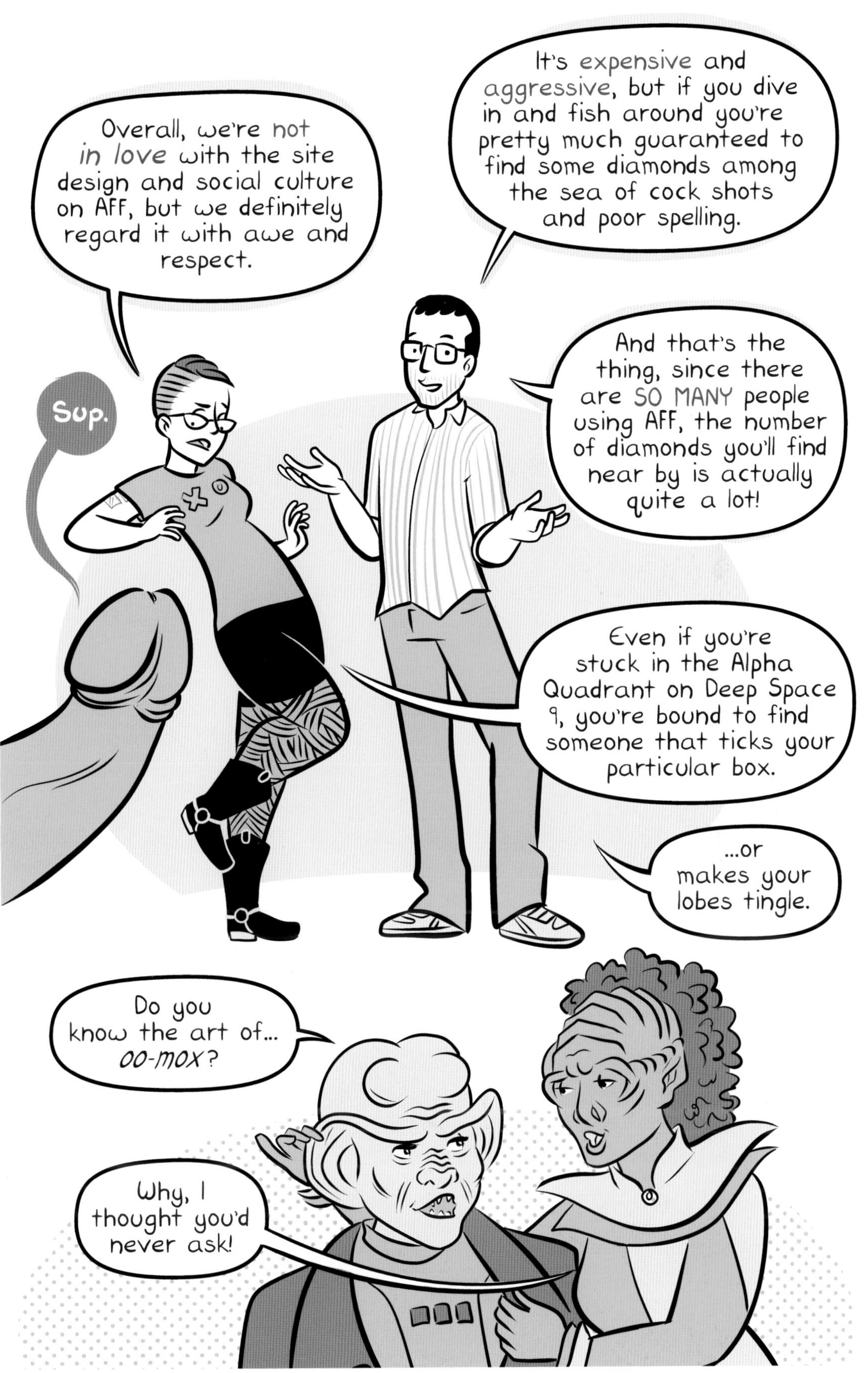
Overall, we're not in love with the site design and social culture on AFF, but we definitely regard it with awe and respect.
It's expensive and aggressive, but if you dive in and fish around you're pretty much guaranteed to find some diamonds among the sea of cock shots and poor spelling.
Sup.
And that's the thing, since there are SO MANY people using AFF, the number of diamonds you'll find near by is actually quite a lot!
Even if you're stuck in the Alpha Quadrant on Deep Space 9, you're bound to find someone that ticks your particular box.
...or makes your lobes tingle.
Do you know the art of... OO-MOX?
Why, I thought you'd never ask!

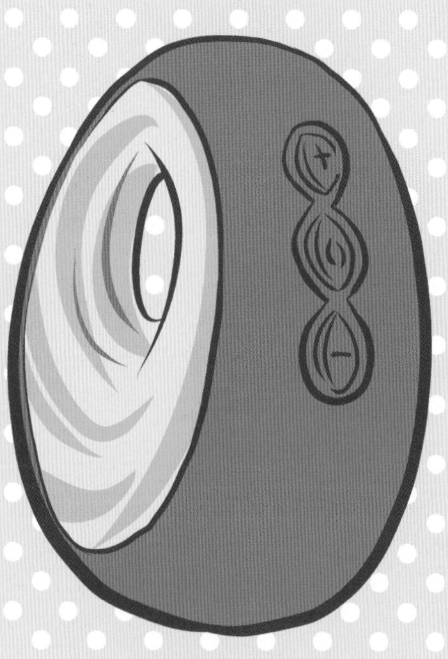

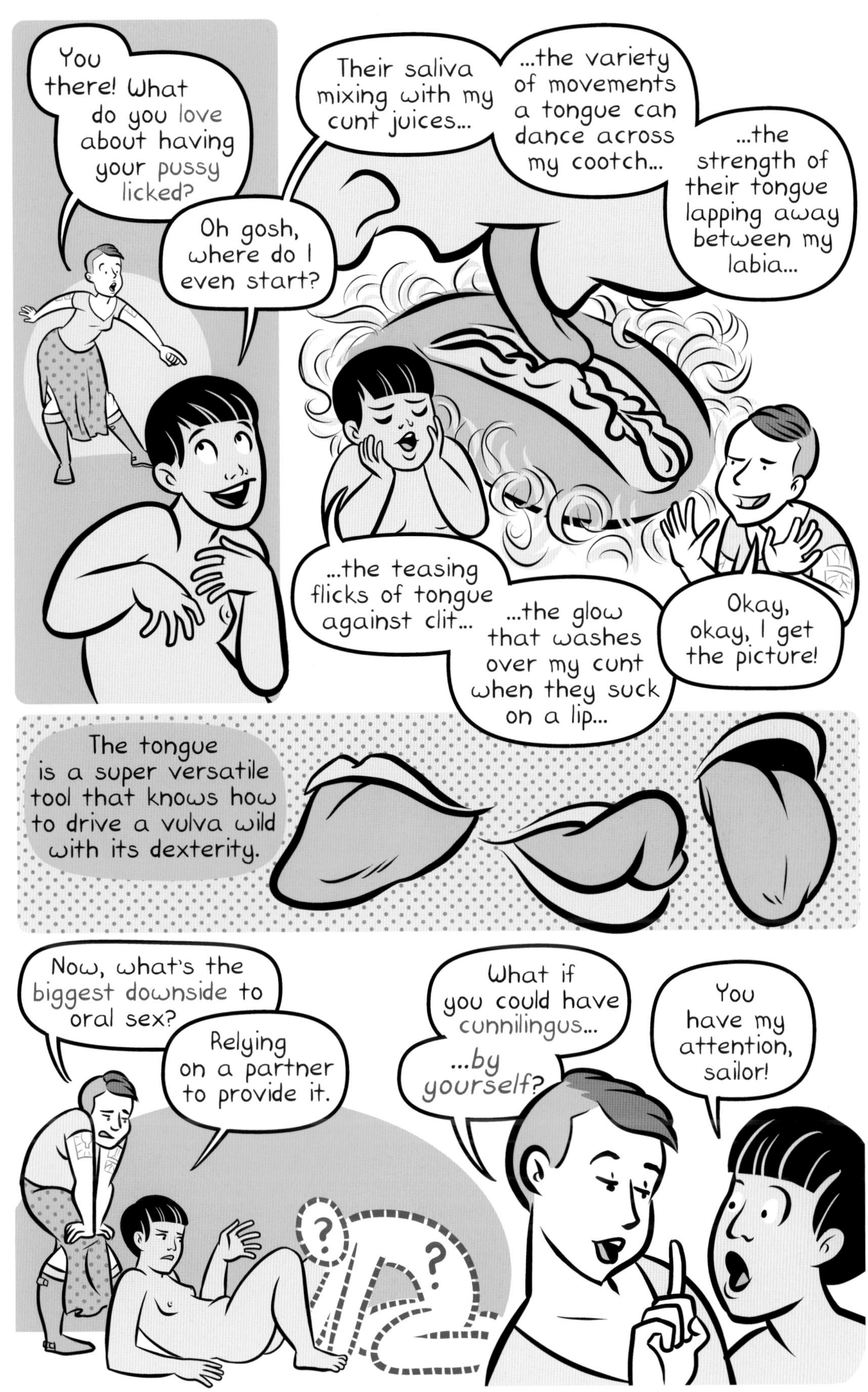
You there! What do you love about having your pussy licked?
Oh gosh, where do I even start?
Their saliva mixing with my cunt juices...
...the variety of movements a tongue can dance across my cootch...
...the strength of their tongue lapping away between my labia...
...the teasing flicks of tongue against clit...
...the glow that washes over my cunt when they suck on a lip...
Okay, okay, I get the picture!
The tongue is a super versatile tool that knows how to drive a vulva wild with its dexterity.
Now, what's the biggest downside to oral sex?
Relying on a partner to provide it.
?
?
What if you could have cunnilingus...
...by yourself?
You have my attention, sailor!

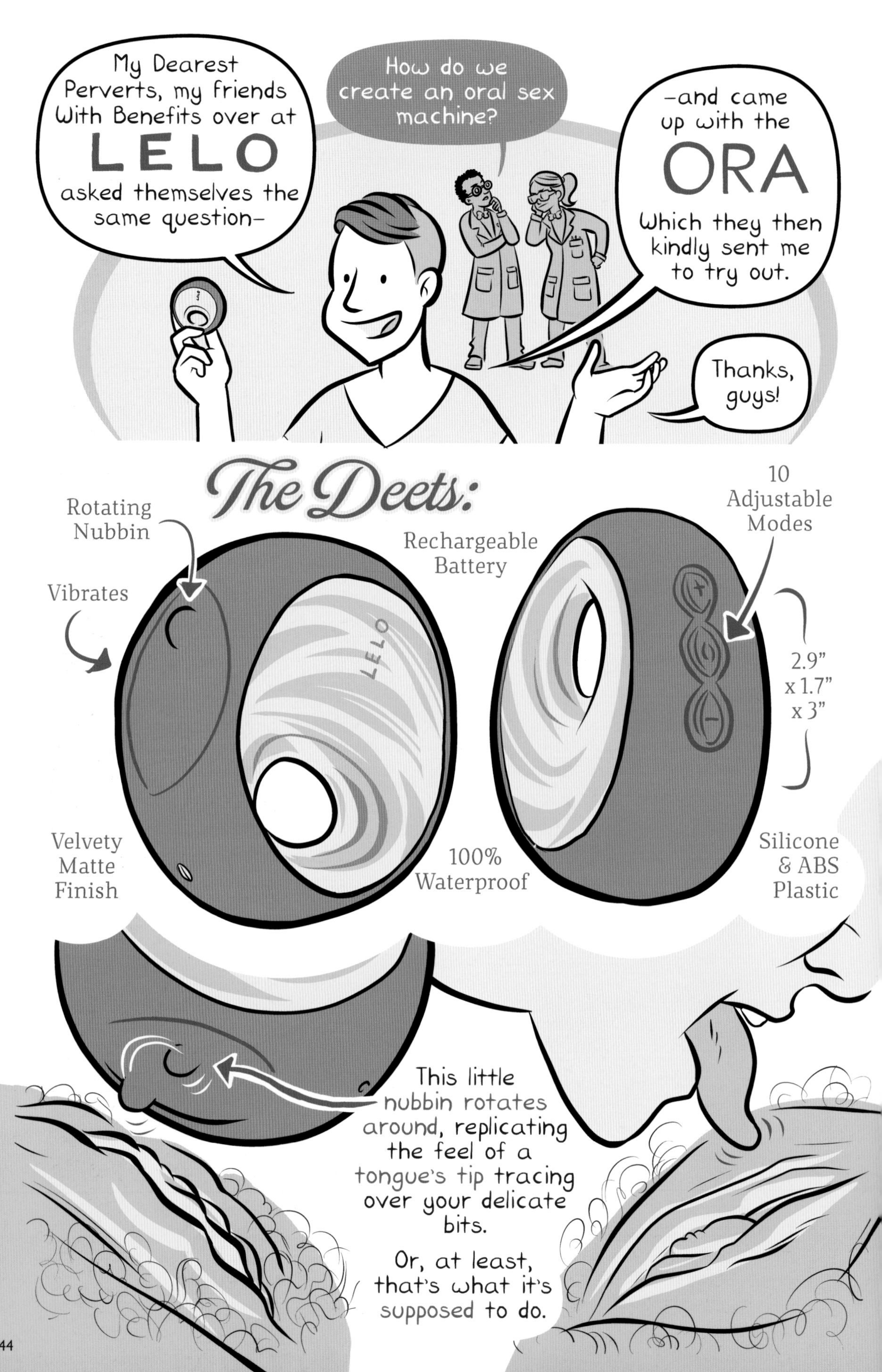
My Dearest Perverts, my friends With Benefits over at
LELO
asked themselves the same question–
How do we create an oral sex machine?
–and came up with the
ORA
Which they then kindly sent me to try out.
Thanks, guys!
The Deets:
Rotating Nubbin
Vibrates
Rechargeable Battery
10 Adjustable Modes
LELO
2.9" x 1.7" x 3"
Velvety Matte Finish
100% Waterproof
Silicone & ABS Plastic
This little nubbin rotates around, replicating the feel of a tongue's tip tracing over your delicate bits.
Or, at least, that's what it's supposed to do.

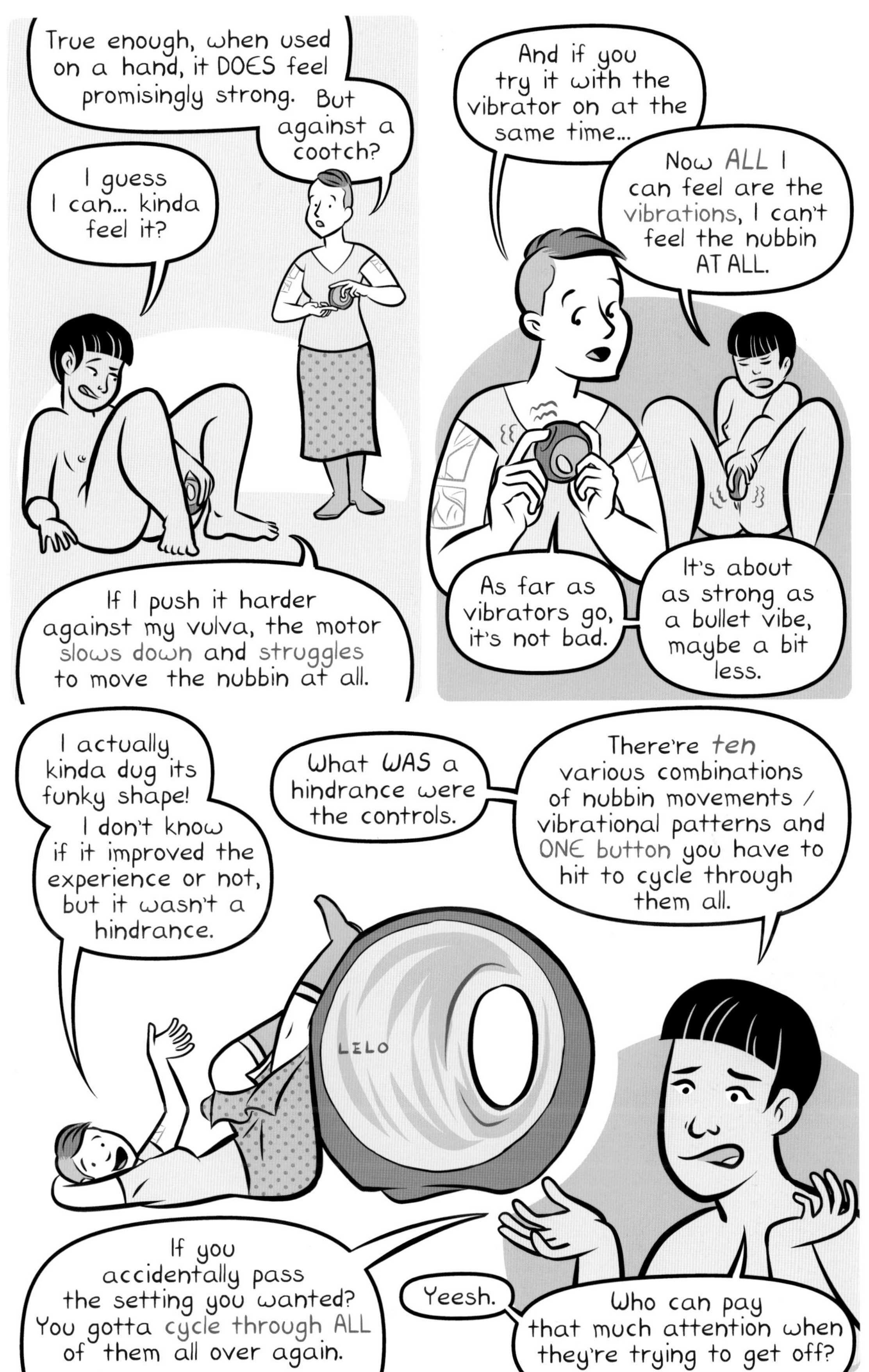
True enough, when used on a hand, it DOES feel promisingly strong. But against a cootch?
I guess I can... kinda feel it?
If I push it harder against my vulva, the motor slows down and struggles to move the nubbin at all.
And if you try it with the vibrator on at the same time...
Now ALL I can feel are the vibrations, I can't feel the nubbin AT ALL.
As far as vibrators go, it's not bad.
It's about as strong as a bullet vibe, maybe a bit less.
I actually kinda dug its funky shape!
I don't know if it improved the experience or not, but it wasn't a hindrance.
What WAS a hindrance were the controls.
There're ten various combinations of nubbin movements / vibrational patterns and ONE button you have to hit to cycle through them all.
LELO
If you accidentally pass the setting you wanted? You gotta cycle through ALL of them all over again.
Yeesh.
Who can pay that much attention when they're trying to get off?

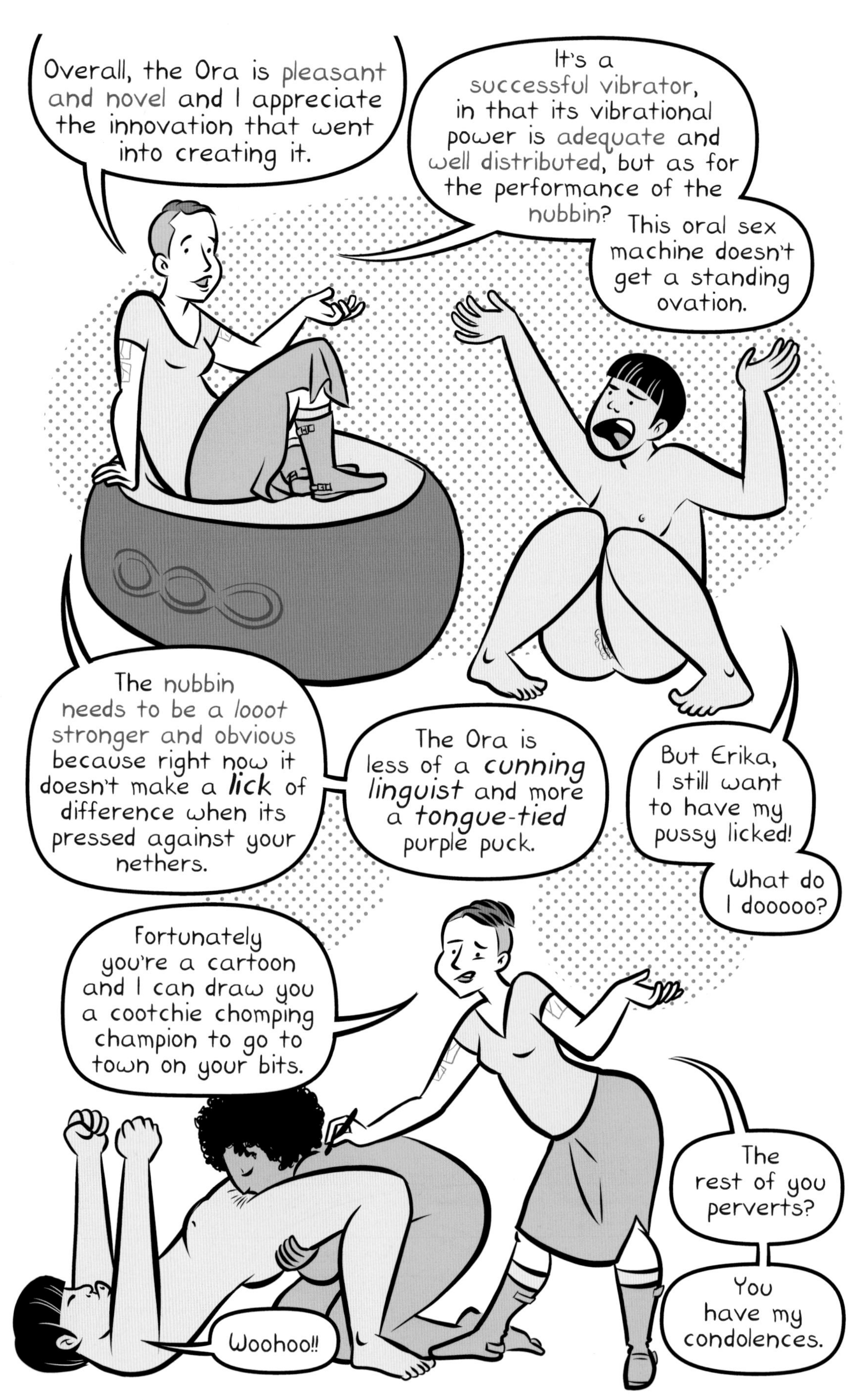

Overall, the Ora is pleasant and novel and I appreciate the innovation that went into creating it.
It's a successful vibrator, in that its vibrational power is adequate and well distributed, but as for the performance of the nubbin?
This oral sex machine doesn't get a standing ovation.
The nubbin needs to be a looot stronger and obvious because right now it doesn't make a *lick* of difference when its pressed against your nethers.
The Ora is less of a *cunning linguist* and more a *tongue-tied* purple puck.
But Erika, I still want to have my pussy licked!
What do I doooooo?
Fortunately you're a cartoon and I can draw you a cootchie chomping champion to go to town on your bits.
Woohoo!!
The rest of you perverts?
You have my condolences.

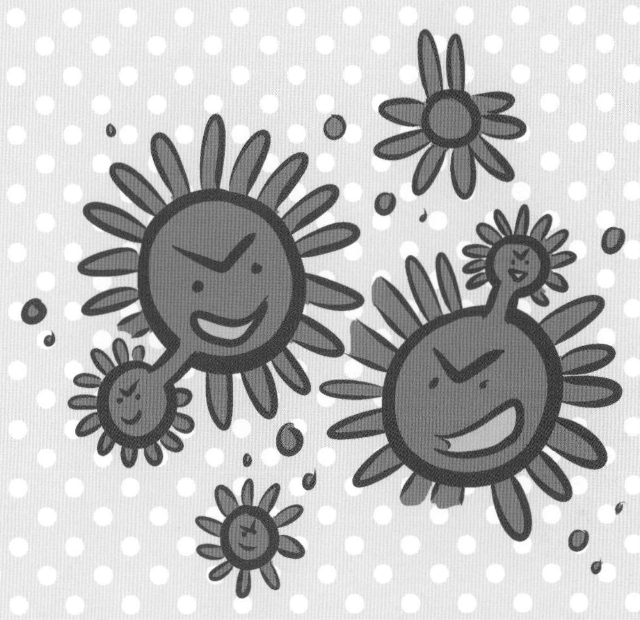

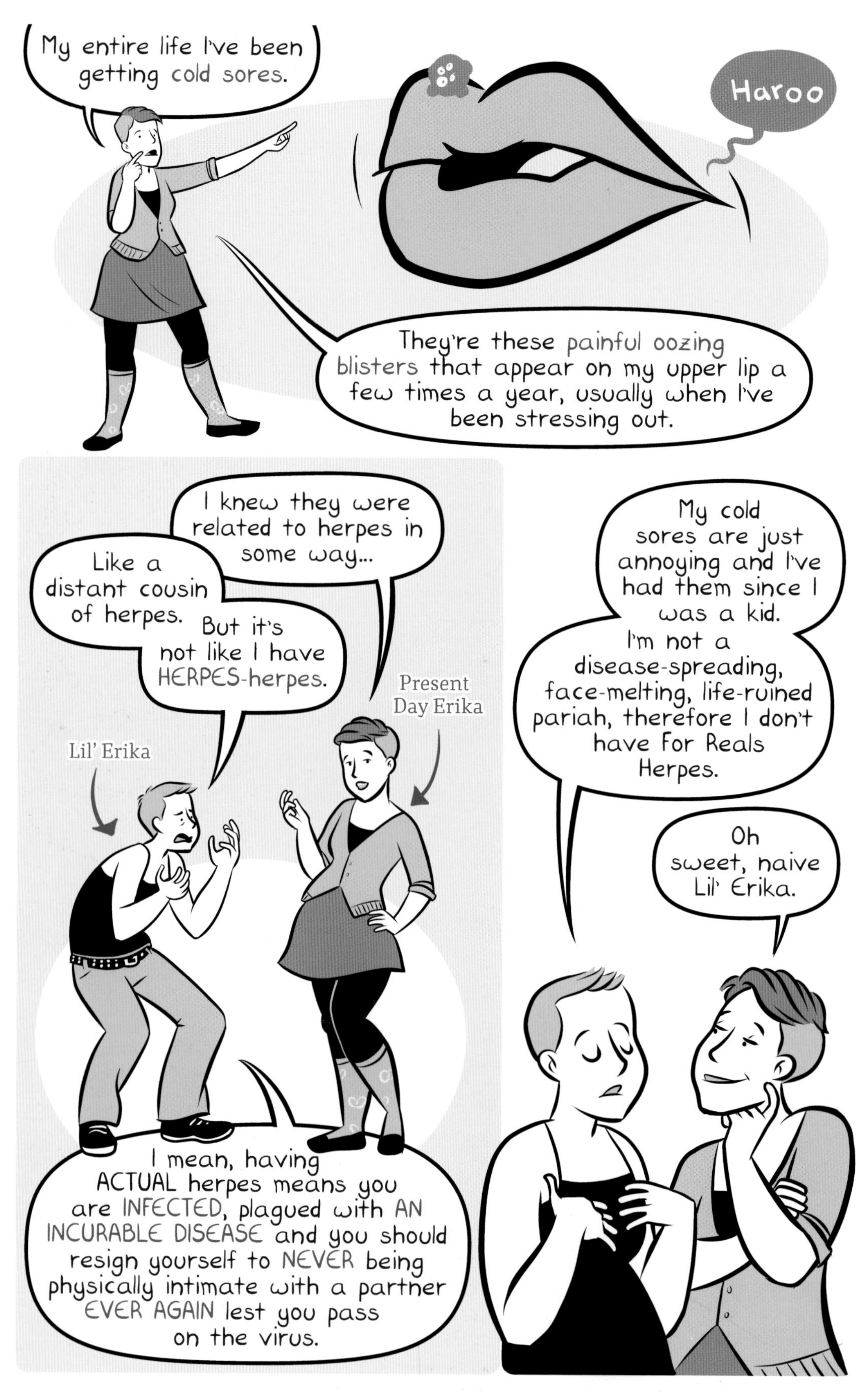
My entire life I've been getting cold sores.
Haroo
They're these painful oozing blisters that appear on my upper lip a few times a year, usually when I've been stressing out.
Like a distant cousin of herpes.
I knew they were related to herpes in some way...
But it's not like I have HERPES-herpes.
Lil' Erika
Present Day Erika
I mean, having ACTUAL herpes means you are INFECTED, plagued with AN INCURABLE DISEASE and you should resign yourself to NEVER being physically intimate with a partner EVER AGAIN lest you pass on the virus.
My cold sores are just annoying and I've had them since I was a kid.
I'm not a disease-spreading, face-melting, life-ruined pariah, therefore I don't have For Reals Herpes.
Oh sweet, naive Lil' Erika.

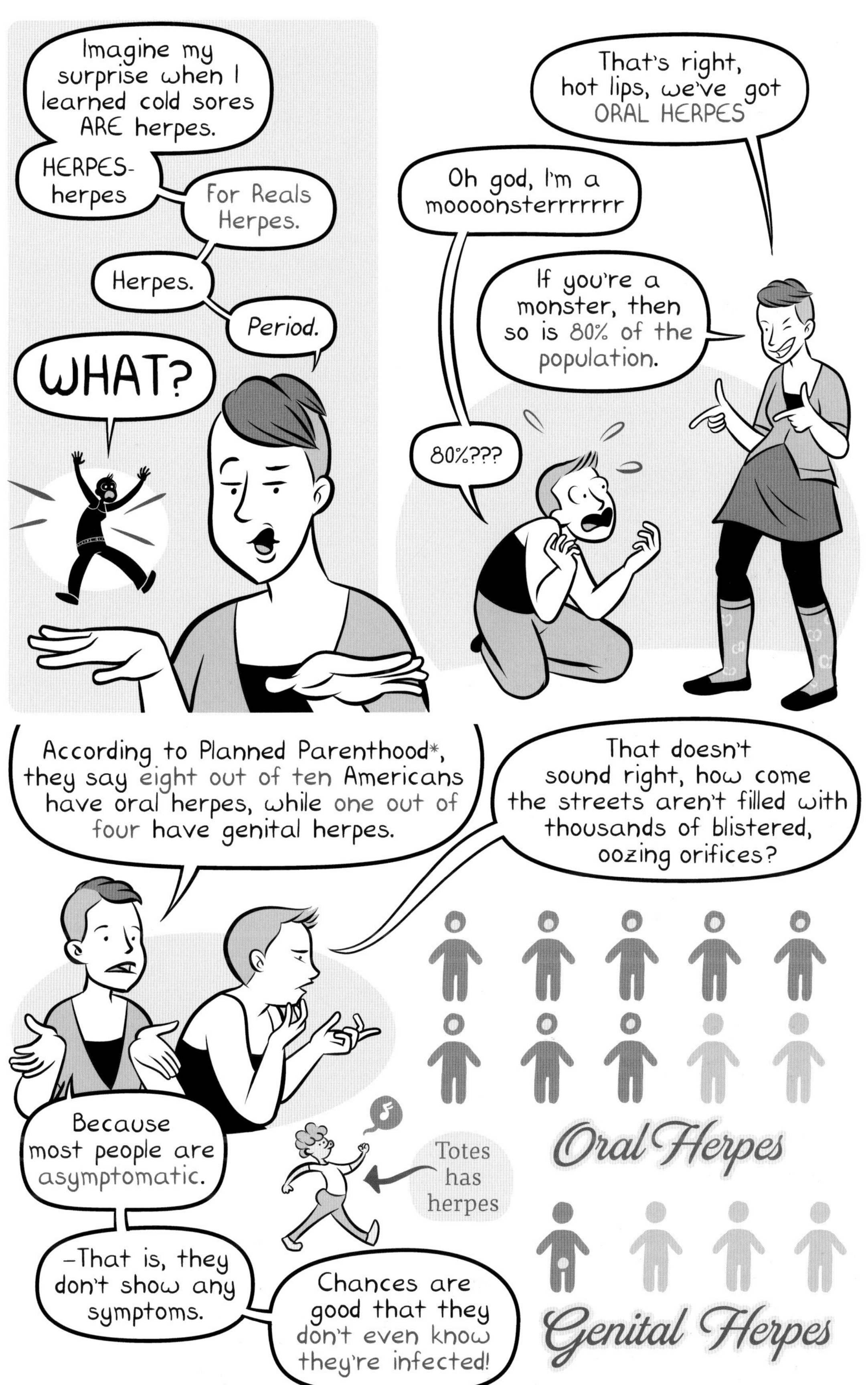
Imagine my surprise when I learned cold sores ARE herpes.
HERPES-herpes
For Reals Herpes.
Herpes.
Period.
WHAT?
That's right, hot lips, we've got ORAL HERPES
Oh god, I'm a moooonsterrrrrr
If you're a monster, then so is 80% of the population.
80%???
According to Planned Parenthood*, they say eight out of ten Americans have oral herpes, while one out of four have genital herpes.
That doesn't sound right, how come the streets aren't filled with thousands of blistered, oozing orifices?
Because most people are asymptomatic.
–That is, they don't show any symptoms.
Chances are good that they don't even know they're infected!
Totes has herpes
Oral Herpes
Genital Herpes

*plannedparenthood.org/health-info/stds-hiv-safer-sex/herpes

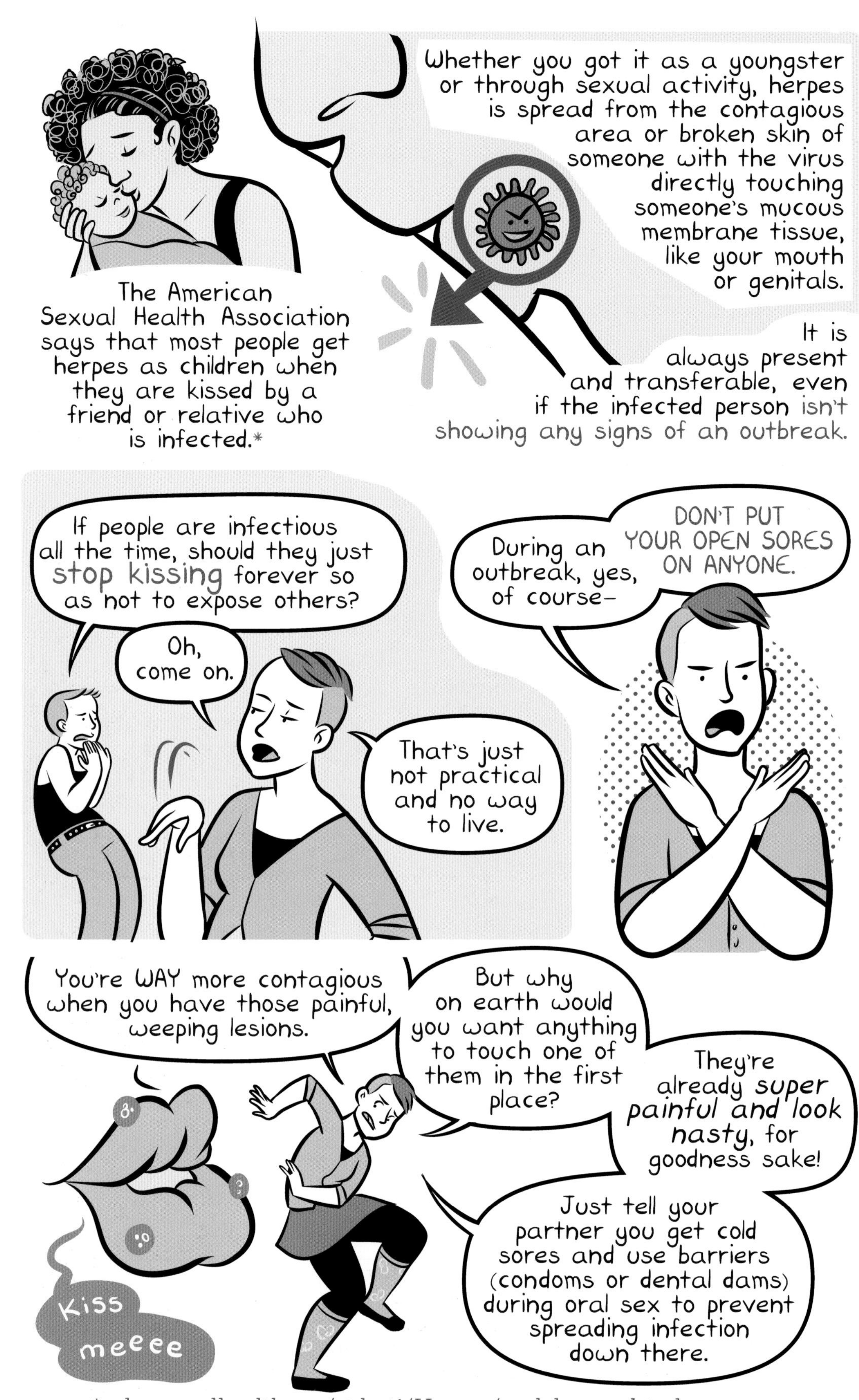
Whether you got it as a youngster or through sexual activity, herpes is spread from the contagious area or broken skin of someone with the virus directly touching someone's mucous membrane tissue, like your mouth or genitals.
The American Sexual Health Association says that most people get herpes as children when they are kissed by a friend or relative who is infected.*
It is always present and transferable, even if the infected person isn't showing any signs of an outbreak.
If people are infectious all the time, should they just stop kissing forever so as not to expose others?
Oh, come on.
That's just not practical and no way to live.
During an outbreak, yes, of course–
DON'T PUT YOUR OPEN SORES ON ANYONE.
You're WAY more contagious when you have those painful, weeping lesions.
But why on earth would you want anything to touch one of them in the first place?
They're already *super painful and look nasty*, for goodness sake!
Just tell your partner you get cold sores and use barriers (condoms or dental dams) during oral sex to prevent spreading infection down there.
Kiss meeee

*ashasexualhealth.org/std-sti/Herpes/oral-herpes.html

The Life and Times of a Herpes Outbreak:*

Remission.

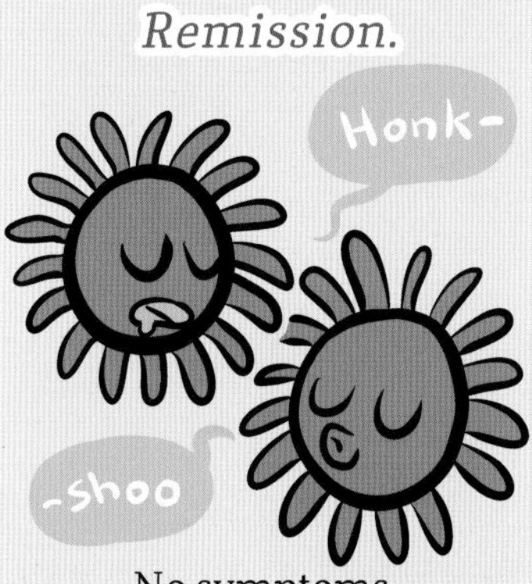

No symptoms, though still contagious, while the virus lives in your sensory nerve ganglia.

Prodromal
Day 0–1

Tingling/itching sensations and reddening skin begin a few hours or days before physical symptoms appear.

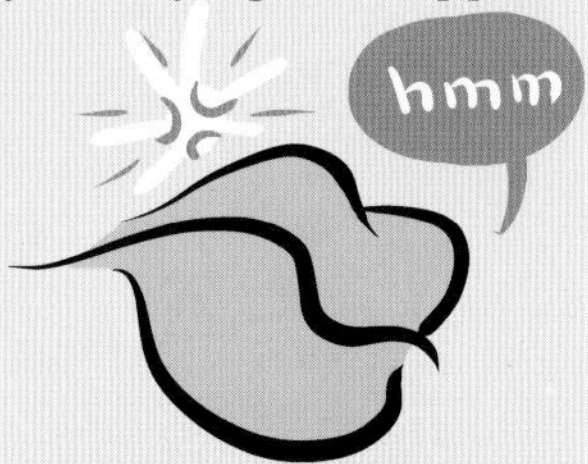

Start treatment, if you have some!

Inflammation
Day 1

The virus begins reproducing and infecting cells at the end of the nerve.

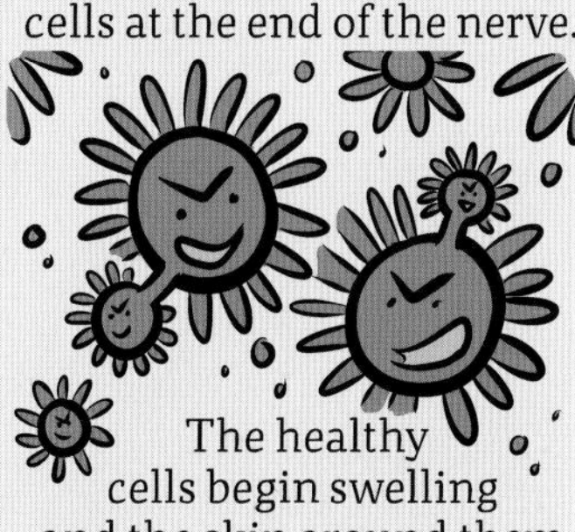

The healthy cells begin swelling and the skin around them becomes reddened.

Pre-sore
Day 2–3

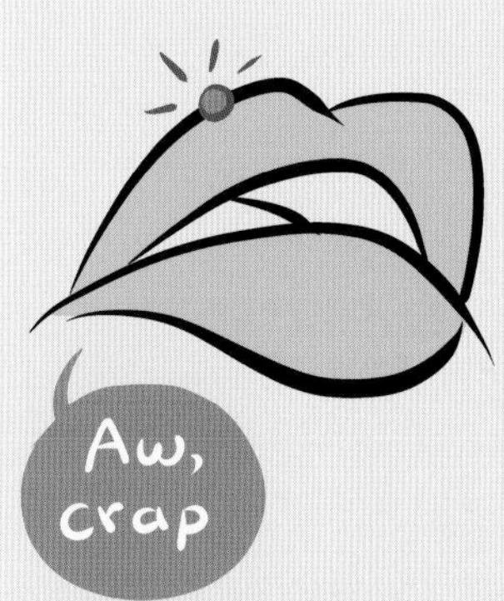

A hard, little, painful bump(s) appears on the skin.

Open lesion
Day 4

Augh, the worst part!

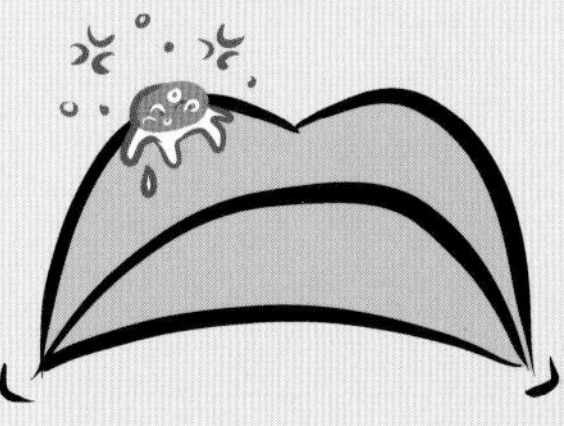

The bump(s) breaks open & create an open, weeping, super painful sore. This fluid is HIGHLY contagious with active viral particles.

Crusting
Day 5–8

A yellow or brown-ish crust develops.

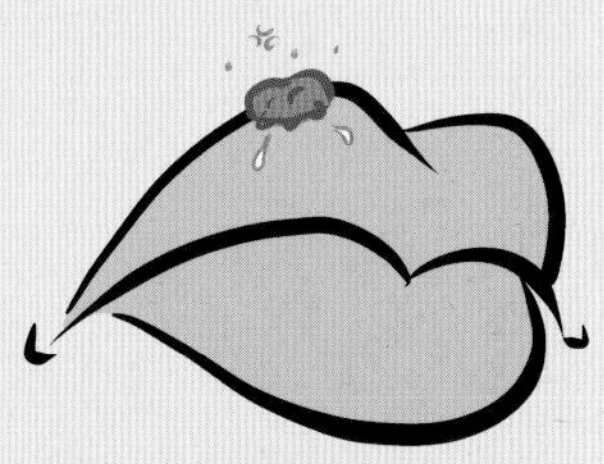

It will crack open regularly from movement, releasing more contagious fluid from within the lesion.

Healing
Day 9–14

As the virus retreats back to dormancy, new skin grows beneath the scab.

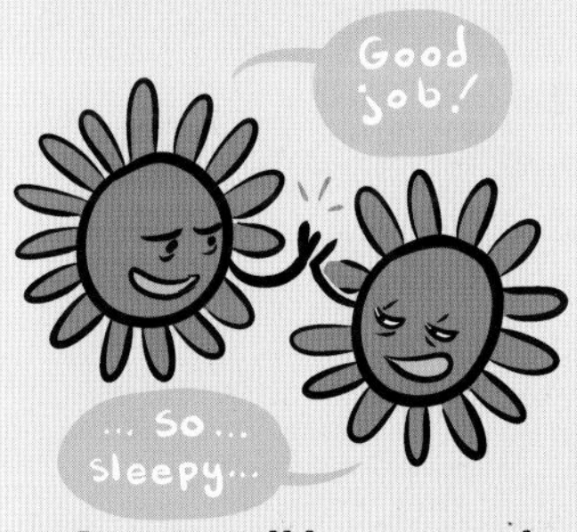

It may still be irritated, itchy, and painful.

Post scab
Day 12–14

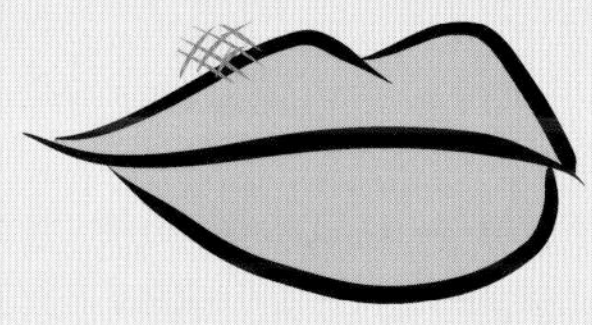

As the destroyed cells regenerate, some redness may linger at the site of the outbreak, and the virus can still shed even at this stage of recovery.

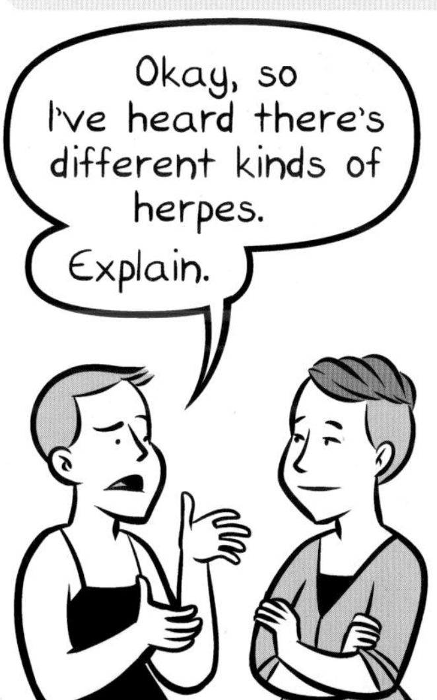

*http://en.wikipedia.org/wiki/Herpes_labialis

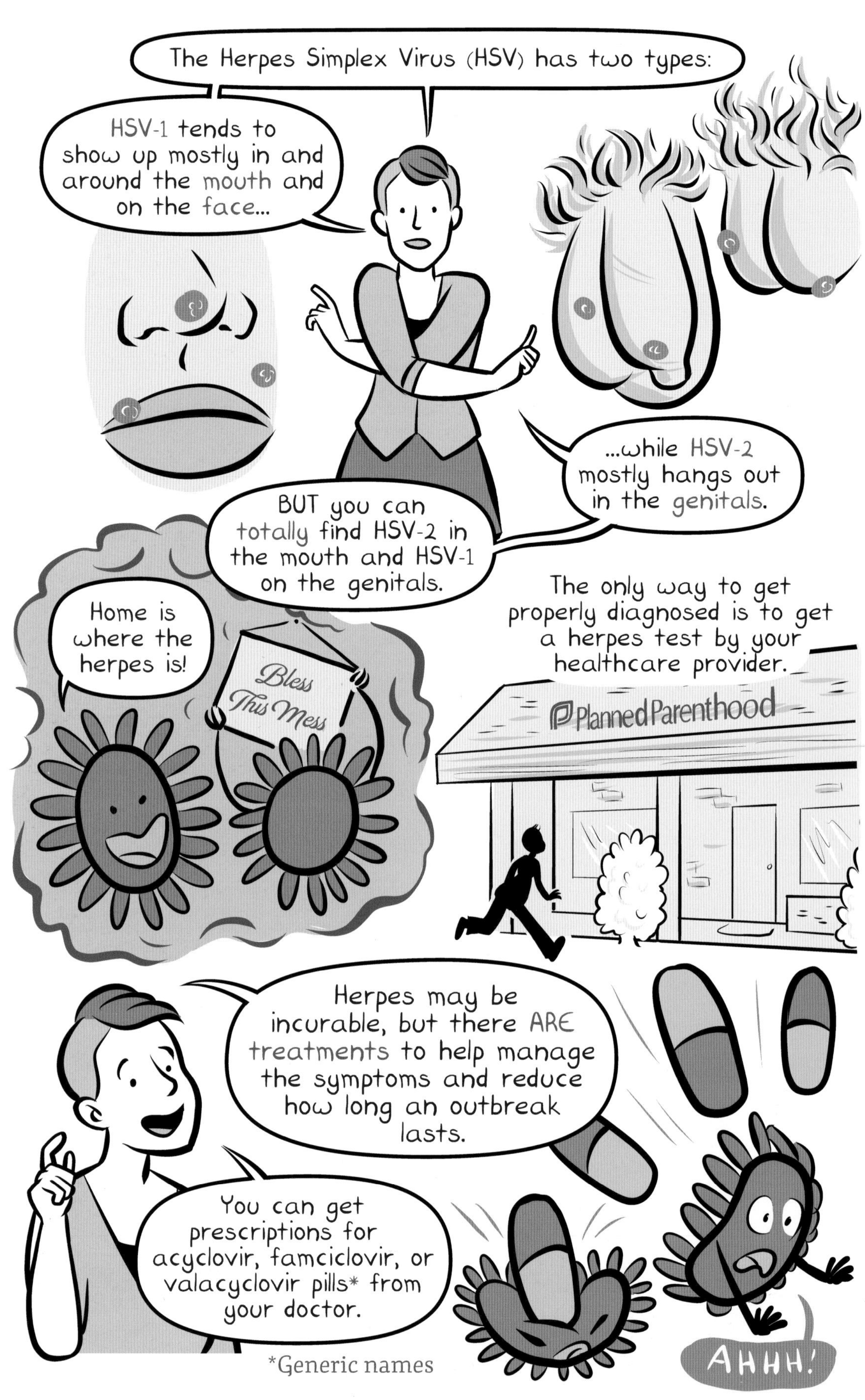
The Herpes Simplex Virus (HSV) has two types:
HSV-1 tends to show up mostly in and around the mouth and on the face...
...while HSV-2 mostly hangs out in the genitals.
BUT you can totally find HSV-2 in the mouth and HSV-1 on the genitals.
Home is where the herpes is!
Bless This Mess
The only way to get properly diagnosed is to get a herpes test by your healthcare provider.
Planned Parenthood
Herpes may be incurable, but there ARE treatments to help manage the symptoms and reduce how long an outbreak lasts.
You can get prescriptions for acyclovir, famciclovir, or valacyclovir pills* from your doctor.
AHHH!

*Generic names

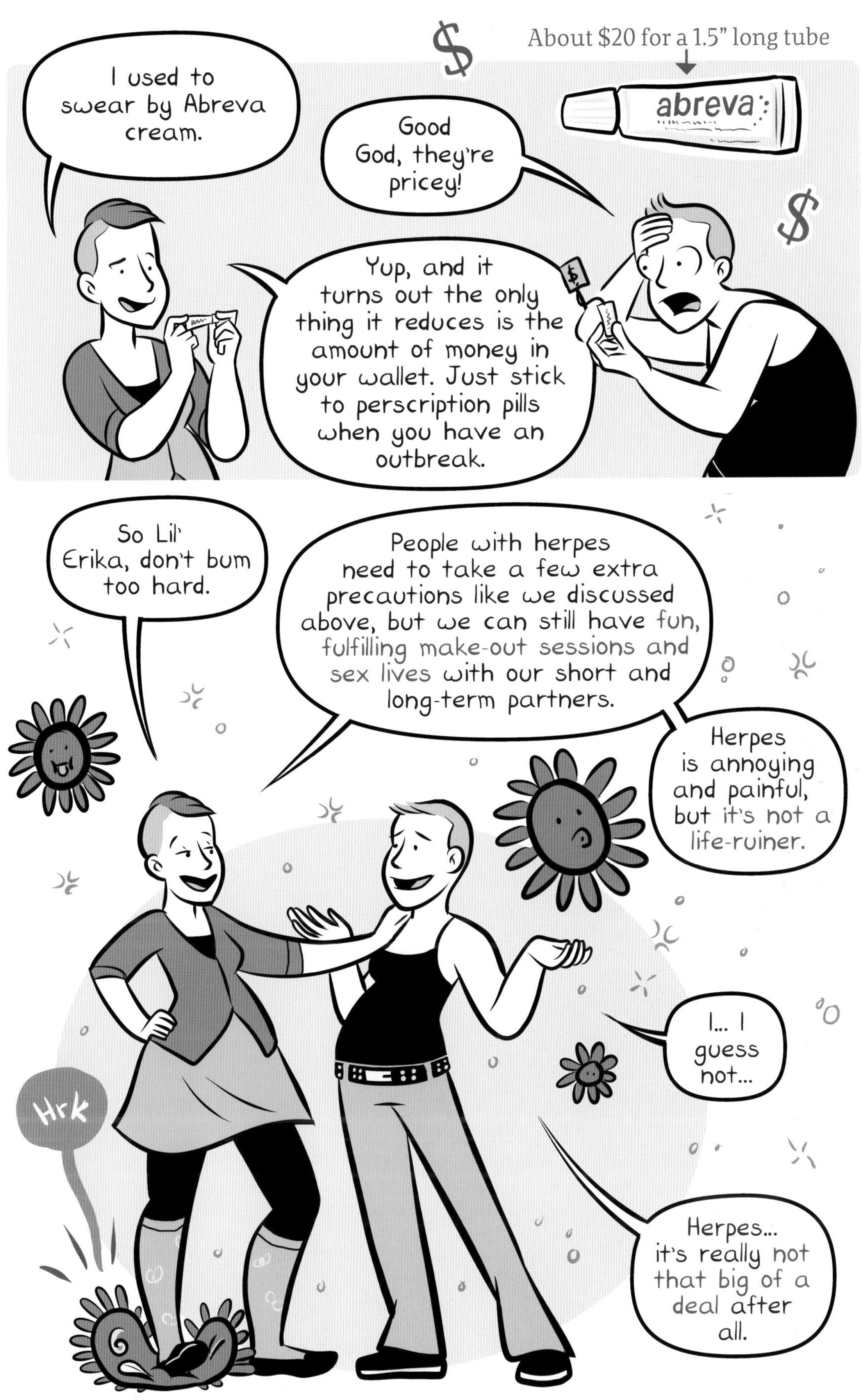
I used to swear by Abreva cream.
About $20 for a 1.5" long tube
abreva
Good God, they're pricey!
Yup, and it turns out the only thing it reduces is the amount of money in your wallet. Just stick to perscription pills when you have an outbreak.
So Lil' Erika, don't bum too hard.
People with herpes need to take a few extra precautions like we discussed above, but we can still have fun, fulfilling make-out sessions and sex lives with our short and long-term partners.
Herpes is annoying and painful, but it's not a life-ruiner.
I... I guess not...
Hrk
Herpes... it's really not that big of a deal after all.

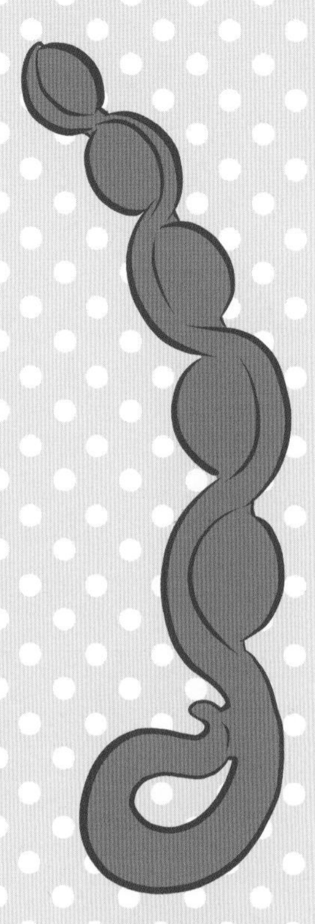

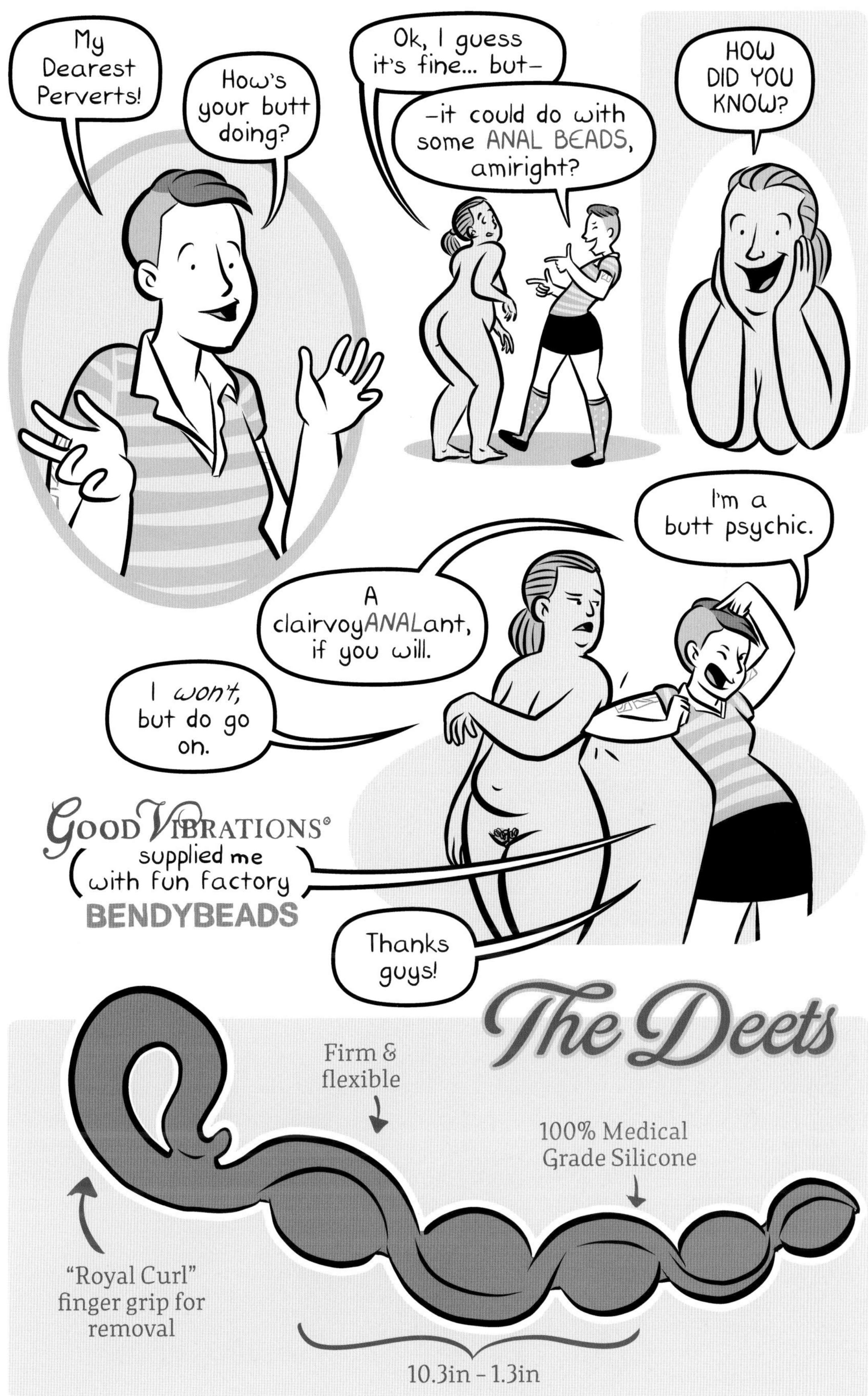
My Dearest Perverts!
How's your butt doing?
Ok, I guess it's fine... but–
–it could do with some ANAL BEADS, amiright?
HOW DID YOU KNOW?
I'm a butt psychic.
A clairvoyANALant, if you will.
I won't, but do go on.
GOOD VIBRATIONS®
supplied me with fun factory
BENDYBEADS
Thanks guys!
The Deets
Firm & flexible
100% Medical Grade Silicone
"Royal Curl" finger grip for removal
10.3in - 1.3in

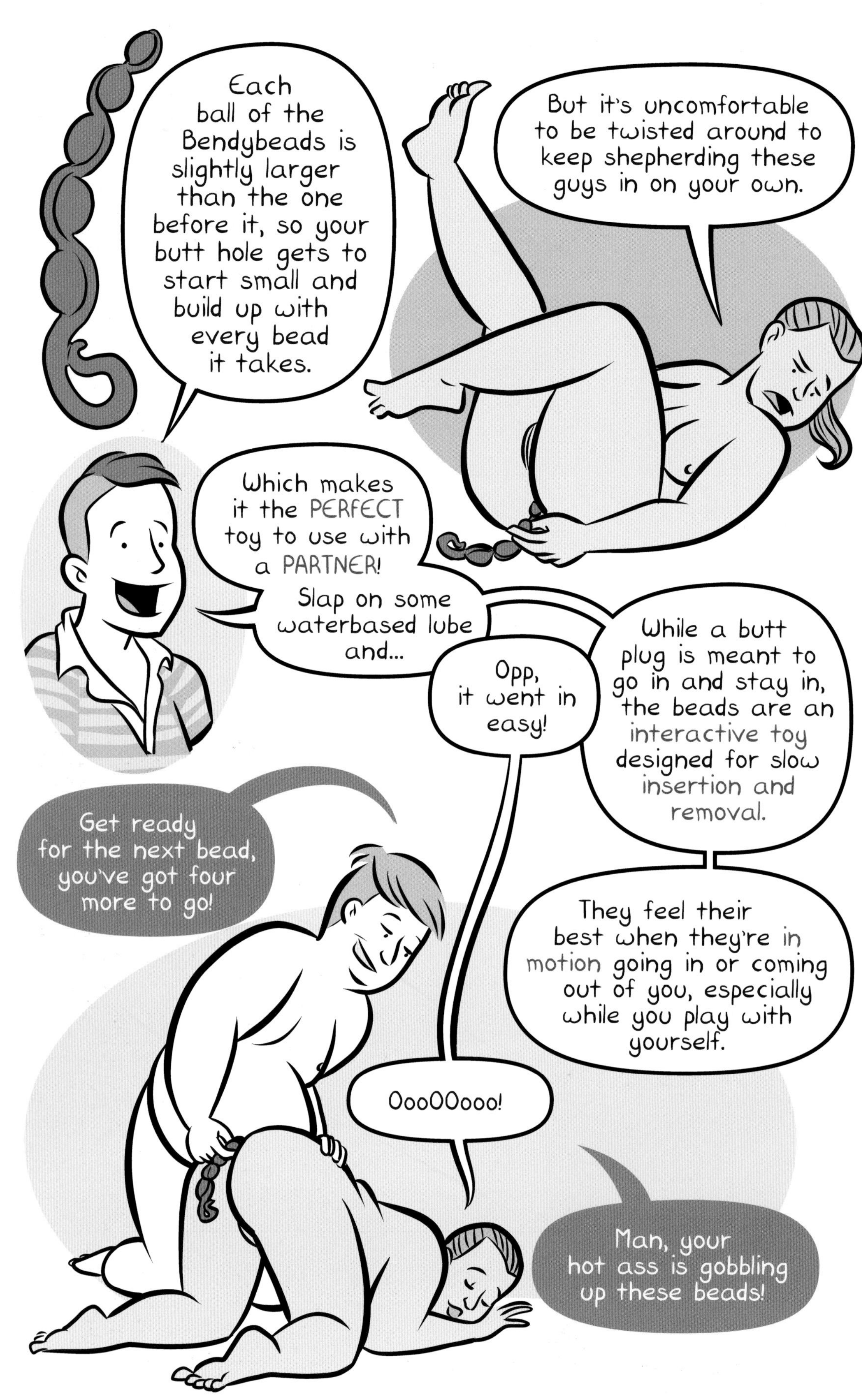
Each ball of the Bendybeads is slightly larger than the one before it, so your butt hole gets to start small and build up with every bead it takes.
But it's uncomfortable to be twisted around to keep shepherding these guys in on your own.
Which makes it the PERFECT toy to use with a PARTNER!
Slap on some waterbased lube and...
Opp, it went in easy!
While a butt plug is meant to go in and stay in, the beads are an interactive toy designed for slow insertion and removal.
They feel their best when they're in motion going in or coming out of you, especially while you play with yourself.
Get ready for the next bead, you've got four more to go!
OooOOooo!
Man, your hot ass is gobbling up these beads!

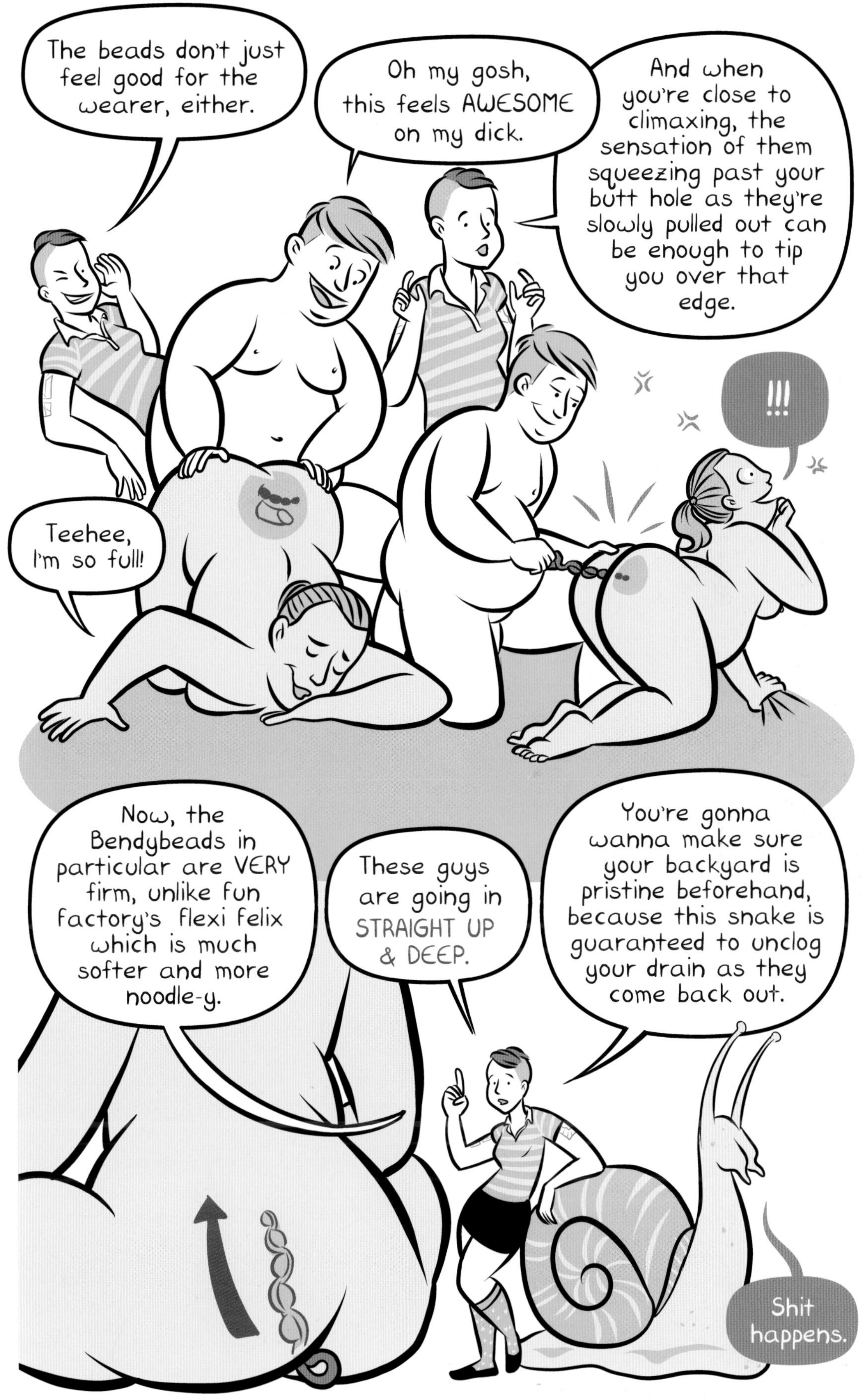
The beads don't just feel good for the wearer, either.
Oh my gosh, this feels AWESOME on my dick.
And when you're close to climaxing, the sensation of them squeezing past your butt hole as they're slowly pulled out can be enough to tip you over that edge.
!!!
Teehee, I'm so full!
Now, the Bendybeads in particular are VERY firm, unlike fun factory's flexi felix which is much softer and more noodle-y.
These guys are going in STRAIGHT UP & DEEP.
You're gonna wanna make sure your backyard is pristine beforehand, because this snake is guaranteed to unclog your drain as they come back out.
Shit happens.

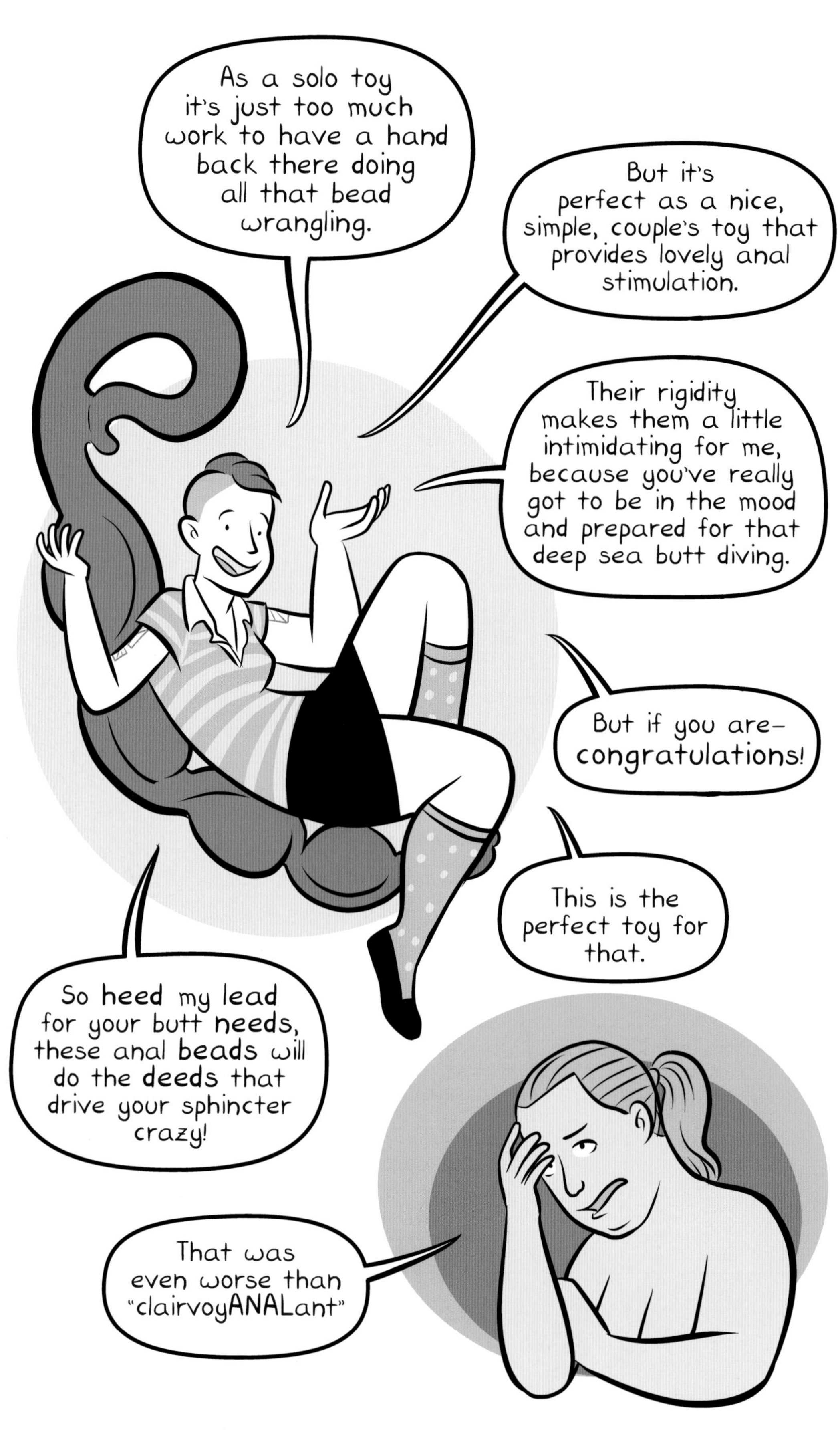
As a solo toy it's just too much work to have a hand back there doing all that bead wrangling.
But it's perfect as a nice, simple, couple's toy that provides lovely anal stimulation.
Their rigidity makes them a little intimidating for me, because you've really got to be in the mood and prepared for that deep sea butt diving.
But if you are– congratulations!
This is the perfect toy for that.
So **heed** my **lead** for your butt **needs**, these anal **beads** will do the **deeds** that drive your sphincter crazy!
That was even worse than "clairvoyANALant"

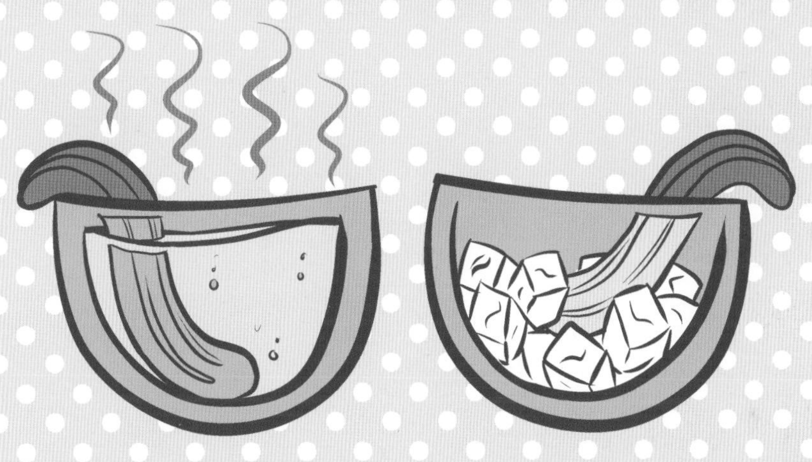

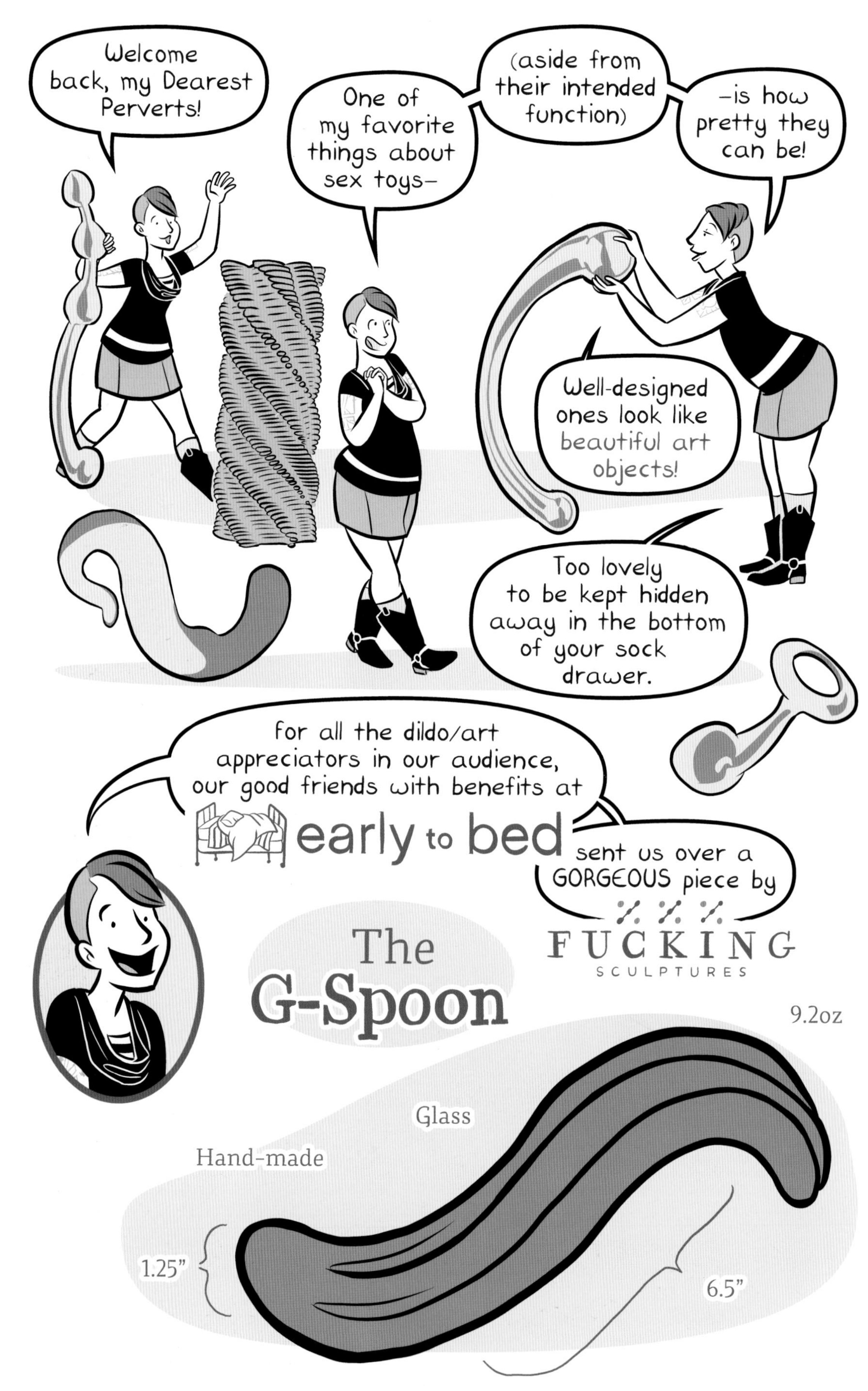
Welcome back, my Dearest Perverts!
One of my favorite things about sex toys–
(aside from their intended function)
–is how pretty they can be!
Well-designed ones look like beautiful art objects!
Too lovely to be kept hidden away in the bottom of your sock drawer.
For all the dildo/art appreciators in our audience, our good friends with benefits at
early to bed
sent us over a GORGEOUS piece by
FUCKING SCULPTURES
The G-Spoon
9.2oz
Glass
Hand-made
1.25"
6.5"

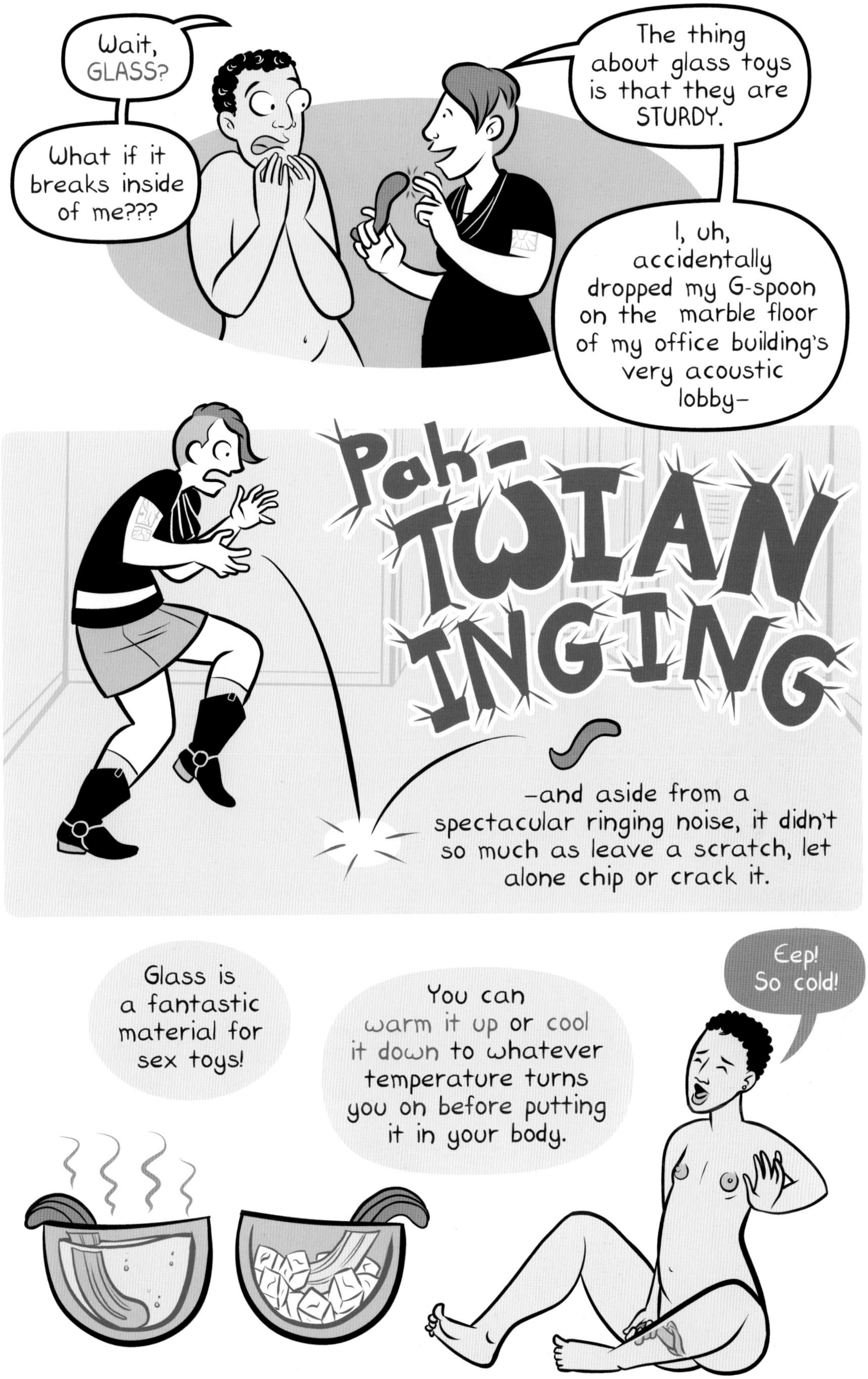

Wait, GLASS?

What if it breaks inside of me???

The thing about glass toys is that they are STURDY.

I, uh, accidentally dropped my G-spoon on the marble floor of my office building's very acoustic lobby–

Pah-TWIAN INGING

–and aside from a spectacular ringing noise, it didn't so much as leave a scratch, let alone chip or crack it.

Glass is a fantastic material for sex toys!

You can warm it up or cool it down to whatever temperature turns you on before putting it in your body.

Eep! So cold!

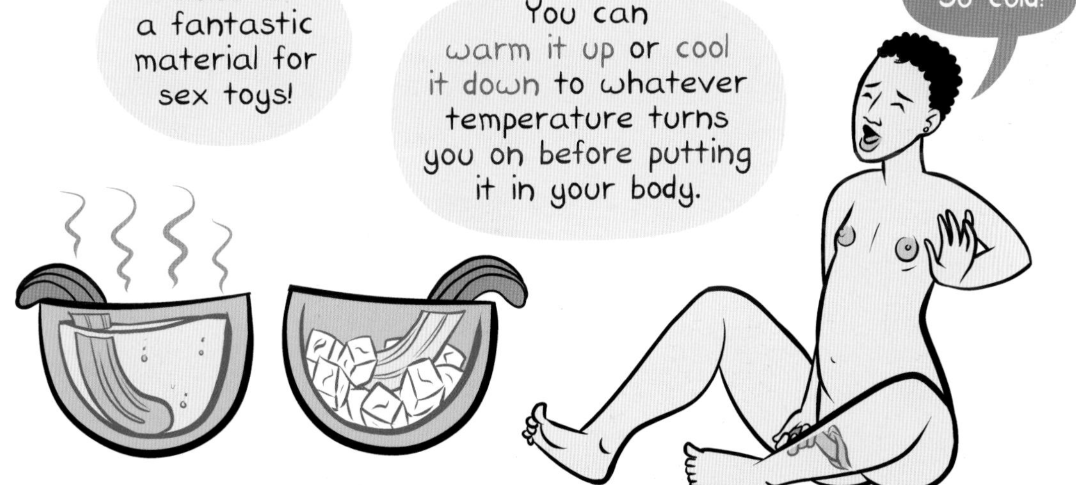

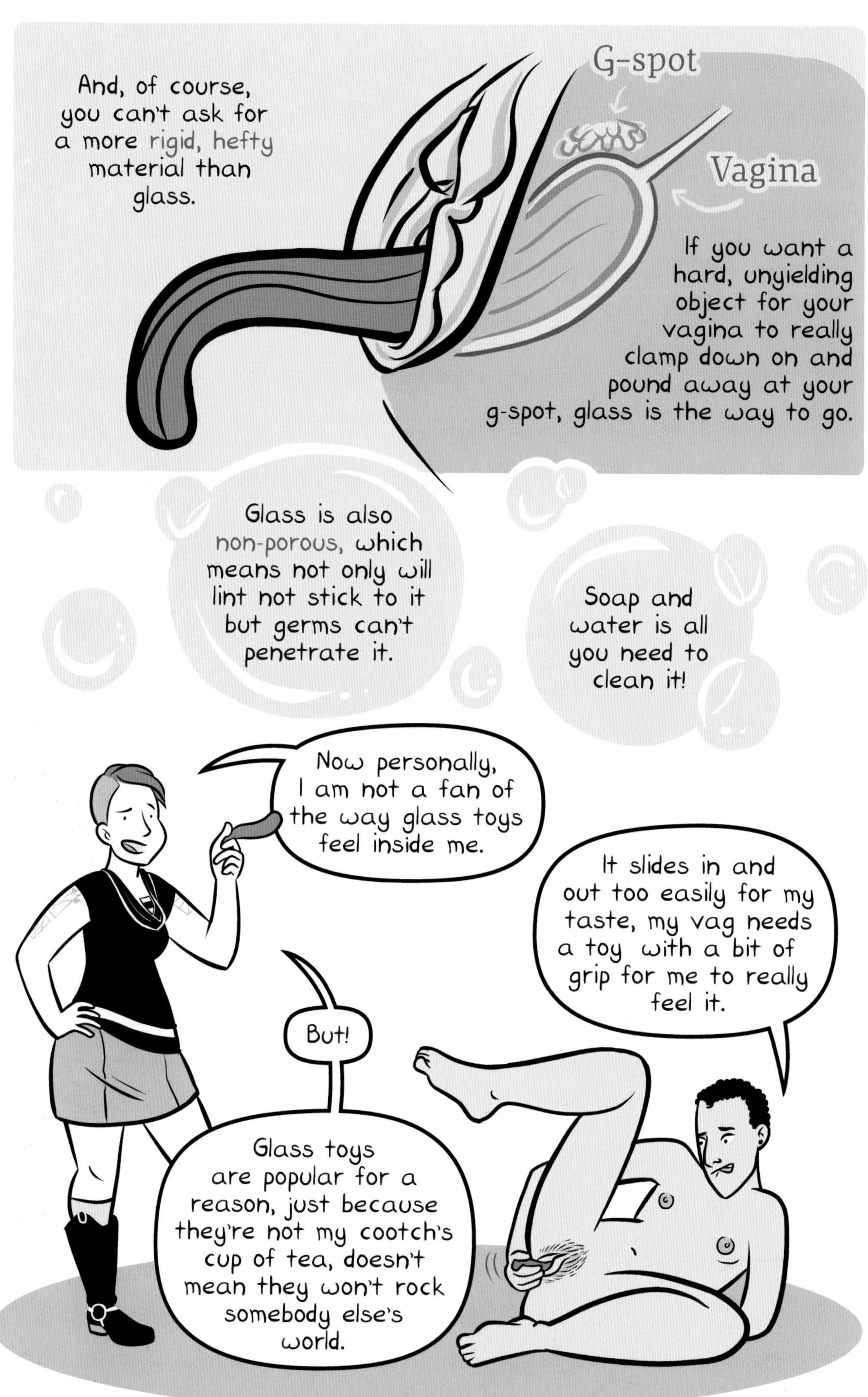
And, of course, you can't ask for a more rigid, hefty material than glass.
G-spot
Vagina
If you want a hard, unyielding object for your vagina to really clamp down on and pound away at your g-spot, glass is the way to go.
Glass is also non-porous, which means not only will lint not stick to it but germs can't penetrate it.
Soap and water is all you need to clean it!
Now personally, I am not a fan of the way glass toys feel inside me.
It slides in and out too easily for my taste, my vag needs a toy with a bit of grip for me to really feel it.
But!
Glass toys are popular for a reason, just because they're not my cootch's cup of tea, doesn't mean they won't rock somebody else's world.

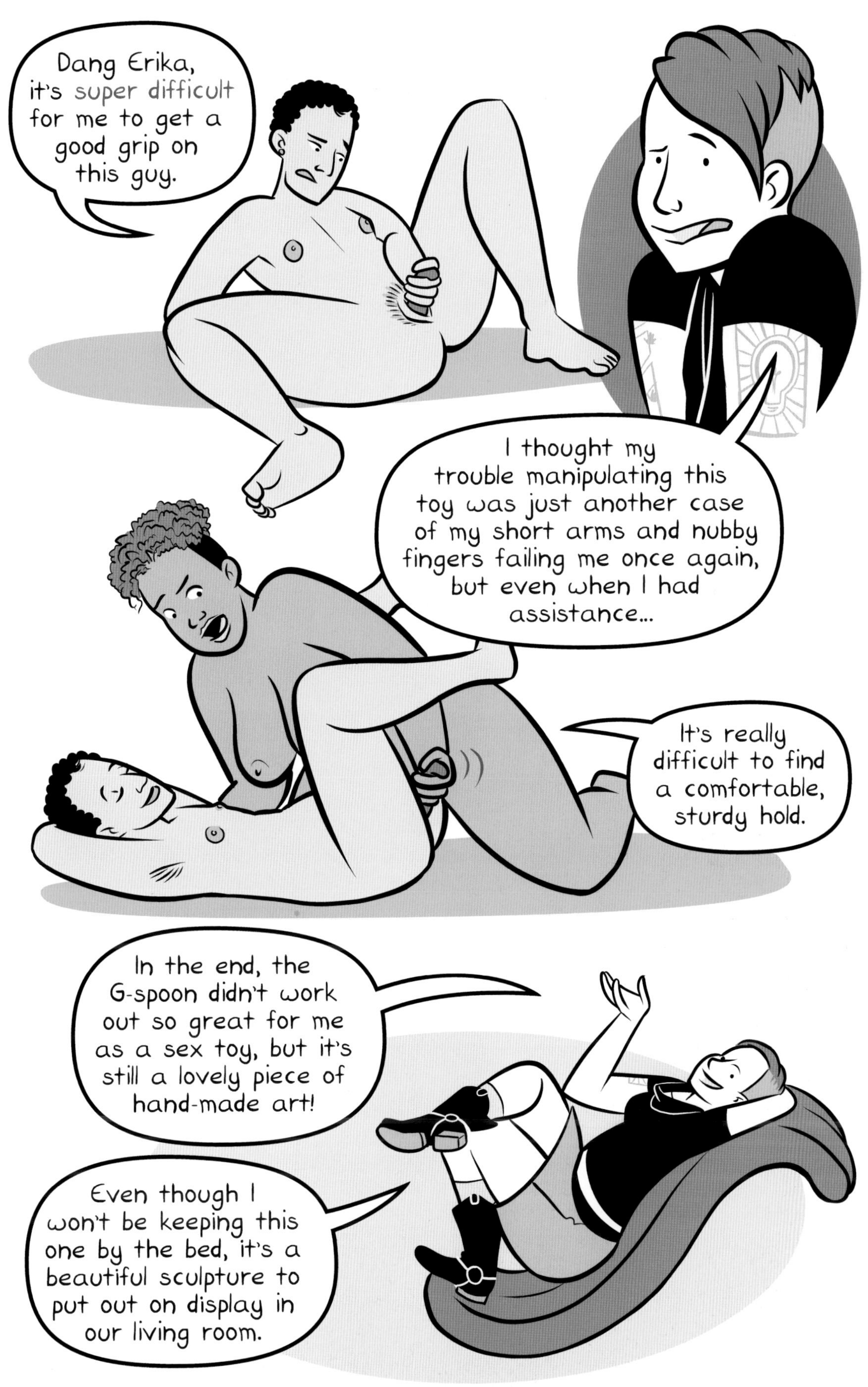
Dang Erika, it's super difficult for me to get a good grip on this guy.
I thought my trouble manipulating this toy was just another case of my short arms and nubby fingers failing me once again, but even when I had assistance...
It's really difficult to find a comfortable, sturdy hold.
In the end, the G-spoon didn't work out so great for me as a sex toy, but it's still a lovely piece of hand-made art!
Even though I won't be keeping this one by the bed, it's a beautiful sculpture to put out on display in our living room.

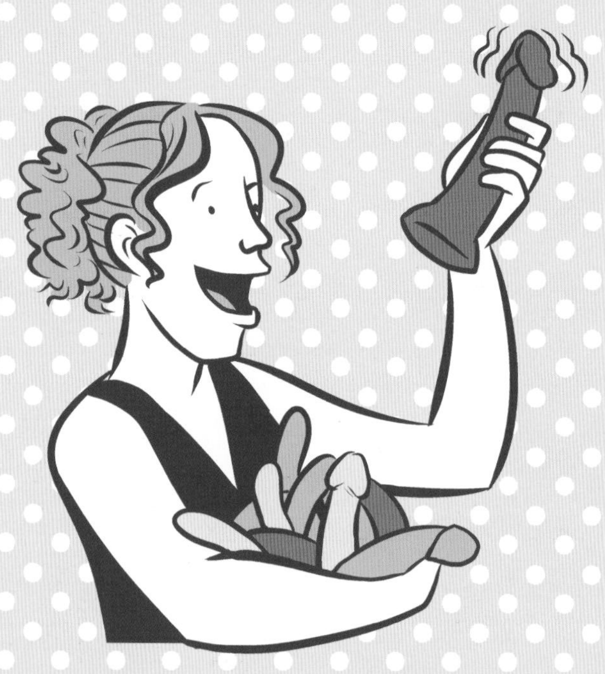

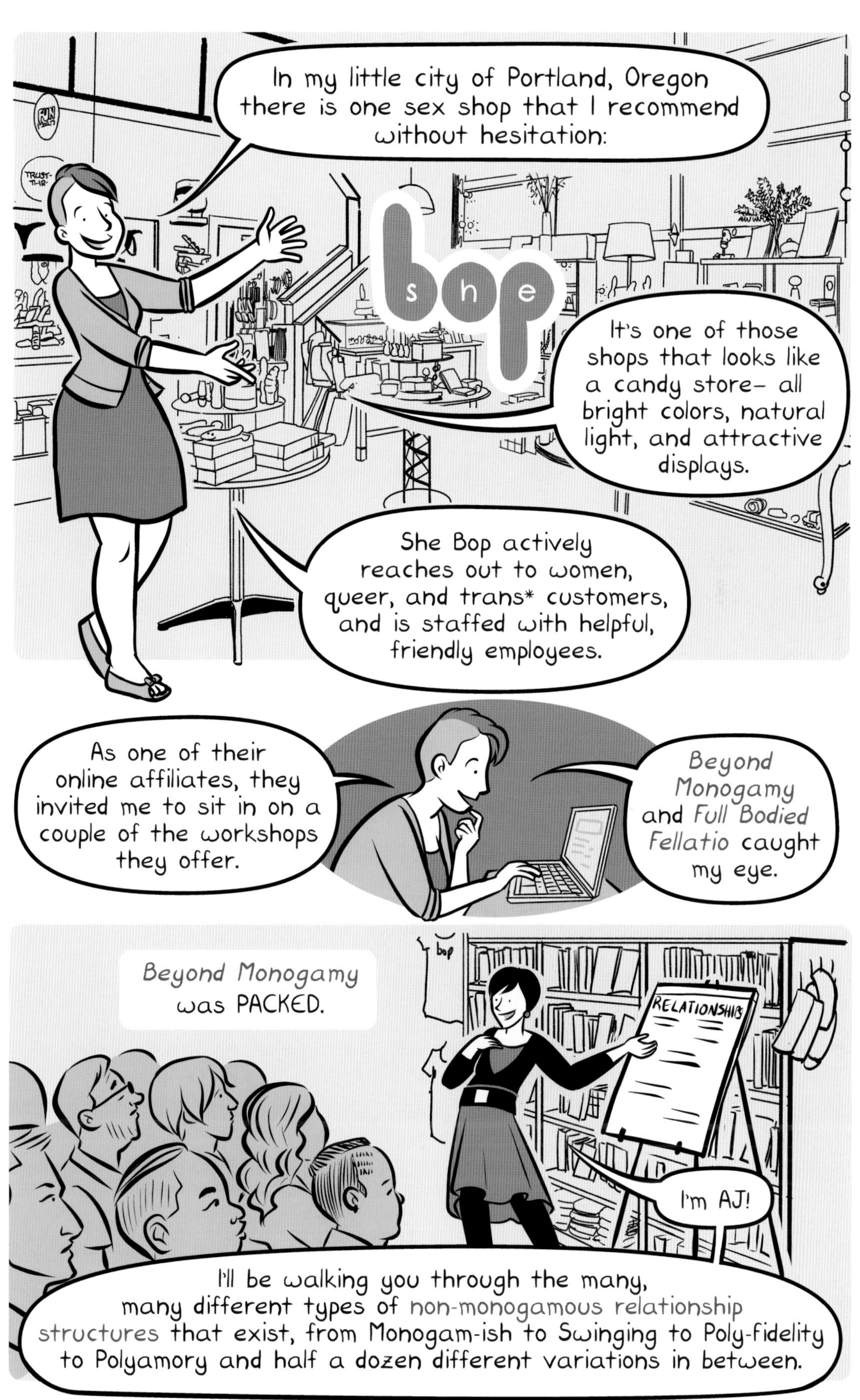
In my little city of Portland, Oregon there is one sex shop that I recommend without hesitation:
she bop
It's one of those shops that looks like a candy store– all bright colors, natural light, and attractive displays.
She Bop actively reaches out to women, queer, and trans* customers, and is staffed with helpful, friendly employees.
As one of their online affiliates, they invited me to sit in on a couple of the workshops they offer.
Beyond Monogamy and Full Bodied Fellatio caught my eye.
Beyond Monogamy was PACKED.
bop
RELATIONSHIPS
I'm AJ!
I'll be walking you through the many, many different types of non-monogamous relationship structures that exist, from Monogam-ish to Swinging to Poly-fidelity to Polyamory and half a dozen different variations in between.

AJ was fun and engaging, packing a TON of information into two hours.

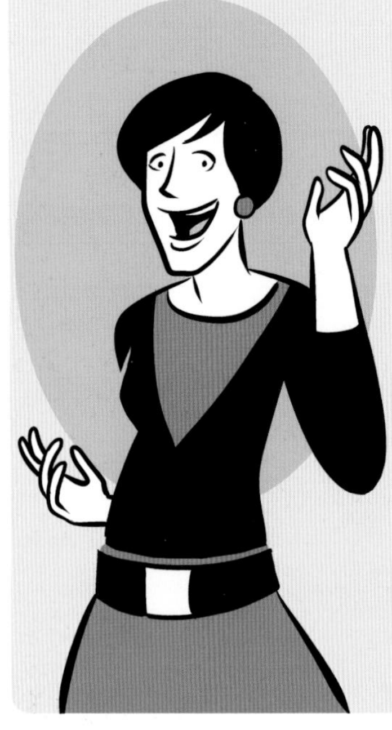

My favorite bit was the Jealousy Jellyfish she used to break down the different components of the ol' Green Eyed Monster.

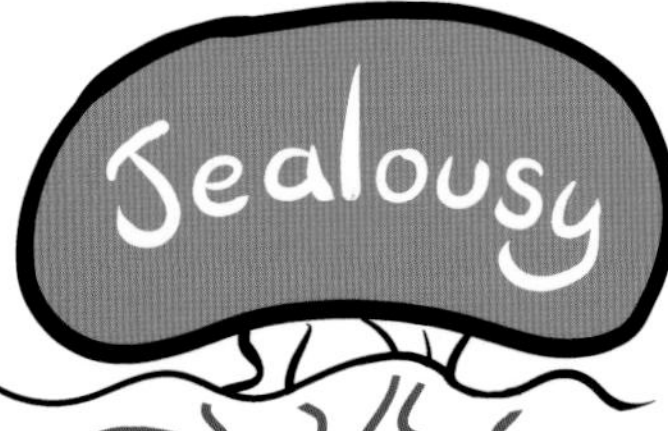

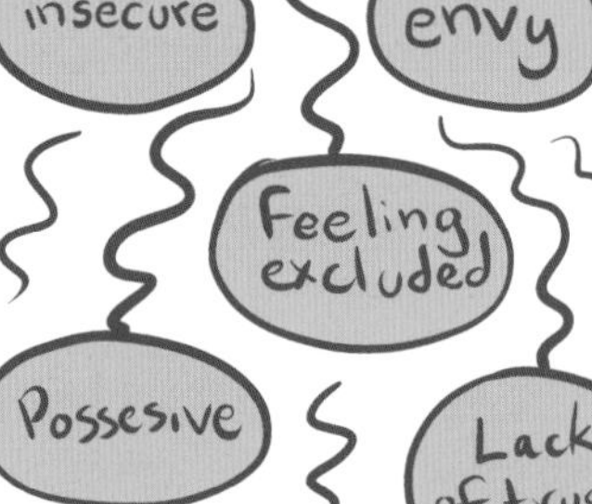

The diversity of the attendees surprised me!

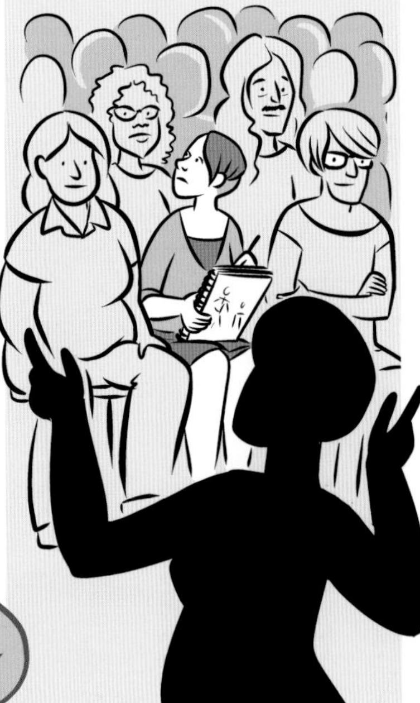

I guess I was expecting middle-aged, heterosexual, cisgender, married couples who've been together a couple decades and are now interested in swinging.

But the ages and genders and sexual orientations of the people who showed up was quite a mix--

--and so were their reasons for attending!

I mean, obviously we were all interested in relationships outside of strict sexual monogamy, but it turns out that means a ton of different options with a zillion nuances unique to each relationship.

It was quite a diverse cross-section of humanity, all trying to navigate love, sex, and relationships with honesty and integrity.

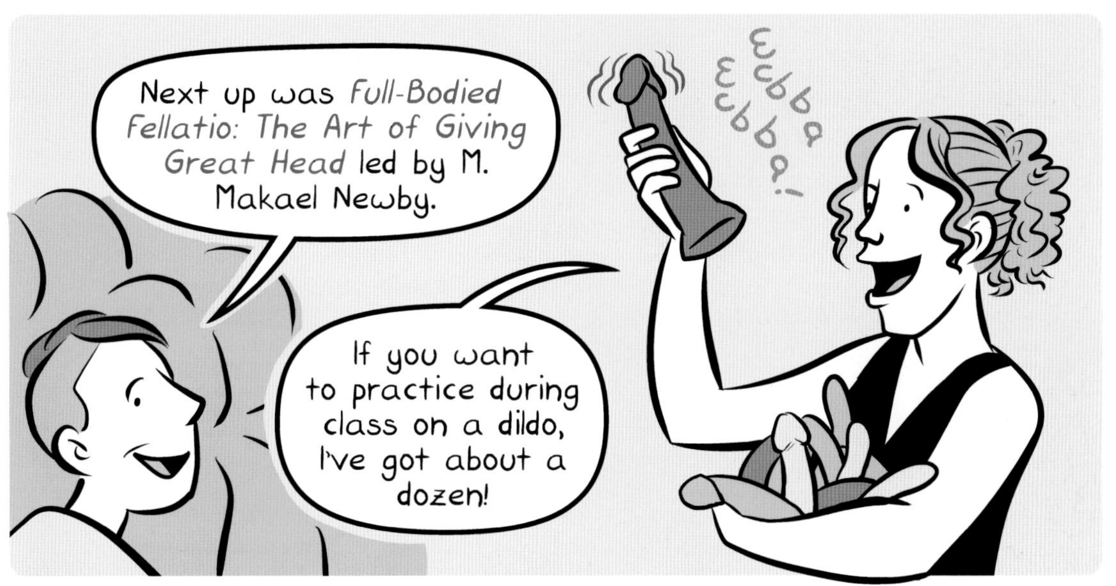
Next up was *Full-Bodied Fellatio: The Art of Giving Great Head* led by M. Makael Newby.
wobba wobba!
If you want to practice during class on a dildo, I've got about a dozen!

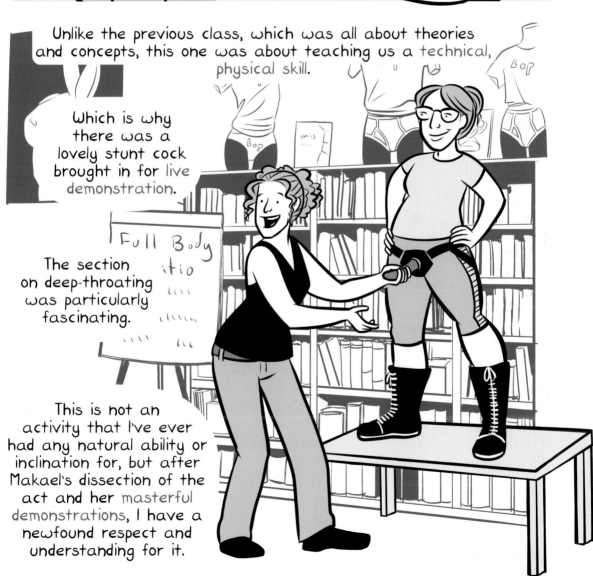

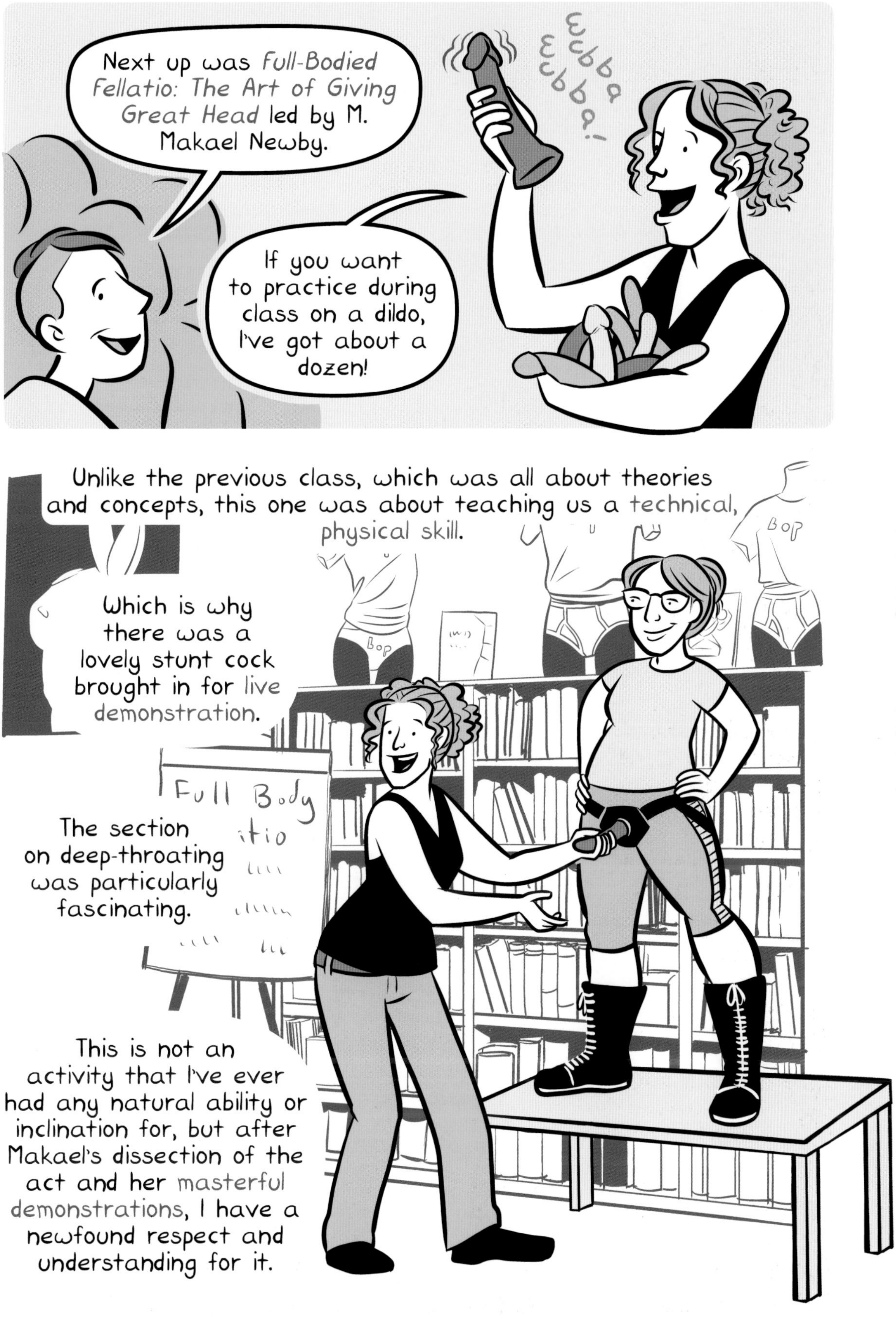

Unlike the previous class, which was all about theories and concepts, this one was about teaching us a technical, physical skill.

Which is why there was a lovely stunt cock brought in for live demonstration.

The section on deep-throating was particularly fascinating.

This is not an activity that I've ever had any natural ability or inclination for, but after Makael's dissection of the act and her masterful demonstrations, I have a newfound respect and understanding for it.

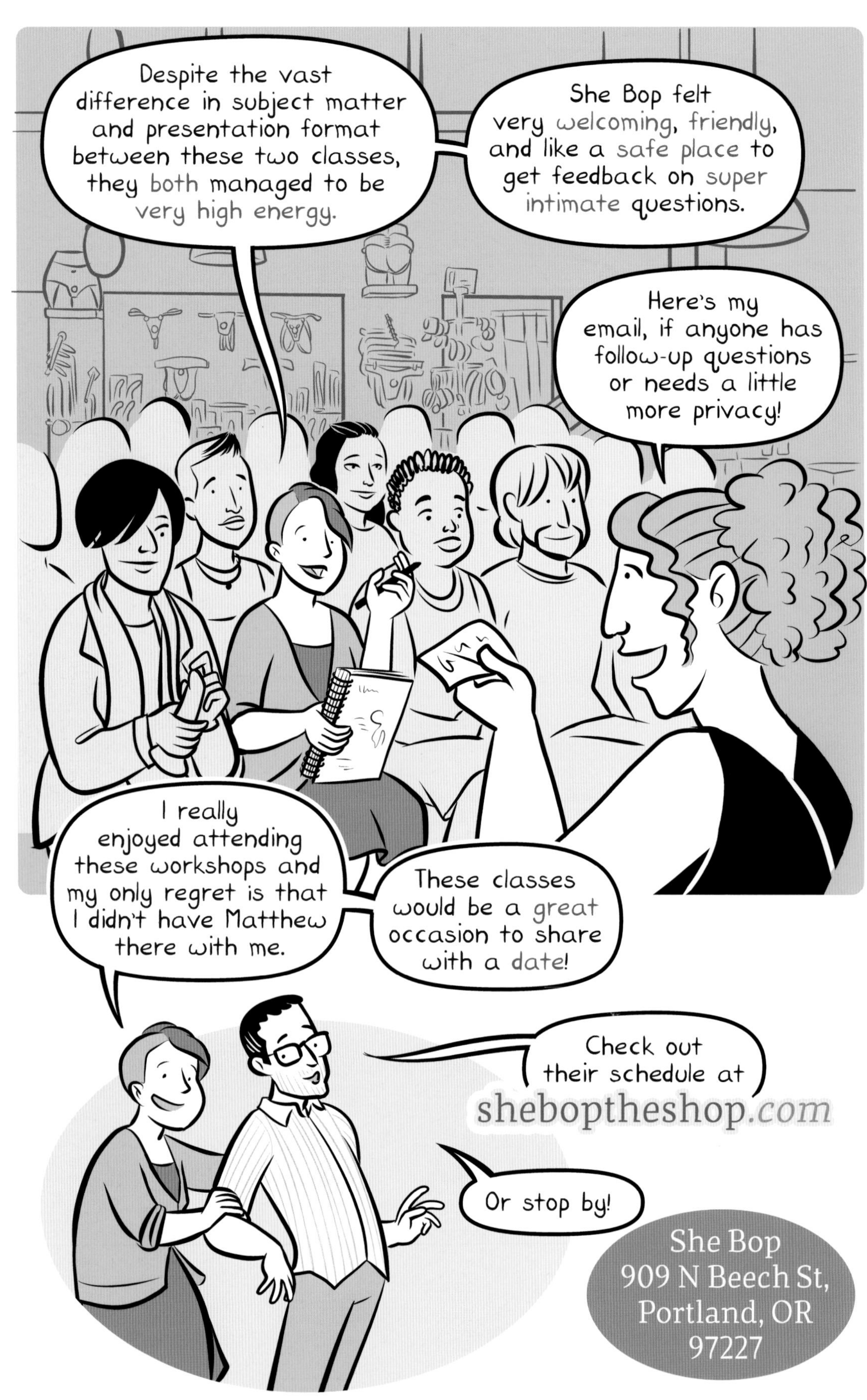
Despite the vast difference in subject matter and presentation format between these two classes, they both managed to be very high energy.
She Bop felt very welcoming, friendly, and like a safe place to get feedback on super intimate questions.
Here's my email, if anyone has follow-up questions or needs a little more privacy!
I really enjoyed attending these workshops and my only regret is that I didn't have Matthew there with me.
These classes would be a great occasion to share with a date!
Check out their schedule at
sheboptheshop.com
Or stop by!
She Bop
909 N Beech St,
Portland, OR
97227

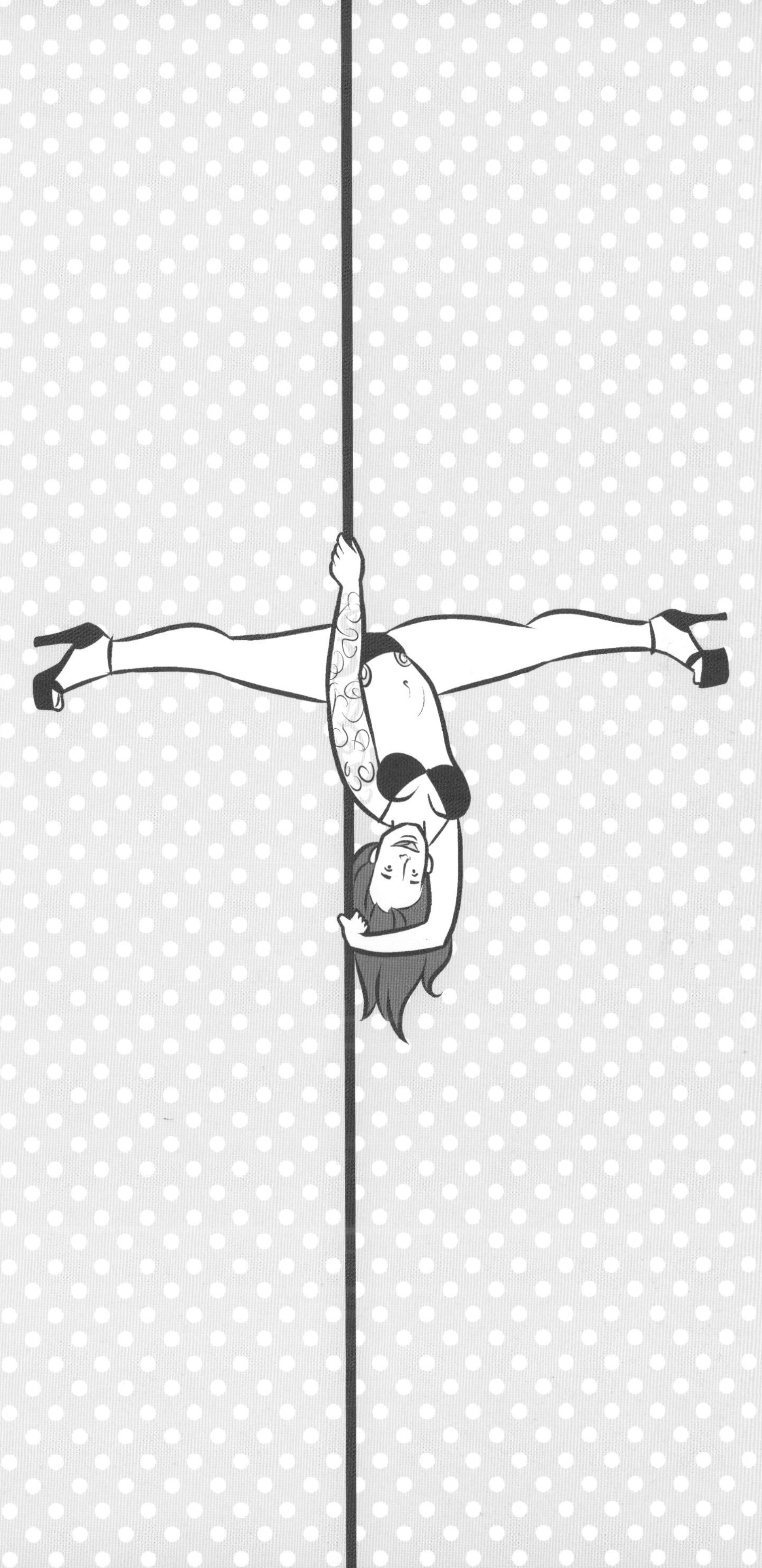

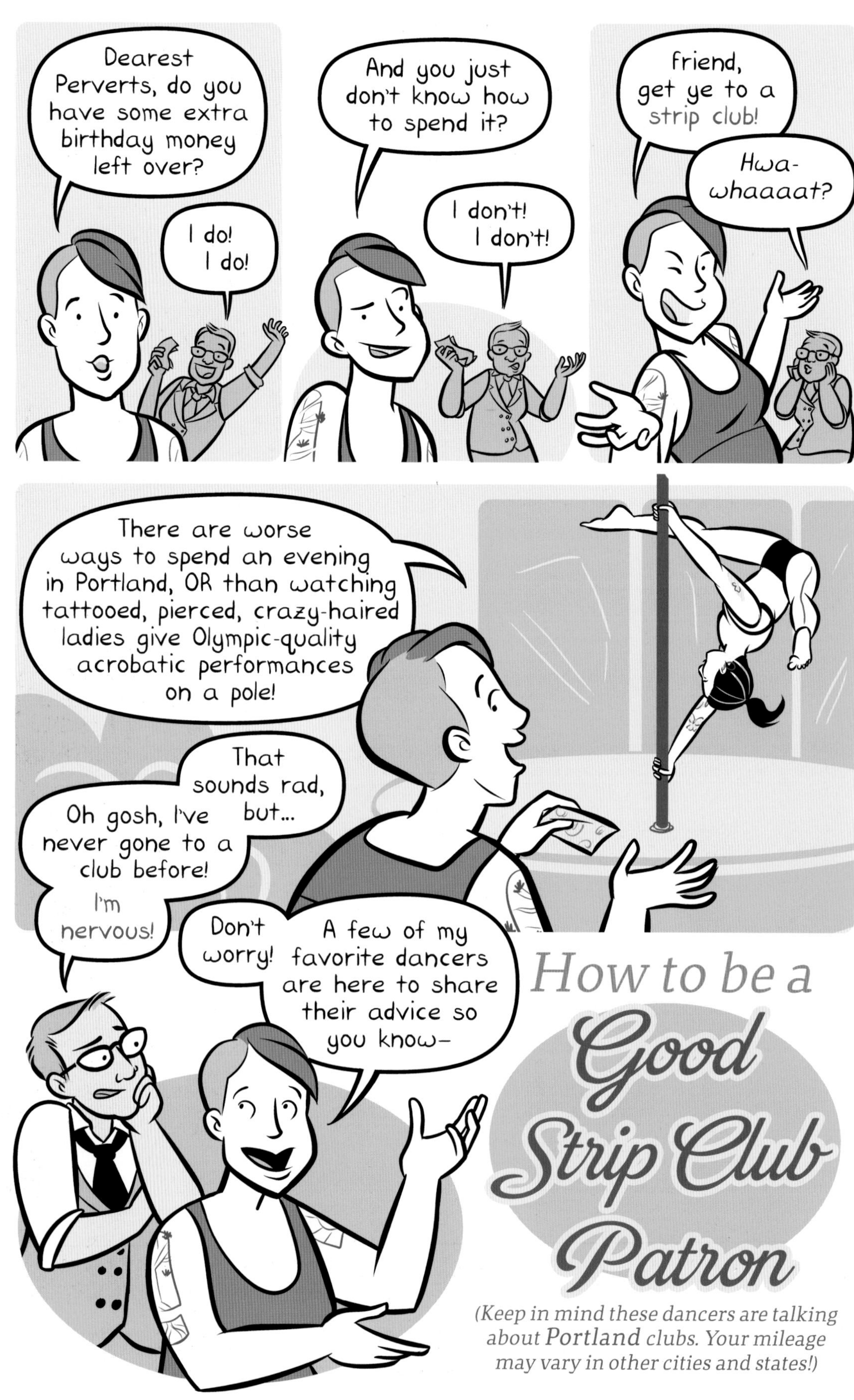
Dearest Perverts, do you have some extra birthday money left over?
I do! I do!
And you just don't know how to spend it?
I don't! I don't!
friend, get ye to a strip club!
Hwa-whaaaat?
There are worse ways to spend an evening in Portland, OR than watching tattooed, pierced, crazy-haired ladies give Olympic-quality acrobatic performances on a pole!
That sounds rad, but...
Oh gosh, I've never gone to a club before!
I'm nervous!
Don't worry!
A few of my favorite dancers are here to share their advice so you know—

How to be a Good Strip Club Patron

*(Keep in mind these dancers are talking about **Portland** clubs. Your mileage may vary in other cities and states!)*

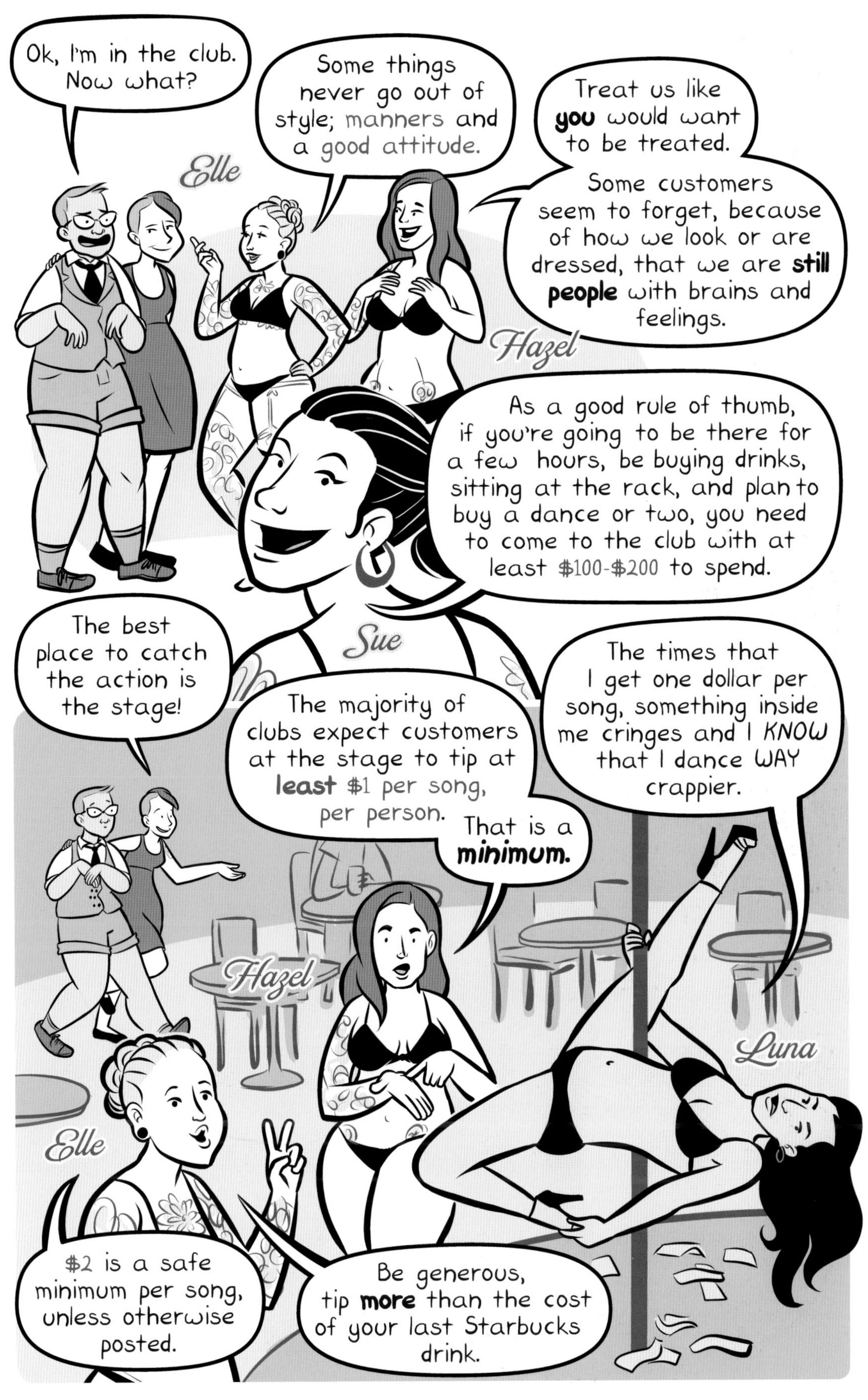
Ok, I'm in the club. Now what?
Some things never go out of style; manners and a good attitude.
Elle
Treat us like **you** would want to be treated.
Some customers seem to forget, because of how we look or are dressed, that we are **still people** with brains and feelings.
Hazel
As a good rule of thumb, if you're going to be there for a few hours, be buying drinks, sitting at the rack, and plan to buy a dance or two, you need to come to the club with at least $100-$200 to spend.
Sue
The best place to catch the action is the stage!
The majority of clubs expect customers at the stage to tip at **least** $1 per song, per person.
That is a **minimum.**
The times that I get one dollar per song, something inside me cringes and I *KNOW* that I dance WAY crappier.
Hazel
Luna
Elle
$2 is a safe minimum per song, unless otherwise posted.
Be generous, tip **more** than the cost of your last Starbucks drink.

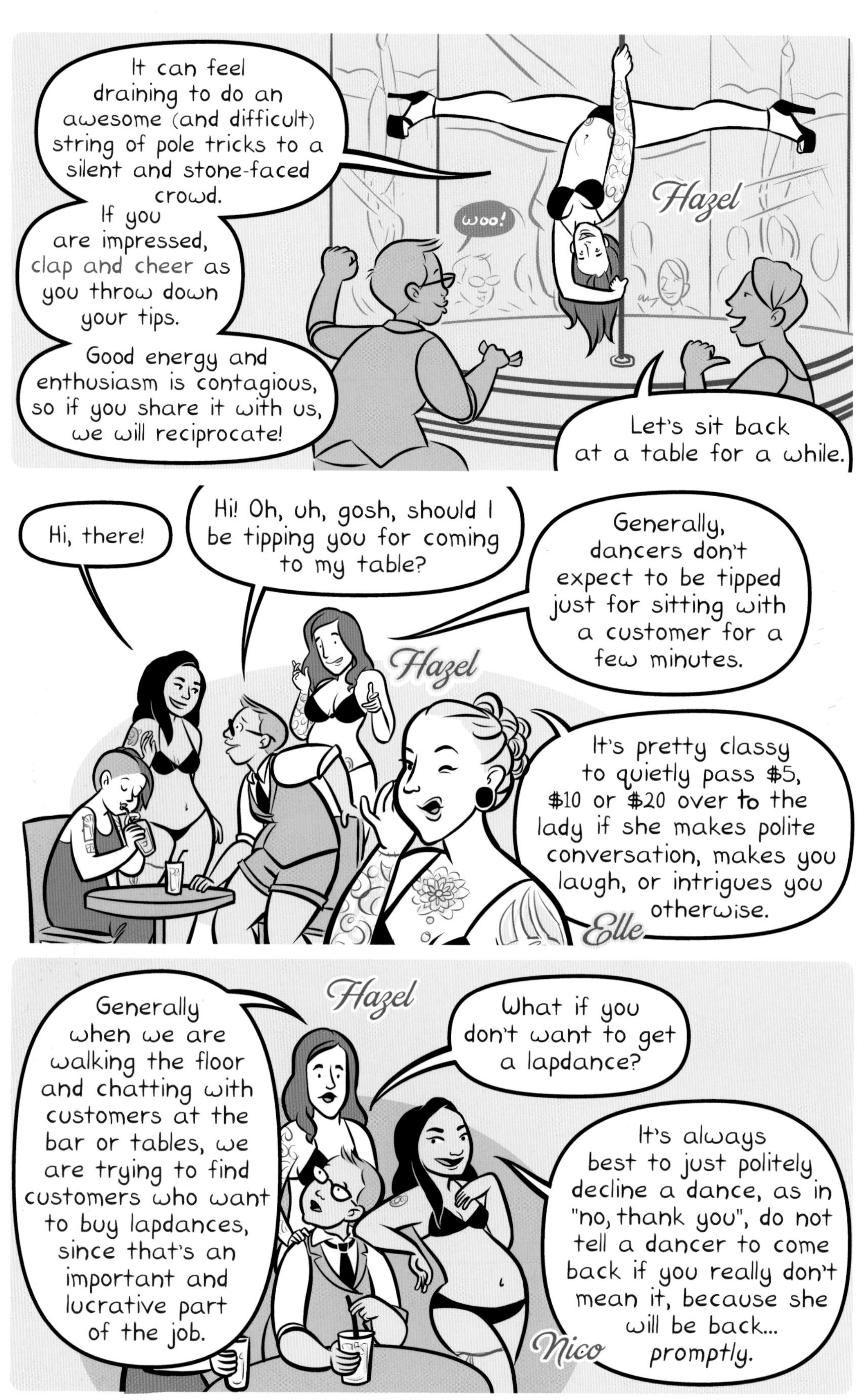

It can feel draining to do an awesome (and difficult) string of pole tricks to a silent and stone-faced crowd.
If you are impressed, clap and cheer as you throw down your tips.
Good energy and enthusiasm is contagious, so if you share it with us, we will reciprocate!
Hazel
woo!
Let's sit back at a table for a while.
Hi, there!
Hi! Oh, uh, gosh, should I be tipping you for coming to my table?
Generally, dancers don't expect to be tipped just for sitting with a customer for a few minutes.
Hazel
It's pretty classy to quietly pass $5, $10 or $20 over to the lady if she makes polite conversation, makes you laugh, or intrigues you otherwise.
Elle
Hazel
Generally when we are walking the floor and chatting with customers at the bar or tables, we are trying to find customers who want to buy lapdances, since that's an important and lucrative part of the job.
What if you don't want to get a lapdance?
It's always best to just politely decline a dance, as in "no, thank you", do not tell a dancer to come back if you really don't mean it, because she will be back... promptly.
Nico

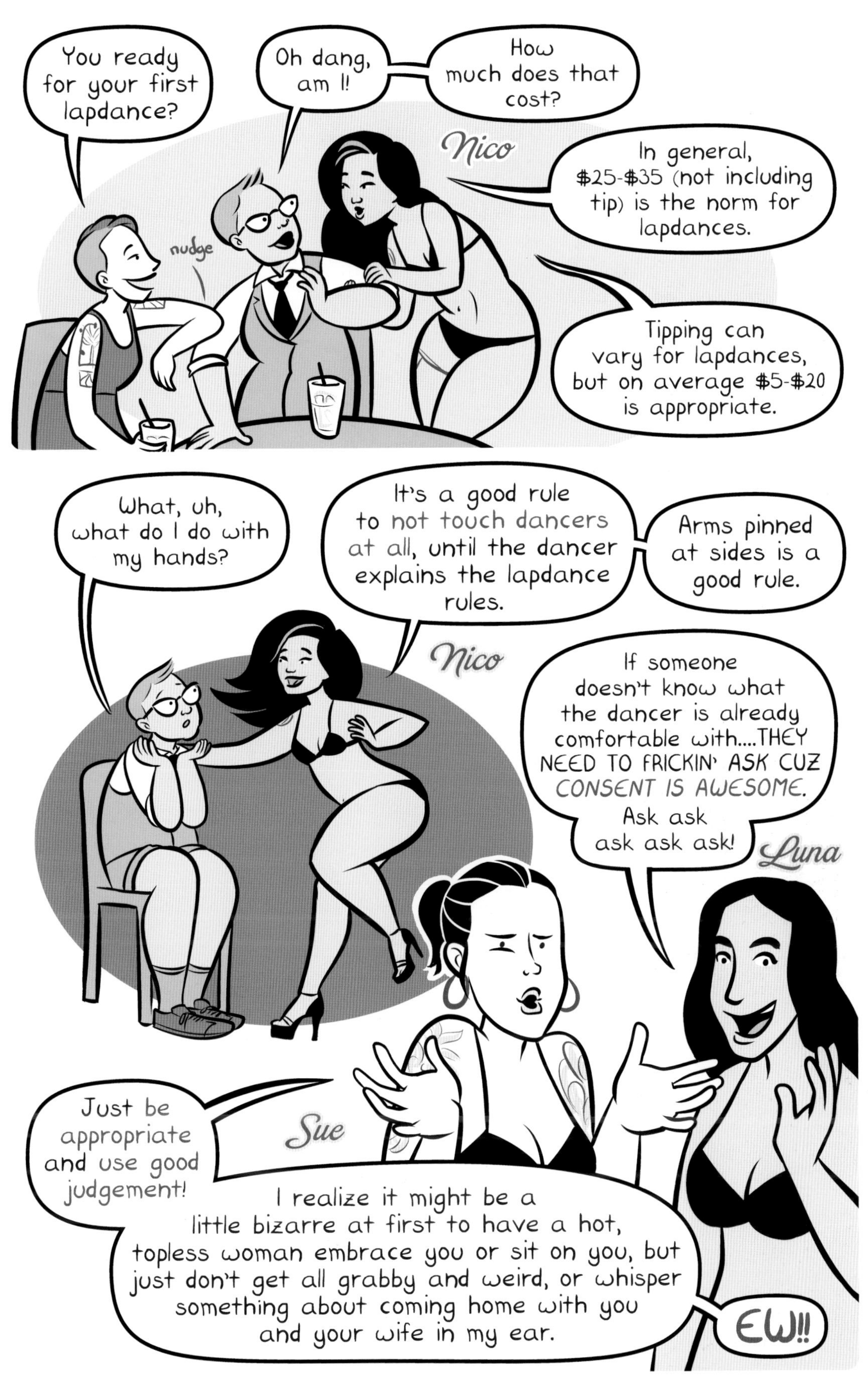
You ready for your first lapdance?
Oh dang, am I!
How much does that cost?
Nico
In general, $25-$35 (not including tip) is the norm for lapdances.
nudge
Tipping can vary for lapdances, but on average $5-$20 is appropriate.
What, uh, what do I do with my hands?
It's a good rule to not touch dancers at all, until the dancer explains the lapdance rules.
Arms pinned at sides is a good rule.
Nico
If someone doesn't know what the dancer is already comfortable with....THEY NEED TO FRICKIN' ASK CUZ CONSENT IS AWESOME. Ask ask ask ask ask!
Luna
Sue
Just be appropriate and use good judgement!
I realize it might be a little bizarre at first to have a hot, topless woman embrace you or sit on you, but just don't get all grabby and weird, or whisper something about coming home with you and your wife in my ear.
EW!!

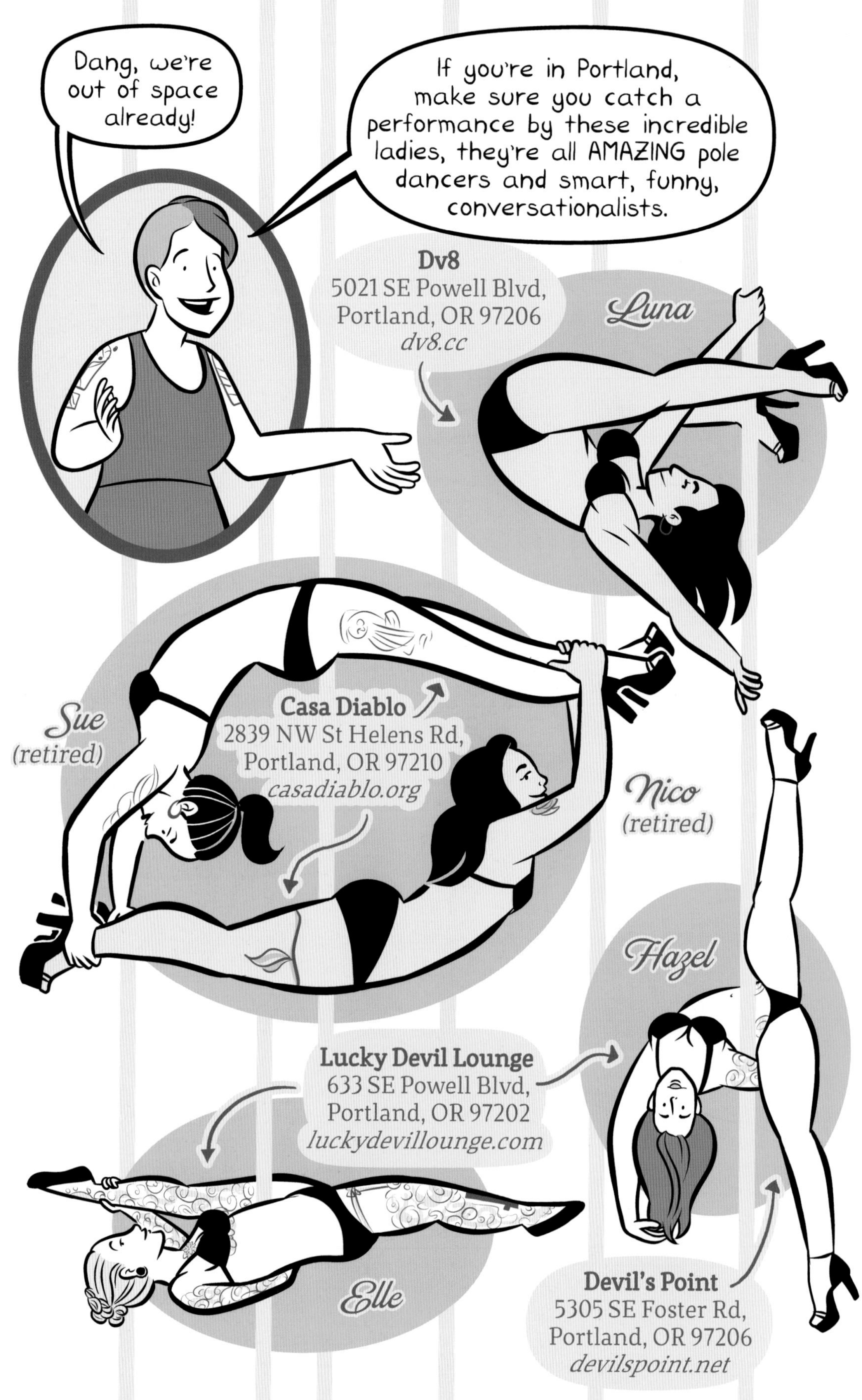
Dang, we're out of space already!
If you're in Portland, make sure you catch a performance by these incredible ladies, they're all AMAZING pole dancers and smart, funny, conversationalists.
Dv8
5021 SE Powell Blvd,
Portland, OR 97206
dv8.cc
Luna
Sue
(retired)
Casa Diablo
2839 NW St Helens Rd,
Portland, OR 97210
casadiablo.org
Nico
(retired)
Hazel
Lucky Devil Lounge
633 SE Powell Blvd,
Portland, OR 97202
luckydevillounge.com
Elle
Devil's Point
5305 SE Foster Rd,
Portland, OR 97206
devilspoint.net

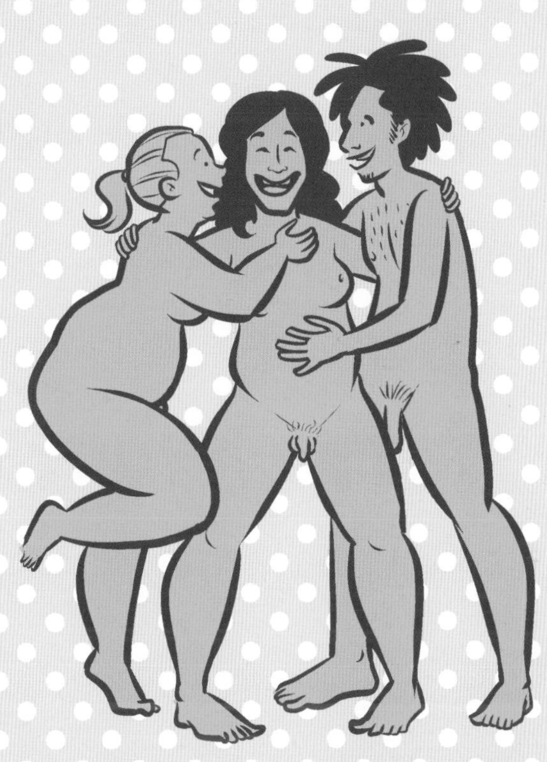

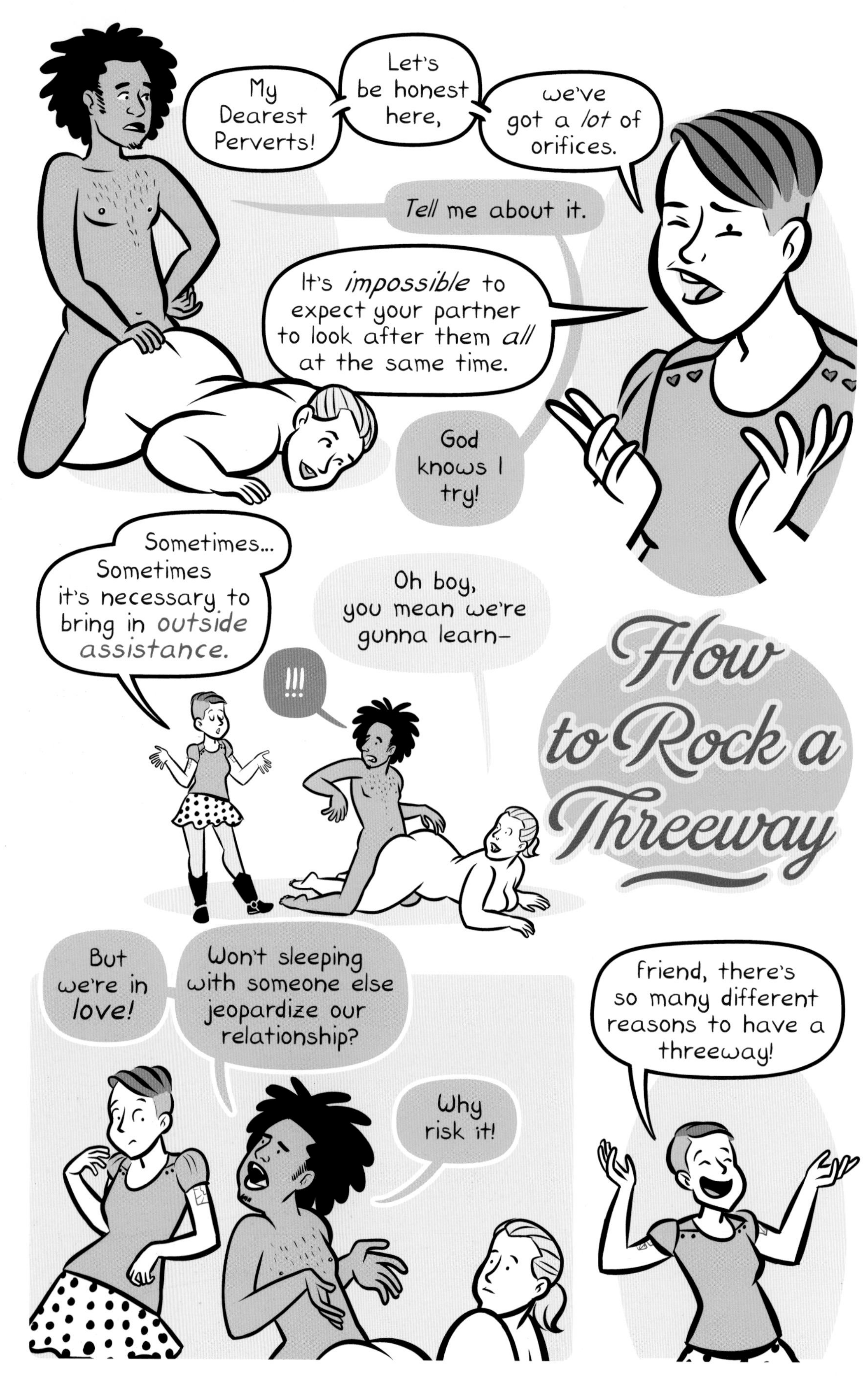
My Dearest Perverts!
Let's be honest here,
we've got a *lot* of orifices.
Tell me about it.
It's *impossible* to expect your partner to look after them *all* at the same time.
God knows I try!
Sometimes... Sometimes it's necessary to bring in outside assistance.
Oh boy, you mean we're gunna learn–
!!!
How to Rock a Threeway
But we're in *love*!
Won't sleeping with someone else jeopardize our relationship?
Why risk it!
friend, there's so many different reasons to have a threeway!

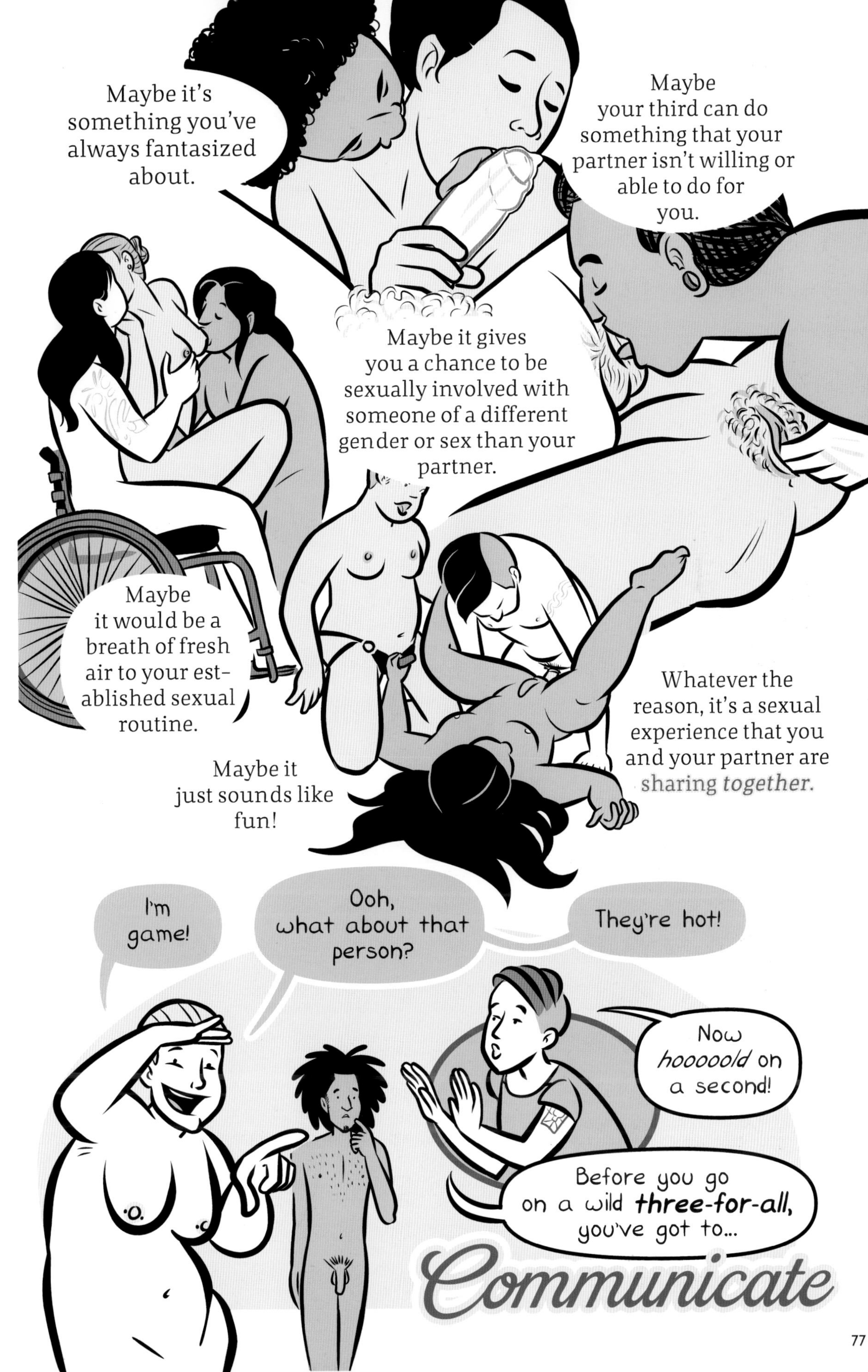
Maybe it's something you've always fantasized about.
Maybe your third can do something that your partner isn't willing or able to do for you.
Maybe it gives you a chance to be sexually involved with someone of a different gender or sex than your partner.
Maybe it would be a breath of fresh air to your est-ablished sexual routine.
Maybe it just sounds like fun!
Whatever the reason, it's a sexual experience that you and your partner are sharing *together*.
I'm game!
Ooh, what about that person?
They're hot!
Now *hoooold* on a second!
Before you go on a wild **three-for-all,** you've got to...
Communicate

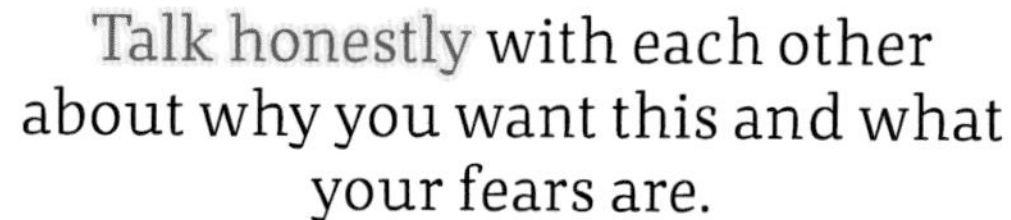

Talk honestly with each other about why you want this and what your fears are.

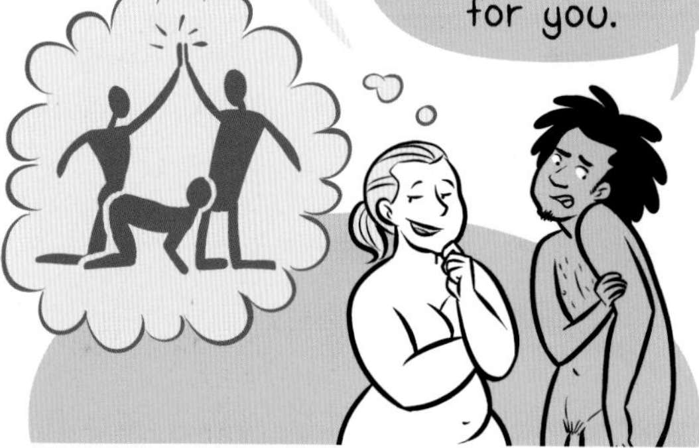

I've always wanted to Eiffel Tower!
I'm scared this means I'm not enough for you.

Address your partner's concerns and reassure them!

Oh honey!

I want to do this WITH you, *together!*

I may have fun with them, but I'm in love with **YOU.**

Generally try to keep an open mind and be up for trying new things *(within reason)* with your partner...

–they just may become your new favorite!

However, if your partner isn't into it right now *–or ever!–* that's *completely* valid and **must be respected.**

Badgering and pressuring them to get your way is *a shitty move!*

If you both *do* decide you wanna give it a go...

NOW we find a third?

...You've got even *MORE* talking to do with each other!

Communicate SOME MORE

Figuring Out the Basics

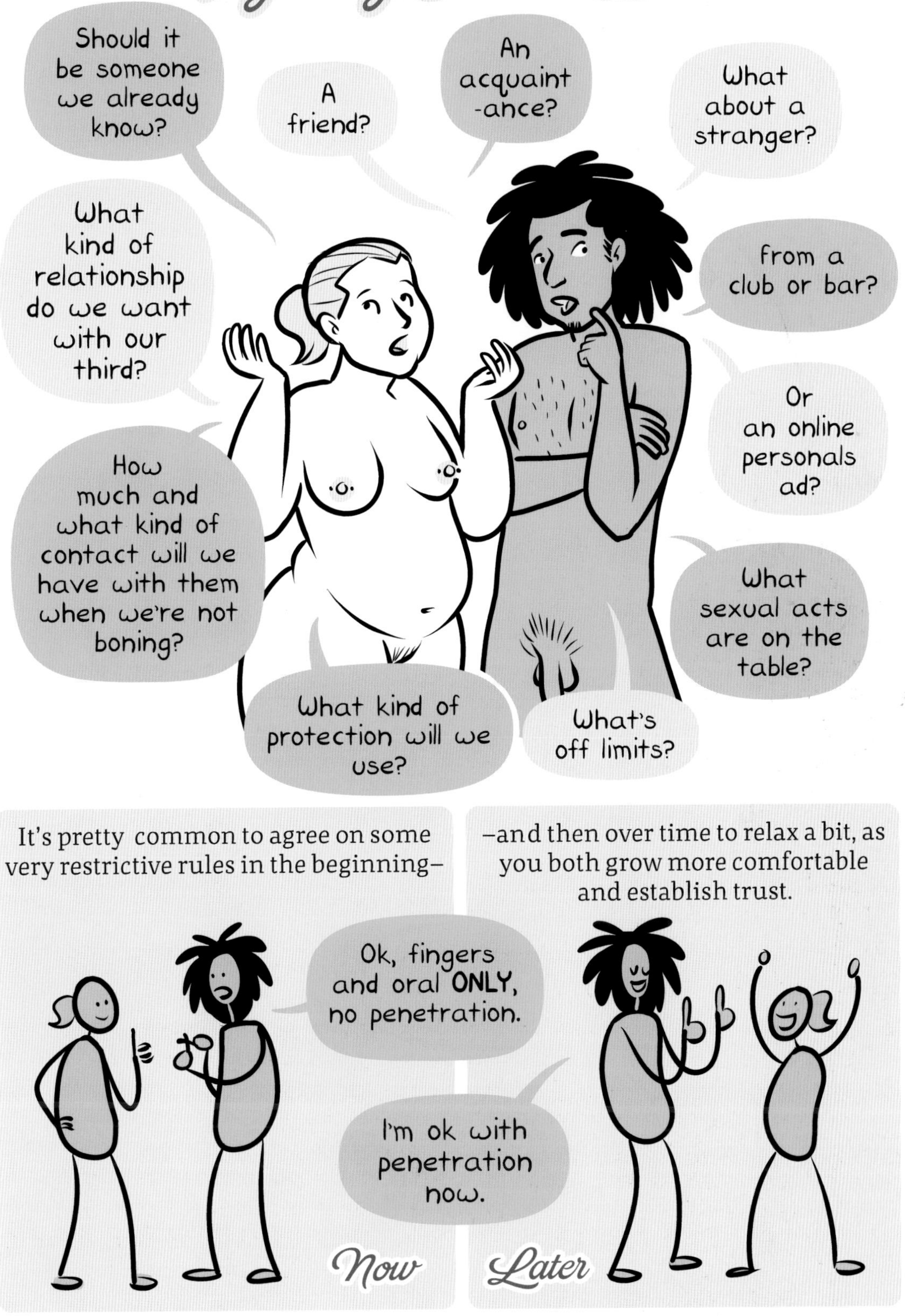

Should it be someone we already know?

A friend?

An acquaint -ance?

What about a stranger?

What kind of relationship do we want with our third?

from a club or bar?

Or an online personals ad?

How much and what kind of contact will we have with them when we're not boning?

What sexual acts are on the table?

What kind of protection will we use?

What's off limits?

It's pretty common to agree on some very restrictive rules in the beginning–

–and then over time to relax a bit, as you both grow more comfortable and establish trust.

Ok, fingers and oral **ONLY**, no penetration.
I'm ok with penetration now.
Now
Later

Talk about these agreement changes between everyone **in advance**, don't make sudden changes right in the middle of fucking!

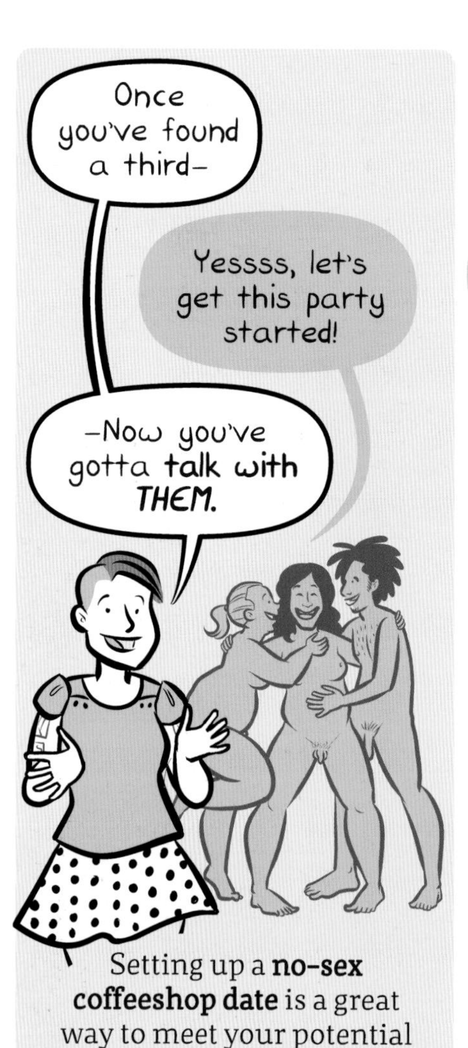
Once you've found a third–
Yessss, let's get this party started!
–Now you've gotta **talk with THEM.**
Setting up a **no-sex coffeeshop date** is a great way to meet your potential sex buddy and get all the deets hammered out **without** any pressure to jump into anything RIGHT NOW.

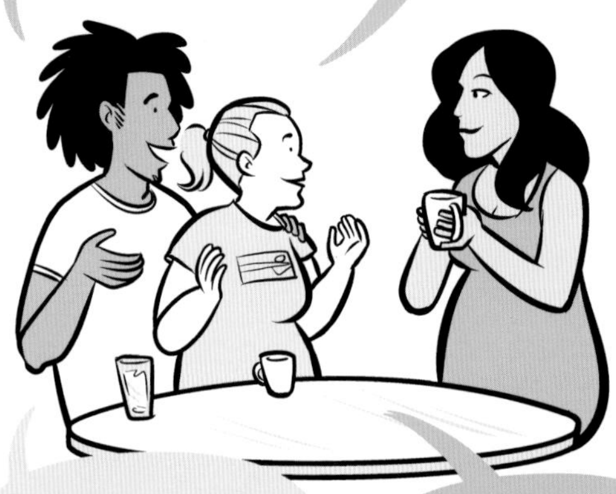
Here is the kind of relationship we have with each other...
When was your last STI testing? Ours was...
Here's what protection we'll be using...
Here's the kind of contact and relationship we want with you afterwards...
We just want to do ***these*** sex acts, but not ***these*** ones...
What are you comfortable with? What's off limits for you?
How do **you** feel? What do **you** want? Do **you** have any questions?

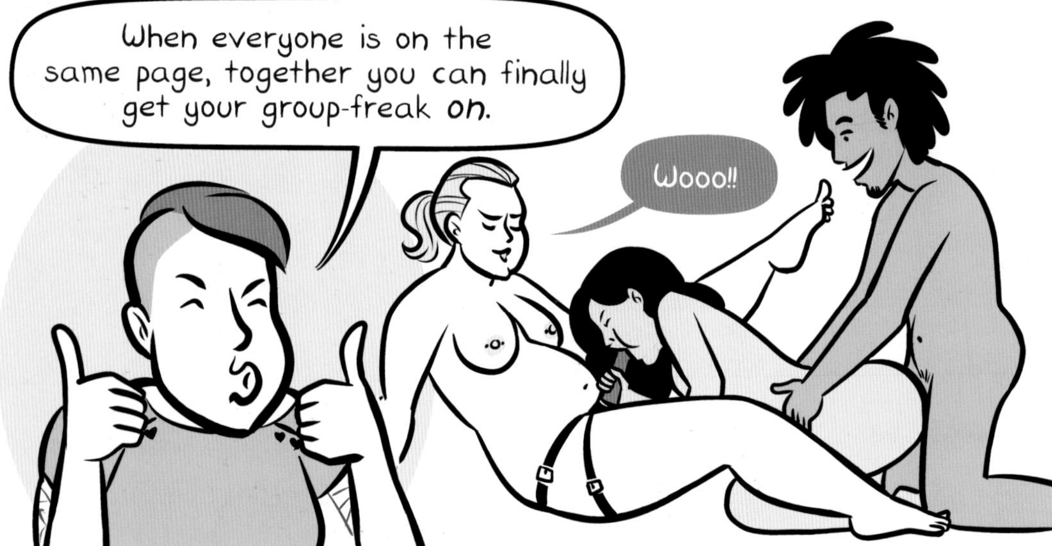
When everyone is on the same page, together you can finally get your group-freak **on**.
Wooo!!

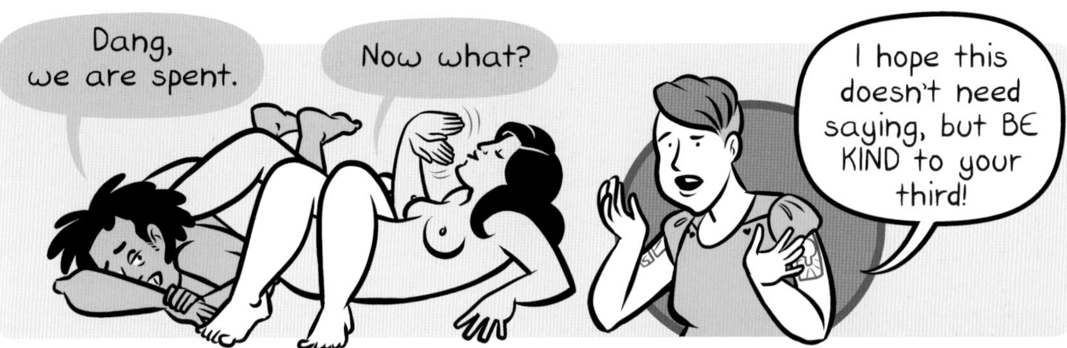
Dang, we are spent.
Now what?
I hope this doesn't need saying, but BE KIND to your third!

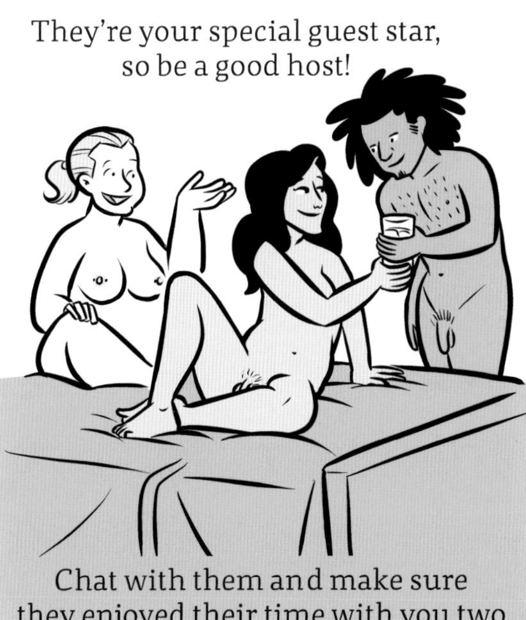
They're your special guest star, so be a good host!
Chat with them and make sure they enjoyed their time with you two.

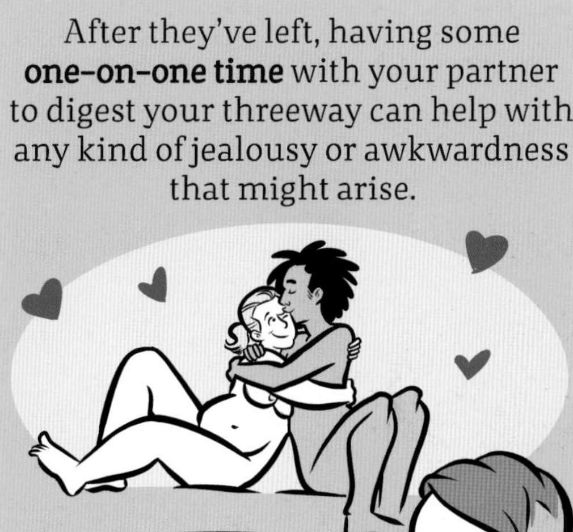
After they've left, having some **one-on-one time** with your partner to digest your threeway can help with any kind of jealousy or awkwardness that might arise.
Or you can just re-cap how awesome it was!

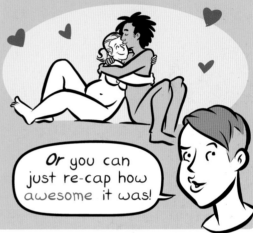

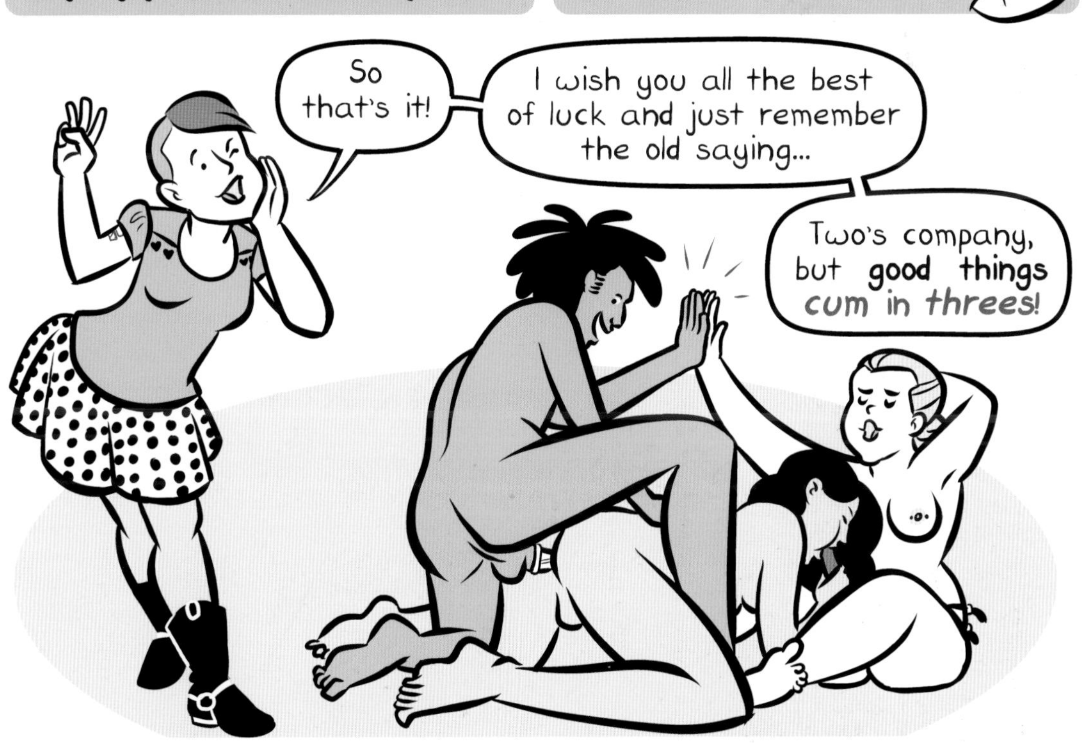
So that's it!
I wish you all the best of luck and just remember the old saying...
Two's company, but **good things cum in threes!**

NOT A
BONER

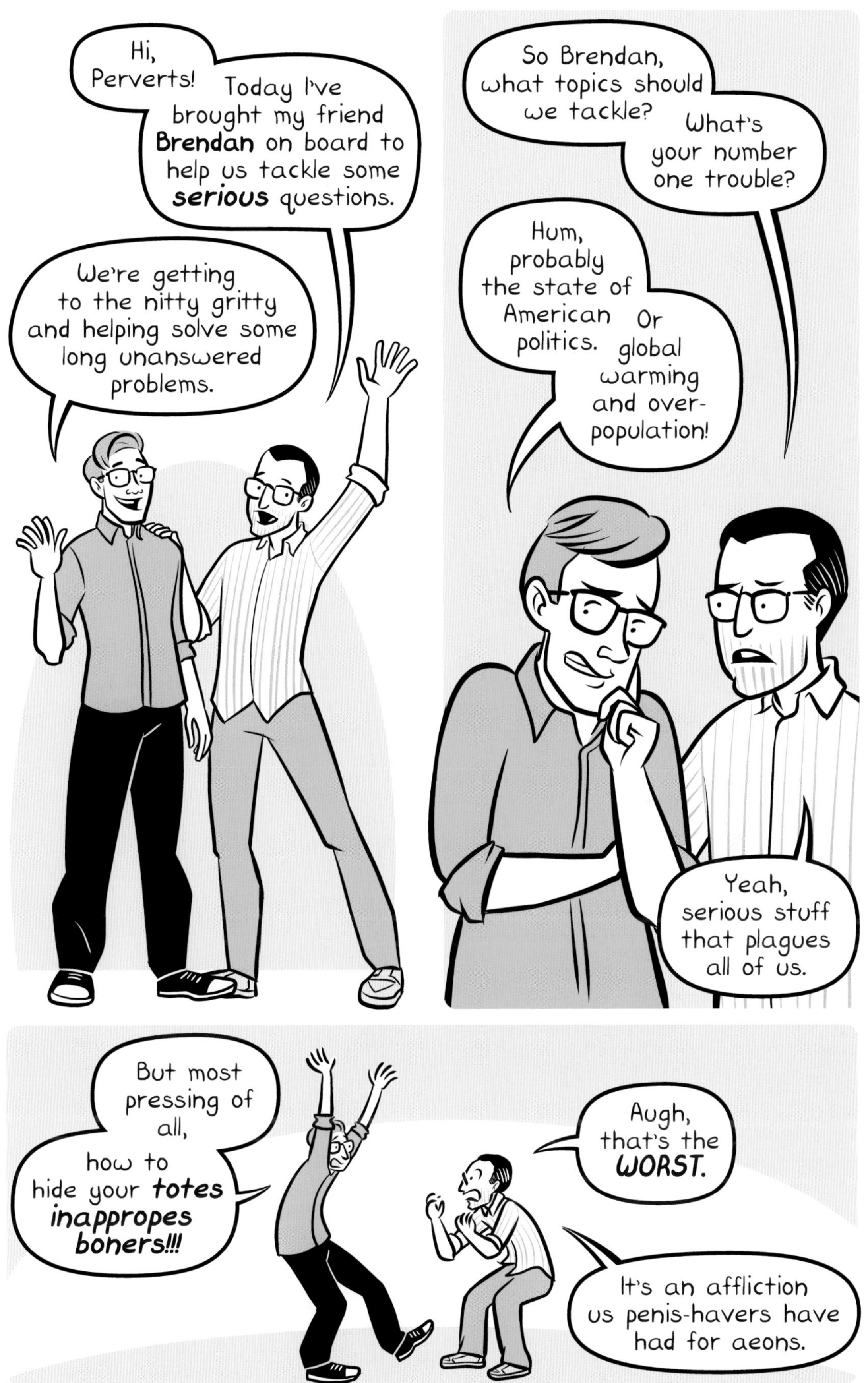
Hi, Perverts!
Today I've brought my friend **Brendan** on board to help us tackle some ***serious*** questions.
We're getting to the nitty gritty and helping solve some long unanswered problems.
So Brendan, what topics should we tackle?
What's your number one trouble?
Hum, probably the state of American politics.
Or global warming and over-population!
Yeah, serious stuff that plagues all of us.
But most pressing of all,
how to hide your ***totes inappropes boners!!!***
Augh, that's the ***WORST.***
It's an affliction us penis-havers have had for aeons.

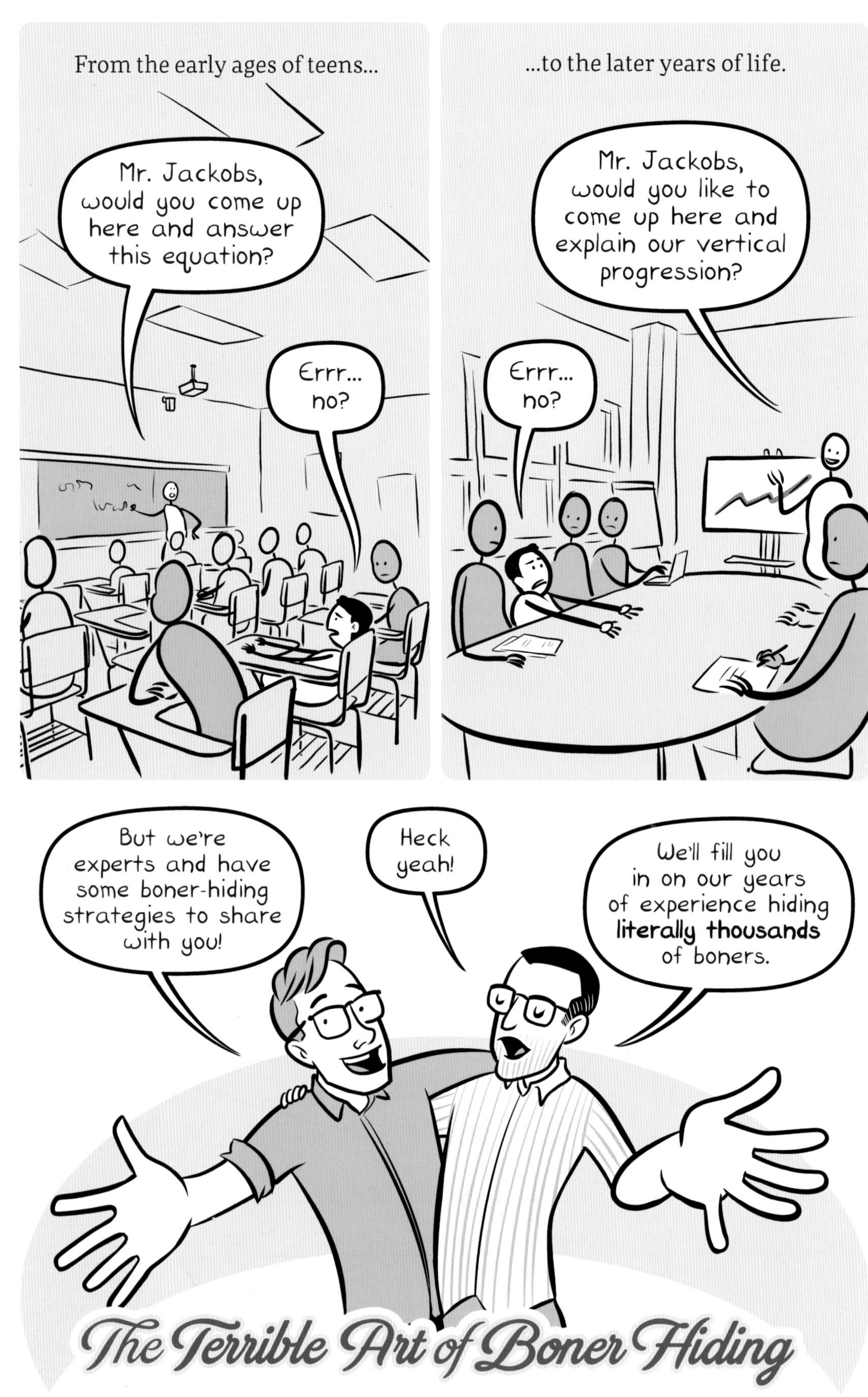

From the early ages of teens...
Mr. Jackobs, would you come up here and answer this equation?
Errr... no?
...to the later years of life.
Mr. Jackobs, would you like to come up here and explain our vertical progression?
Errr... no?
But we're experts and have some boner-hiding strategies to share with you!
Heck yeah!
We'll fill you in on our years of experience hiding **literally thousands** of boners.
The Terrible Art of Boner Hiding

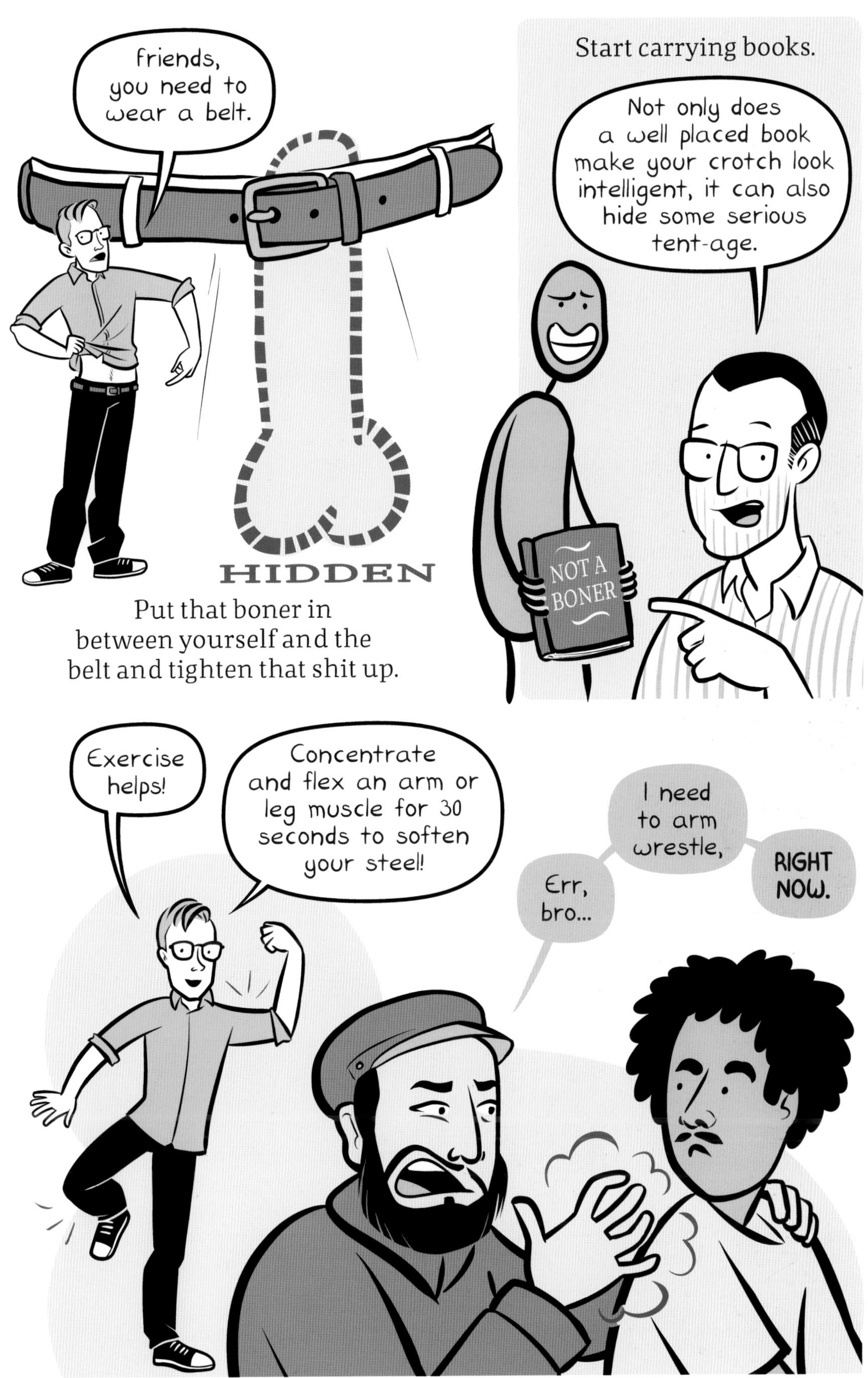
friends, you need to wear a belt.
HIDDEN
Put that boner in between yourself and the belt and tighten that shit up.
Start carrying books.
Not only does a well placed book make your crotch look intelligent, it can also hide some serious tent-age.
NOT A BONER
Exercise helps!
Concentrate and flex an arm or leg muscle for 30 seconds to soften your steel!
Err, bro...
I need to arm wrestle,
RIGHT NOW.

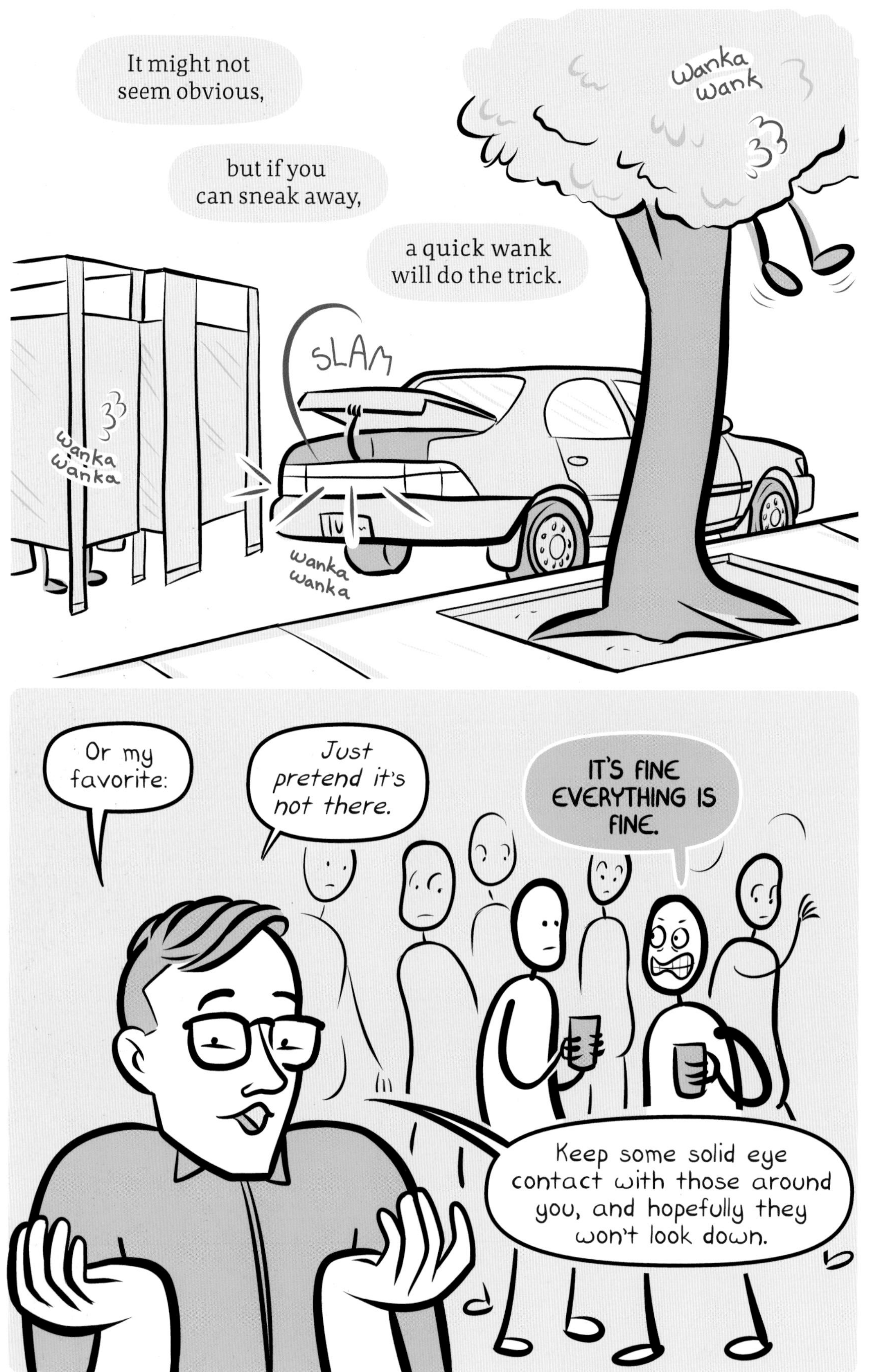
It might not seem obvious,
but if you can sneak away,
a quick wank will do the trick.
Wanka wank
SLAM
Wanka Wanka
wanka wanka
Or my favorite:
Just pretend it's not there.
IT'S FINE EVERYTHING IS FINE.
Keep some solid eye contact with those around you, and hopefully they won't look down.

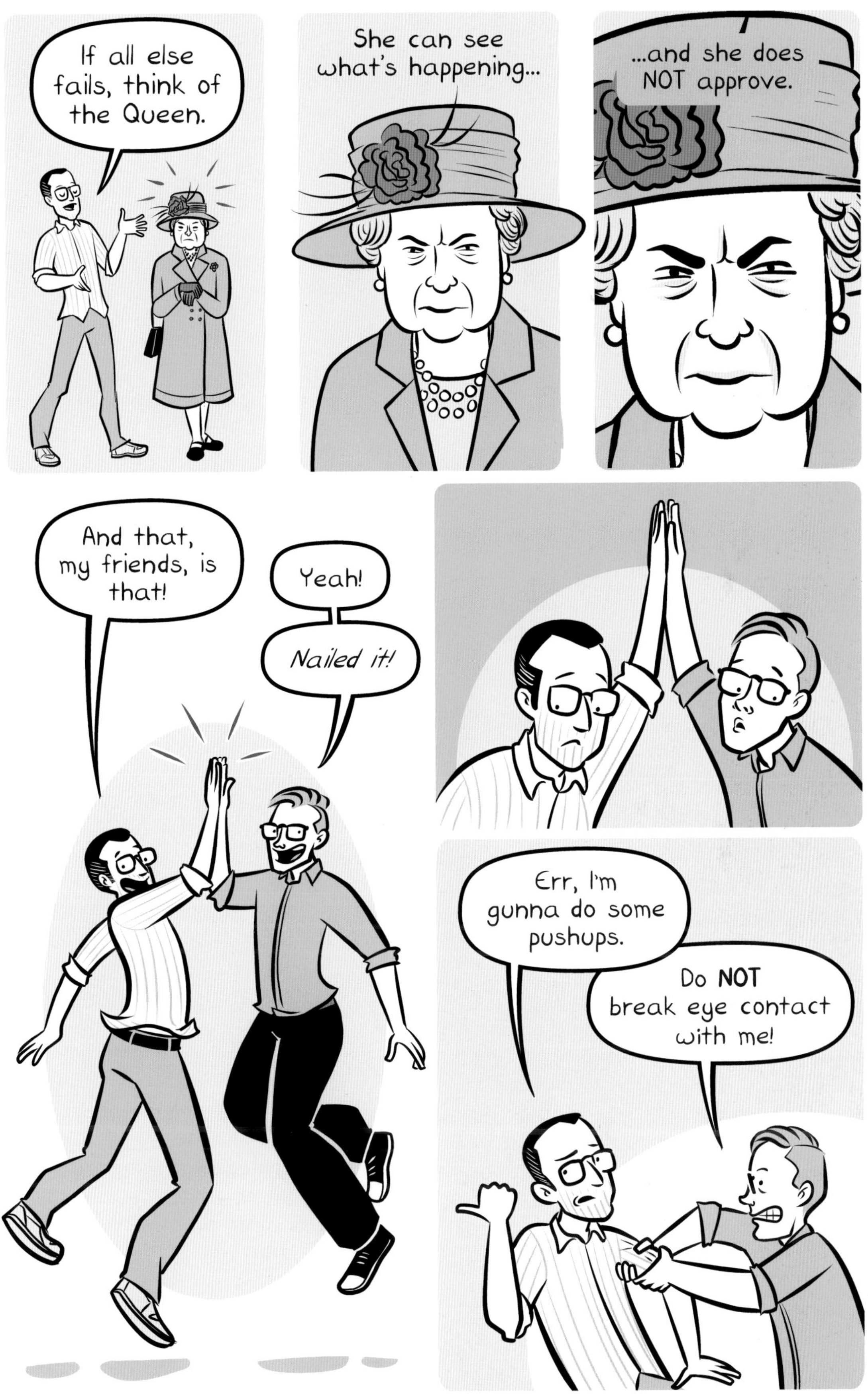
If all else fails, think of the Queen.
She can see what's happening...
...and she does NOT approve.
And that, my friends, is that!
Yeah!
Nailed it!
Err, I'm gunna do some pushups.
Do **NOT** break eye contact with me!

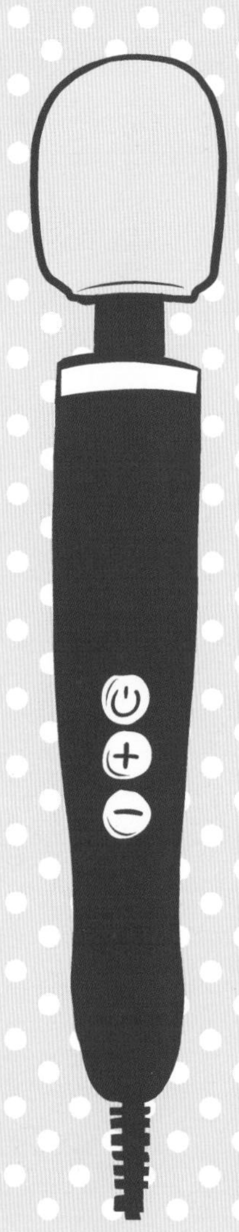

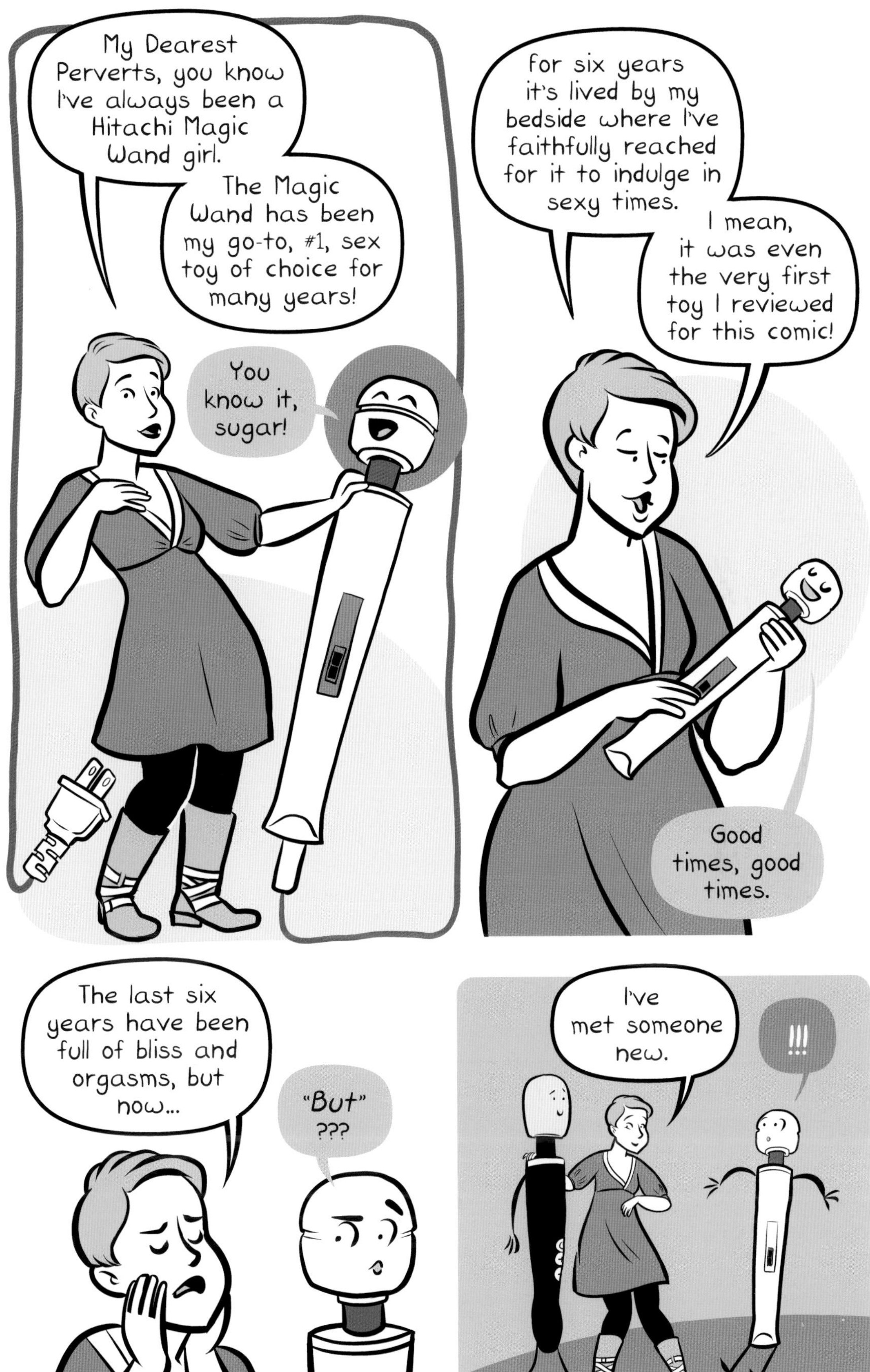
My Dearest Perverts, you know I've always been a Hitachi Magic Wand girl.
The Magic Wand has been my go-to, #1, sex toy of choice for many years!
You know it, sugar!
For six years it's lived by my bedside where I've faithfully reached for it to indulge in sexy times.
I mean, it was even the very first toy I reviewed for this comic!
Good times, good times.
The last six years have been full of bliss and orgasms, but now...
"But" ???
I've met someone new.
!!!

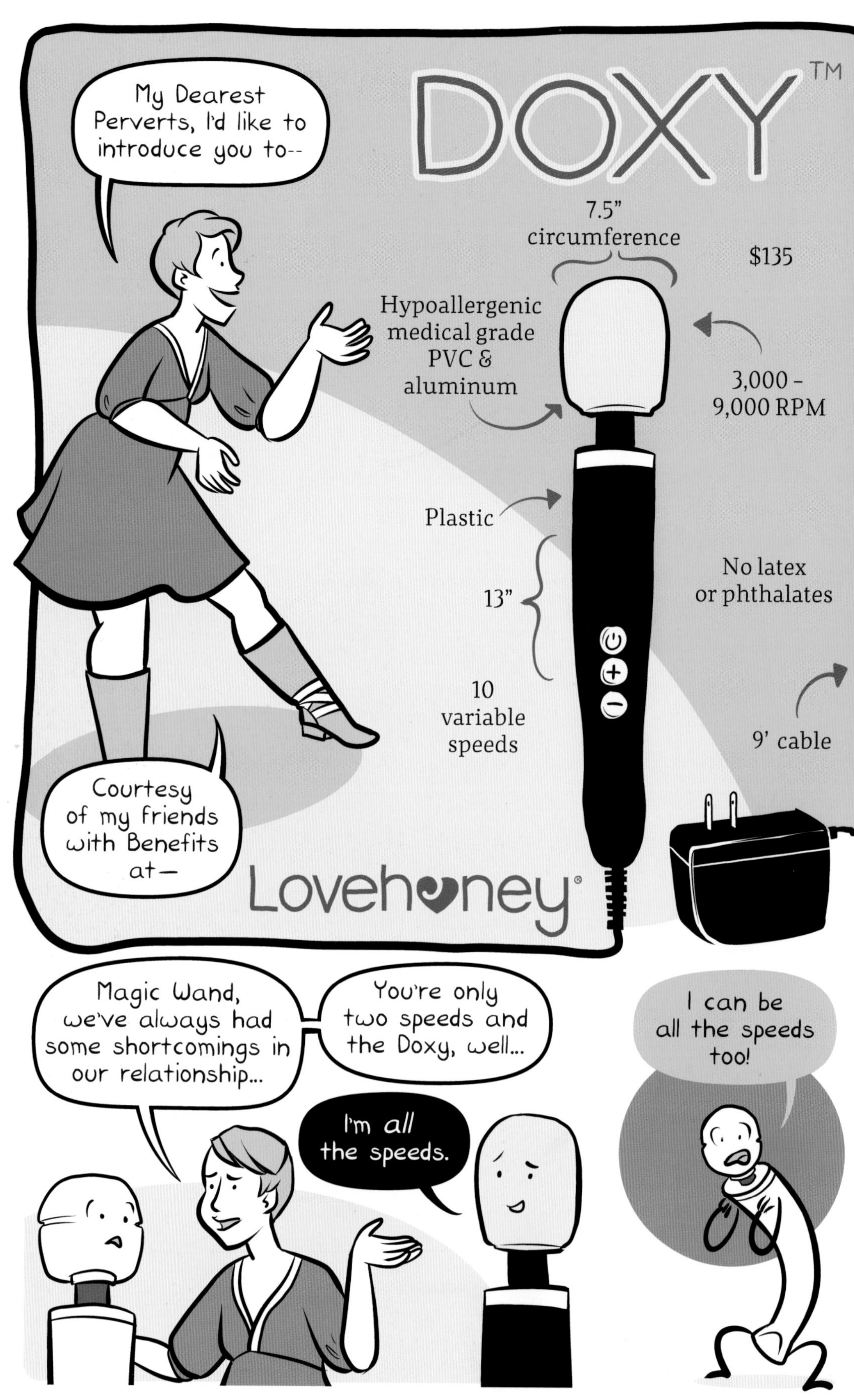
My Dearest Perverts, I'd like to introduce you to--
DOXY™
7.5" circumference
$135
Hypoallergenic medical grade PVC & aluminum
3,000 - 9,000 RPM
Plastic
13"
No latex or phthalates
10 variable speeds
9' cable
Courtesy of my friends with Benefits at—
Lovehoney®
Magic Wand, we've always had some shortcomings in our relationship...
You're only two speeds and the Doxy, well...
I'm *all* the speeds.
I can be all the speeds too!

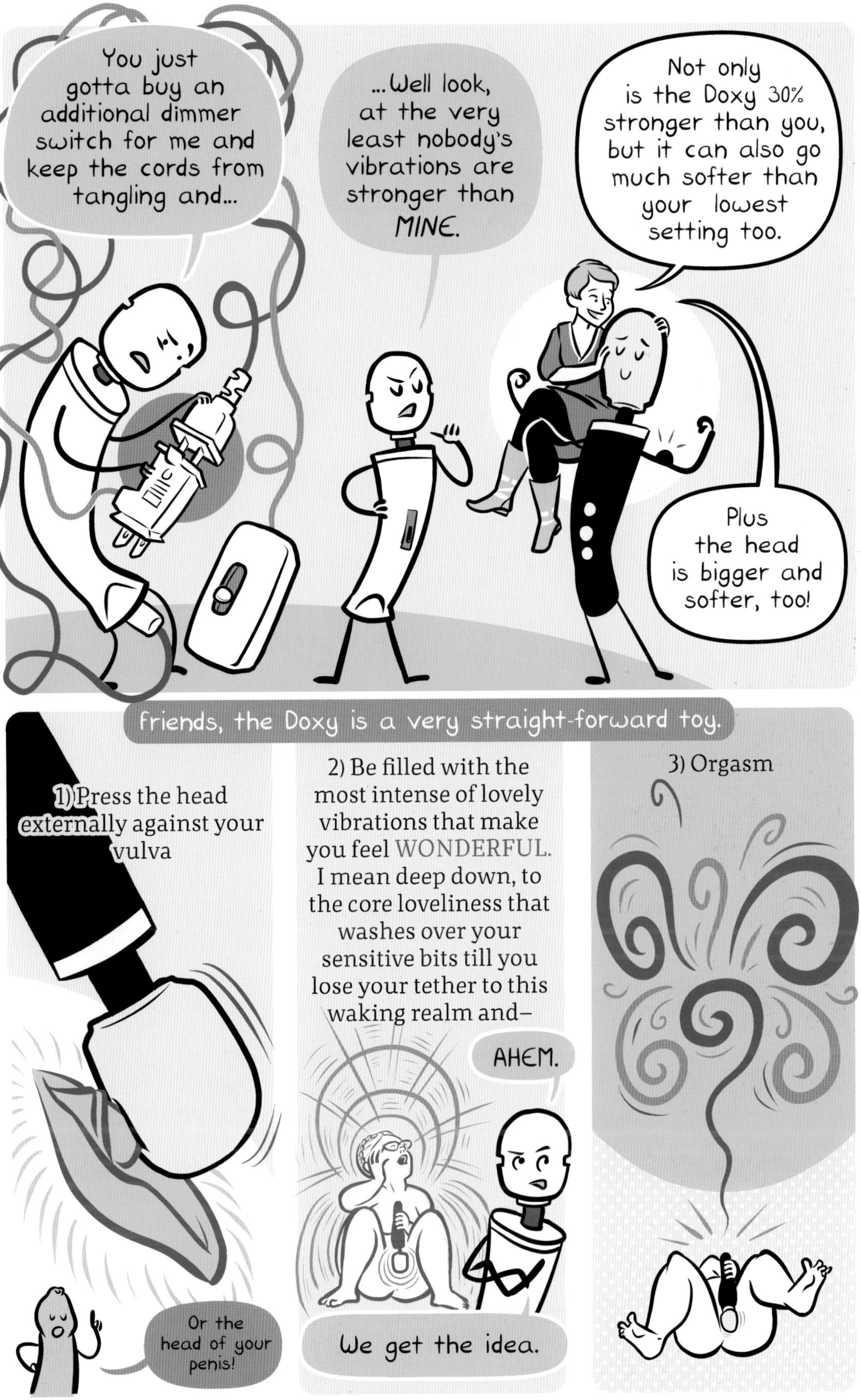

You just gotta buy an additional dimmer switch for me and keep the cords from tangling and...

...Well look, at the very least nobody's vibrations are stronger than MINE.

Not only is the Doxy 30% stronger than you, but it can also go much softer than your lowest setting too.

Plus the head is bigger and softer, too!

friends, the Doxy is a very straight-forward toy.

1) Press the head externally against your vulva

Or the head of your penis!

2) Be filled with the most intense of lovely vibrations that make you feel WONDERFUL. I mean deep down, to the core loveliness that washes over your sensitive bits till you lose your tether to this waking realm and—

AHEM.

We get the idea.

3) Orgasm

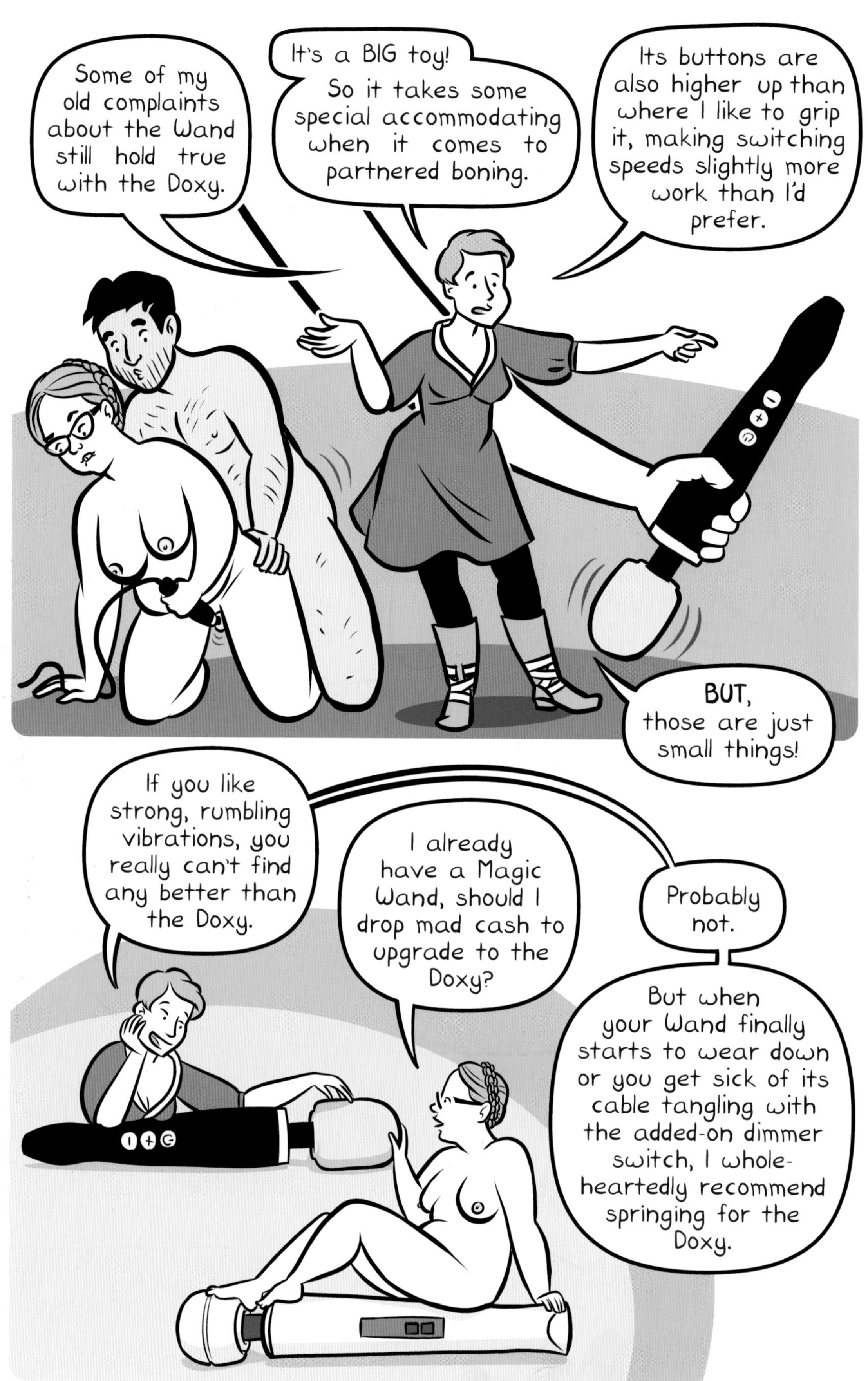
Some of my old complaints about the Wand still hold true with the Doxy.
It's a BIG toy!
So it takes some special accommodating when it comes to partnered boning.
Its buttons are also higher up than where I like to grip it, making switching speeds slightly more work than I'd prefer.
BUT, those are just small things!
If you like strong, rumbling vibrations, you really can't find any better than the Doxy.
I already have a Magic Wand, should I drop mad cash to upgrade to the Doxy?
Probably not.
But when your Wand finally starts to wear down or you get sick of its cable tangling with the added-on dimmer switch, I wholeheartedly recommend springing for the Doxy.

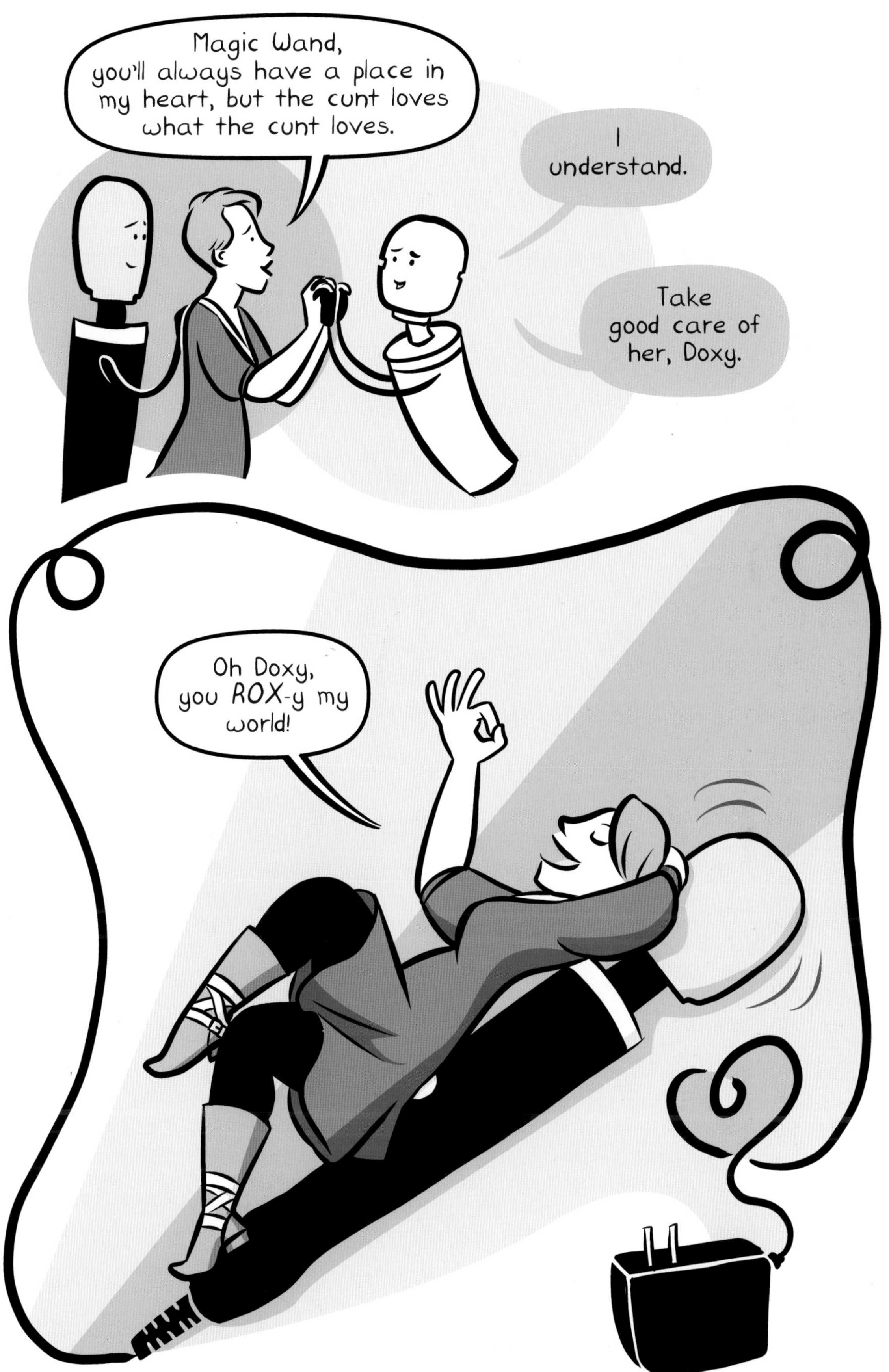
Magic Wand, you'll always have a place in my heart, but the cunt loves what the cunt loves.
I understand.
Take good care of her, Doxy.
Oh Doxy, you ROX-y my world!

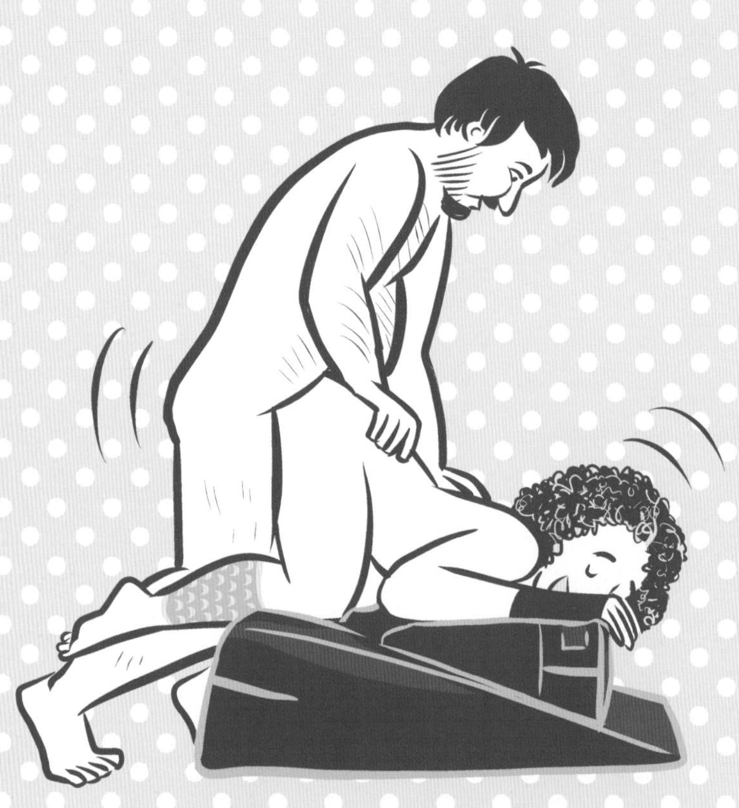

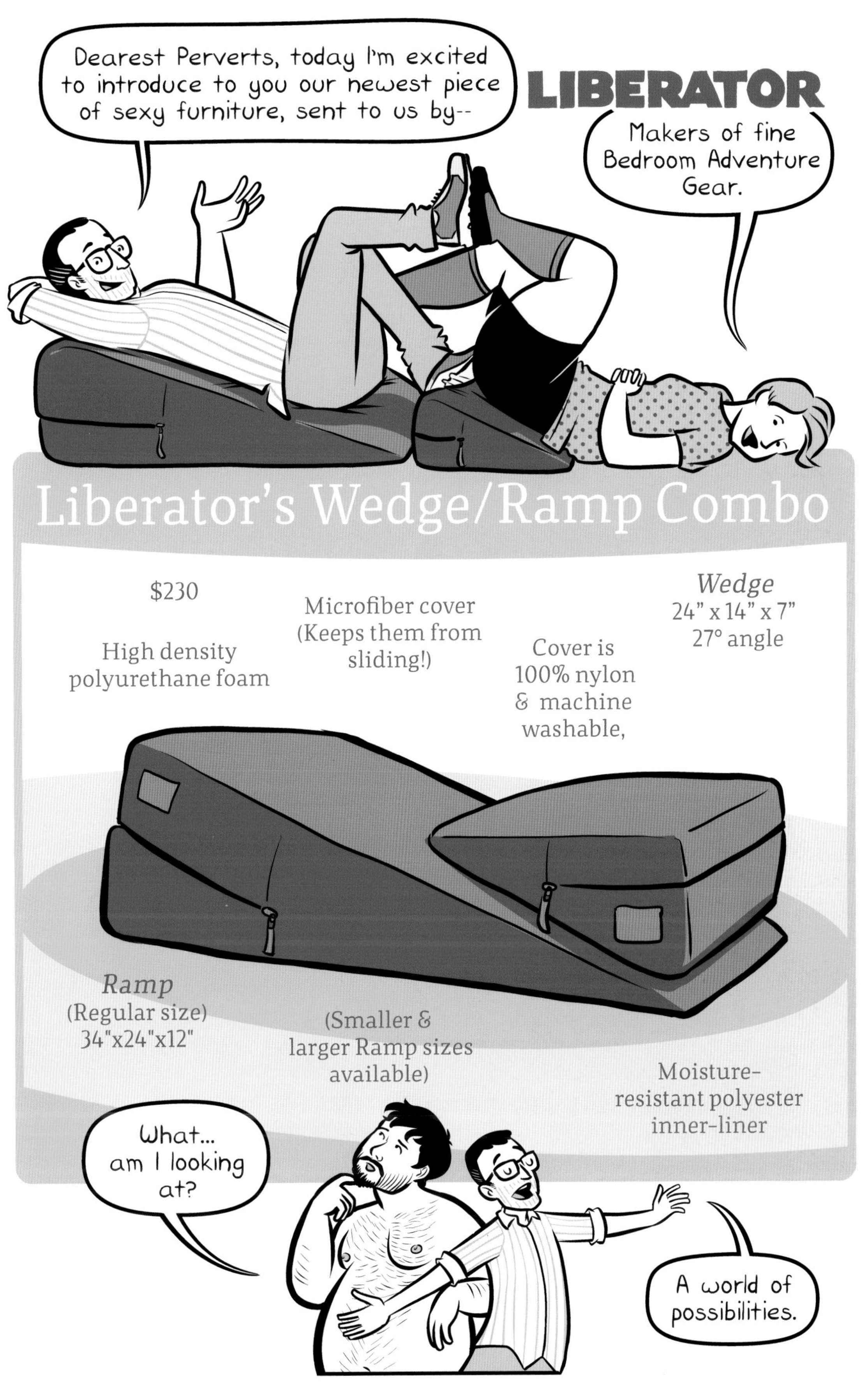
Dearest Perverts, today I'm excited to introduce to you our newest piece of sexy furniture, sent to us by--
LIBERATOR
Makers of fine Bedroom Adventure Gear.
Liberator's Wedge/Ramp Combo
$230
High density polyurethane foam
Microfiber cover (Keeps them from sliding!)
Cover is 100% nylon & machine washable,
Wedge
24" x 14" x 7"
27° angle
Ramp
(Regular size)
34"x24"x12"
(Smaller & larger Ramp sizes available)
Moisture-resistant polyester inner-liner
What... am I looking at?
A world of possibilities.

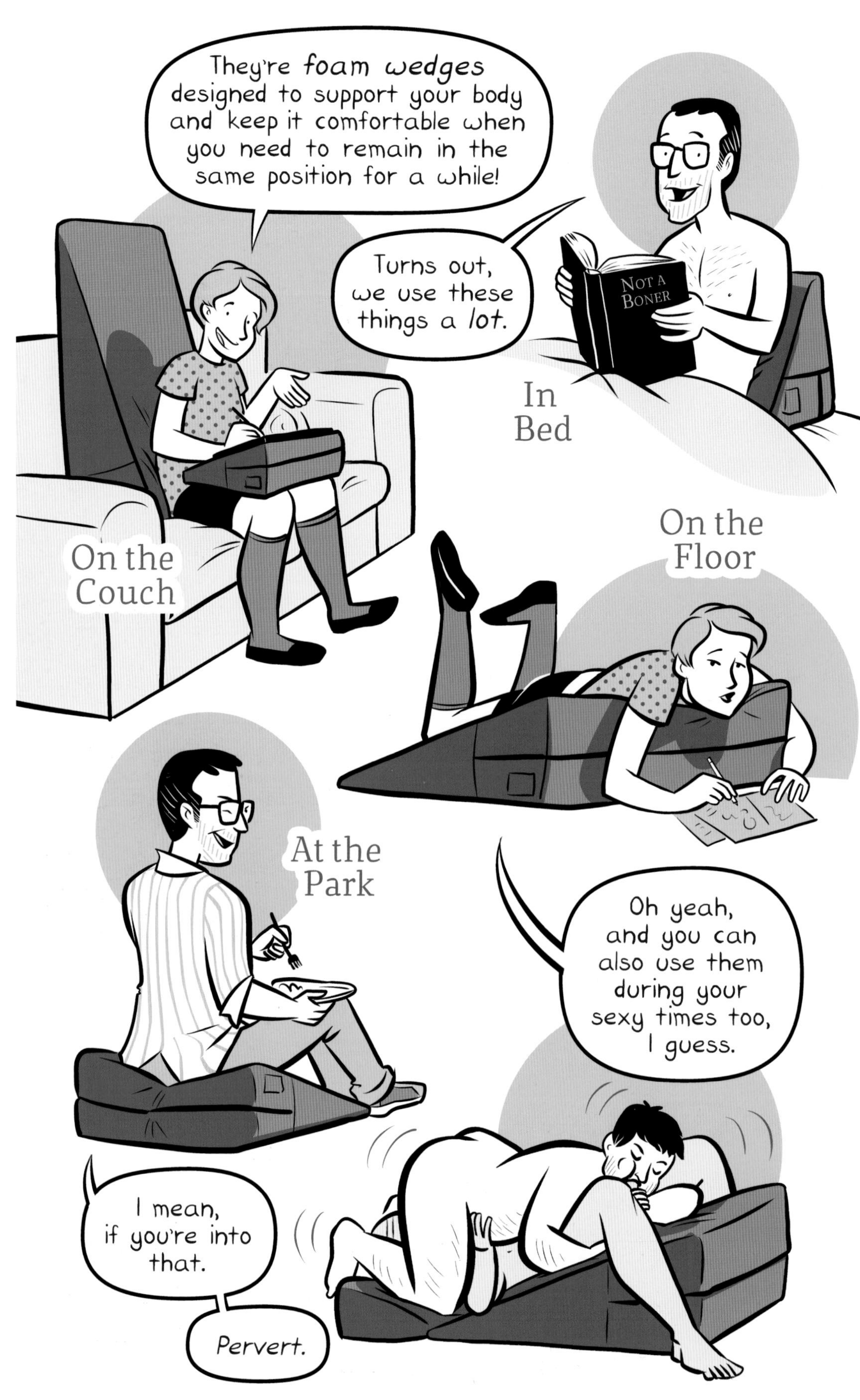
They're foam wedges designed to support your body and keep it comfortable when you need to remain in the same position for a while!
Turns out, we use these things a lot.
NOT A BONER
In Bed
On the Couch
On the Floor
At the Park
Oh yeah, and you can also use them during your sexy times too, I guess.
I mean, if you're into that.
Pervert.

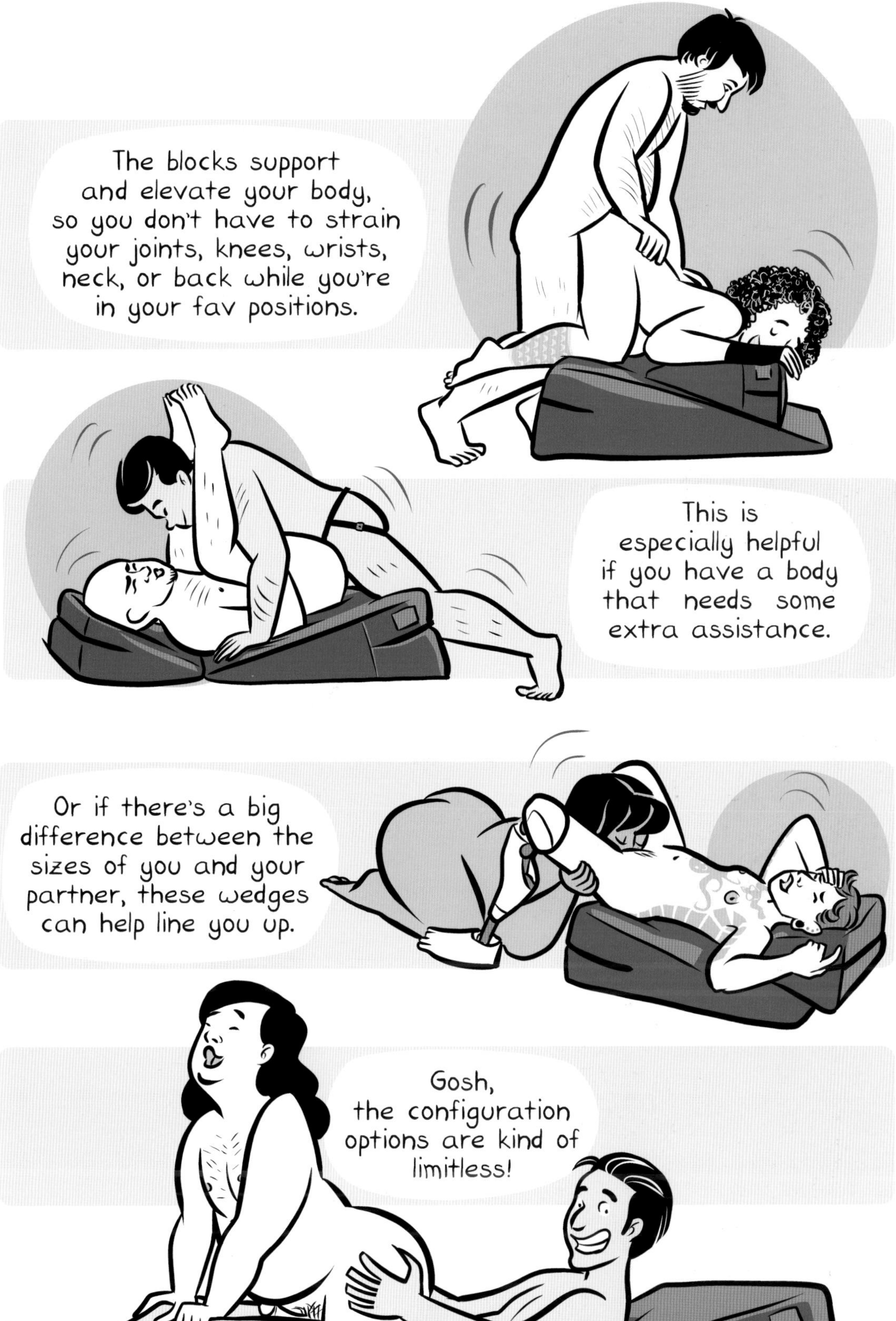
The blocks support and elevate your body, so you don't have to strain your joints, knees, wrists, neck, or back while you're in your fav positions.
This is especially helpful if you have a body that needs some extra assistance.
Or if there's a big difference between the sizes of you and your partner, these wedges can help line you up.
Gosh, the configuration options are kind of limitless!

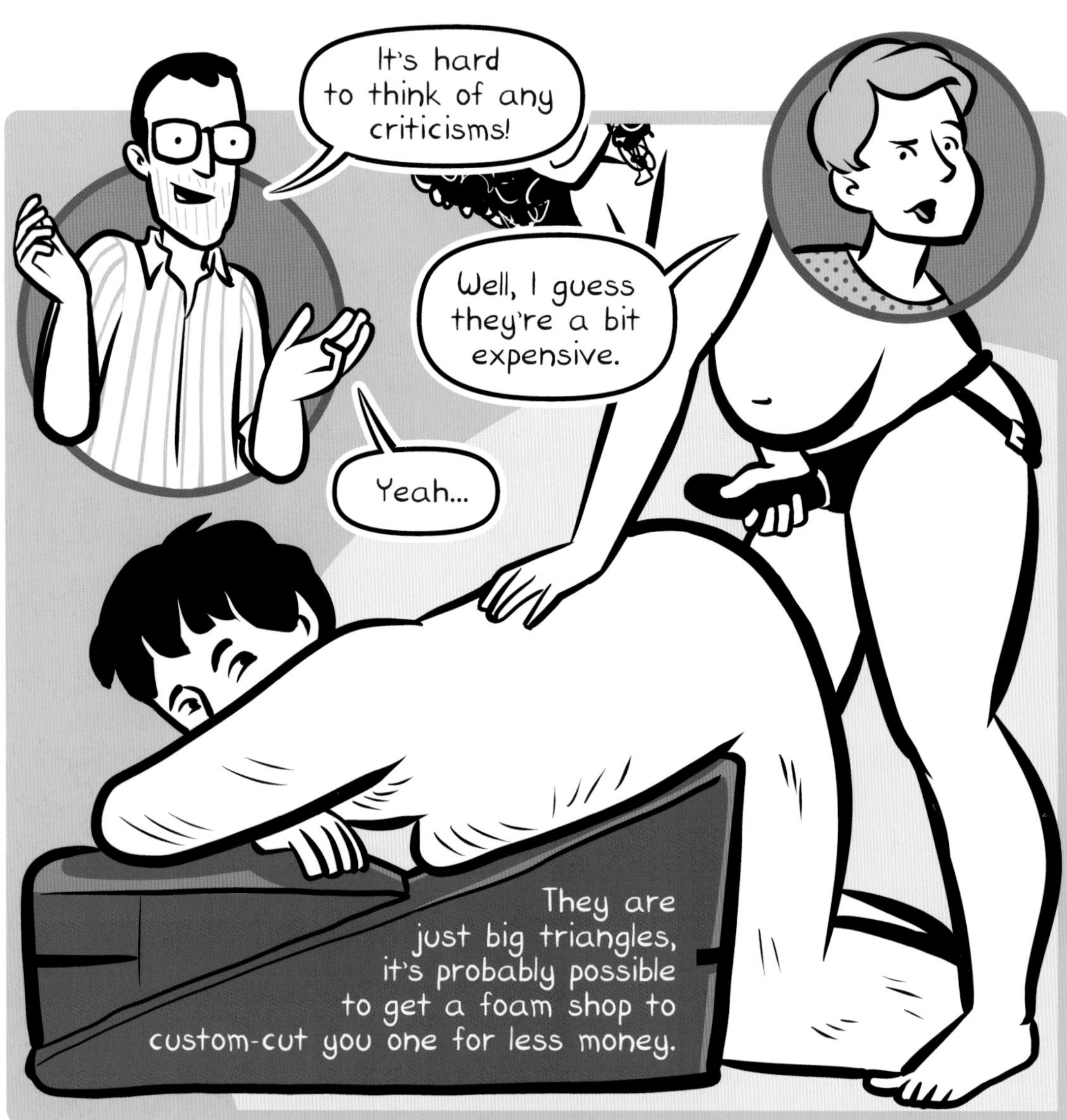
It's hard to think of any criticisms!
Well, I guess they're a bit expensive.
Yeah...
They are just big triangles, it's probably possible to get a foam shop to custom-cut you one for less money.

But Liberator has already picked out the perfect foam density...

...cut it to the comfiest angles to support your body positions...

...and provided you with easily removable and washable coverings...

...so the price doesn't feel *too* criminal.

It may be a touch pricey, but the quality of what you're getting in exchange seems worth it.

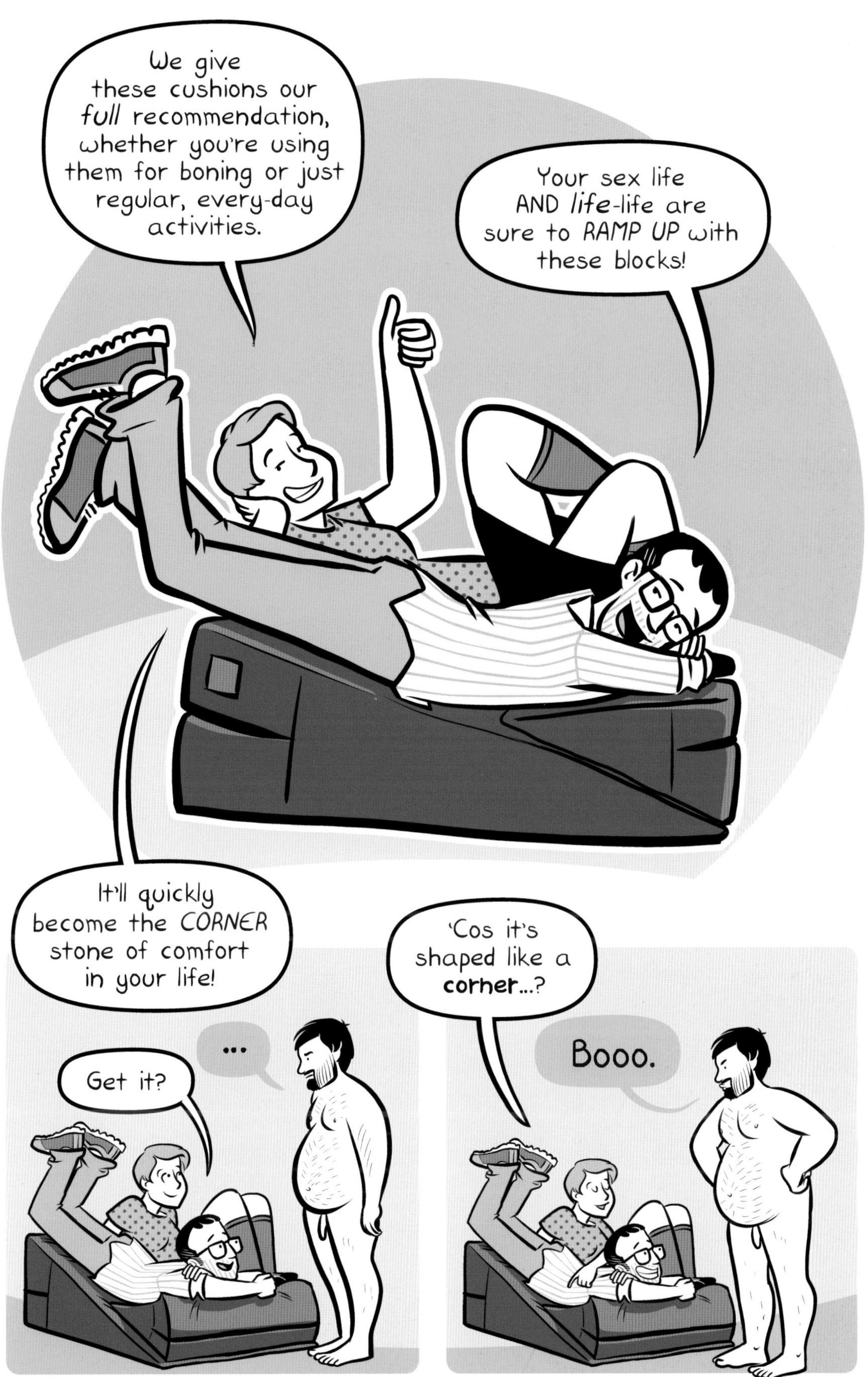
We give these cushions our *full* recommendation, whether you're using them for boning or just regular, every-day activities.
Your sex life AND *life*-life are sure to *RAMP UP* with these blocks!
It'll quickly become the CORNER stone of comfort in your life!
Get it?
...
'Cos it's shaped like a **corner**...?
Booo.

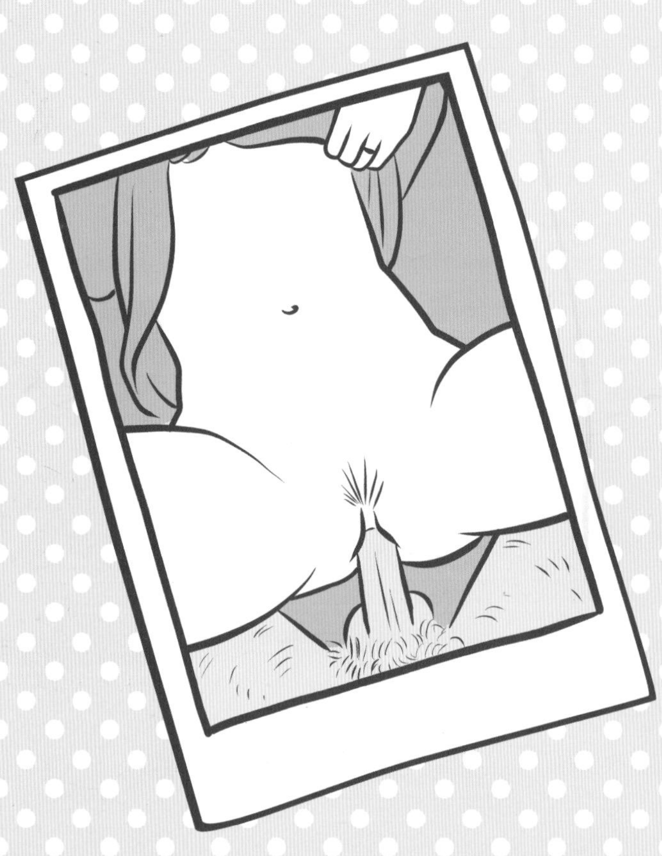

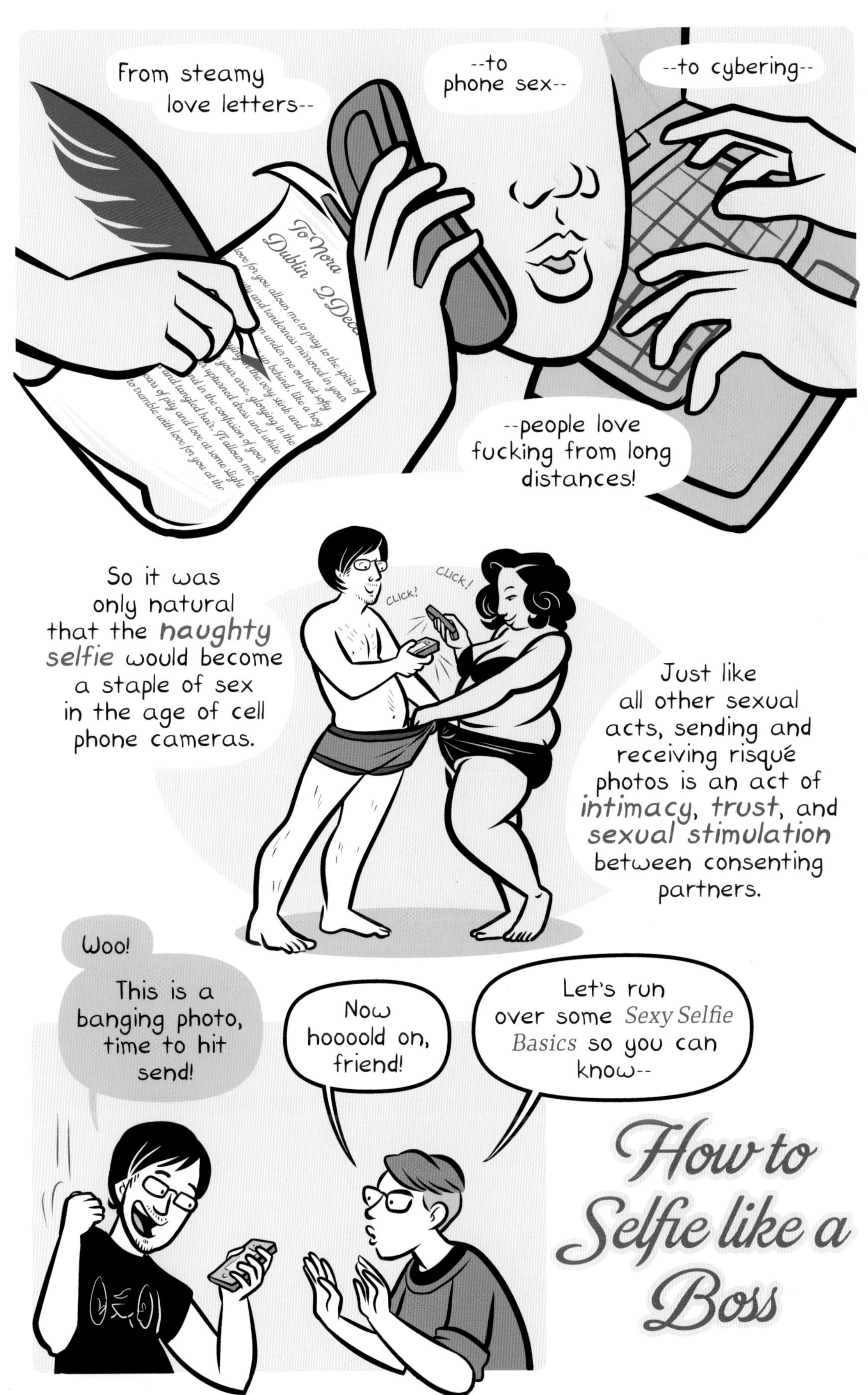
From steamy love letters--
To Nora
--to phone sex--
--to cybering--
--people love fucking from long distances!
So it was only natural that the naughty selfie would become a staple of sex in the age of cell phone cameras.
CLICK!
CLICK!
Just like all other sexual acts, sending and receiving risqué photos is an act of intimacy, trust, and sexual stimulation between consenting partners.
Woo!
This is a banging photo, time to hit send!
Now hoooold on, friend!
Let's run over some Sexy Selfie Basics so you can know--
How to Selfie like a Boss

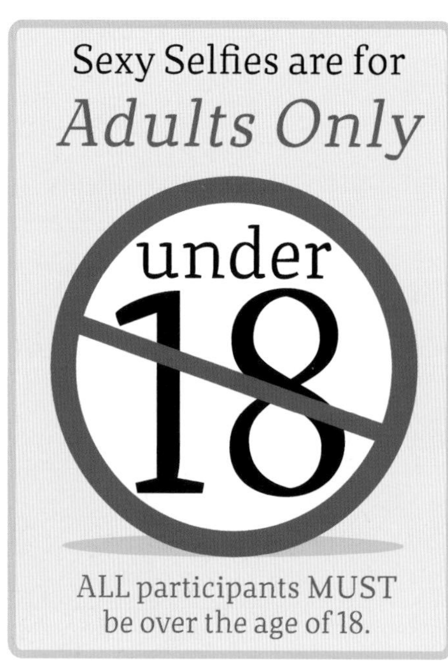

Sexy Selfies are for
Adults Only
under
18
ALL participants MUST
be over the age of 18.

There are *serious legal consequences* for any naked photos that are exchanged between people where anyone is under 18.

Creating/sharing/possessing any photos of a minor is legally *CHILD PORNOGRAPHY*, a *felony*!

(Even if it's consensually from one 17-and-a-half year old to another.)

Don't get incarcerated or have to register as a sex offender because you swapped naughty pictures with your high school sweetie!

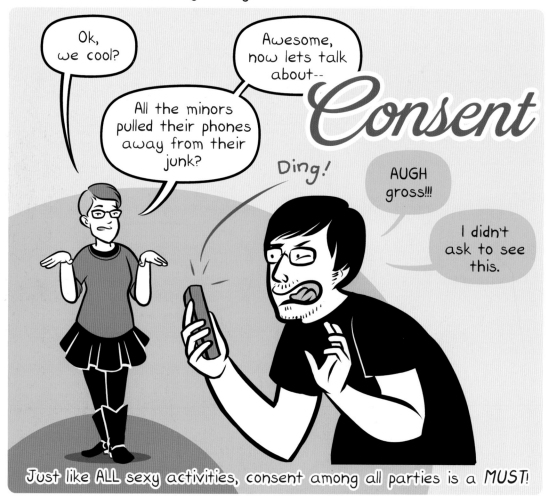

Ok, we cool?

All the minors pulled their phones away from their junk?

Awesome, now lets talk about--

Consent

Ding!

AUGH gross!!!

I didn't ask to see this.

Just like ALL sexy activities, consent among all parties is a *MUST*!

You want that special someone to be *HAPPY* when they get a picture of your goods--

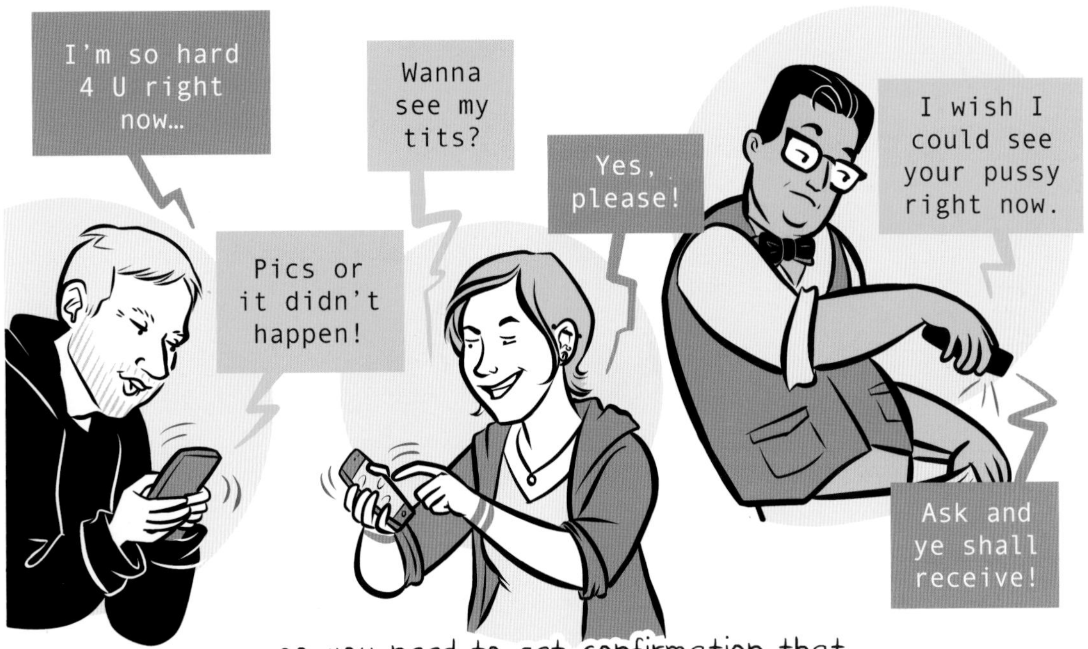

I'm so hard 4 U right now...
Pics or it didn't happen!
Wanna see my tits?
Yes, please!
I wish I could see your pussy right now.
Ask and ye shall receive!

--so you need to get confirmation that they want to see 'em before you send 'em.

NO SHARING

NEVER EVER share a naked photo that you received consensually unless you have explicit permission.

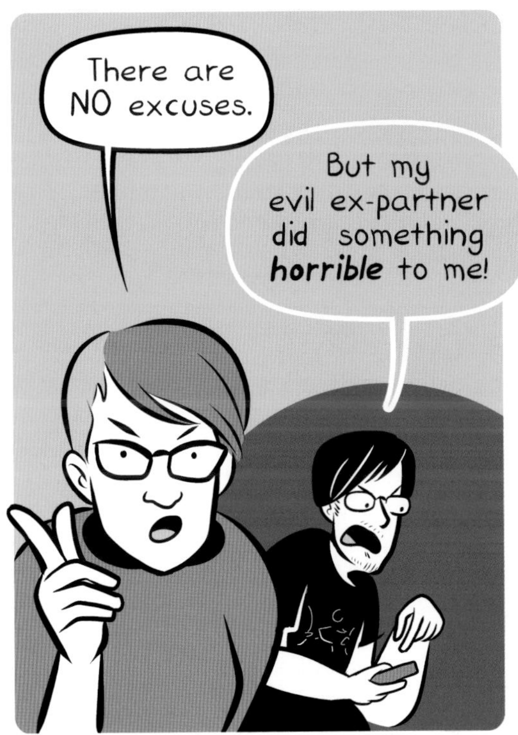

There are NO excuses.
But my evil ex-partner did something ***horrible*** to me!

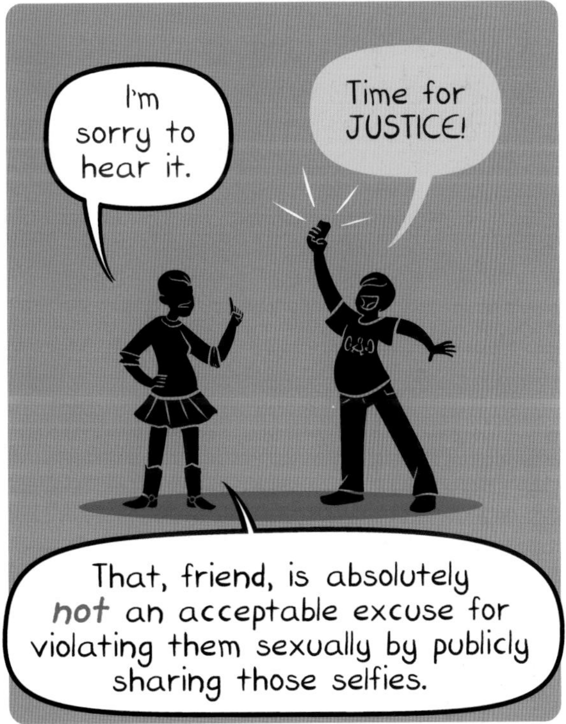

I'm sorry to hear it.
Time for JUSTICE!
That, friend, is absolutely ***not*** an acceptable excuse for violating them sexually by publicly sharing those selfies.

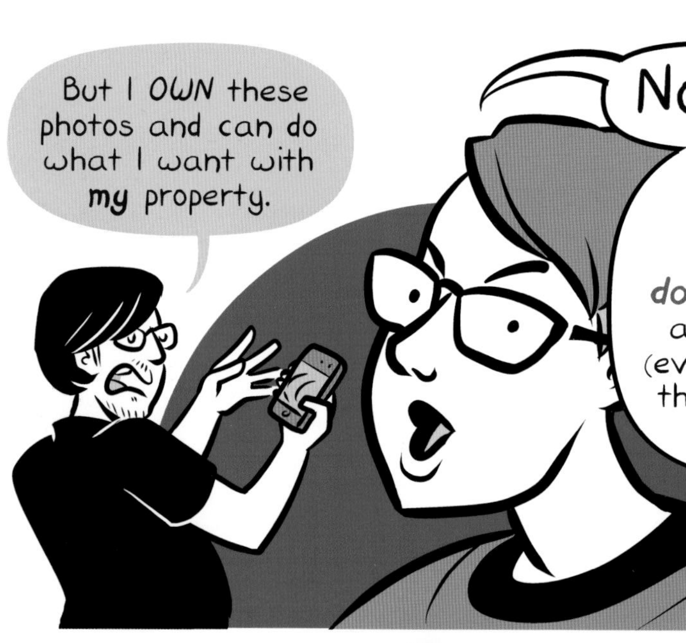

But I *OWN* these photos and can do what I want with **my** property.
Nope!
They shared that with you as an act of intimacy and trust, but you ***do not own their body*** and making it available (even photos of it) without their consent is not only a ***sexual violation*** but also means you are a ***garbage person!***

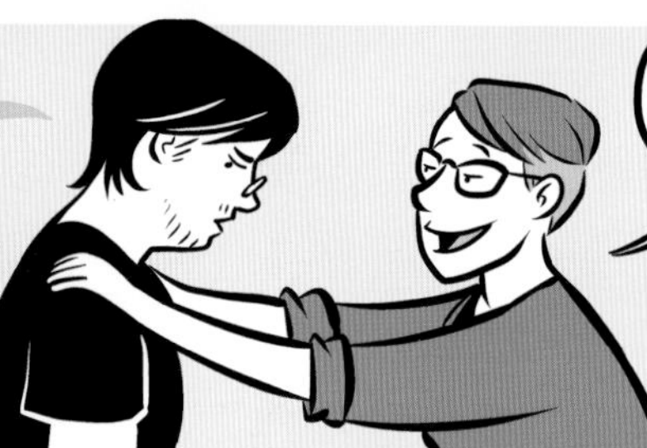

You're right, I'm mad and hurt but I'm not a garbage person.
I didn't think so!
Also, if you're ever asked to delete those pictures, **DO IT.**

Use your noggin and take

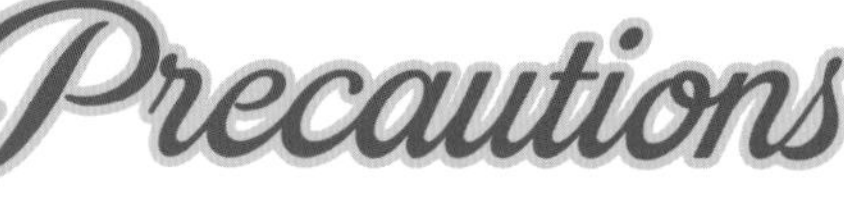

Listen, shit happens.

There is risk to this activity.

If your life will have profoundly negative consequences if a naughty selfie of you gets shared, then hide your distinguishing characteristics.

No face shots!

Leave out the obvious birth marks!

Photoshop out them tattoos and piercings!

But EVEN THEN. Photos can have hidden information in their data that may still lead back to you, so realize there's ALWAYS gonna be risk.

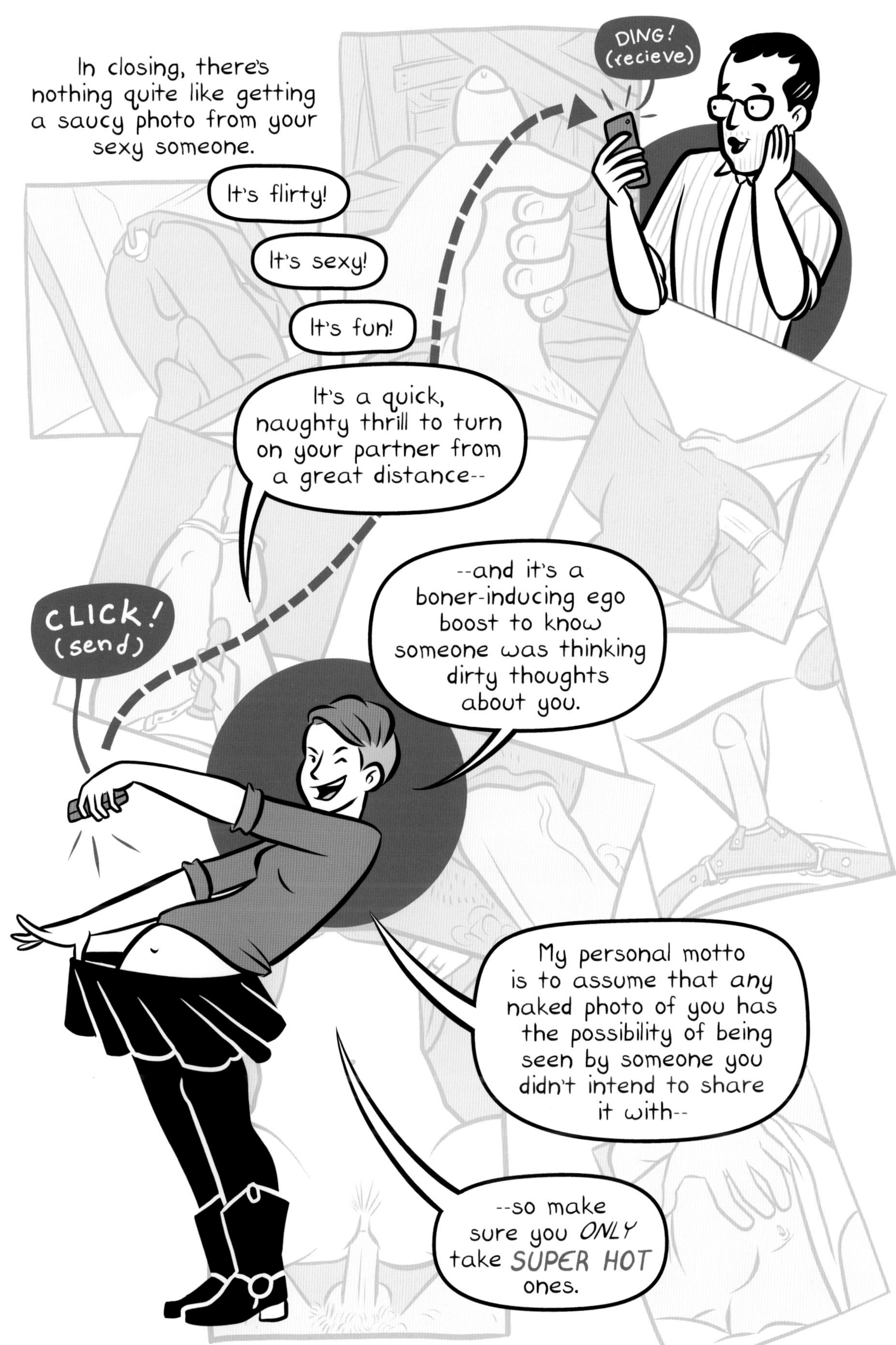

In closing, there's nothing quite like getting a saucy photo from your sexy someone.
It's flirty!
It's sexy!
It's fun!
DING! (recieve)
It's a quick, naughty thrill to turn on your partner from a great distance--
CLICK! (send)
--and it's a boner-inducing ego boost to know someone was thinking dirty thoughts about you.
My personal motto is to assume that *any* naked photo of you has the possibility of being seen by someone you didn't intend to share it with--
--so make sure you *ONLY* take **SUPER HOT** ones.

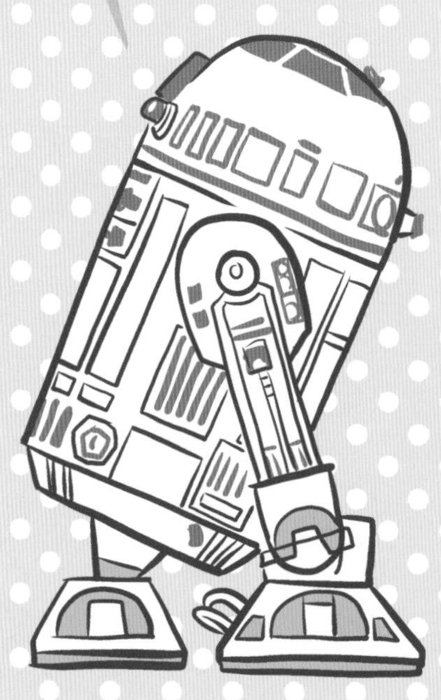
broop
doo!

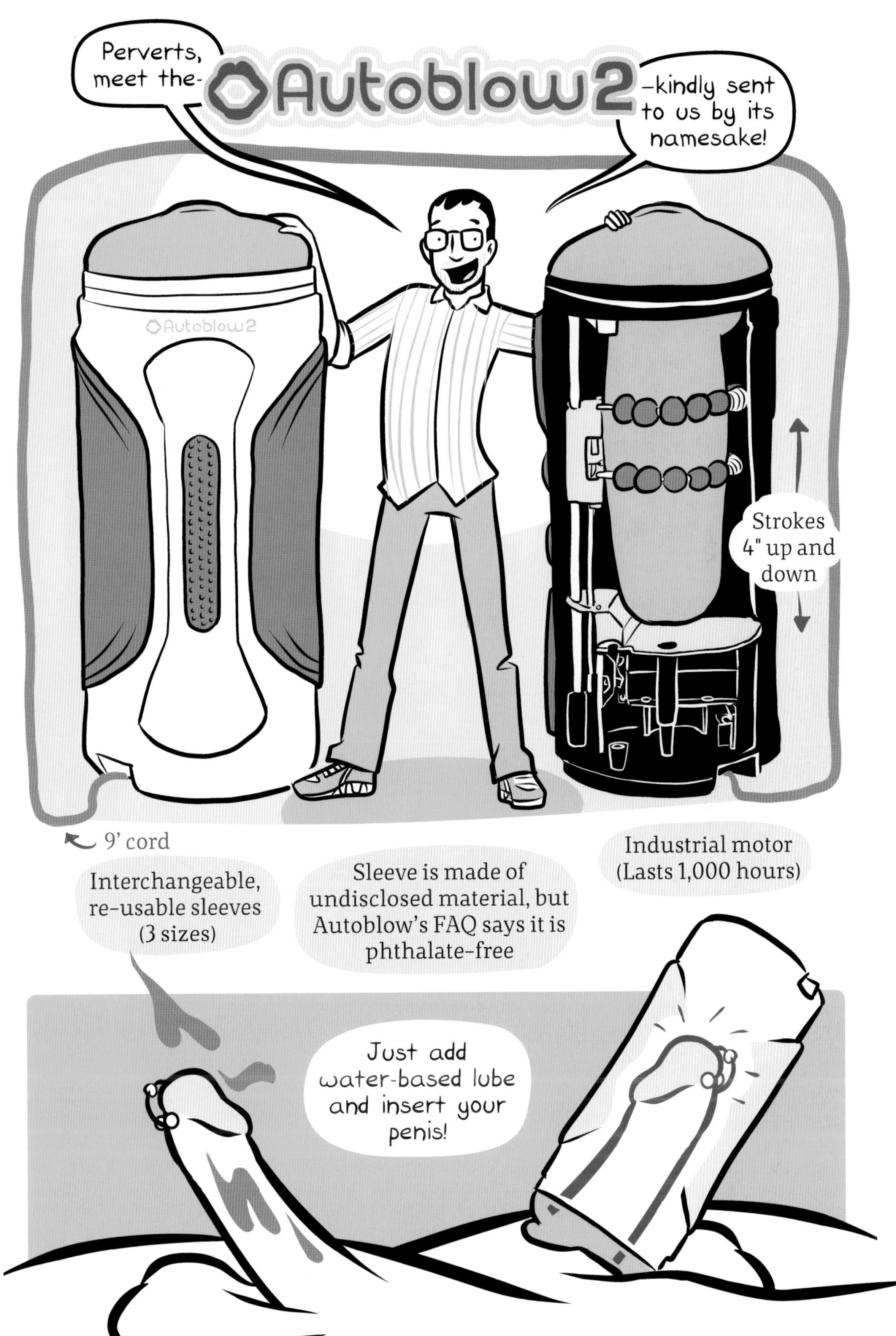
Perverts, meet the-
Autoblow 2
-kindly sent to us by its namesake!
Autoblow 2
Strokes 4" up and down
9' cord
Interchangeable, re-usable sleeves (3 sizes)
Sleeve is made of undisclosed material, but Autoblow's FAQ says it is phthalate-free
Industrial motor (Lasts 1,000 hours)
Just add water-based lube and insert your penis!

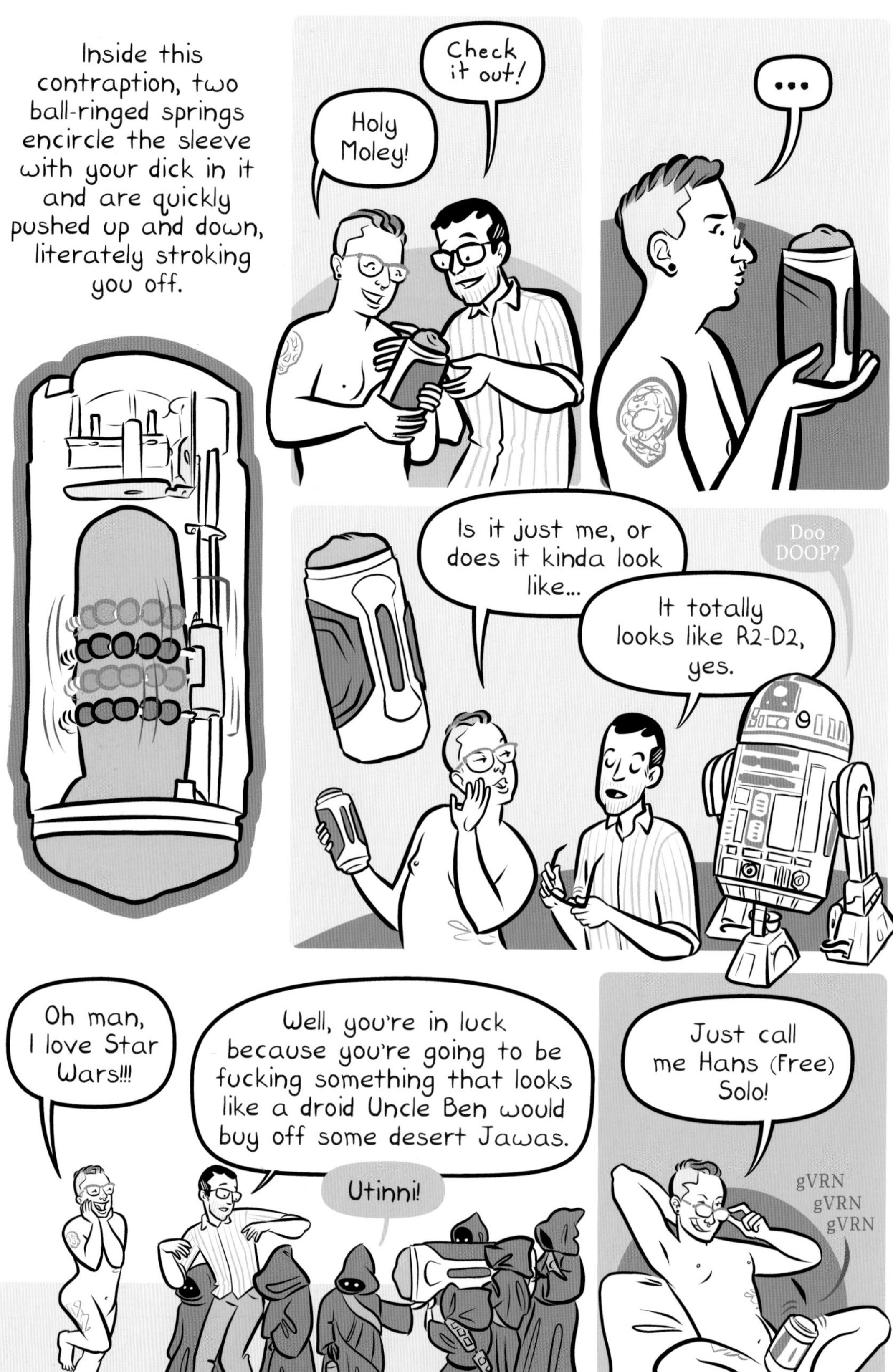
Inside this contraption, two ball-ringed springs encircle the sleeve with your dick in it and are quickly pushed up and down, literately stroking you off.
Check it out!
Holy Moley!
...
Is it just me, or does it kinda look like...
Doo DOOP?
It totally looks like R2-D2, yes.
Oh man, I love Star Wars!!!
Well, you're in luck because you're going to be fucking something that looks like a droid Uncle Ben would buy off some desert Jawas.
Utinni!
Just call me Hans (Free) Solo!
gVRN
gVRN
gVRN

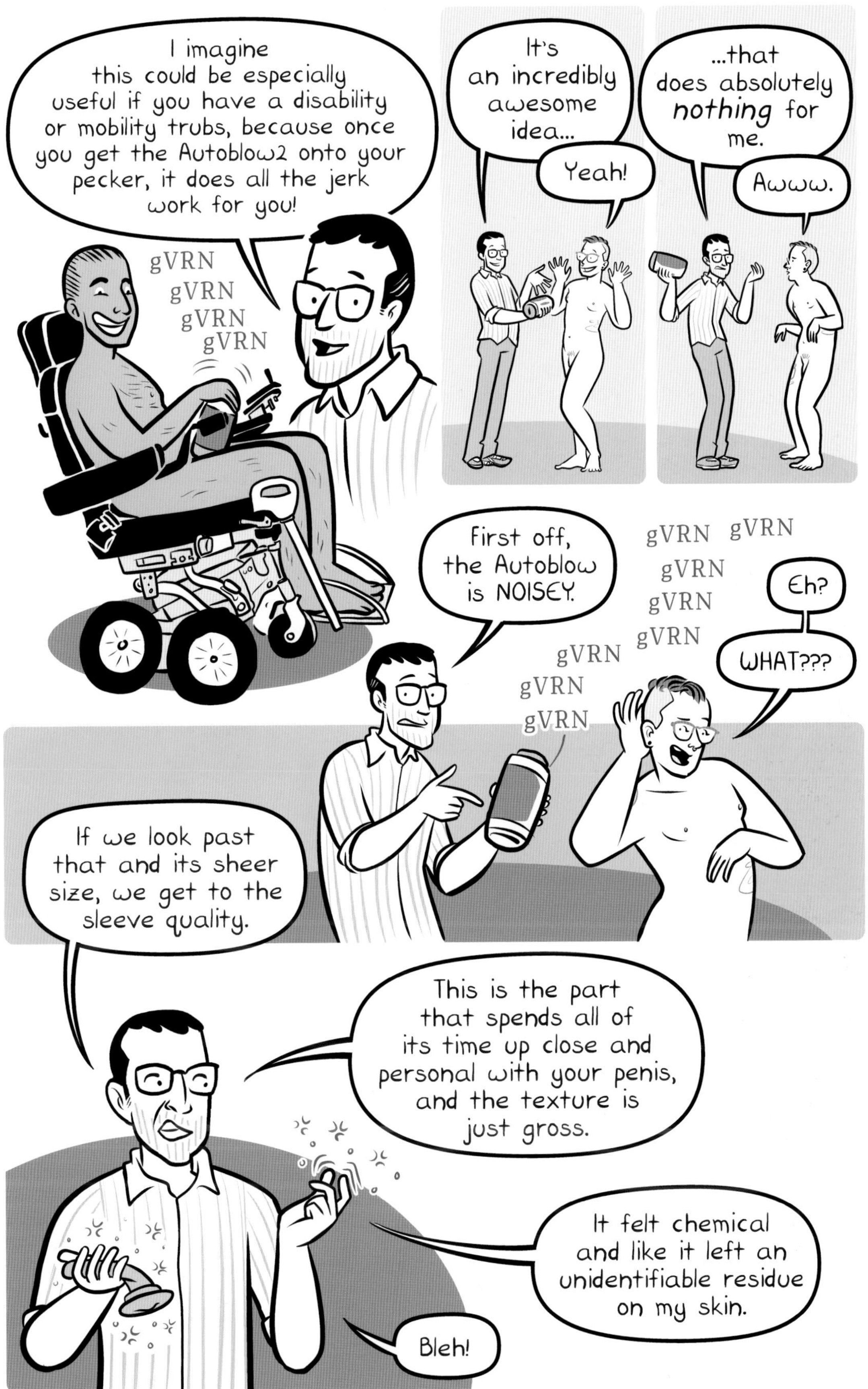
I imagine this could be especially useful if you have a disability or mobility trubs, because once you get the Autoblow2 onto your pecker, it does all the jerk work for you!
gVRN
gVRN
gVRN
gVRN
It's an incredibly awesome idea...
Yeah!
...that does absolutely *nothing* for me.
Awww.
First off, the Autoblow is NOISEY.
gVRN gVRN
gVRN
gVRN
gVRN
gVRN
gVRN
gVRN
Eh?
WHAT???
If we look past that and its sheer size, we get to the sleeve quality.
This is the part that spends all of its time up close and personal with your penis, and the texture is just gross.
It felt chemical and like it left an unidentifiable residue on my skin.
Bleh!

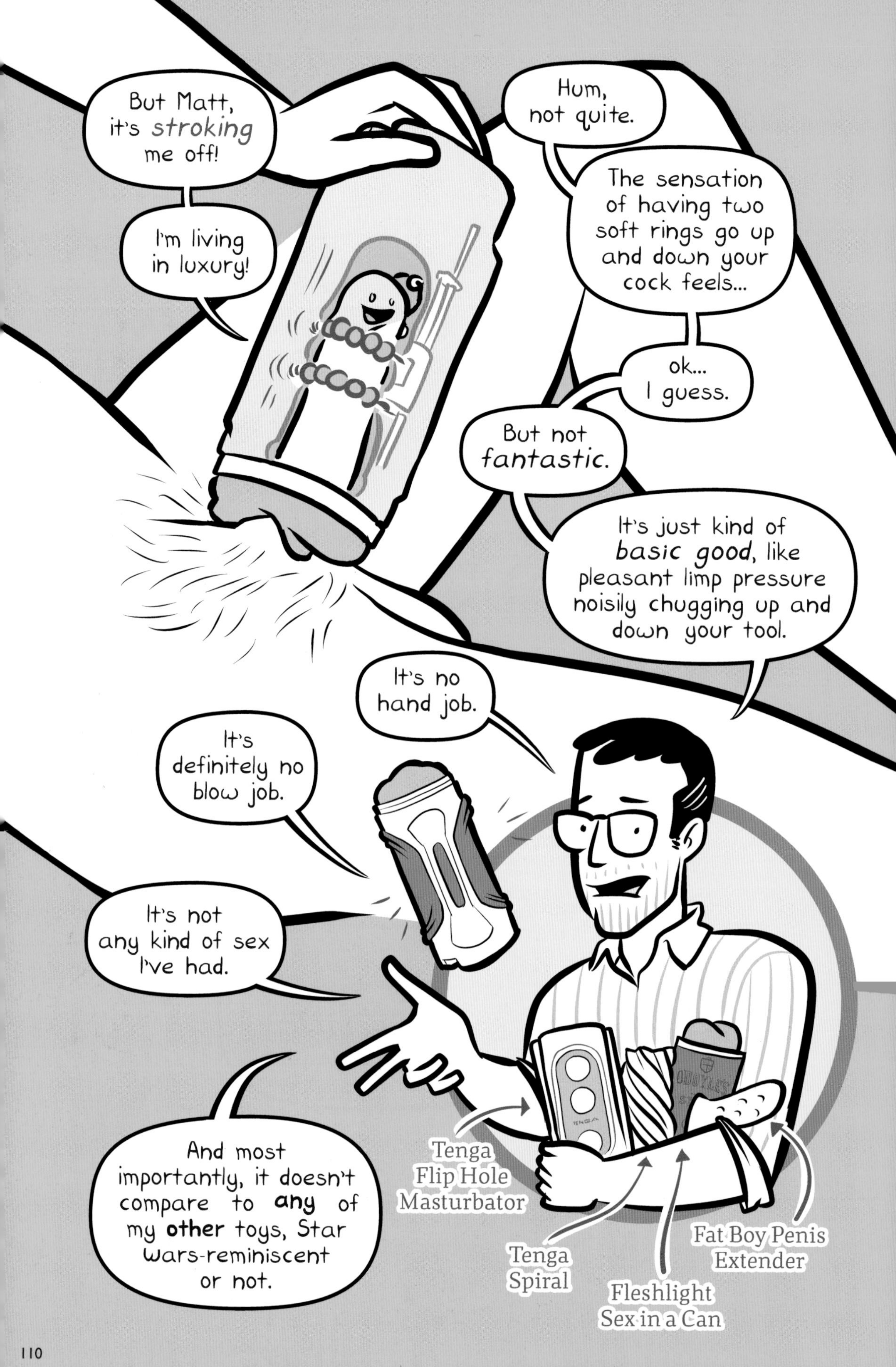
But Matt, it's stroking me off!
I'm living in luxury!
Hum, not quite.
The sensation of having two soft rings go up and down your cock feels...
ok... I guess.
But not fantastic.
It's just kind of basic good, like pleasant limp pressure noisily chugging up and down your tool.
It's no hand job.
It's definitely no blow job.
It's not any kind of sex I've had.
And most importantly, it doesn't compare to any of my other toys, Star Wars-reminiscent or not.
Tenga Flip Hole Masturbator
Tenga Spiral
Fleshlight Sex in a Can
Fat Boy Penis Extender

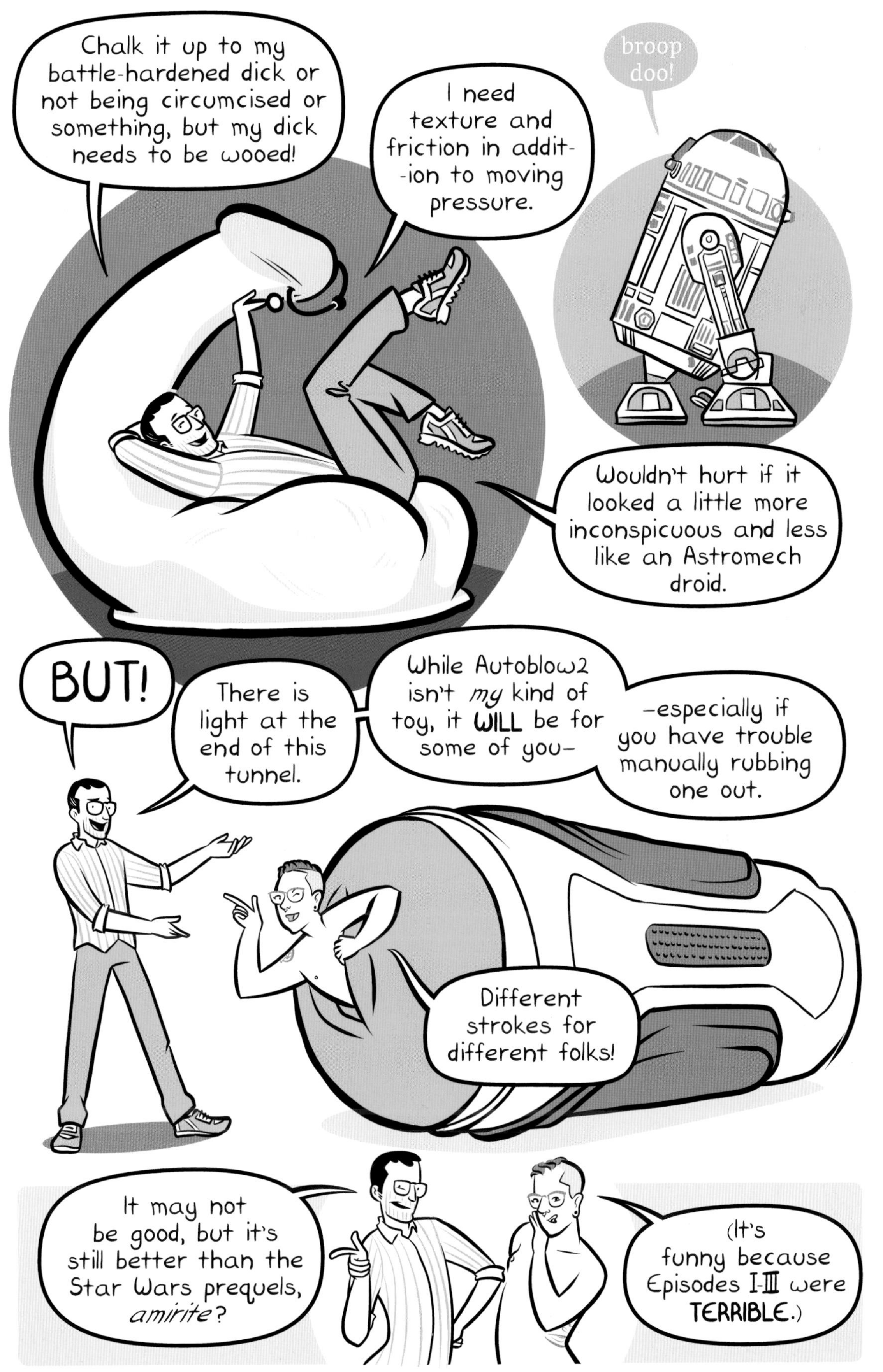
Chalk it up to my battle-hardened dick or not being circumcised or something, but my dick needs to be wooed!
I need texture and friction in addit- -ion to moving pressure.
broop doo!
Wouldn't hurt if it looked a little more inconspicuous and less like an Astromech droid.
BUT!
There is light at the end of this tunnel.
While Autoblow2 isn't *my* kind of toy, it **WILL** be for some of you–
–especially if you have trouble manually rubbing one out.
Different strokes for different folks!
It may not be good, but it's still better than the Star Wars prequels, *amirite*?
(It's funny because Episodes I-III were **TERRIBLE**.)

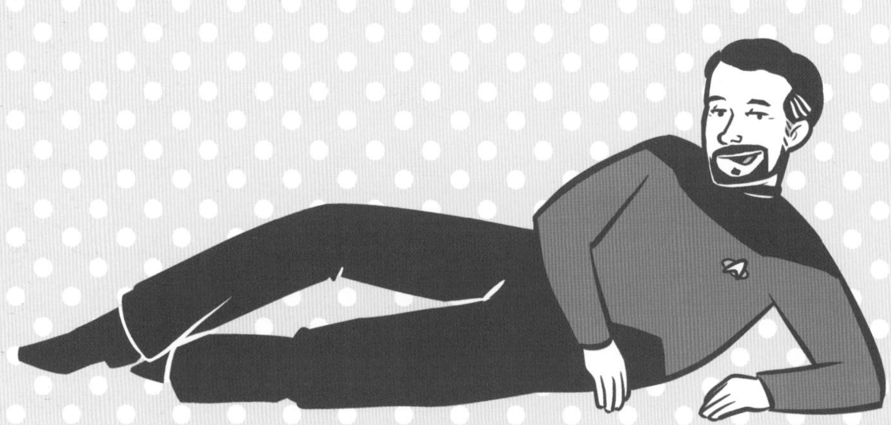

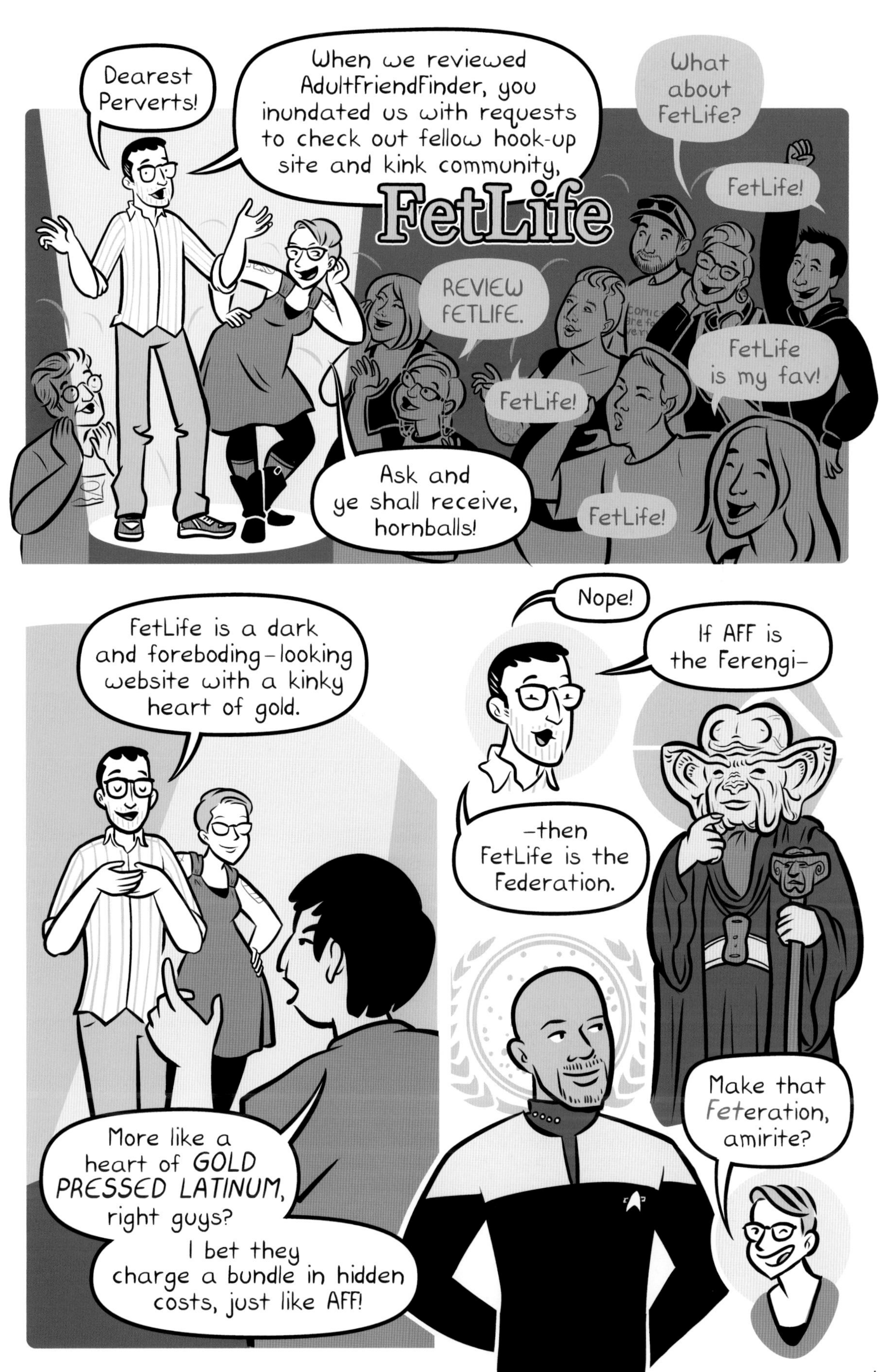
Dearest Perverts!
When we reviewed AdultFriendFinder, you inundated us with requests to check out fellow hook-up site and kink community,
FetLife
What about FetLife?
FetLife!
REVIEW FETLIFE.
FetLife is my fav!
FetLife!
Ask and ye shall receive, hornballs!
FetLife!
FetLife is a dark and foreboding-looking website with a kinky heart of gold.
More like a heart of GOLD PRESSED LATINUM, right guys?
I bet they charge a bundle in hidden costs, just like AFF!
Nope!
If AFF is the Ferengi-
-then FetLife is the Federation.
Make that Feteration, amirite?

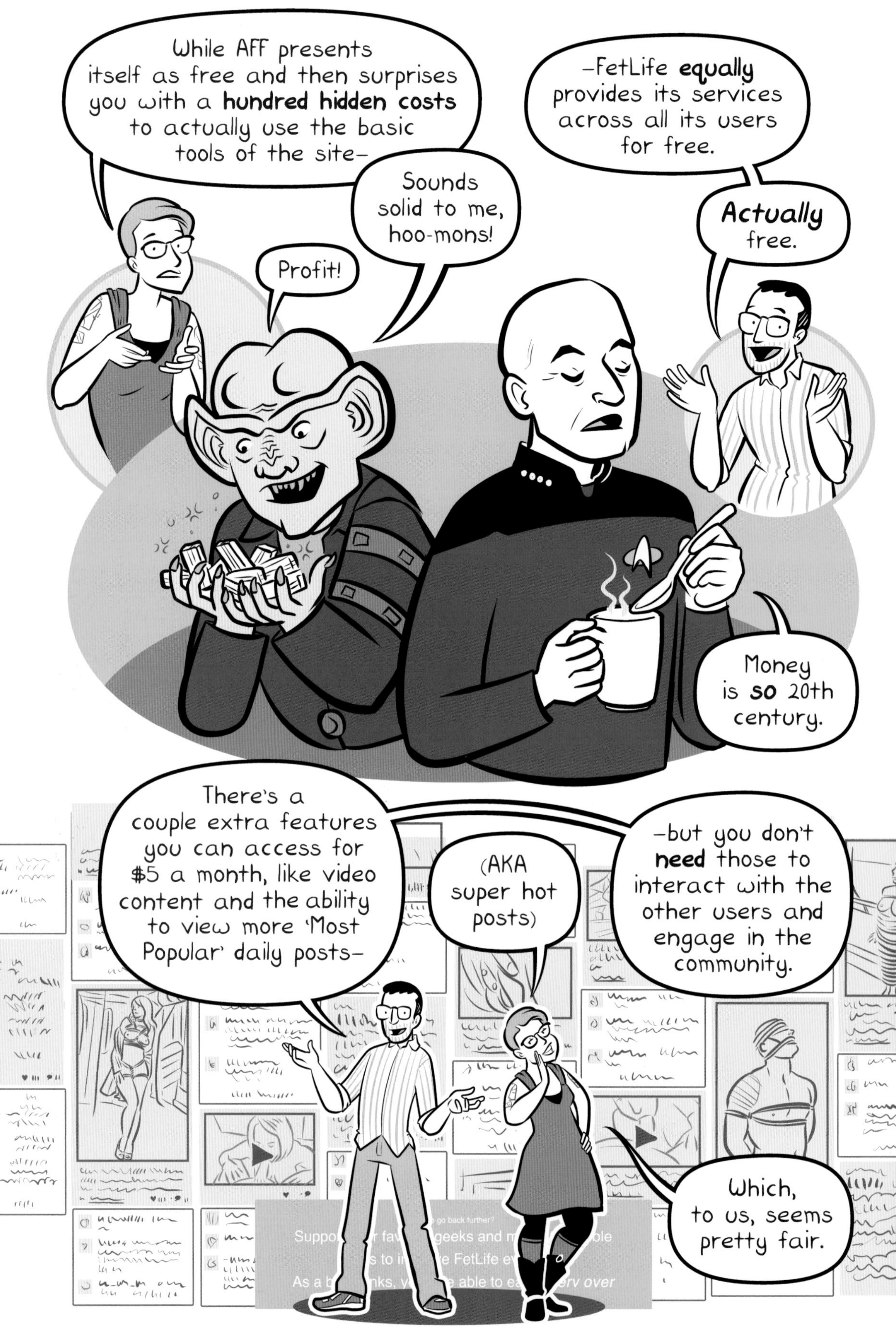
While AFF presents itself as free and then surprises you with a **hundred hidden costs** to actually use the basic tools of the site–
Sounds solid to me, hoo-mons!
Profit!
–FetLife **equally** provides its services across all its users for free.
Actually free.
Money is **so** 20th century.
There's a couple extra features you can access for $5 a month, like video content and the ability to view more 'Most Popular' daily posts–
(AKA super hot posts)
–but you don't **need** those to interact with the other users and engage in the community.
Which, to us, seems pretty fair.

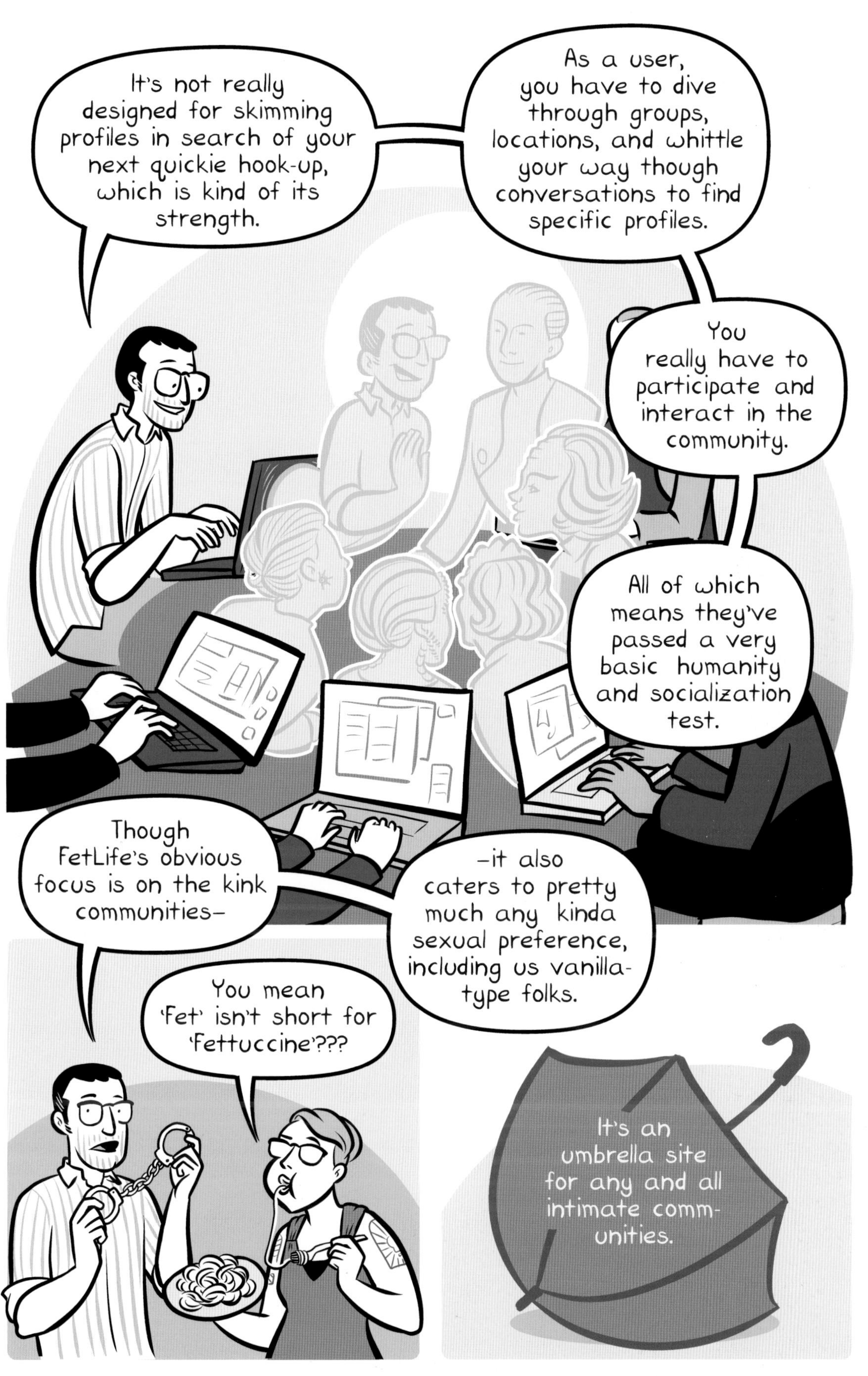
It's not really designed for skimming profiles in search of your next quickie hook-up, which is kind of its strength.
As a user, you have to dive through groups, locations, and whittle your way though conversations to find specific profiles.
You really have to participate and interact in the community.
All of which means they've passed a very basic humanity and socialization test.
Though FetLife's obvious focus is on the kink communities–
–it also caters to pretty much any kinda sexual preference, including us vanilla-type folks.
You mean 'Fet' isn't short for 'Fettuccine'???
It's an umbrella site for any and all intimate comm-unities.

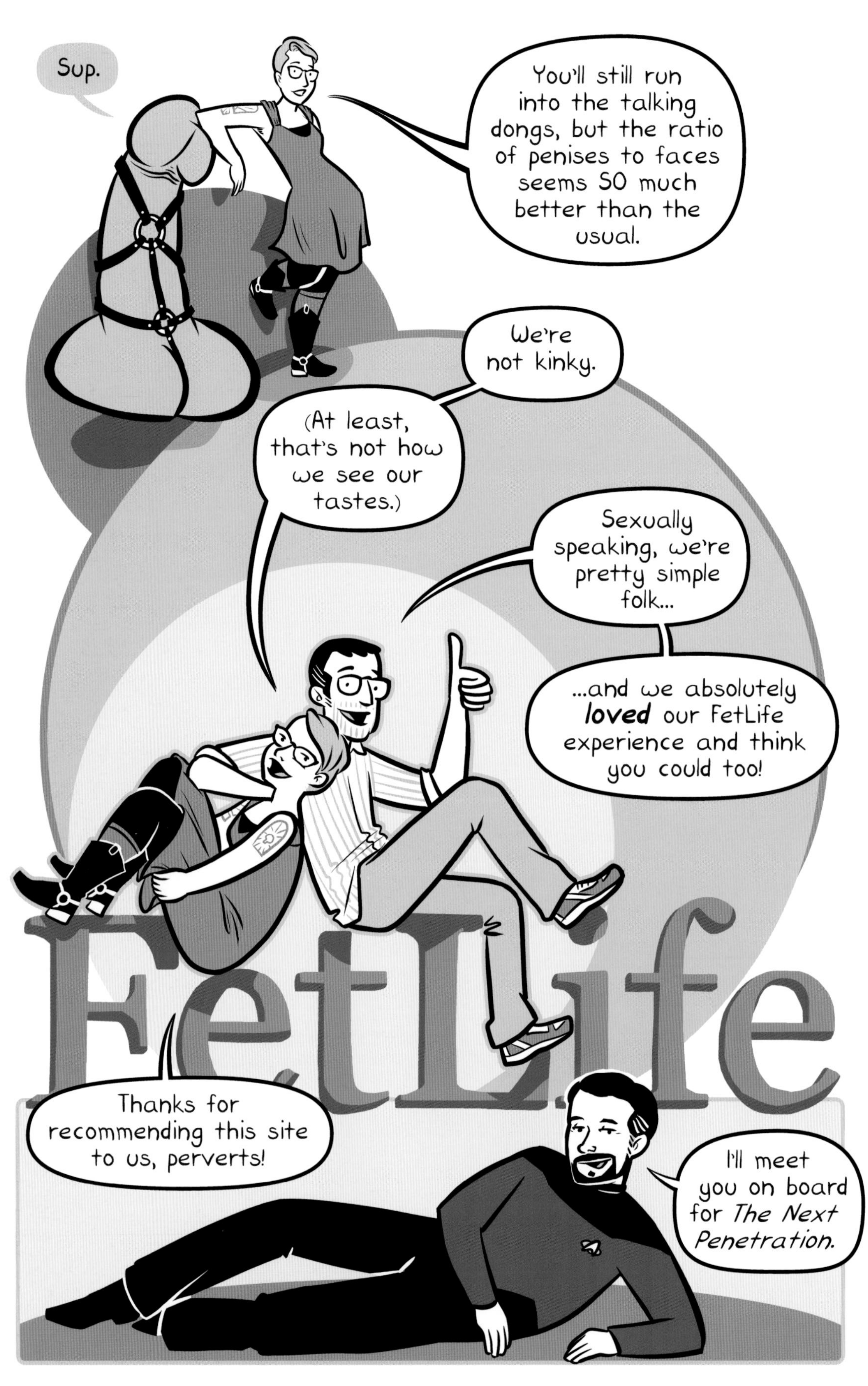
Sup.
You'll still run into the talking dongs, but the ratio of penises to faces seems SO much better than the usual.
We're not kinky.
(At least, that's not how we see our tastes.)
Sexually speaking, we're pretty simple folk...
...and we absolutely **loved** our FetLife experience and think you could too!
FetLife
Thanks for recommending this site to us, perverts!
I'll meet you on board for *The Next Penetration*.

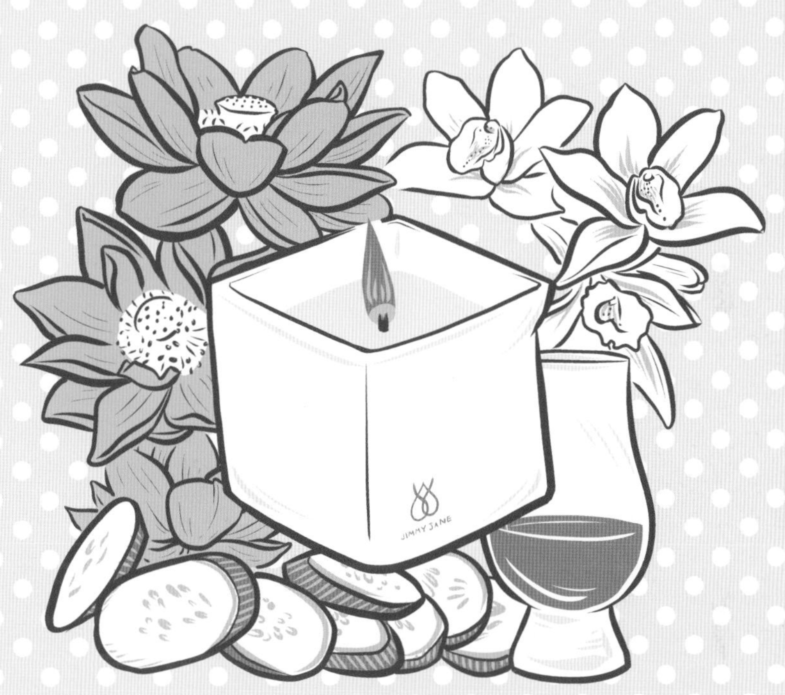
JIMMY JANE

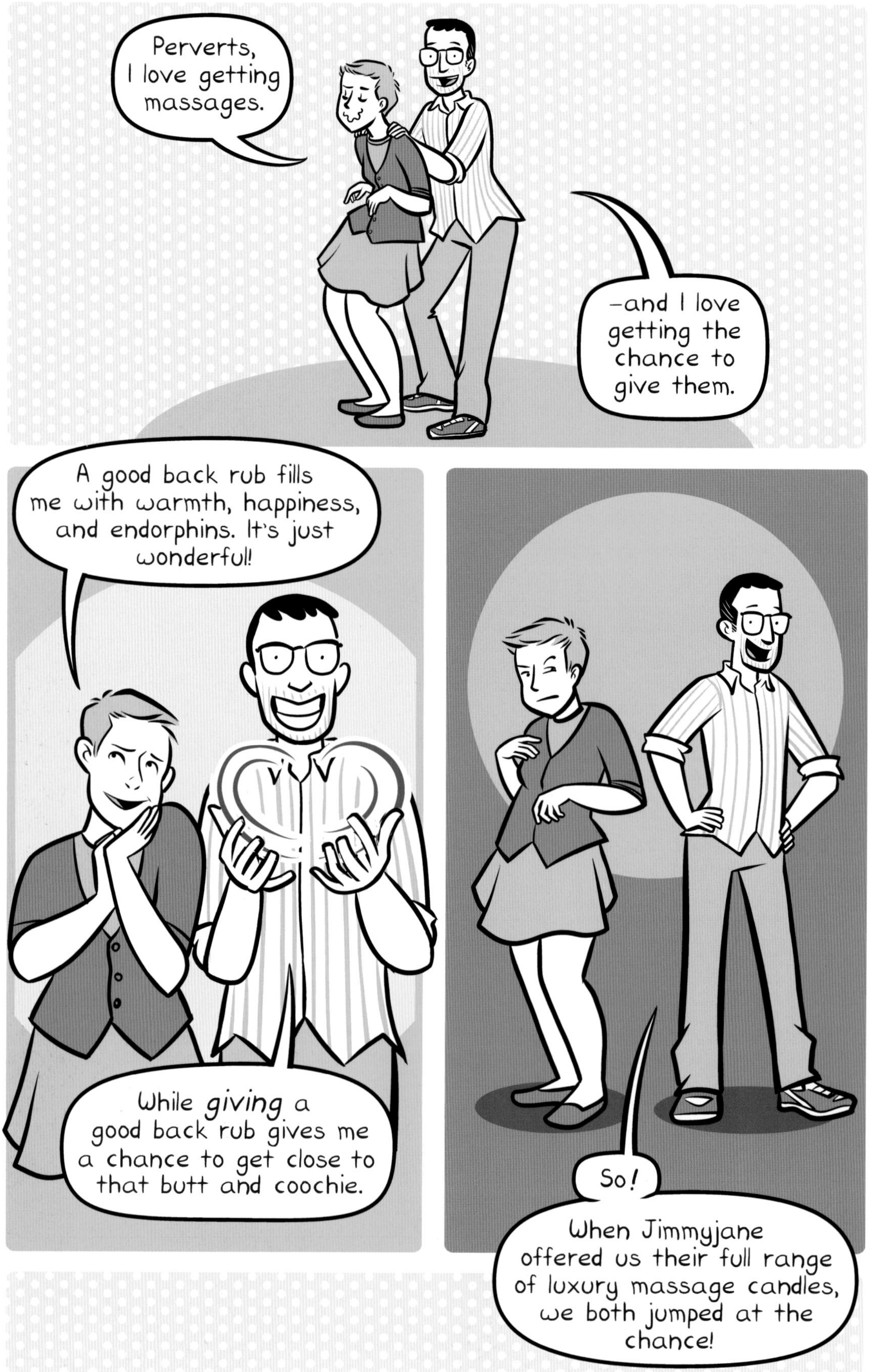

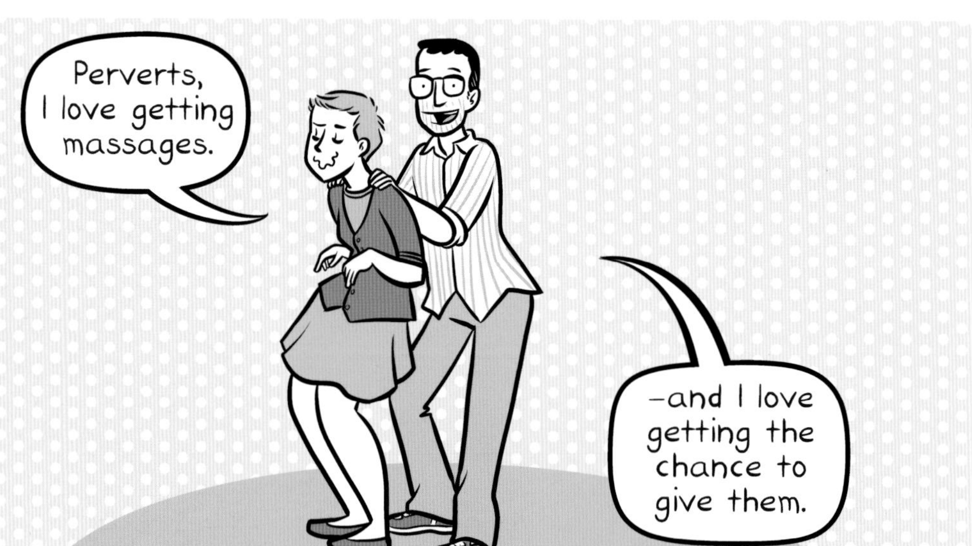
Perverts, I love getting massages.
–and I love getting the chance to give them.

A good back rub fills me with warmth, happiness, and endorphins. It's just wonderful!

While *giving* a good back rub gives me a chance to get close to that butt and coochie.

So!

When Jimmyjane offered us their full range of luxury massage candles, we both jumped at the chance!

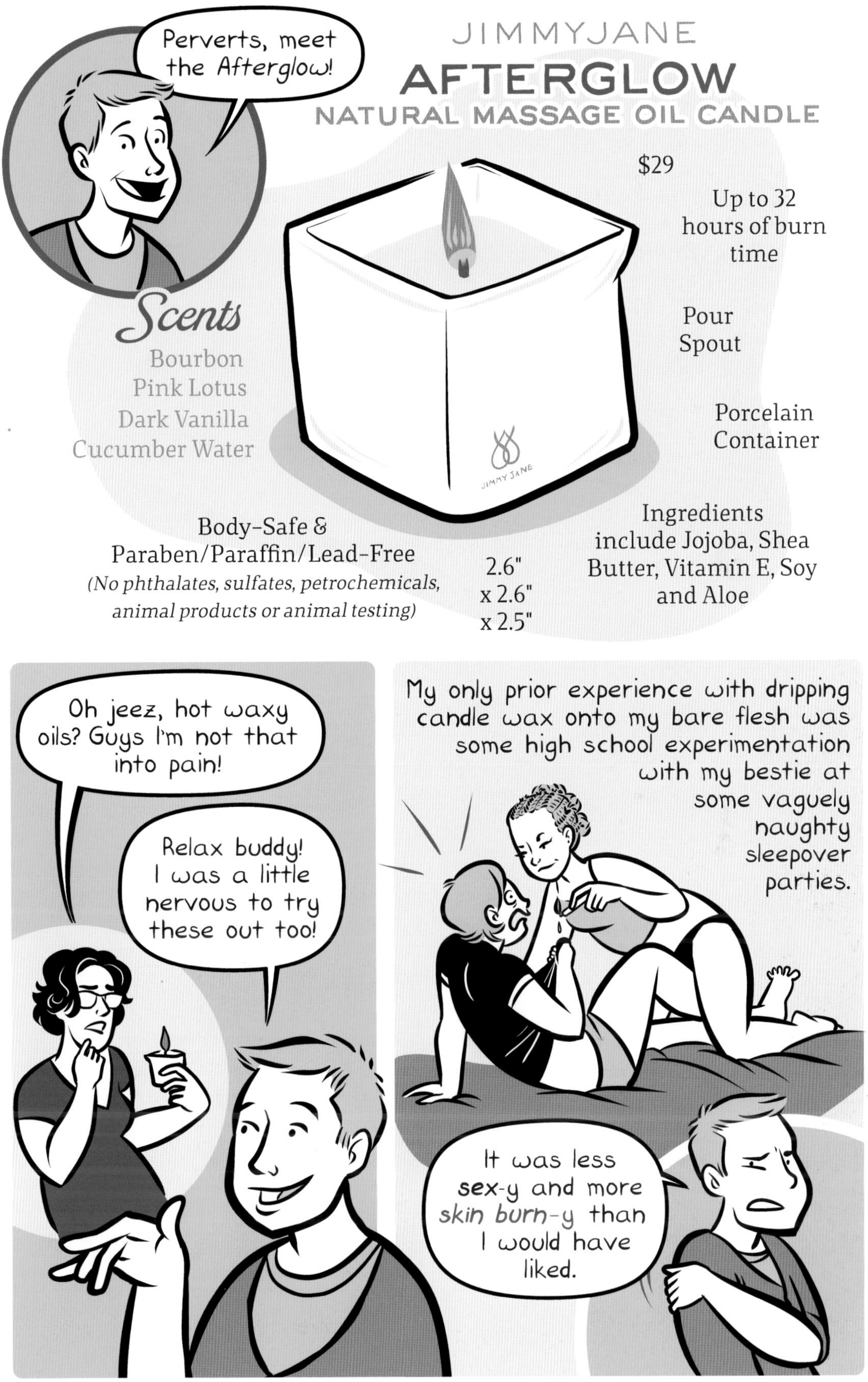

Perverts, meet the Afterglow!

JIMMYJANE AFTERGLOW NATURAL MASSAGE OIL CANDLE

$29

Up to 32 hours of burn time

Pour Spout

Porcelain Container

Ingredients include Jojoba, Shea Butter, Vitamin E, Soy and Aloe

2.6" x 2.6" x 2.5"

Body-Safe & Paraben/Paraffin/Lead-Free
(No phthalates, sulfates, petrochemicals, animal products or animal testing)

Scents

Bourbon
Pink Lotus
Dark Vanilla
Cucumber Water

JIMMY JANE

Oh jeez, hot waxy oils? Guys I'm not that into pain!

Relax buddy! I was a little nervous to try these out too!

My only prior experience with dripping candle wax onto my bare flesh was some high school experimentation with my bestie at some vaguely naughty sleepover parties.

It was less **sex**-y and more *skin burn*-y than I would have liked.

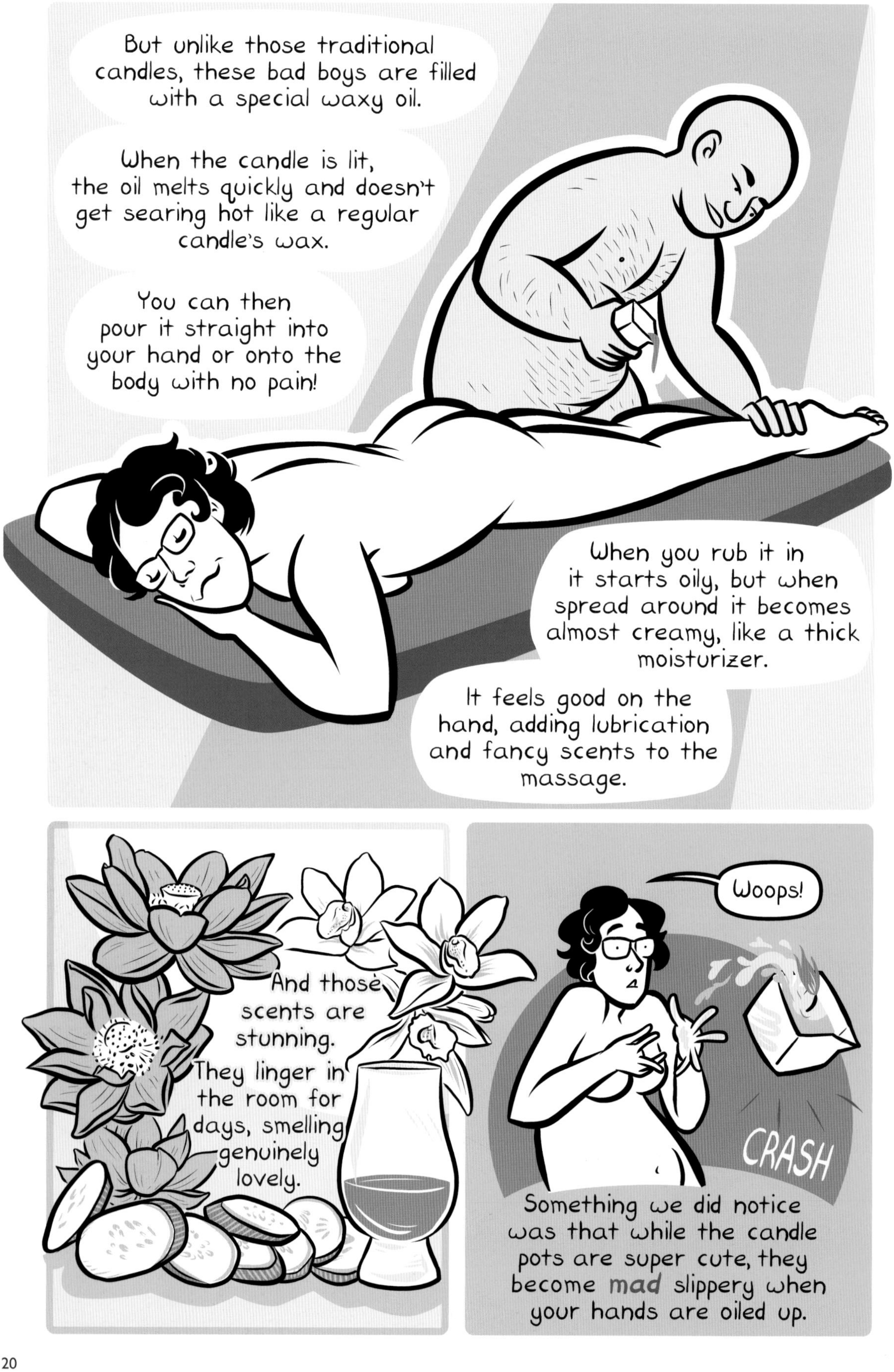

But unlike those traditional candles, these bad boys are filled with a special waxy oil.

When the candle is lit, the oil melts quickly and doesn't get searing hot like a regular candle's wax.

You can then pour it straight into your hand or onto the body with no pain!

When you rub it in it starts oily, but when spread around it becomes almost creamy, like a thick moisturizer.

It feels good on the hand, adding lubrication and fancy scents to the massage.

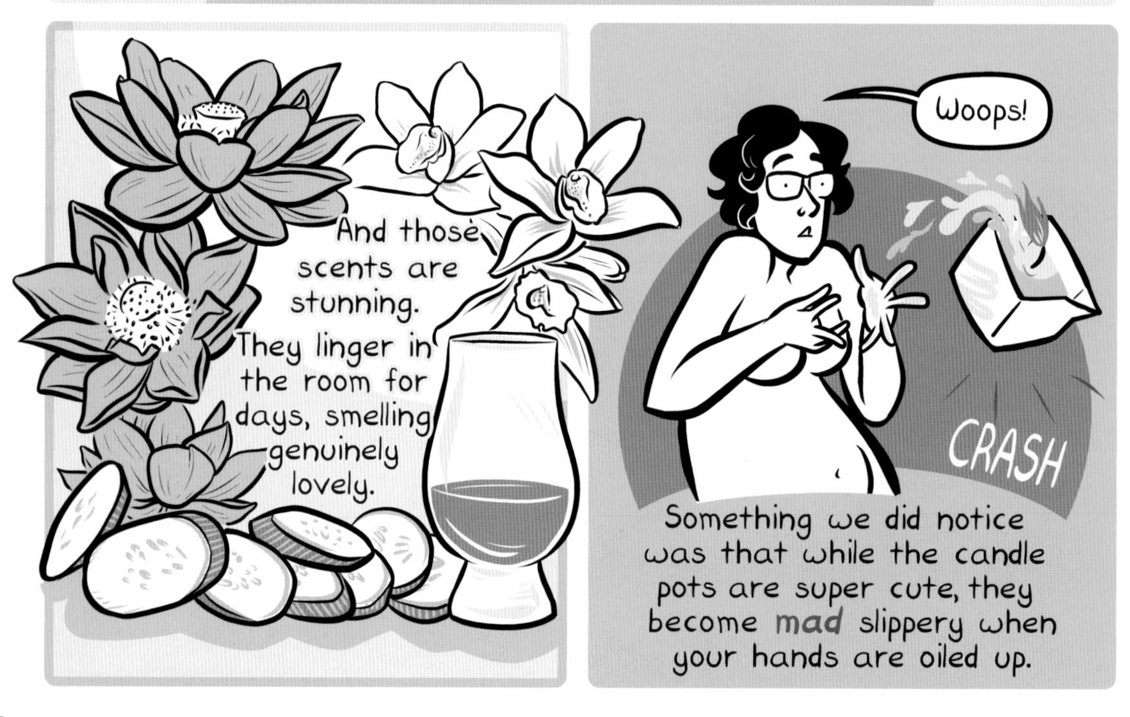

And those scents are stunning. They linger in the room for days, smelling genuinely lovely.
Woops!
CRASH
Something we did notice was that while the candle pots are super cute, they become mad slippery when your hands are oiled up.

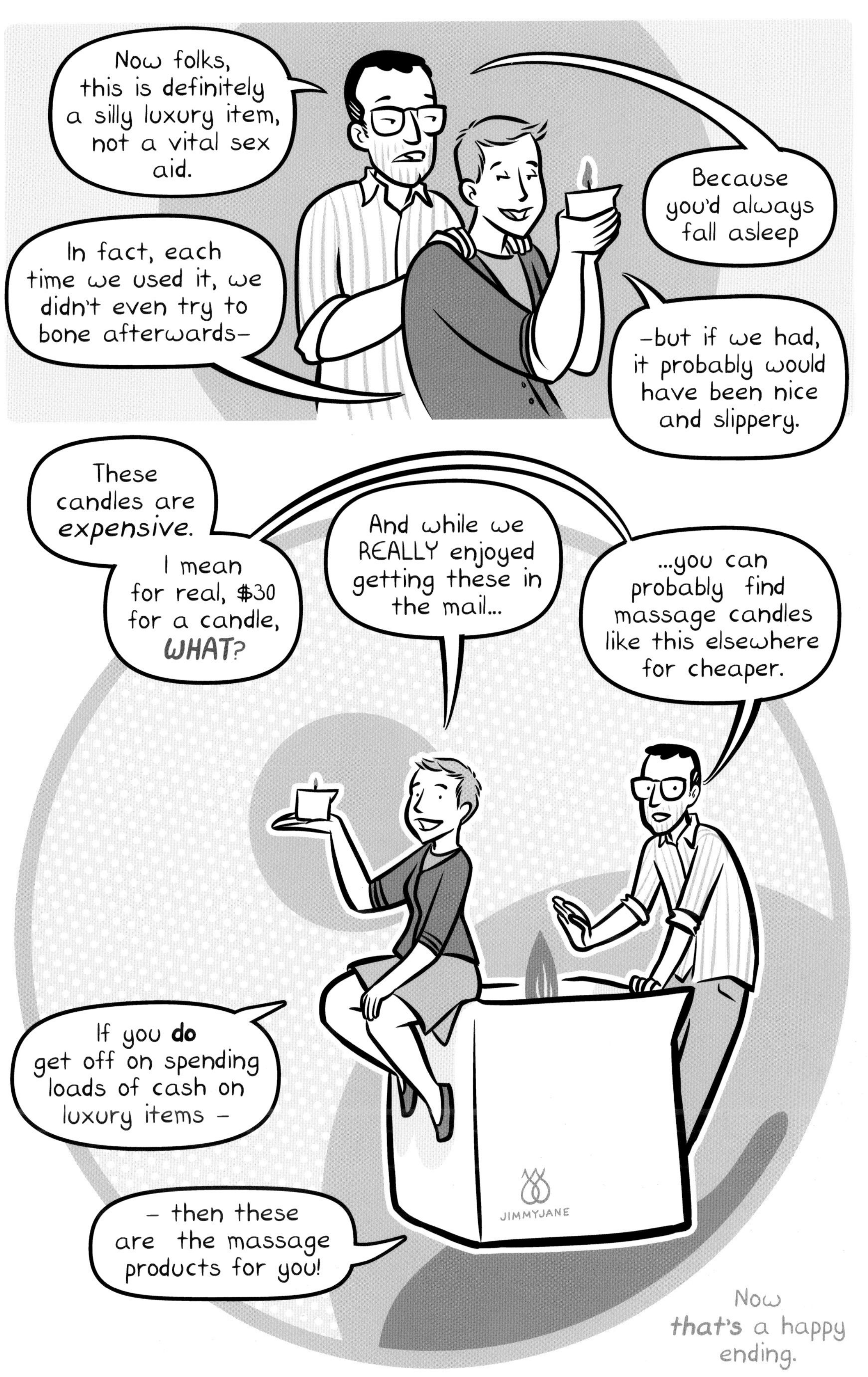
Now folks, this is definitely a silly luxury item, not a vital sex aid.
Because you'd always fall asleep
In fact, each time we used it, we didn't even try to bone afterwards–
–but if we had, it probably would have been nice and slippery.
These candles are *expensive*.
I mean for real, $30 for a candle, **WHAT**?
And while we REALLY enjoyed getting these in the mail...
...you can probably find massage candles like this elsewhere for cheaper.
If you **do** get off on spending loads of cash on luxury items –
– then these are the massage products for you!
JIMMYJANE
Now *that's* a happy ending.

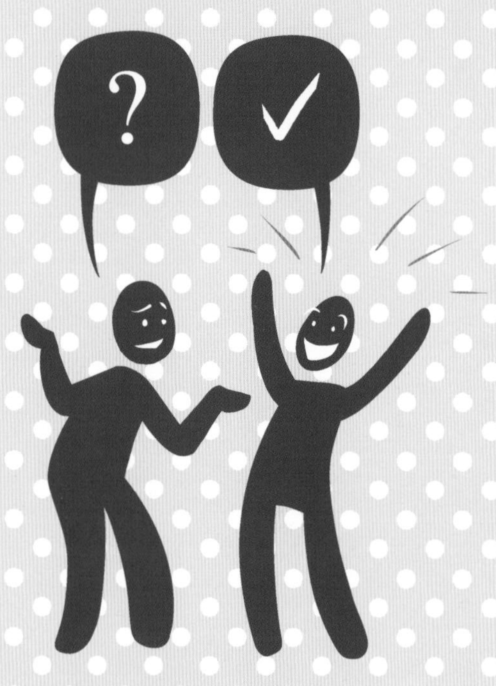

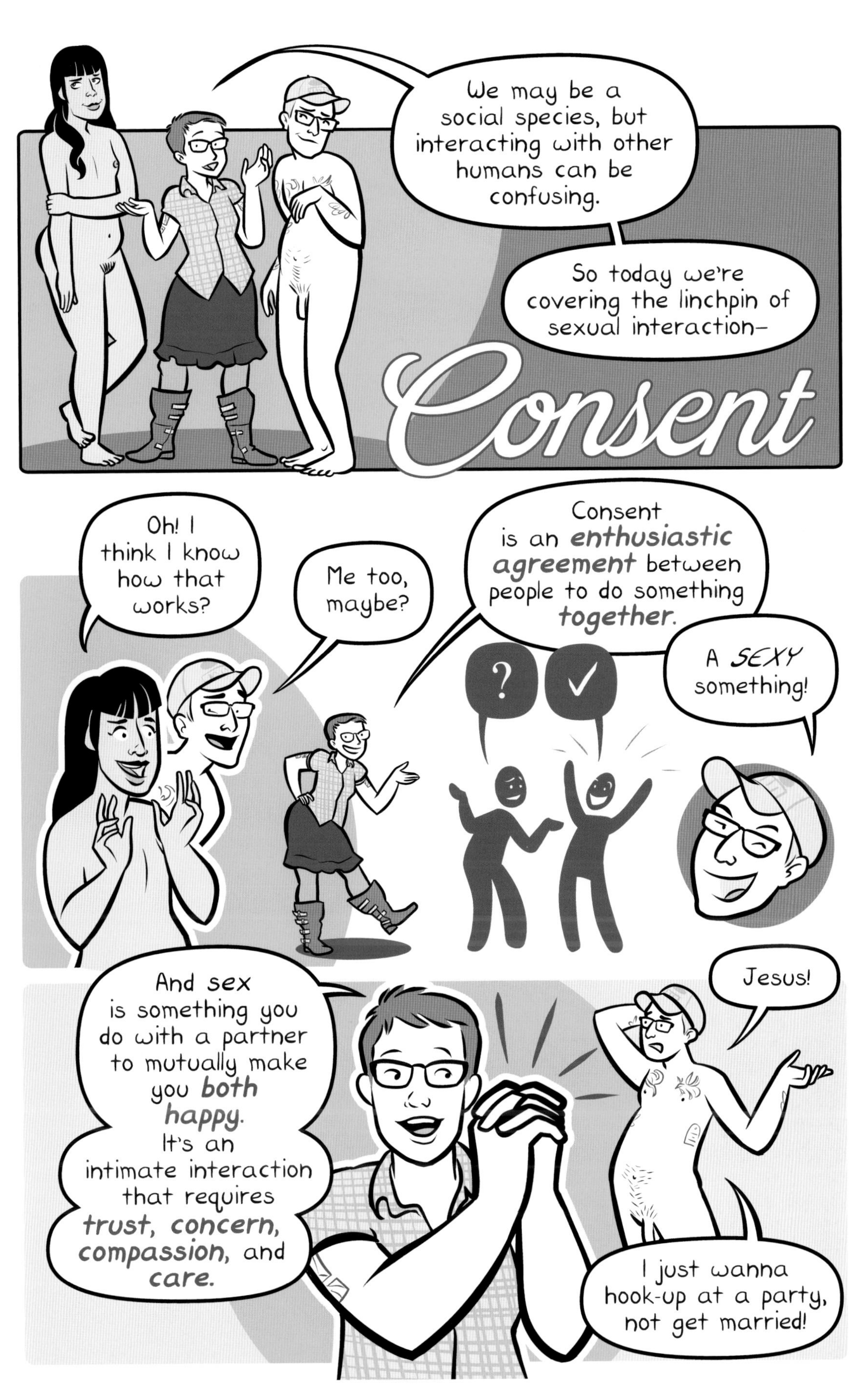
We may be a social species, but interacting with other humans can be confusing.
So today we're covering the linchpin of sexual interaction–
Consent
Oh! I think I know how that works?
Me too, maybe?
Consent is an **enthusiastic agreement** between people to do something **together**.
?
✓
A *SEXY* something!
And sex is something you do with a partner to mutually make you **both happy**. It's an intimate interaction that requires **trust, concern, compassion**, and **care**.
Jesus!
I just wanna hook-up at a party, not get married!

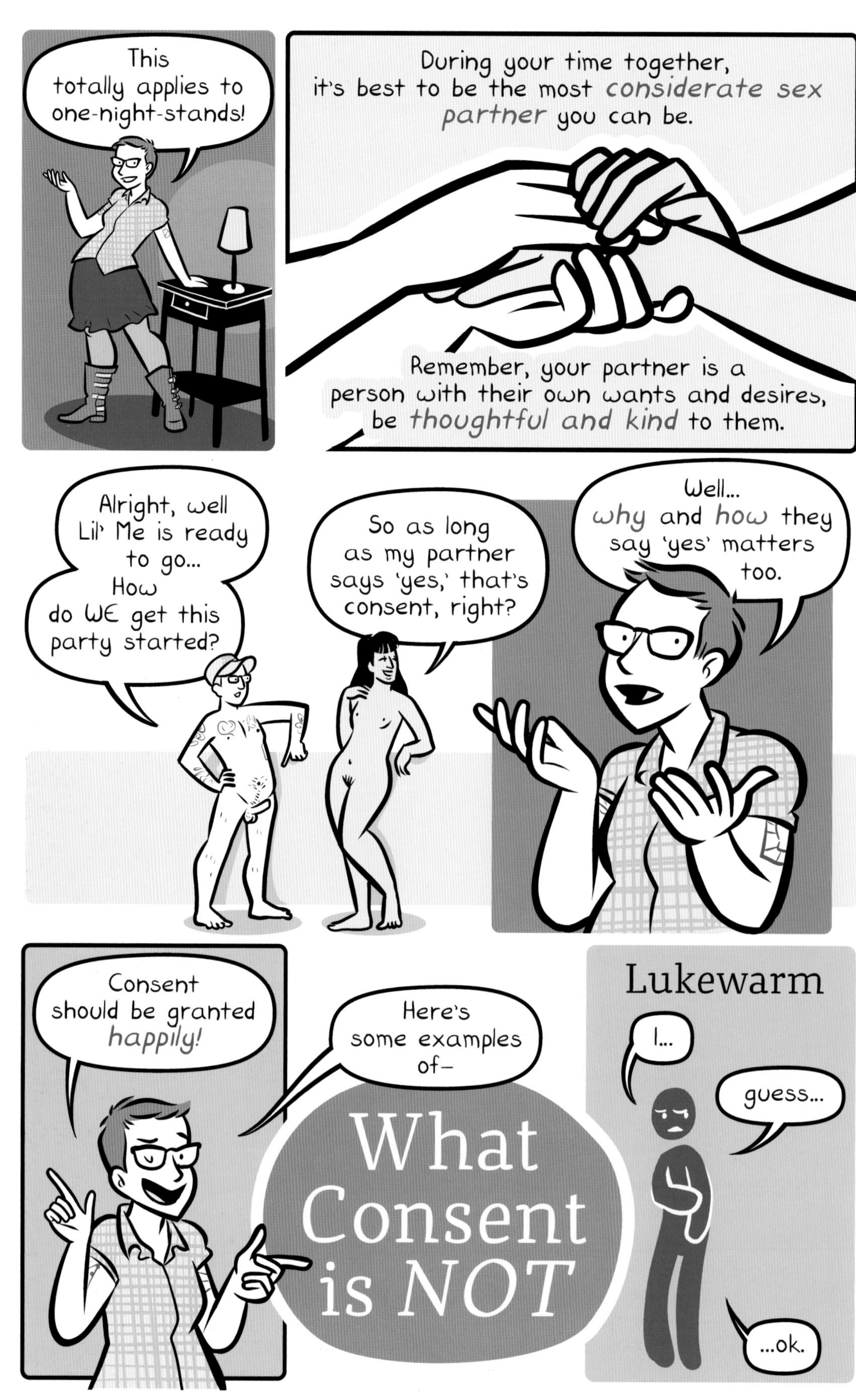
This totally applies to one-night-stands!
During your time together, it's best to be the most considerate sex partner you can be.
Remember, your partner is a person with their own wants and desires, be thoughtful and kind to them.
Alright, well Lil' Me is ready to go... How do WE get this party started?
So as long as my partner says 'yes,' that's consent, right?
Well... why and how they say 'yes' matters too.
Consent should be granted happily!
Here's some examples of–
What Consent is NOT
Lukewarm
I...
guess...
...ok.

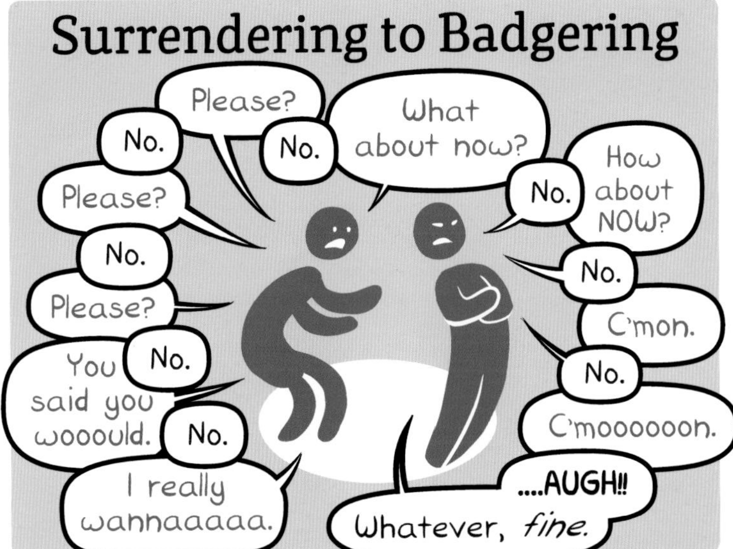

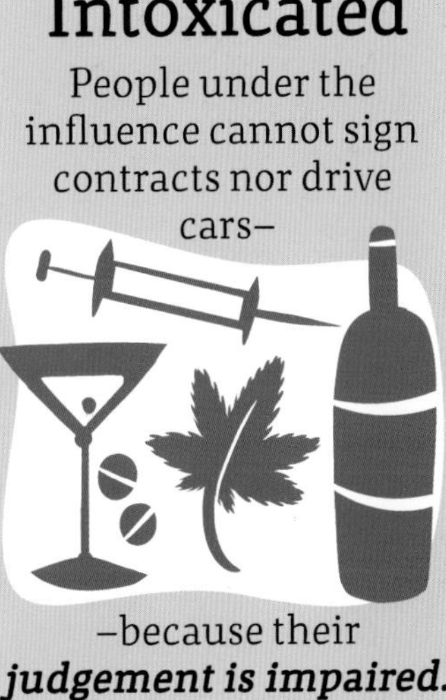
Intoxicated
People under the influence cannot sign contracts nor drive cars–
–because their ***judgement is impaired.***

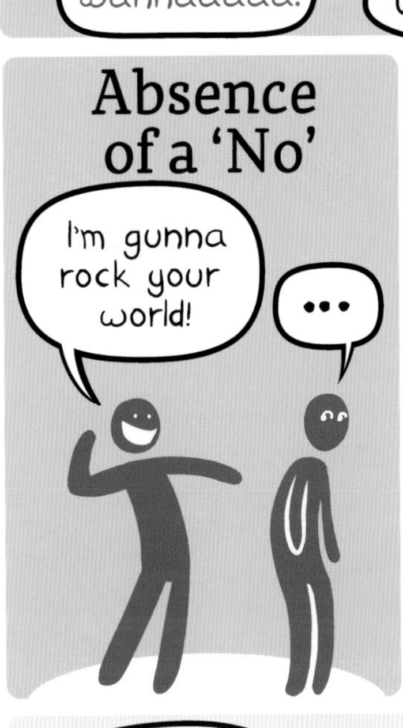
Absence of a 'No'
I'm gunna rock your world!
...

Unconscious

If someone's unconscious, consent is ***IMPOSSIBLE.***

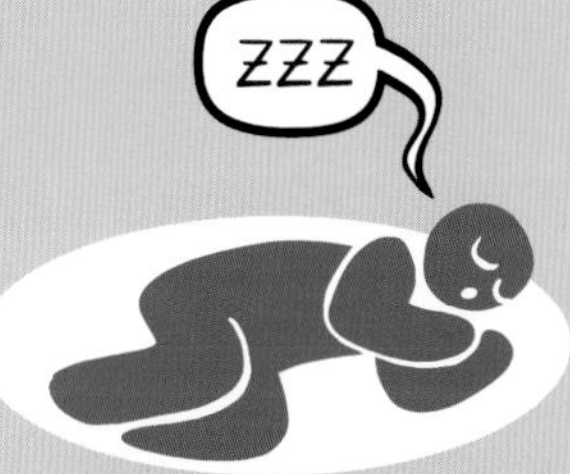
ZZZ

Prior consent does not apply once they're no longer awake.

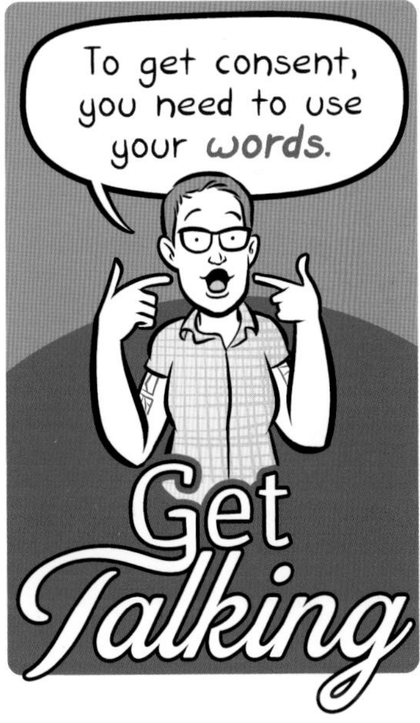
To get consent, you need to use your **words**.
Get Talking

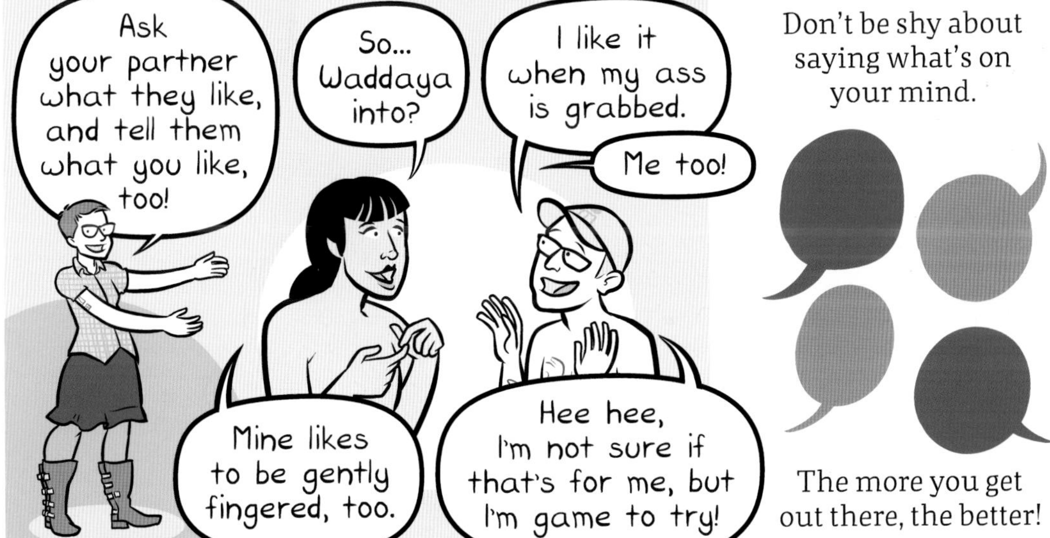
Ask your partner what they like, and tell them what you like, too!
So... Waddaya into?
I like it when my ass is grabbed.
Me too!
Mine likes to be gently fingered, too.
Hee hee, I'm not sure if that's for me, but I'm game to try!
Don't be shy about saying what's on your mind.
The more you get out there, the better!

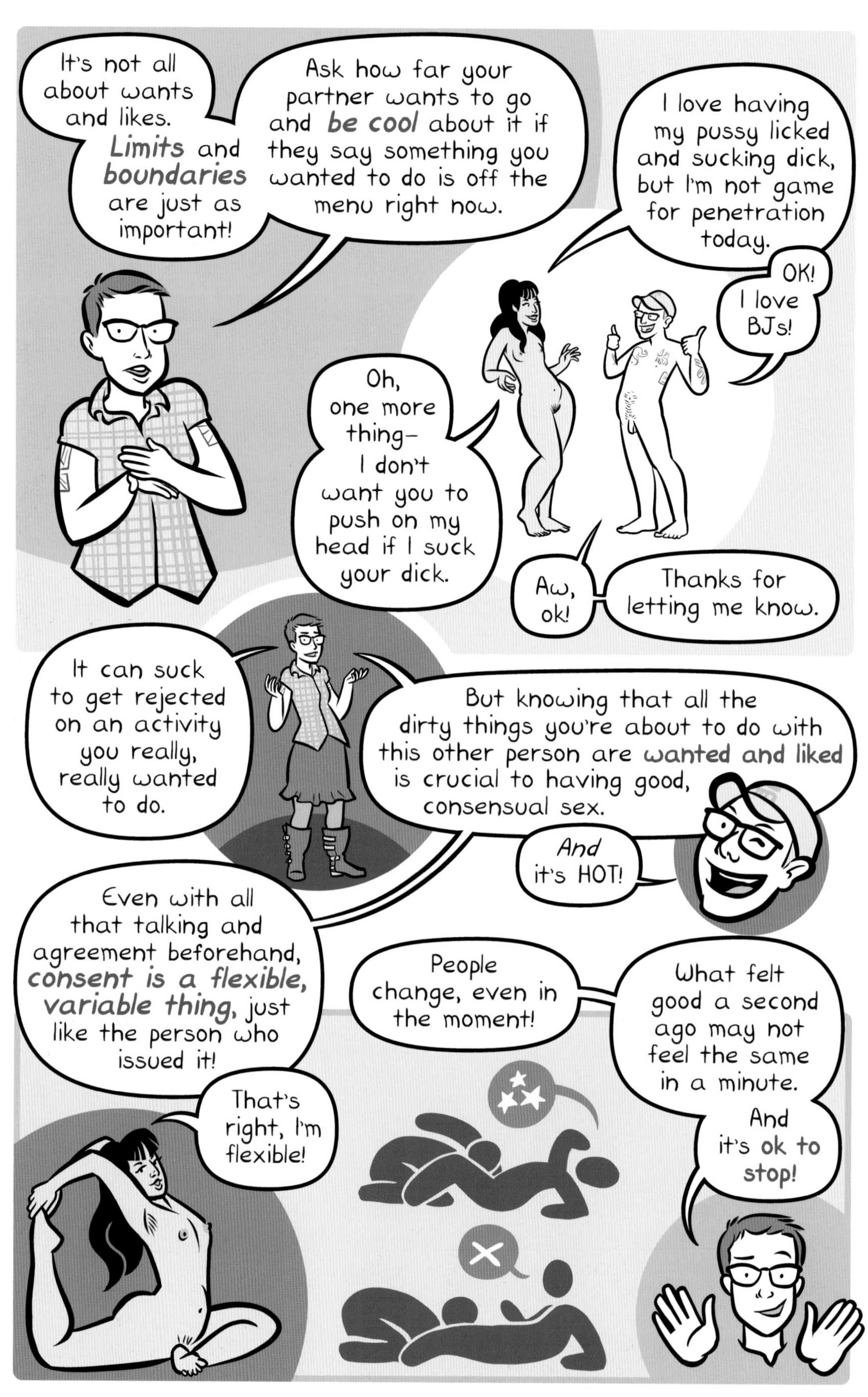
It's not all about wants and likes. Limits and boundaries are just as important!
Ask how far your partner wants to go and be cool about it if they say something you wanted to do is off the menu right now.
I love having my pussy licked and sucking dick, but I'm not game for penetration today.
OK! I love BJs!
Oh, one more thing— I don't want you to push on my head if I suck your dick.
Aw, ok!
Thanks for letting me know.
It can suck to get rejected on an activity you really, really wanted to do.
But knowing that all the dirty things you're about to do with this other person are wanted and liked is crucial to having good, consensual sex.
And it's HOT!
Even with all that talking and agreement beforehand, consent is a flexible, variable thing, just like the person who issued it!
That's right, I'm flexible!
People change, even in the moment!
What felt good a second ago may not feel the same in a minute.
And it's ok to stop!

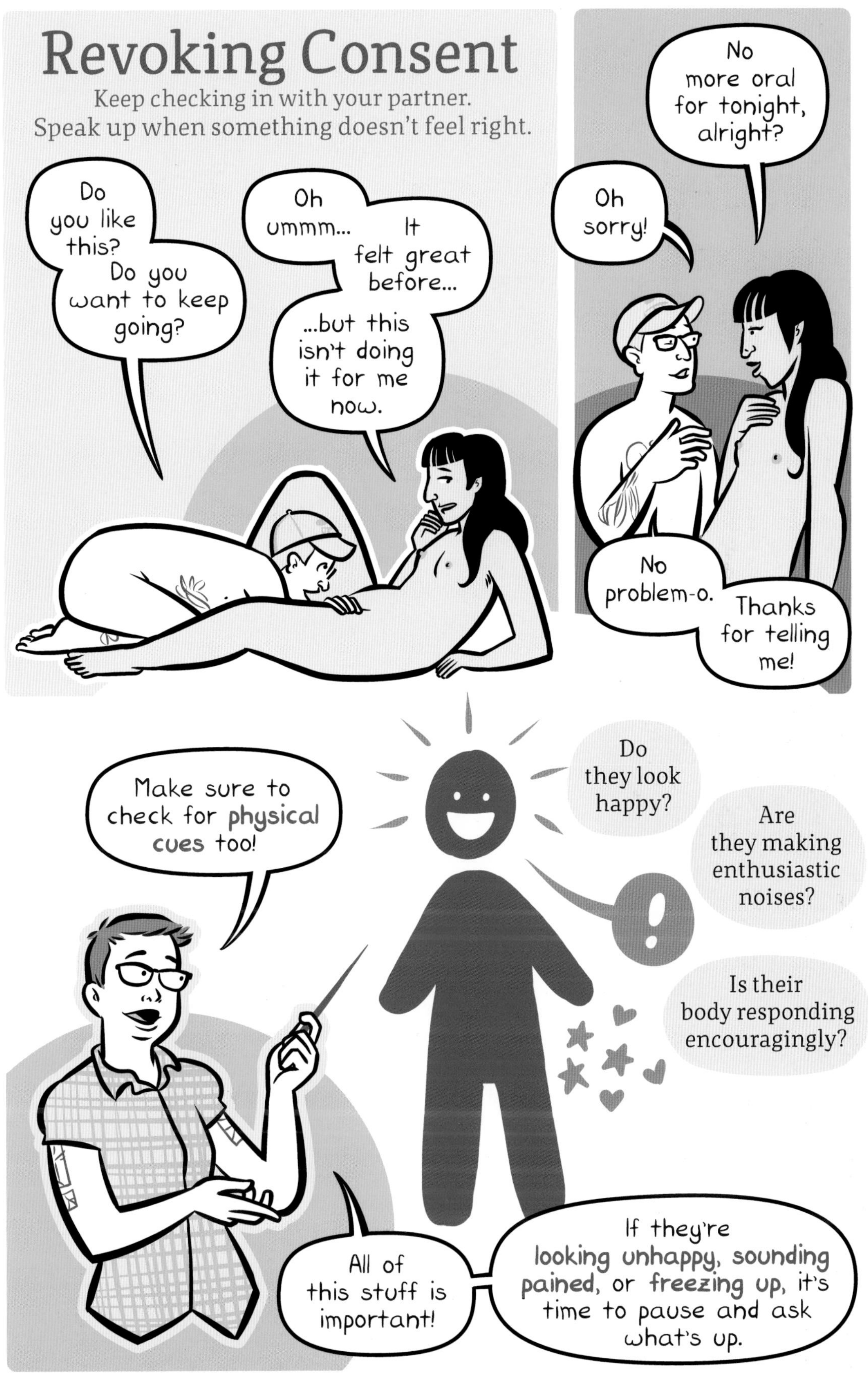

Revoking Consent
Keep checking in with your partner.
Speak up when something doesn't feel right.
Do you like this? Do you want to keep going?
Oh ummm... It felt great before...
...but this isn't doing it for me now.
No more oral for tonight, alright?
Oh sorry!
No problem-o.
Thanks for telling me!
Make sure to check for physical cues too!
Do they look happy?
Are they making enthusiastic noises?
Is their body responding encouragingly?
All of this stuff is important!
If they're looking unhappy, sounding pained, or freezing up, it's time to pause and ask what's up.

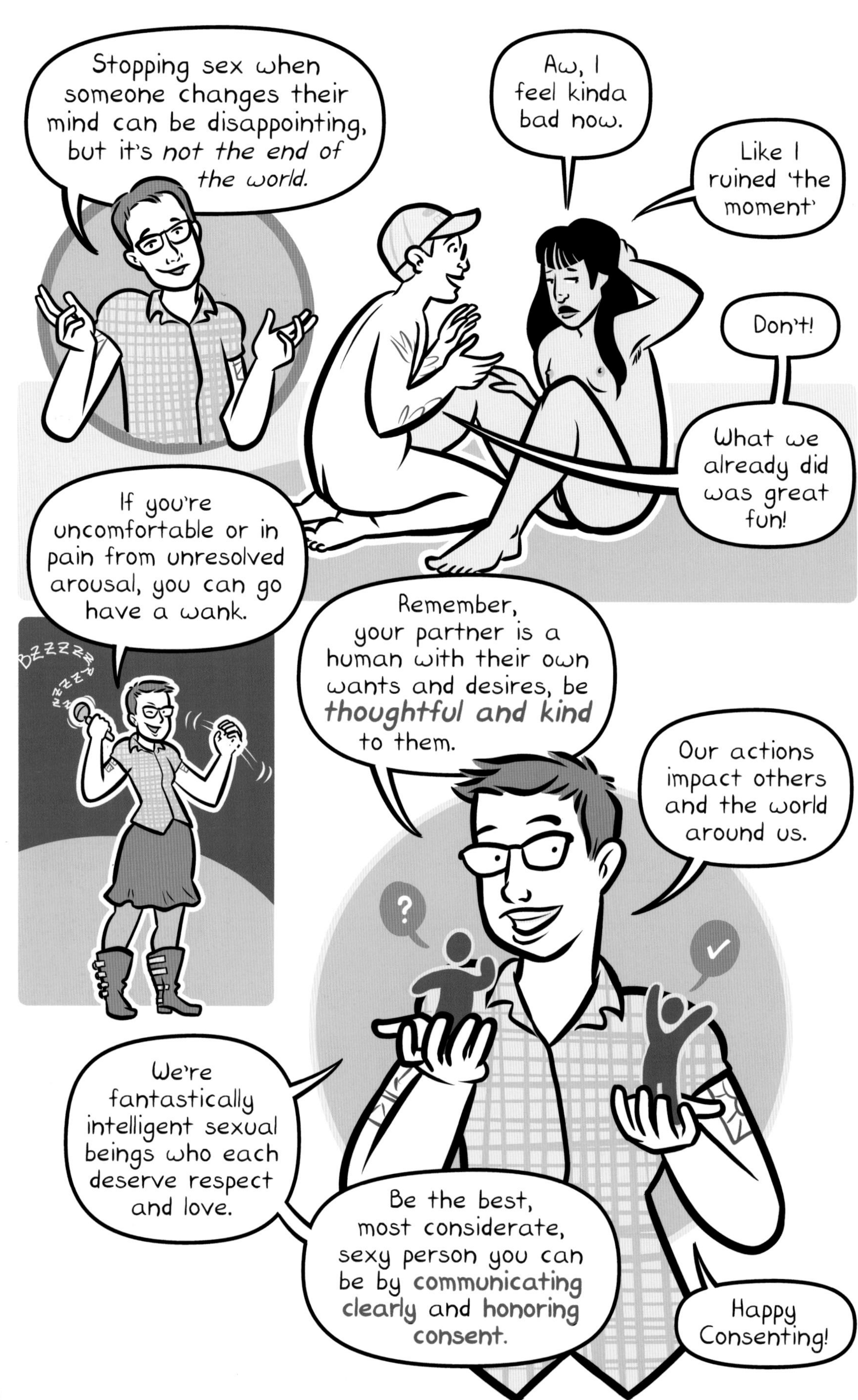
Stopping sex when someone changes their mind can be disappointing, but it's *not the end of the world.*
Aw, I feel kinda bad now.
Like I ruined 'the moment'
Don't!
What we already did was great fun!
If you're uncomfortable or in pain from unresolved arousal, you can go have a wank.
BZZZZZZ
ZZZZZZ
Remember, your partner is a human with their own wants and desires, be **thoughtful and kind** to them.
Our actions impact others and the world around us.
?
We're fantastically intelligent sexual beings who each deserve respect and love.
Be the best, most considerate, sexy person you can be by **communicating clearly** and **honoring consent**.
Happy Consenting!

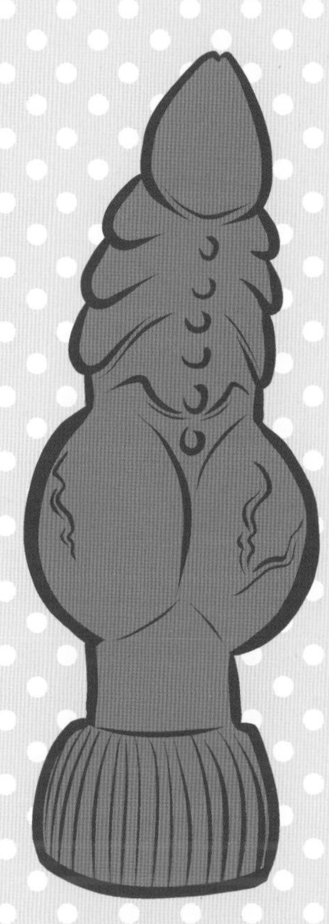

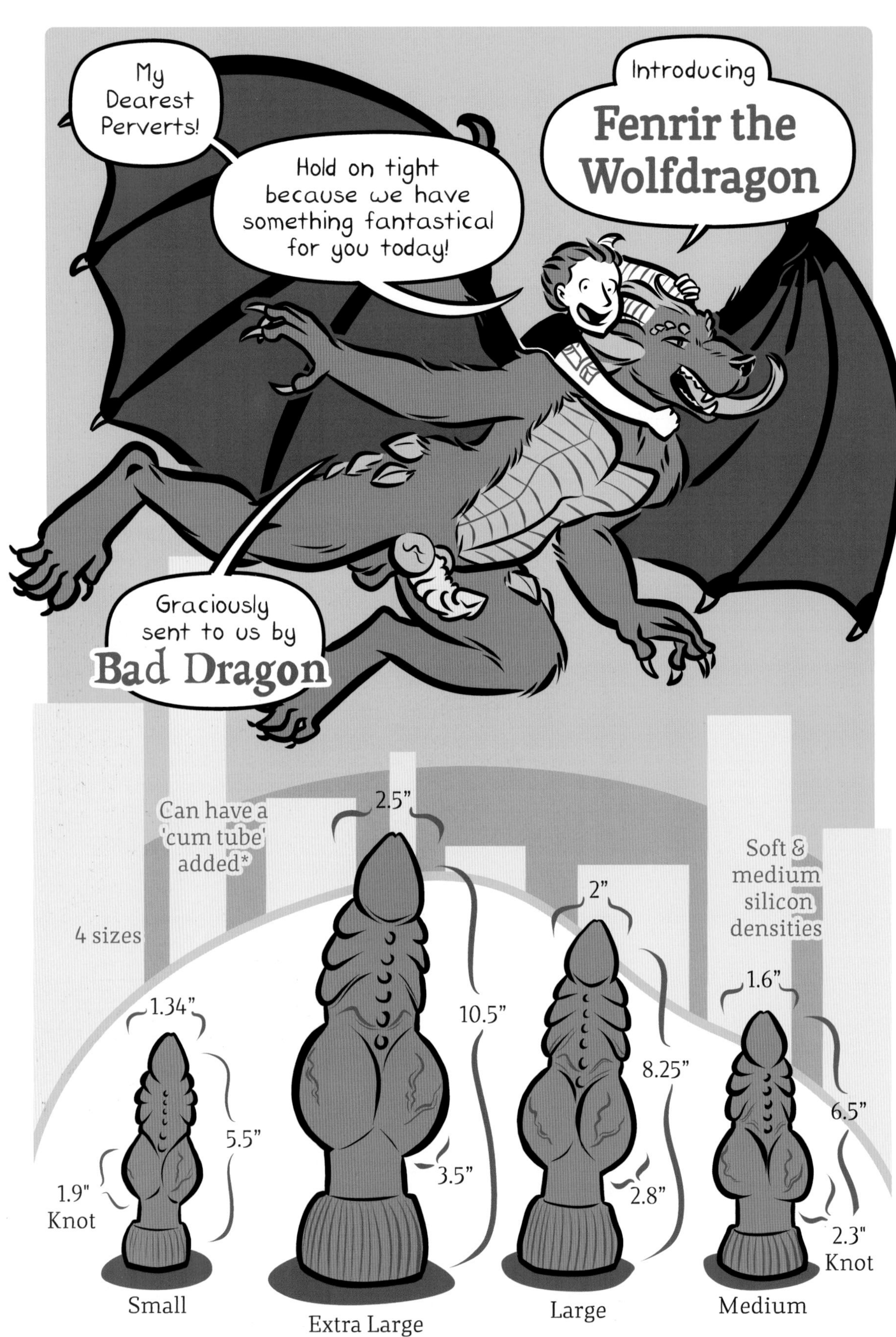

My Dearest Perverts!
Hold on tight because we have something fantastical for you today!
Introducing
Fenrir the Wolfdragon
Graciously sent to us by
Bad Dragon
Can have a 'cum tube' added*
4 sizes
Soft & medium silicon densities
2.5"
10.5"
3.5"
2"
8.25"
2.8"
1.6"
6.5"
2.3" Knot
1.34"
5.5"
1.9" Knot
Small
Extra Large
Large
Medium

*(A tube that shoots lube out of the shaft)

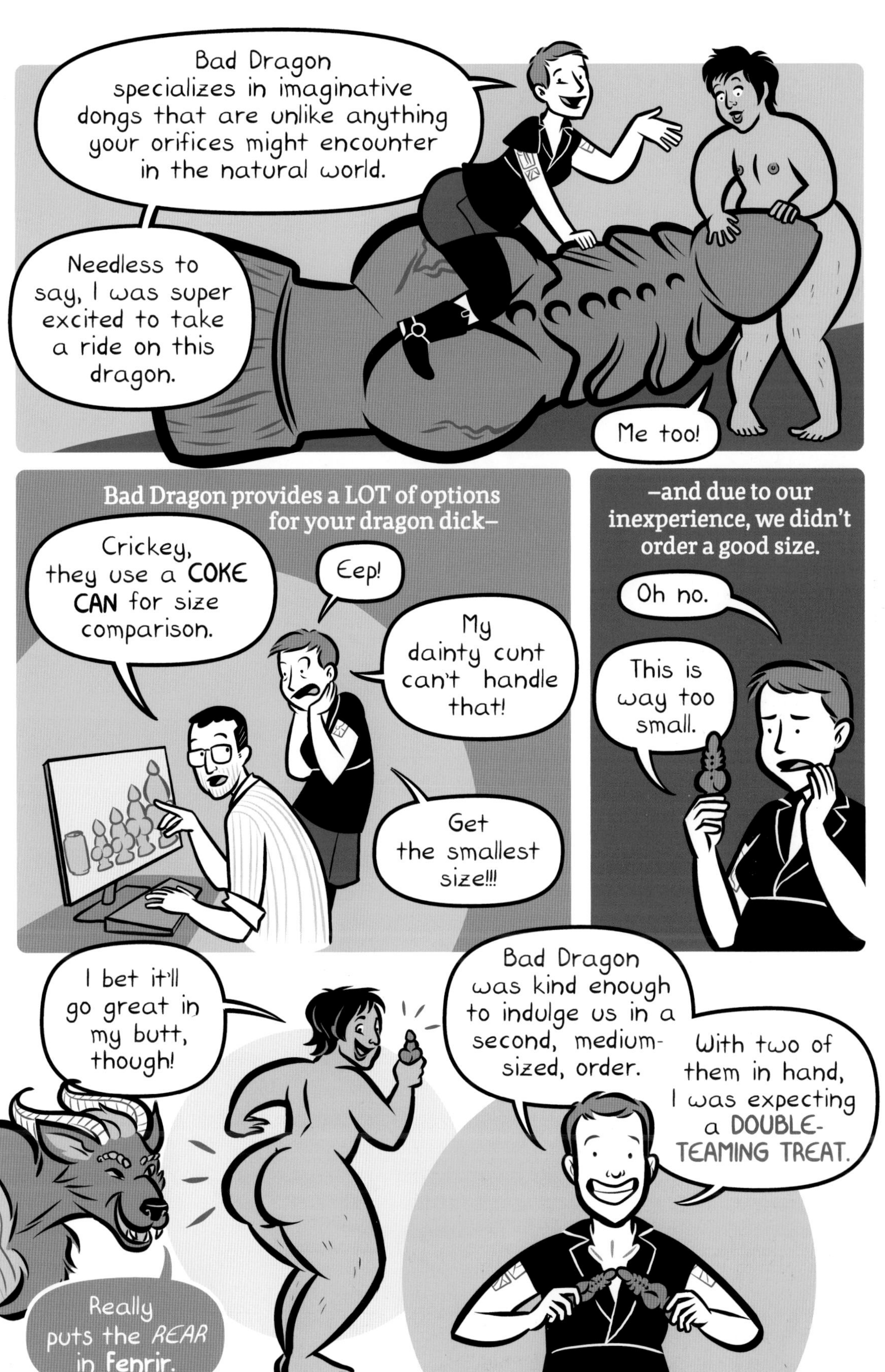
Bad Dragon specializes in imaginative dongs that are unlike anything your orifices might encounter in the natural world.
Needless to say, I was super excited to take a ride on this dragon.
Me too!
Bad Dragon provides a LOT of options for your dragon dick–
Crickey, they use a **COKE CAN** for size comparison.
Eep!
My dainty cunt can't handle that!
Get the smallest size!!!
–and due to our inexperience, we didn't order a good size.
Oh no.
This is way too small.
I bet it'll go great in my butt, though!
Really puts the *REAR* in **Fenrir**.
Bad Dragon was kind enough to indulge us in a second, medium-sized, order.
With two of them in hand, I was expecting a **DOUBLE-TEAMING TREAT.**

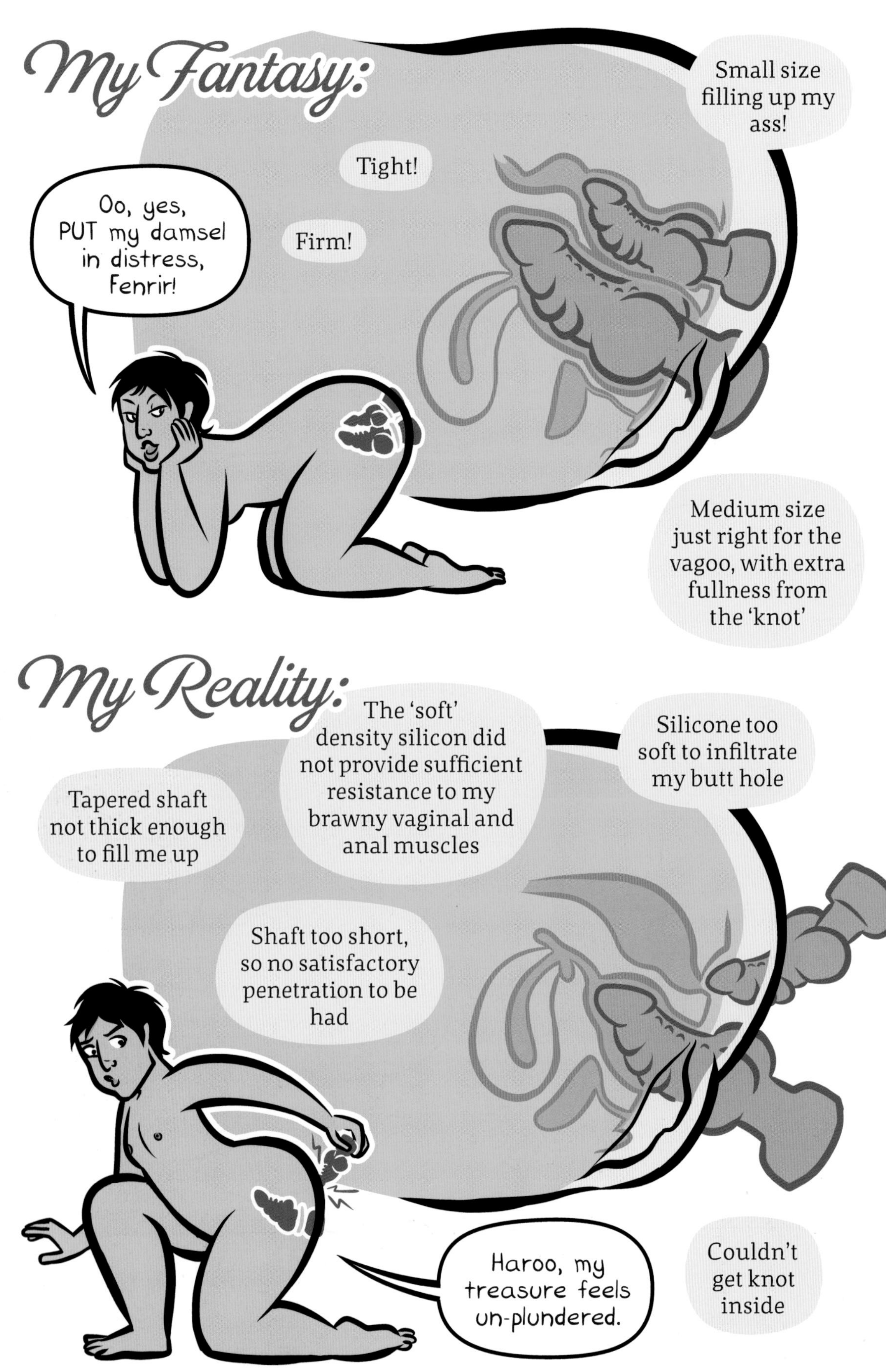
My Fantasy:
Oo, yes, PUT my damsel in distress, Fenrir!
Tight!
Firm!
Small size filling up my ass!
Medium size just right for the vagoo, with extra fullness from the 'knot'
My Reality:
Tapered shaft not thick enough to fill me up
The 'soft' density silicon did not provide sufficient resistance to my brawny vaginal and anal muscles
Silicone too soft to infiltrate my butt hole
Shaft too short, so no satisfactory penetration to be had
Haroo, my treasure feels un-plundered.
Couldn't get knot inside

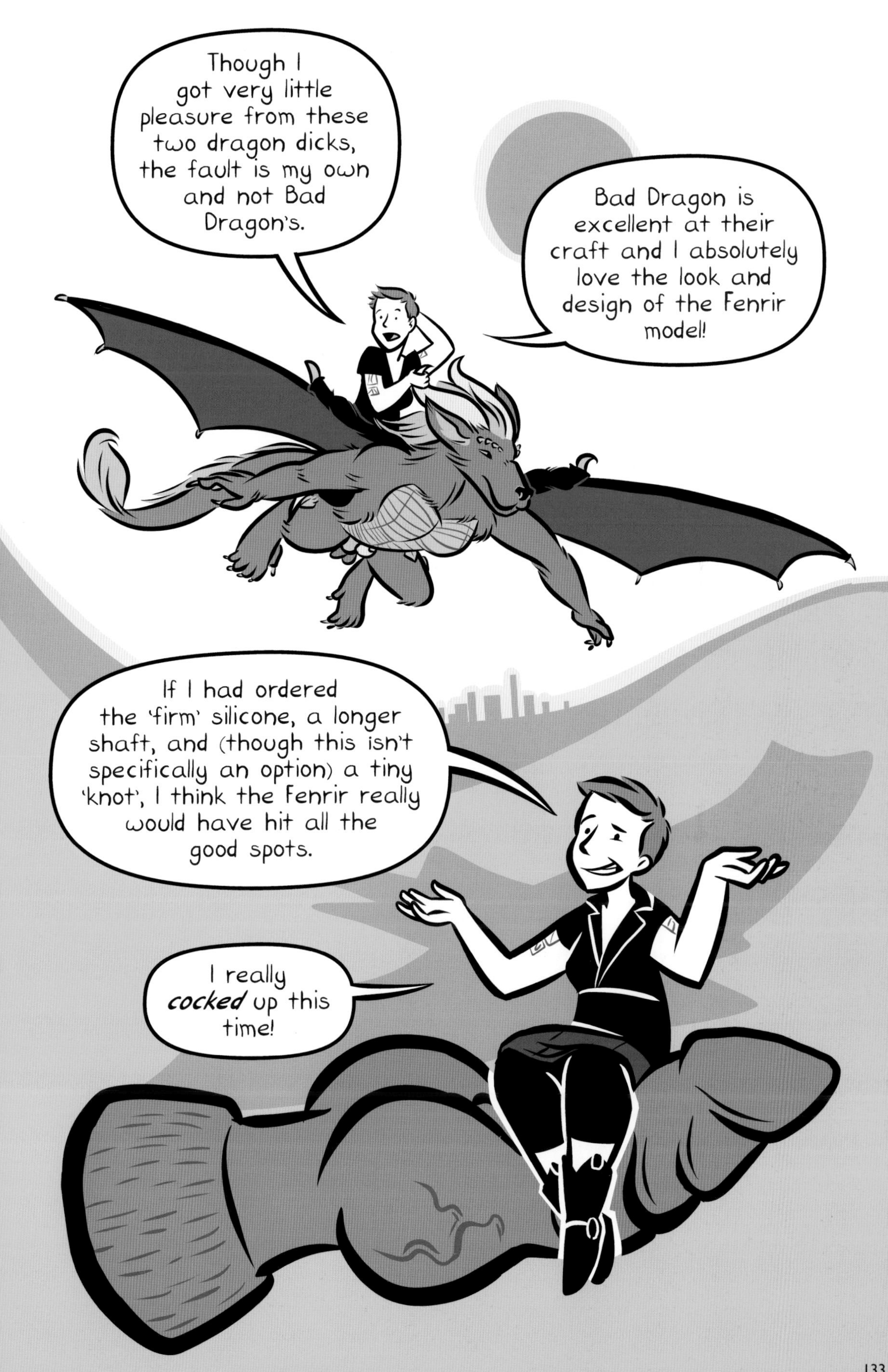
Though I got very little pleasure from these two dragon dicks, the fault is my own and not Bad Dragon's.
Bad Dragon is excellent at their craft and I absolutely love the look and design of the Fenrir model!
If I had ordered the 'firm' silicone, a longer shaft, and (though this isn't specifically an option) a tiny 'knot', I think the Fenrir really would have hit all the good spots.
I really ***cocked*** up this time!

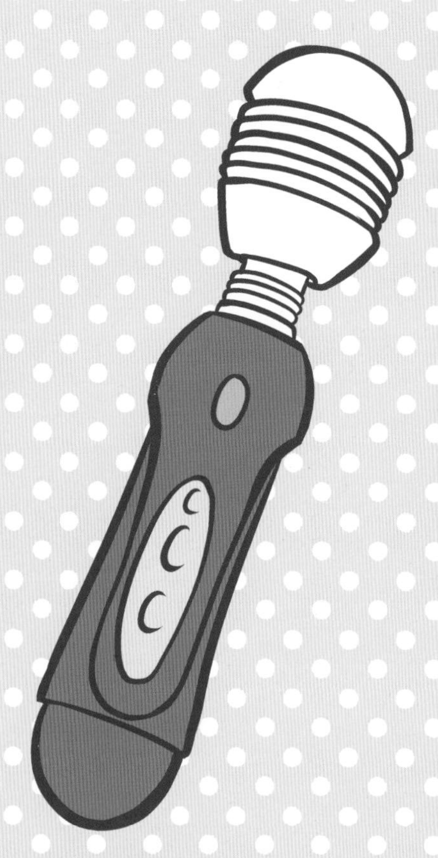

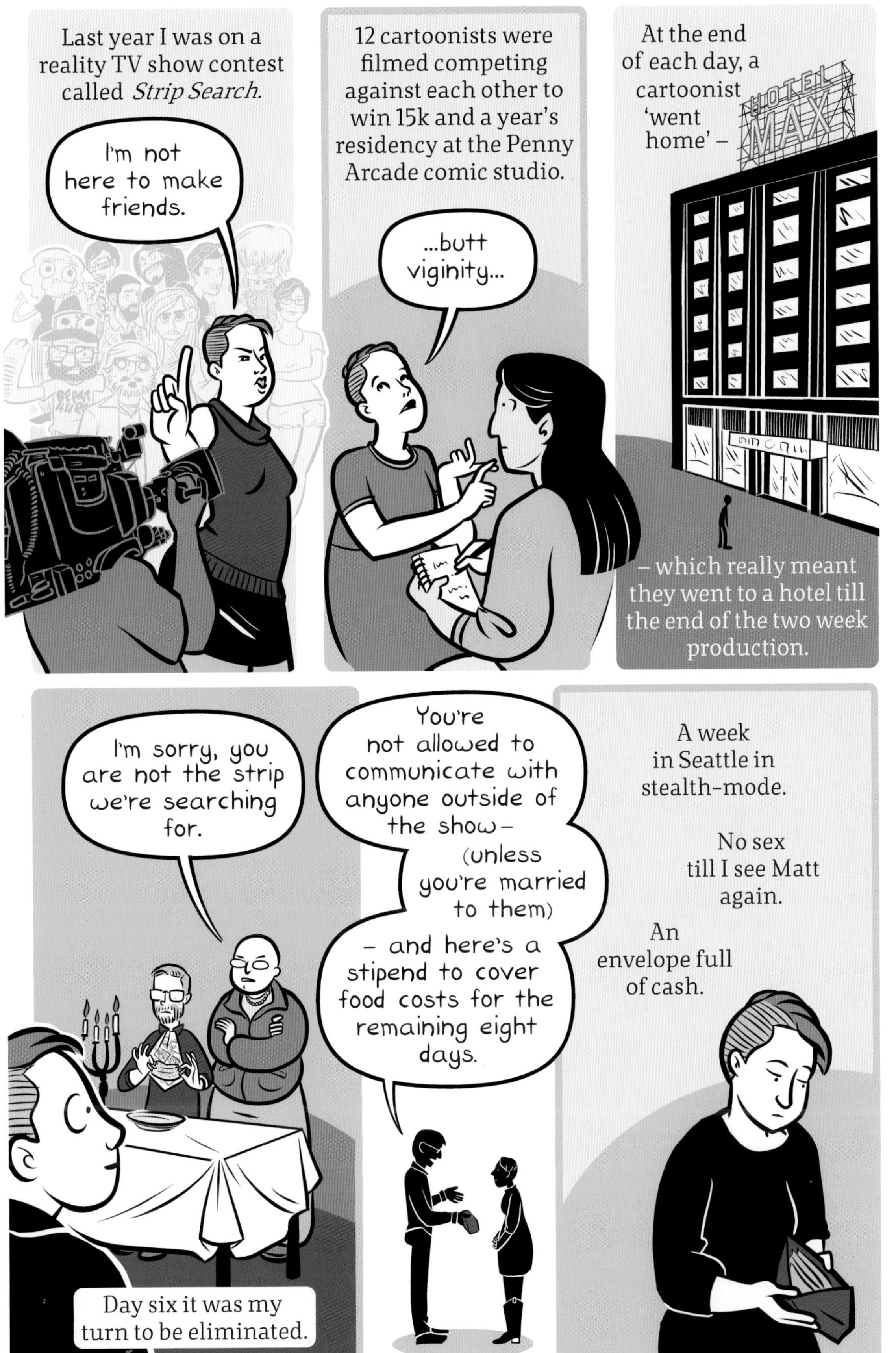
Last year I was on a reality TV show contest called *Strip Search*.
I'm not here to make friends.
BEAST AURY
12 cartoonists were filmed competing against each other to win 15k and a year's residency at the Penny Arcade comic studio.
...butt viginity...
At the end of each day, a cartoonist 'went home' –
HOTEL MAX
– which really meant they went to a hotel till the end of the two week production.
I'm sorry, you are not the strip we're searching for.
Day six it was my turn to be eliminated.
You're not allowed to communicate with anyone outside of the show – (unless you're married to them)
– and here's a stipend to cover food costs for the remaining eight days.
A week in Seattle in stealth-mode.
No sex till I see Matt again.
An envelope full of cash.

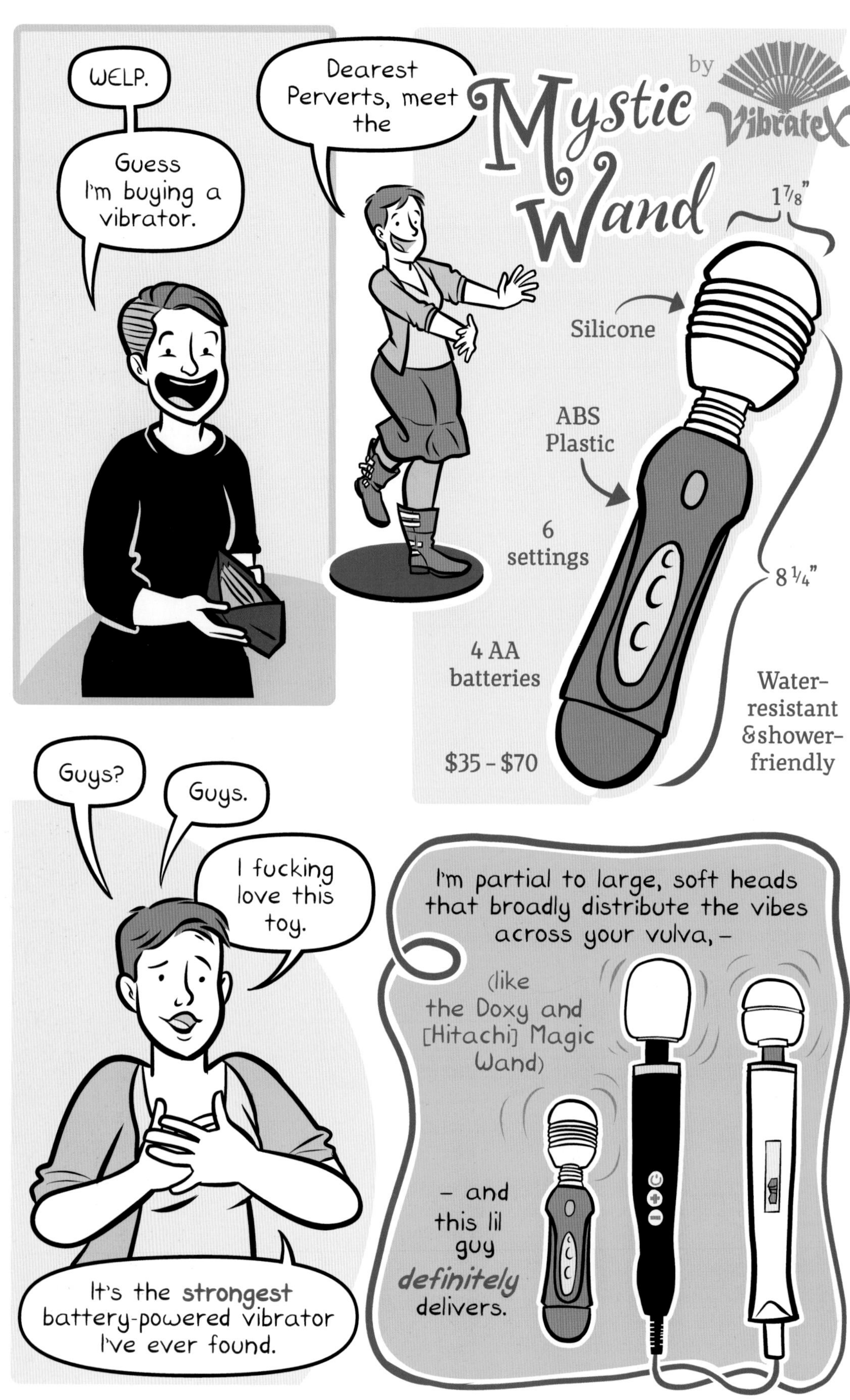
WELP.
Guess I'm buying a vibrator.
Dearest Perverts, meet the
Mystic Wand
by Vibratex
1 7/8"
Silicone
ABS Plastic
6 settings
8 1/4"
4 AA batteries
Water-resistant & shower-friendly
$35 - $70
Guys?
Guys.
I fucking love this toy.
It's the strongest battery-powered vibrator I've ever found.
I'm partial to large, soft heads that broadly distribute the vibes across your vulva, –
(like the Doxy and [Hitachi] Magic Wand)
– and this lil guy *definitely* delivers.

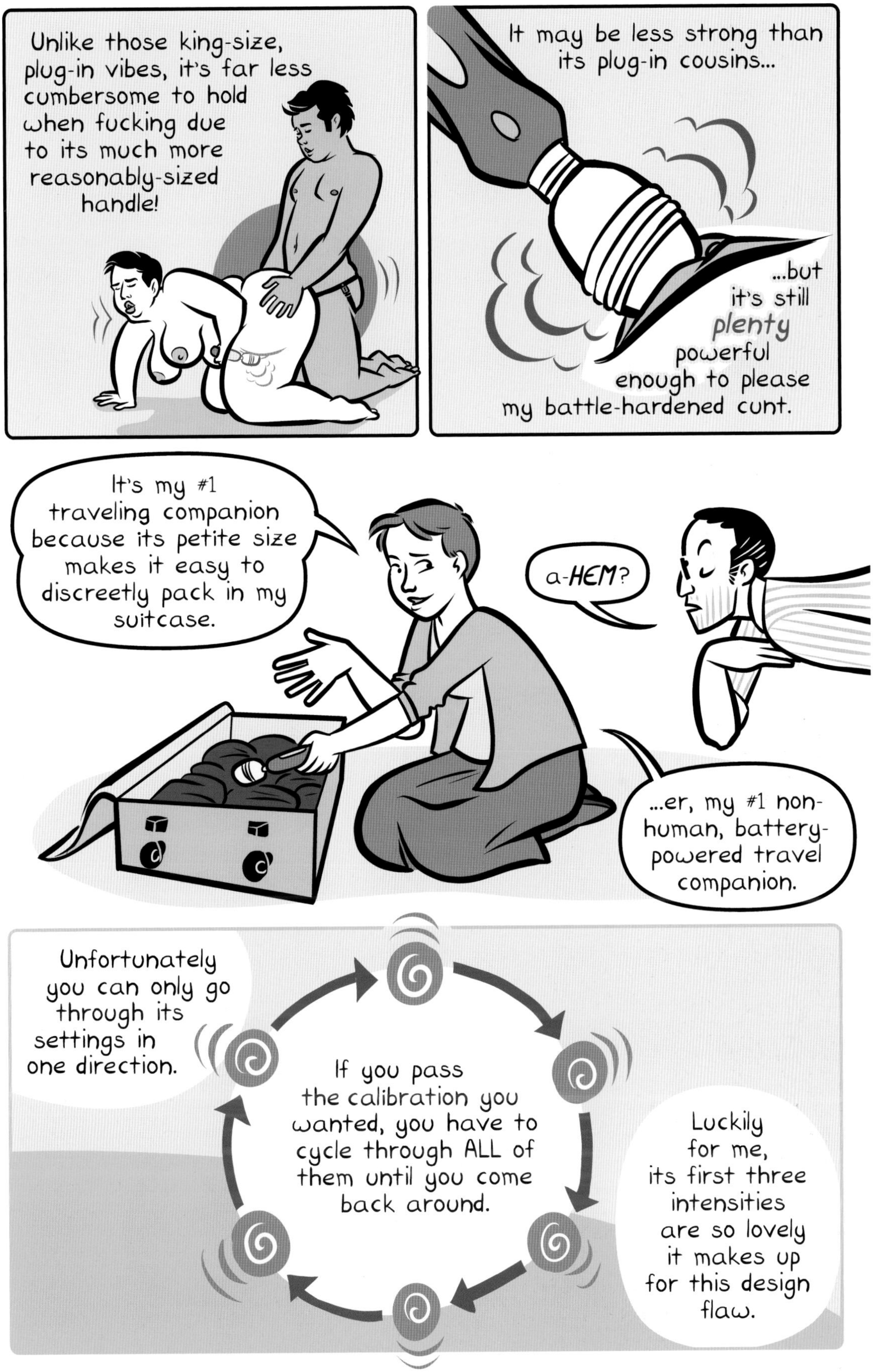

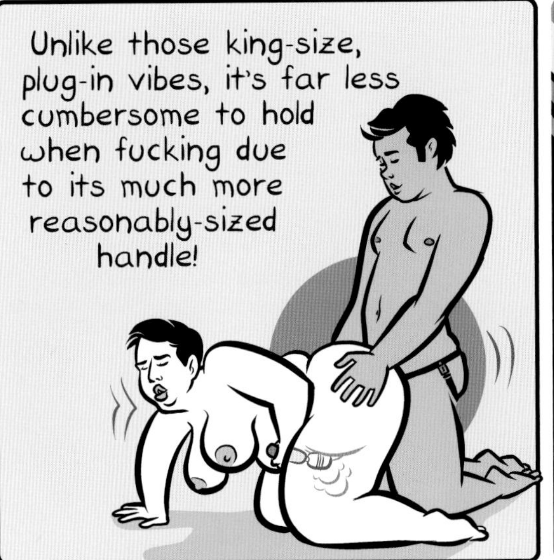

Unlike those king-size, plug-in vibes, it's far less cumbersome to hold when fucking due to its much more reasonably-sized handle!

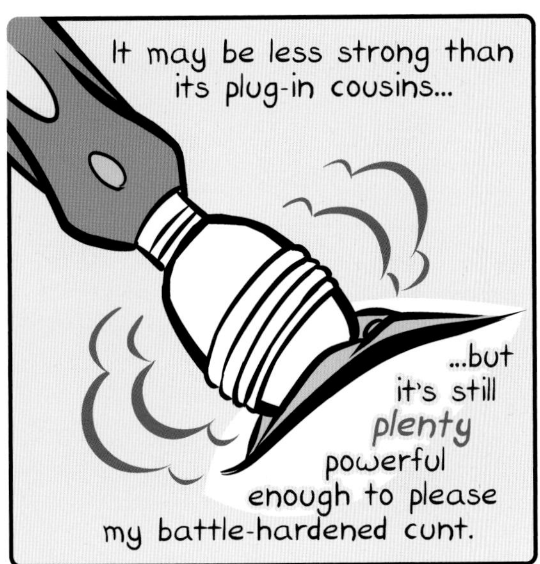

It may be less strong than its plug-in cousins...
...but it's still plenty powerful enough to please my battle-hardened cunt.

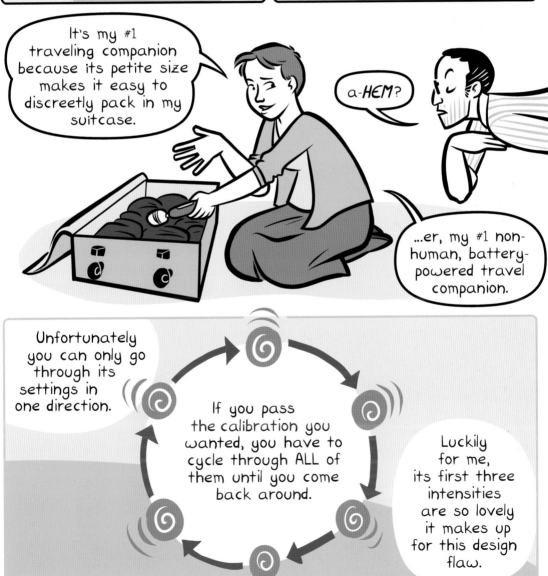

It's my #1 traveling companion because its petite size makes it easy to discreetly pack in my suitcase.

a-HEM?

...er, my #1 non-human, battery-powered travel companion.

Unfortunately you can only go through its settings in one direction.

If you pass the calibration you wanted, you have to cycle through ALL of them until you come back around.

Luckily for me, its first three intensities are so lovely it makes up for this design flaw.

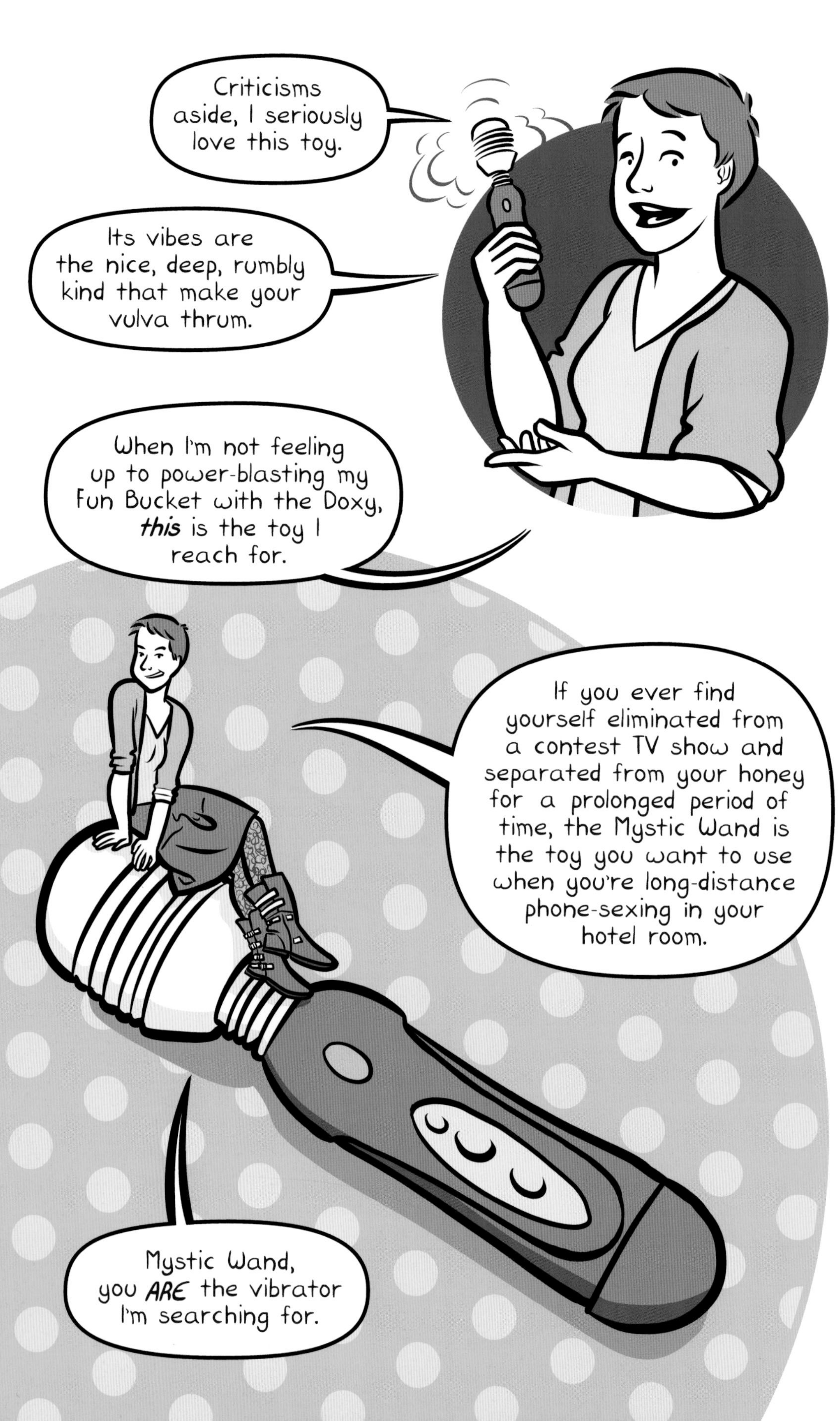
Criticisms aside, I seriously love this toy.
Its vibes are the nice, deep, rumbly kind that make your vulva thrum.
When I'm not feeling up to power-blasting my Fun Bucket with the Doxy, *this* is the toy I reach for.
If you ever find yourself eliminated from a contest TV show and separated from your honey for a prolonged period of time, the Mystic Wand is the toy you want to use when you're long-distance phone-sexing in your hotel room.
Mystic Wand, you *ARE* the vibrator I'm searching for.

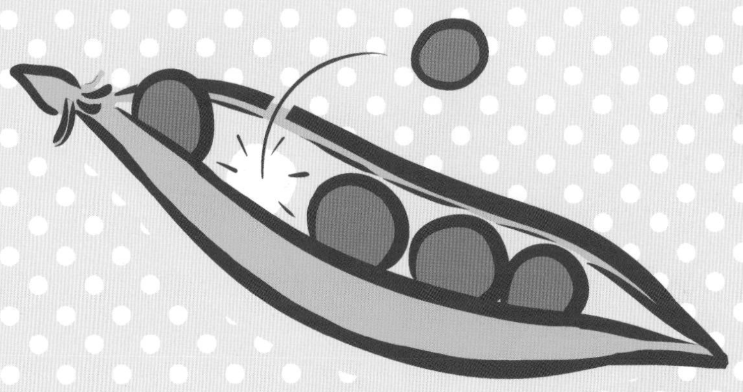

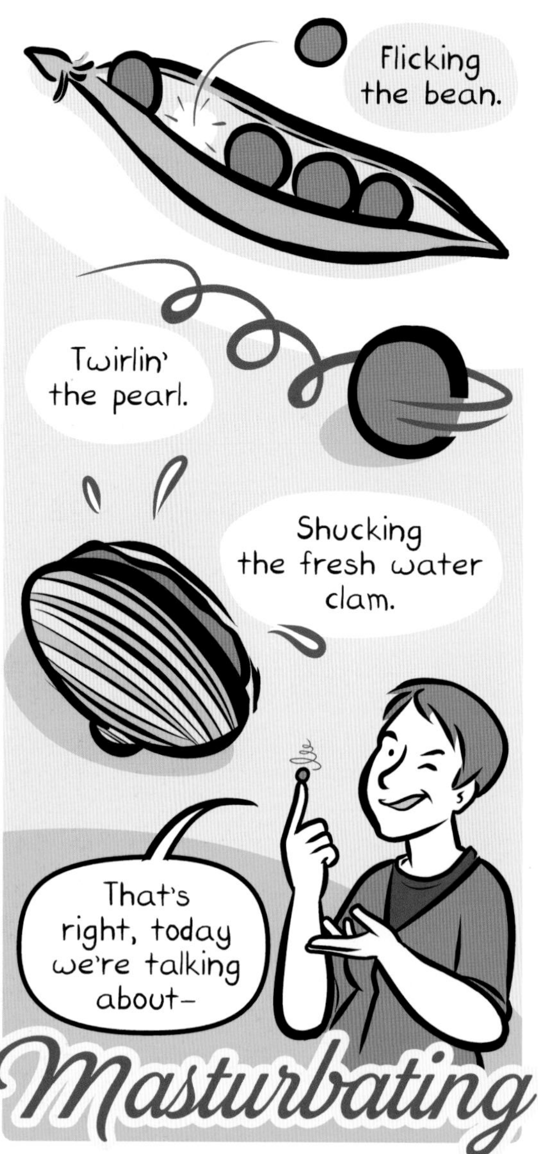
Flicking the bean.
Twirlin' the pearl.
Shucking the fresh water clam.
That's right, today we're talking about–
Masturbating

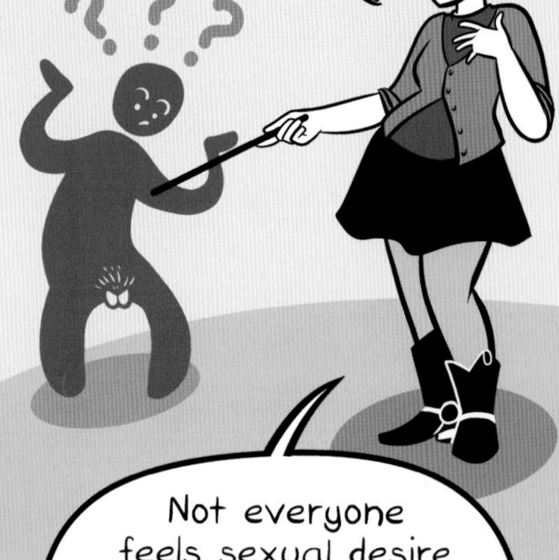
Personally, I was a pretty late bloomer myself when it came to masturbation and orgasms, which is a fairly common phenomena among us folks with vulvas.
Not everyone feels sexual desire or arousal, but if you do, understanding how your genitals work and how to please your body are important sex life skills.

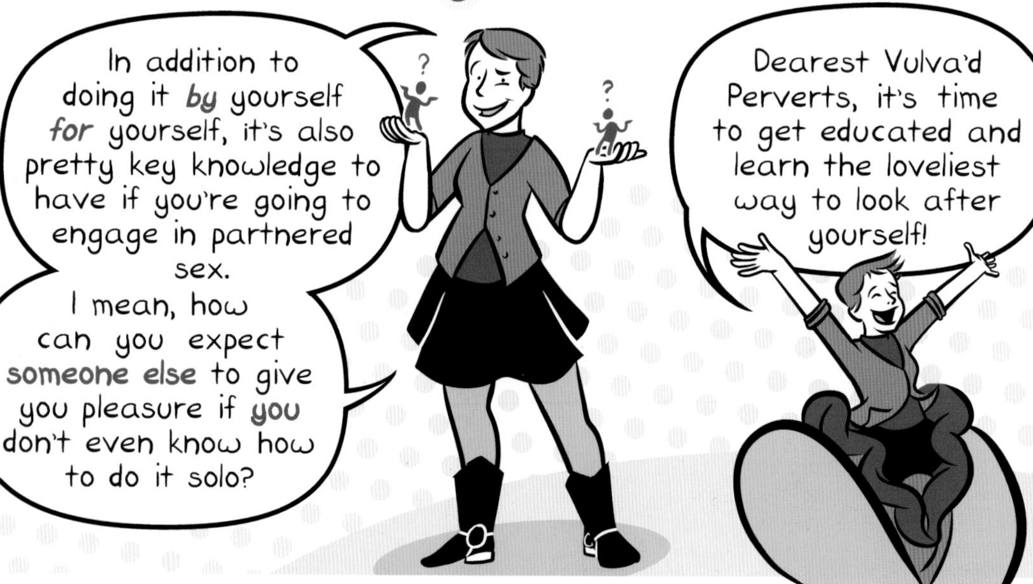
In addition to doing it *by* yourself *for* yourself, it's also pretty key knowledge to have if you're going to engage in partnered sex.
I mean, how can you expect **someone else** to give you pleasure if **you** don't even know how to do it solo?
Dearest Vulva'd Perverts, it's time to get educated and learn the loveliest way to look after yourself!

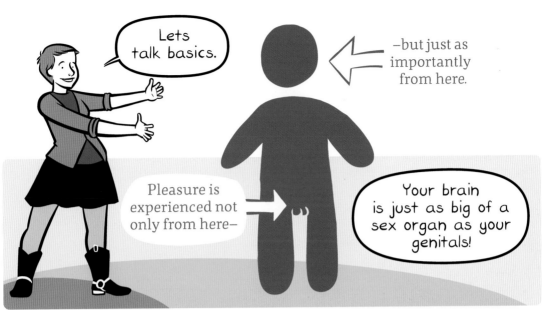

Where you are emotionally and mentally plays a vital role in allowing your body to feel pleasure.

Meditate

Take a bath

Check out some smut

Stress and worry are arousal-killers, so set aside some time where you can relax and indulge yourself.

Social Media

Family

Homework

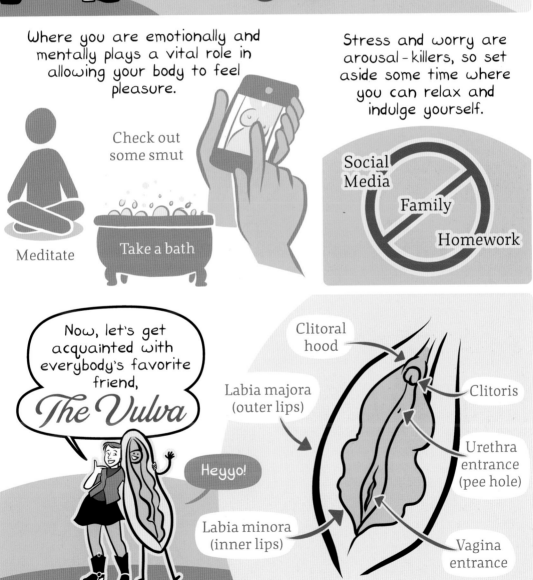

Now, let's get acquainted with everybody's favorite friend, *The Vulva*

Heyyo!

Clitoral hood

Clitoris

Labia majora (outer lips)

Urethra entrance (pee hole)

Labia minora (inner lips)

Vagina entrance

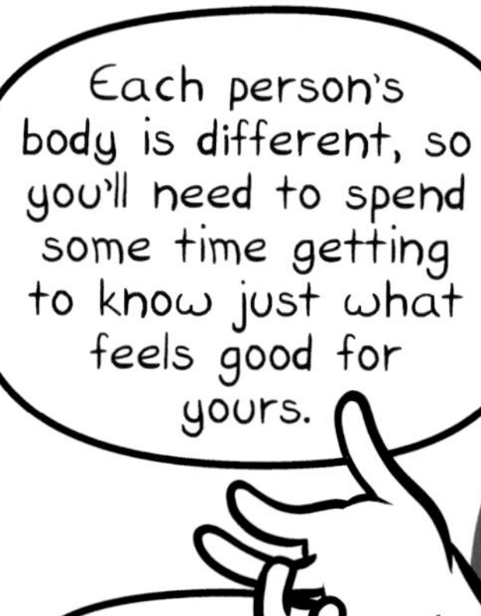
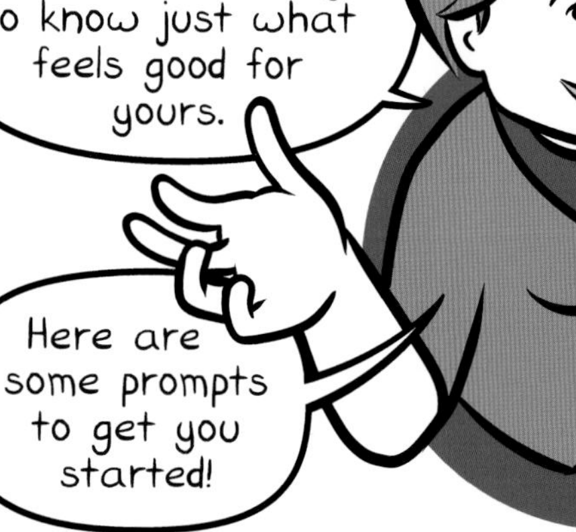
Each person's body is different, so you'll need to spend some time getting to know just what feels good for yours.
Here are some prompts to get you started!

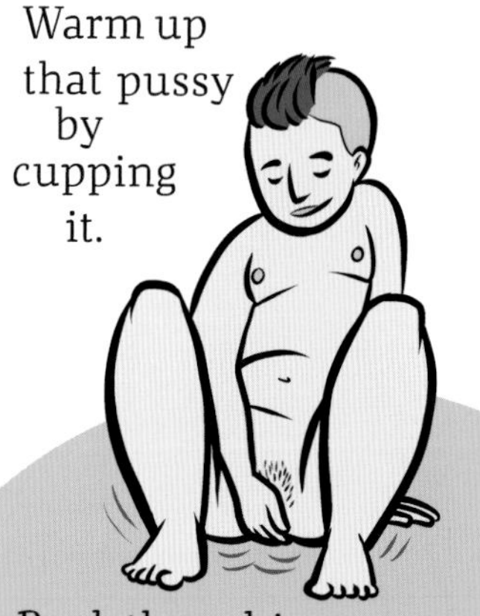
Warm up that pussy by cupping it.
Rock those hips so your outer lips are massaged against your hand.

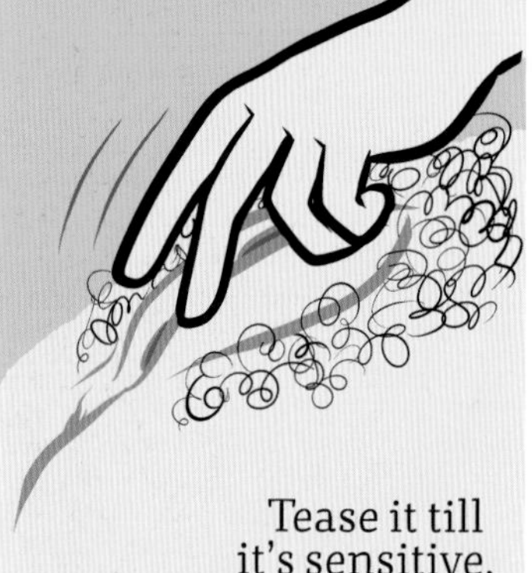
Trail your fingers along the edge of your vulva and across the surface.
Tease it till it's sensitive.

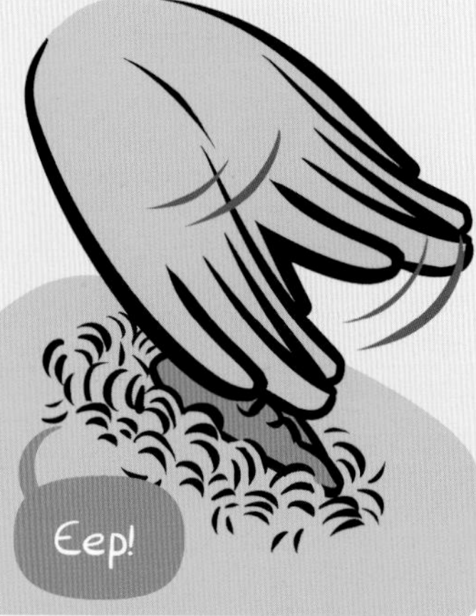
Give it some gentle pats or a friendly whack to wake it up.
Eep!

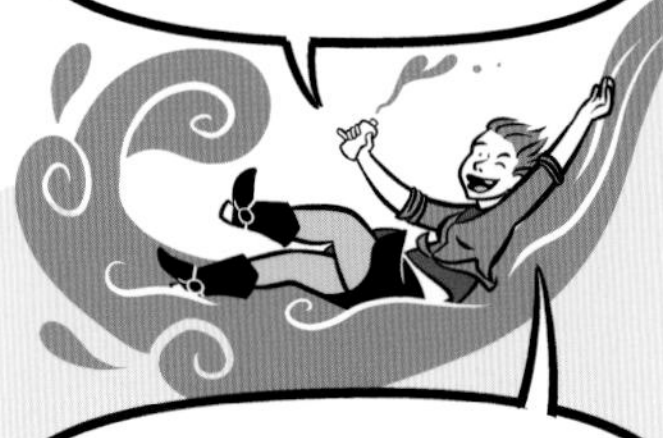
Generally speaking, a slippery vulva is a happy vulva.
If you're not naturally wet, then it's time to reach for your favorite lube.

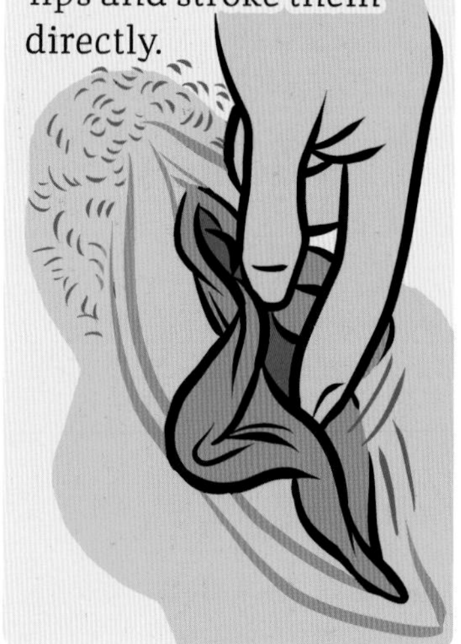
Trace around your inner lips and stroke them directly.

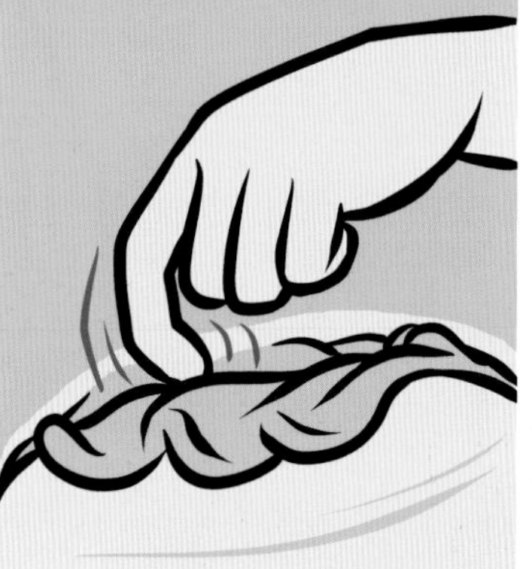
Try fluttering your finger in one specific spot before moving on to another.

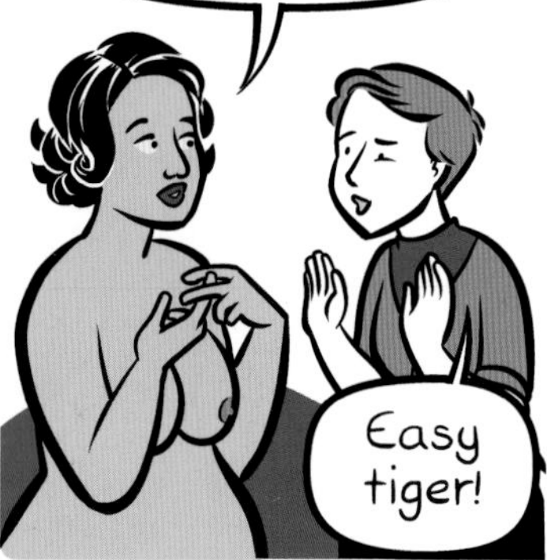
And then to orgasm I just push my fingers in the hole, right?
Easy tiger!

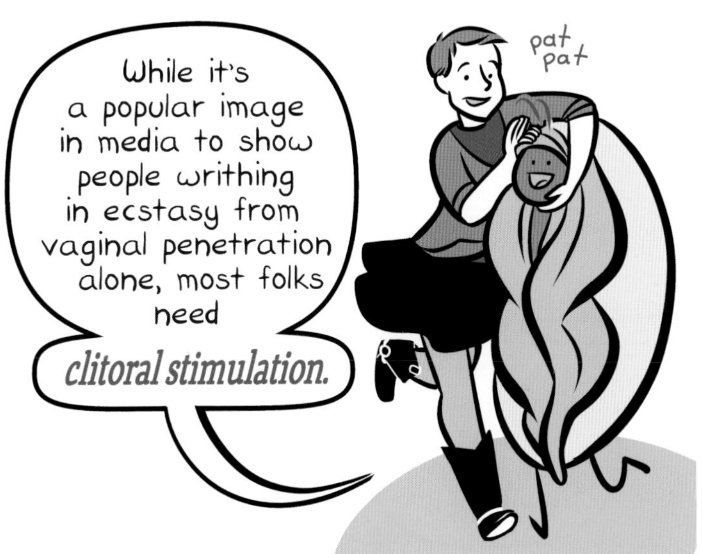

While it's a popular image in media to show people writhing in ecstasy from vaginal penetration alone, most folks need
clitoral stimulation.
pat pat

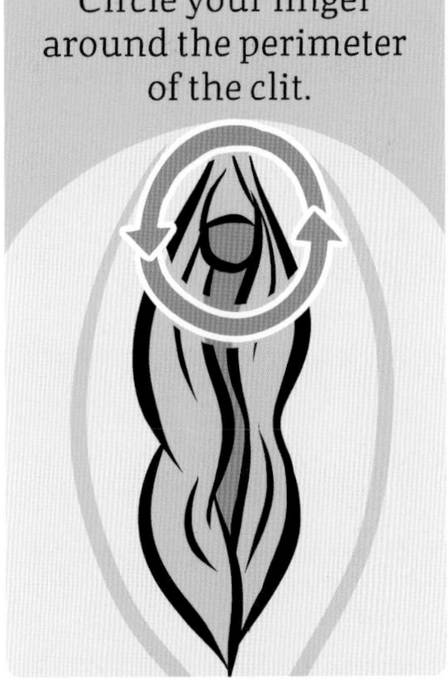

Circle your finger around the perimeter of the clit.

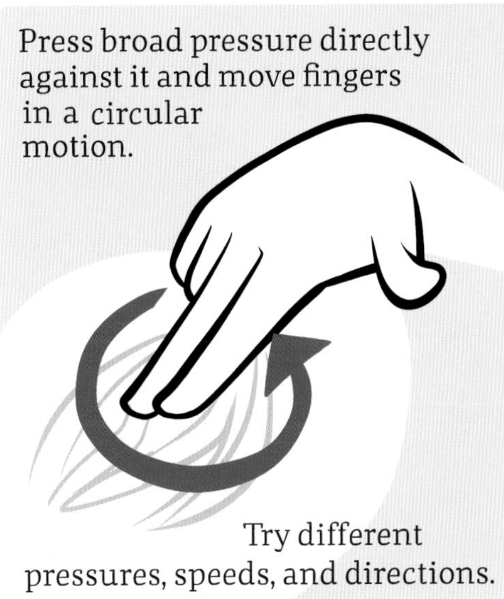

Press broad pressure directly against it and move fingers in a circular motion.
Try different pressures, speeds, and directions.

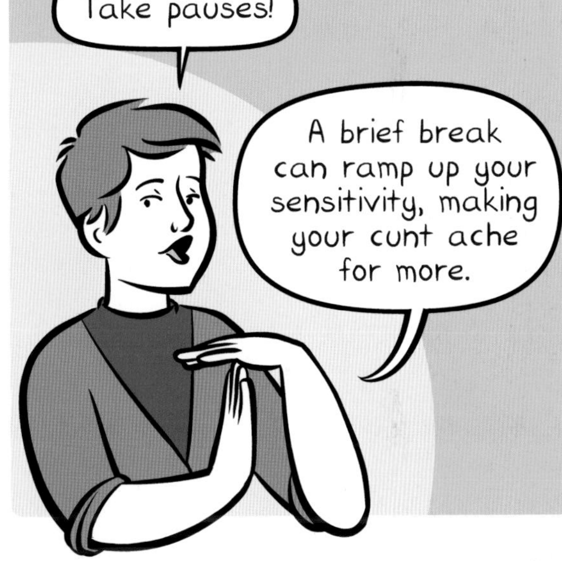

Take pauses!
A brief break can ramp up your sensitivity, making your cunt ache for more.

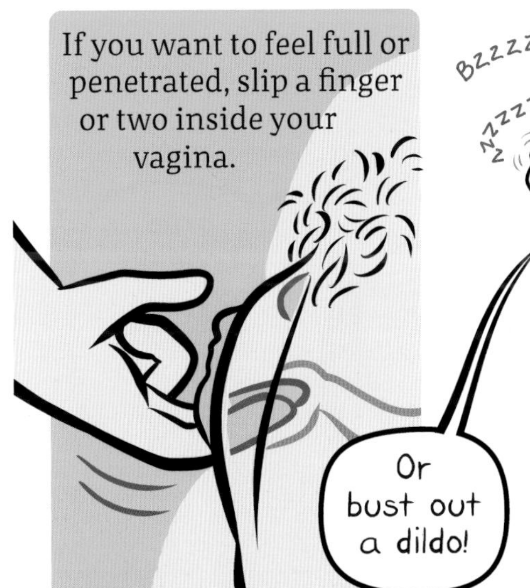

If you want to feel full or penetrated, slip a finger or two inside your vagina.
Or bust out a dildo!

BZZZZZZZ ZZZZZZZ

If manual stimulation just doesn't seem to cut it for you, try out a vibrator!

I thought I couldn't enjoy masturbation (let alone orgasm) until I added vibrations to the mix.

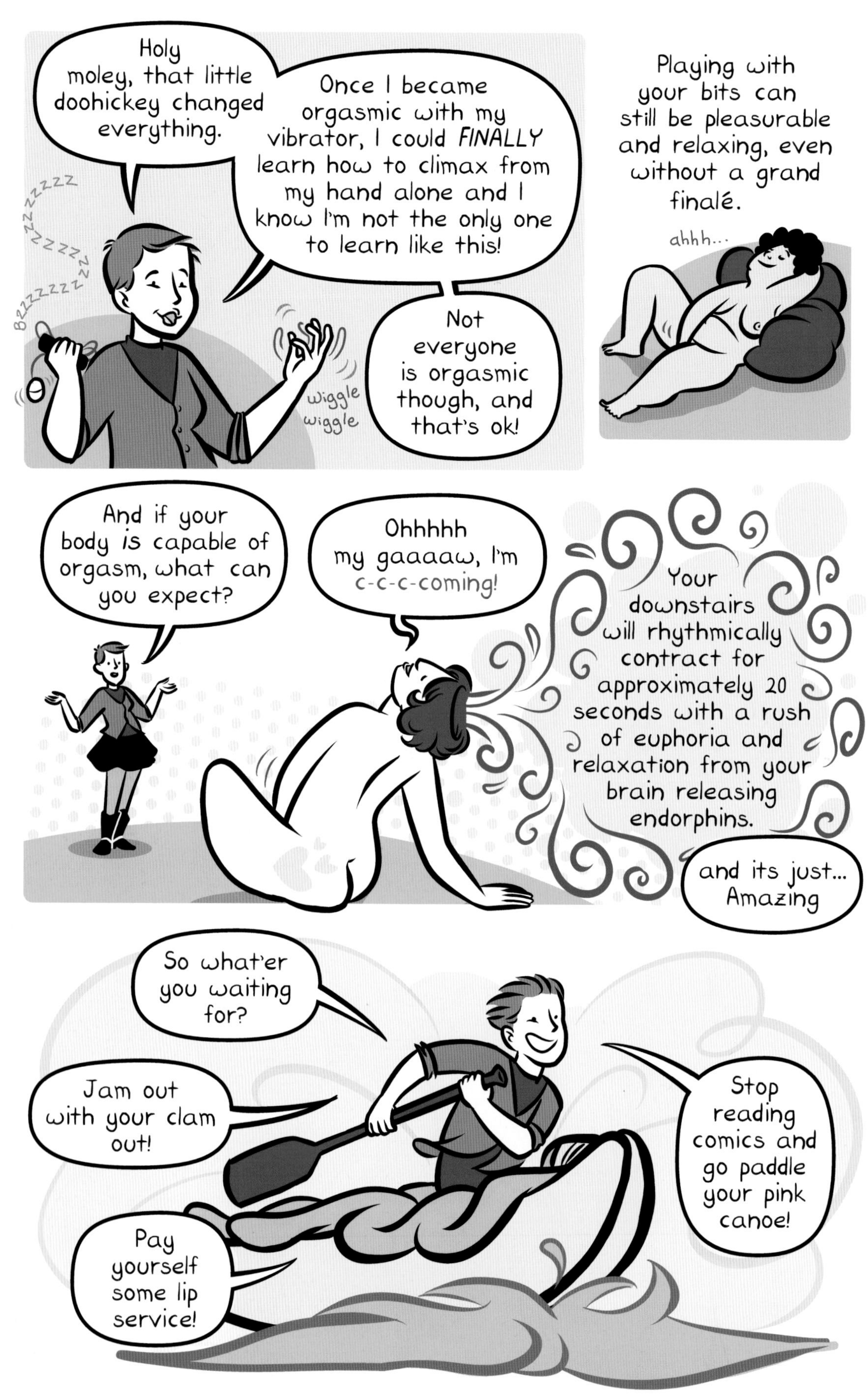
Holy moley, that little doohickey changed everything.
Bzzzzzzzz
Once I became orgasmic with my vibrator, I could FINALLY learn how to climax from my hand alone and I know I'm not the only one to learn like this!
wiggle wiggle
Not everyone is orgasmic though, and that's ok!
Playing with your bits can still be pleasurable and relaxing, even without a grand finalé.
ahhh...
And if your body is capable of orgasm, what can you expect?
Ohhhhh my gaaaaw, I'm c-c-c-coming!
Your downstairs will rhythmically contract for approximately 20 seconds with a rush of euphoria and relaxation from your brain releasing endorphins.
and its just... Amazing
So what'er you waiting for?
Jam out with your clam out!
Stop reading comics and go paddle your pink canoe!
Pay yourself some lip service!

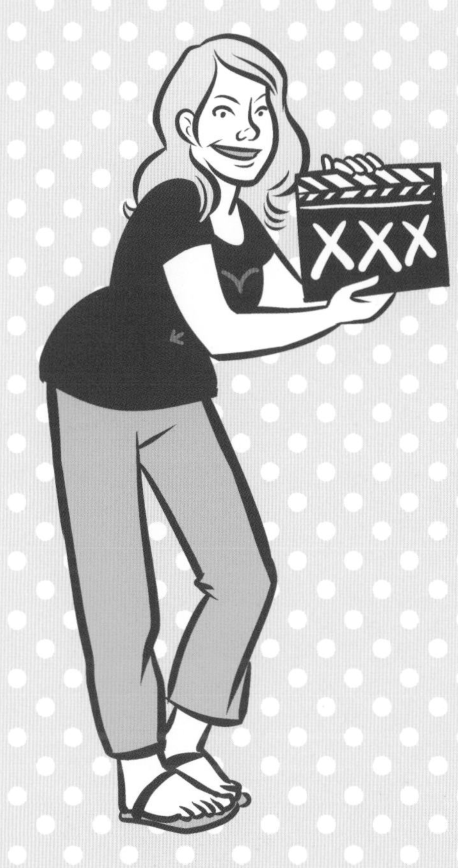
XXX

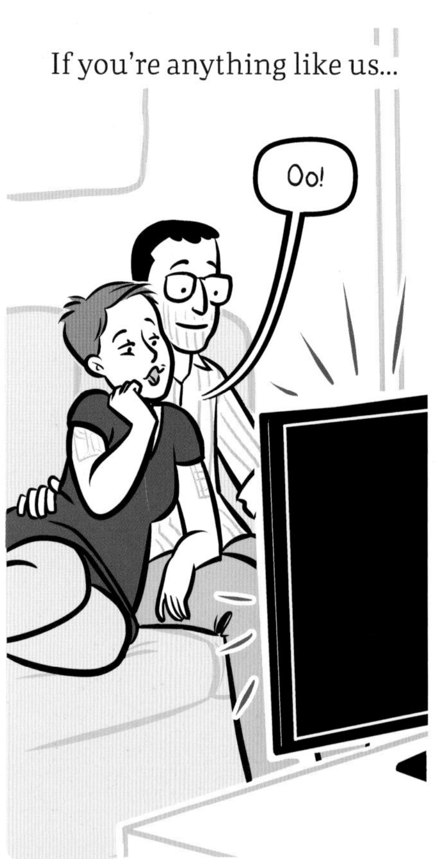
If you're anything like us...
Oo!

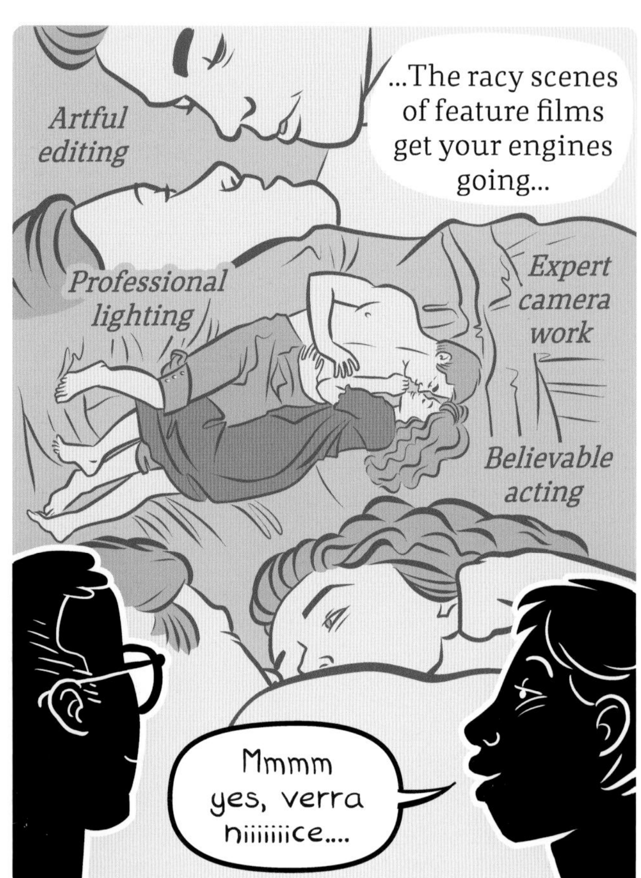
...The racy scenes of feature films get your engines going...
Artful editing
Professional lighting
Expert camera work
Believable acting
Mmmm yes, verra niiiiiice....

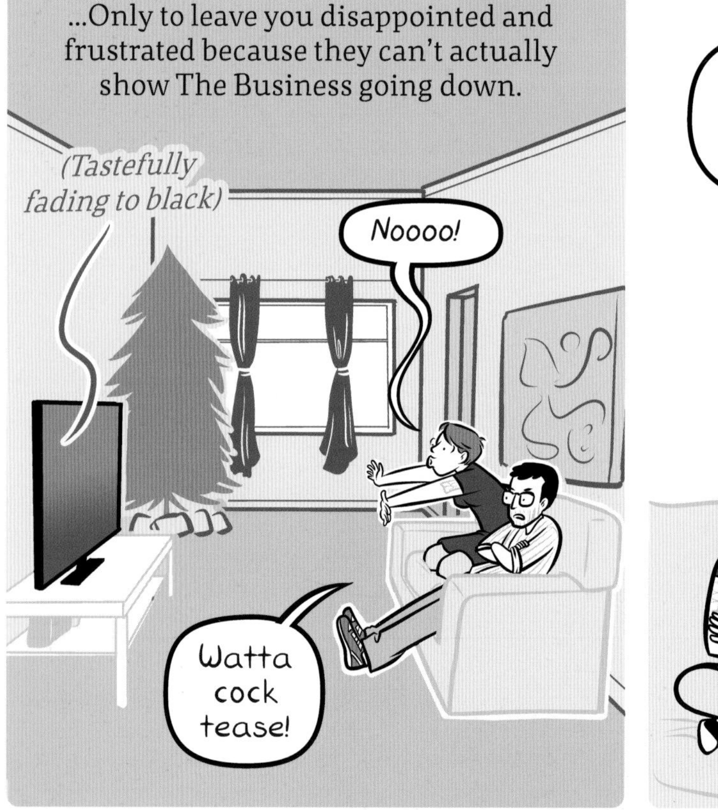
...Only to leave you disappointed and frustrated because they can't actually show The Business going down.
(Tastefully fading to black)
Noooo!
Watta cock tease!

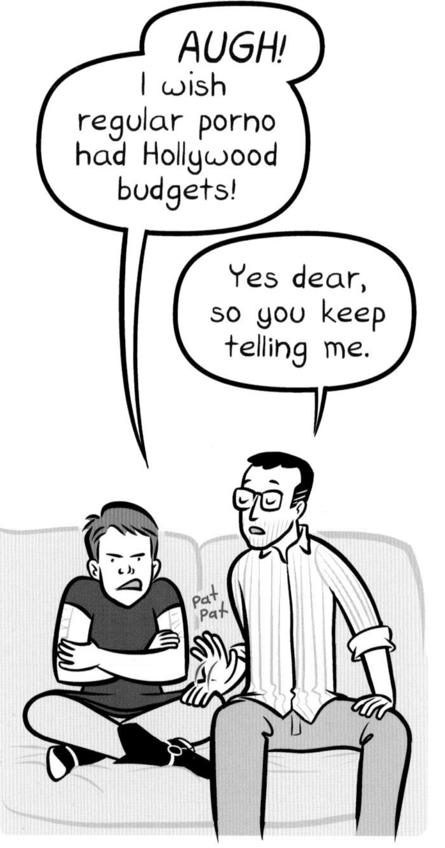
AUGH! I wish regular porno had Hollywood budgets!
Yes dear, so you keep telling me.
Pat Pat

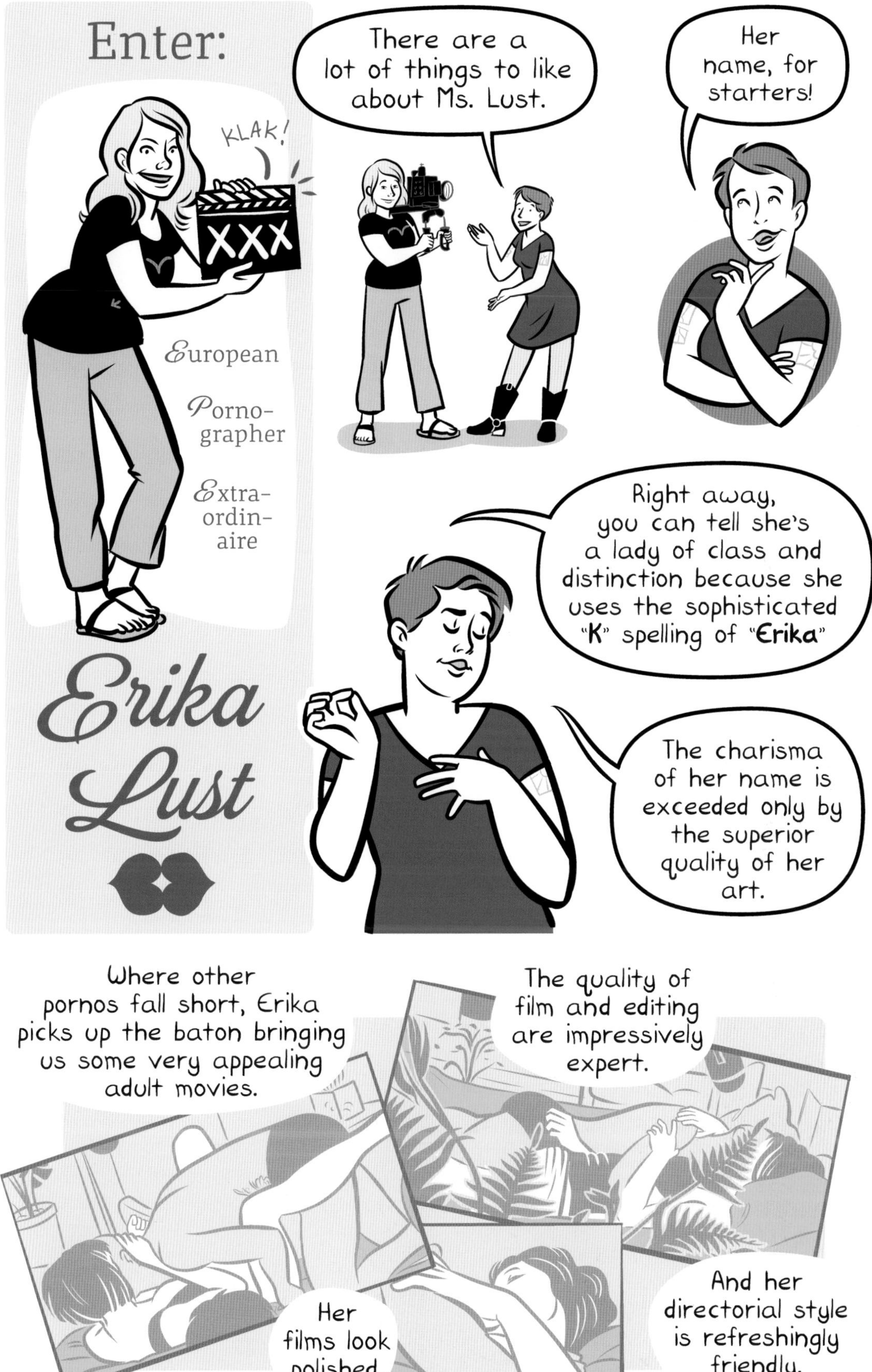
Enter:
KLAK!
XXX
European
Pornographer
Extraordinaire
Erika Lust
There are a lot of things to like about Ms. Lust.
Her name, for starters!
Right away, you can tell she's a lady of class and distinction because she uses the sophisticated "K" spelling of "Erika"
The charisma of her name is exceeded only by the superior quality of her art.
Where other pornos fall short, Erika picks up the baton bringing us some very appealing adult movies.
The quality of film and editing are impressively expert.
Her films look polished.
And her directorial style is refreshingly friendly.

*Stills from "*Let's Make a Porno*"

Her aim is to--

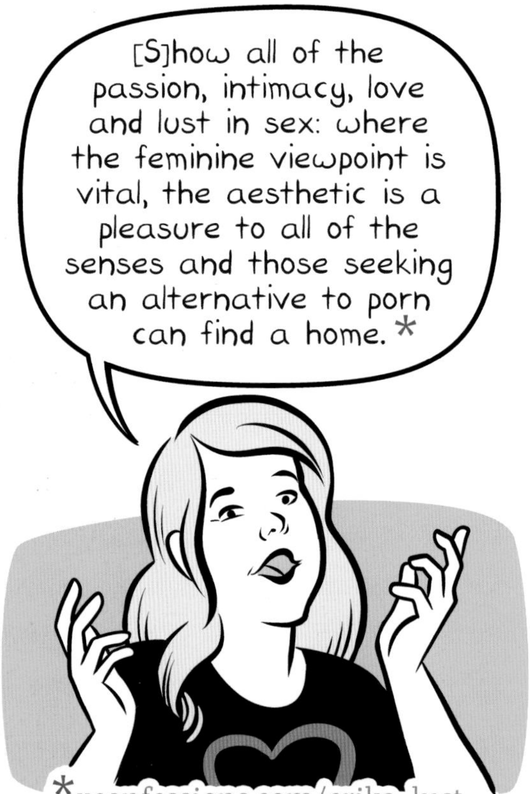

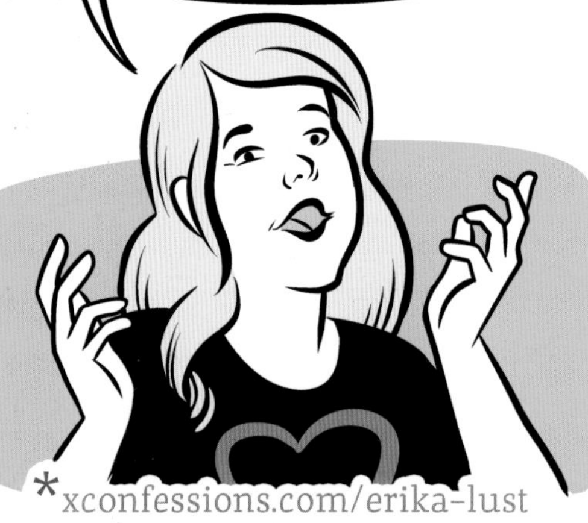
[S]how all of the passion, intimacy, love and lust in sex: where the feminine viewpoint is vital, the aesthetic is a pleasure to all of the senses and those seeking an alternative to porn can find a home. *

*xconfessions.com/erika-lust

Erika invited us to review her curated catalogue of movies,

LUST CINEMA

lustcinema.com

- $35 a month
- Updates ~twice a month
- Full Erika Lust Library
- Other films by Lust's favorite directors
- Downloadable HD content

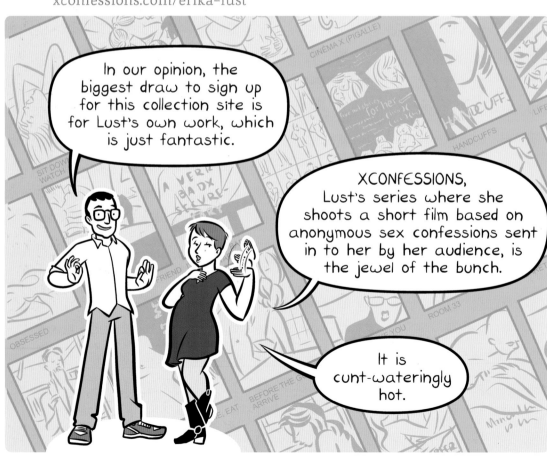

In our opinion, the biggest draw to sign up for this collection site is for Lust's own work, which is just fantastic.

XCONFESSIONS, Lust's series where she shoots a short film based on anonymous sex confessions sent in to her by her audience, is the jewel of the bunch.

It is cunt-wateringly hot.

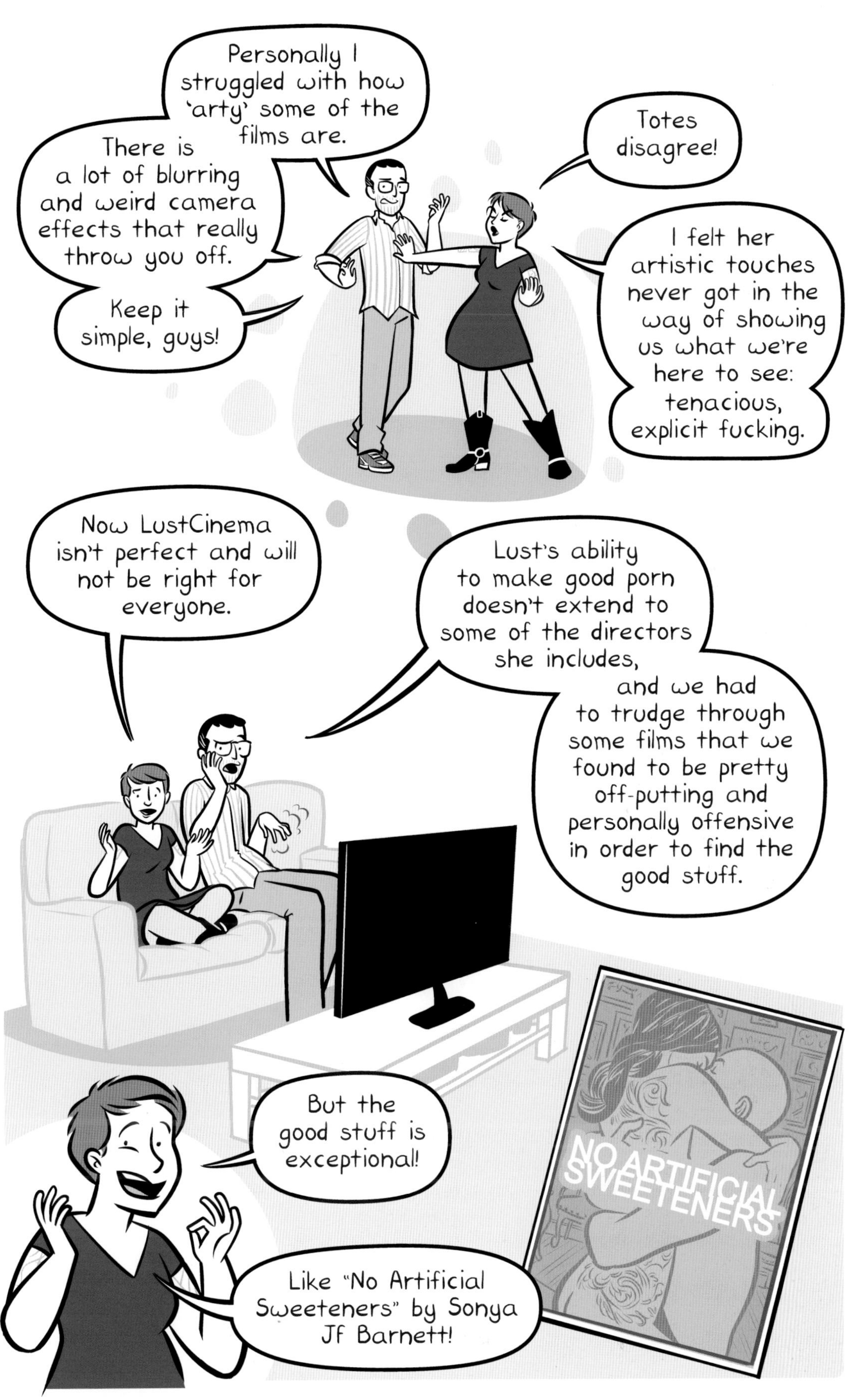
Personally I struggled with how 'arty' some of the films are.
There is a lot of blurring and weird camera effects that really throw you off.
Keep it simple, guys!
Totes disagree!
I felt her artistic touches never got in the way of showing us what we're here to see: tenacious, explicit fucking.
Now LustCinema isn't perfect and will not be right for everyone.
Lust's ability to make good porn doesn't extend to some of the directors she includes,
and we had to trudge through some films that we found to be pretty off-putting and personally offensive in order to find the good stuff.
But the good stuff is exceptional!
NO ARTIFICIAL SWEETENERS
Like "No Artificial Sweeteners" by Sonya Jf Barnett!

Another nitpick of ours is the lack of body diversity across the site.

It skews towards portraying white, trim, cisgender bodies and it'd be nice to see a bit more variety.

On a technical note, the site *struggles* to load

even with a good internet connection.

But the positives outweigh the negatives!

Lust is an impressive director and we had a ton of fun watching her porn together.

If you're looking for skin flicks that deliver on the pretty without stepping on the depiction of good old fashioned fucking, then give LustCinema a try and seek out Erika Lust's films in particular.

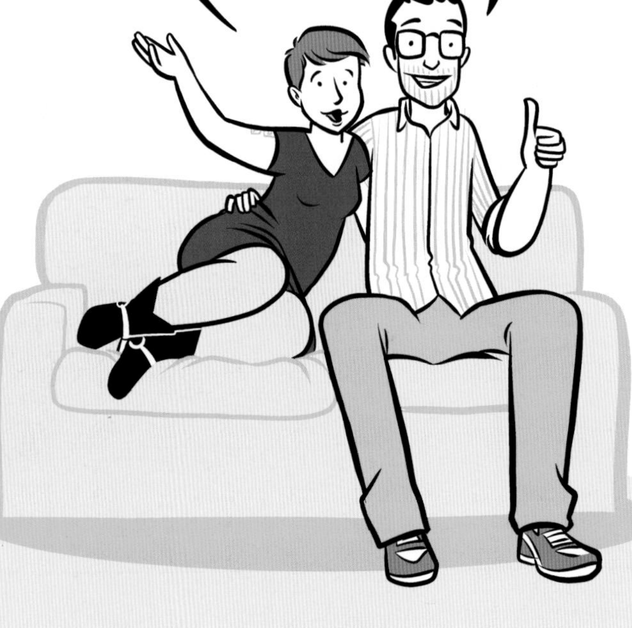

With a name like **Erika** you *know* it's going to be good.

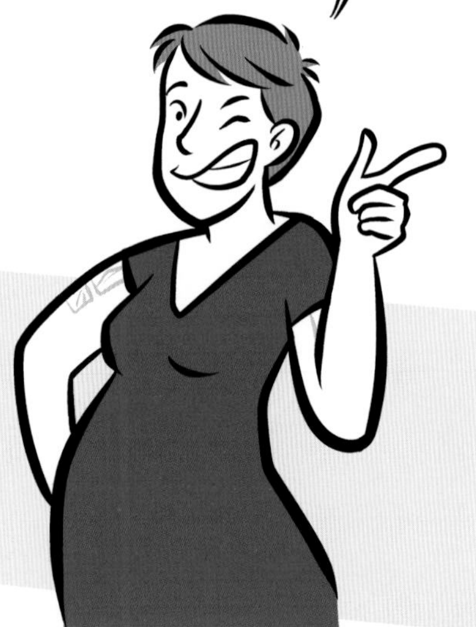

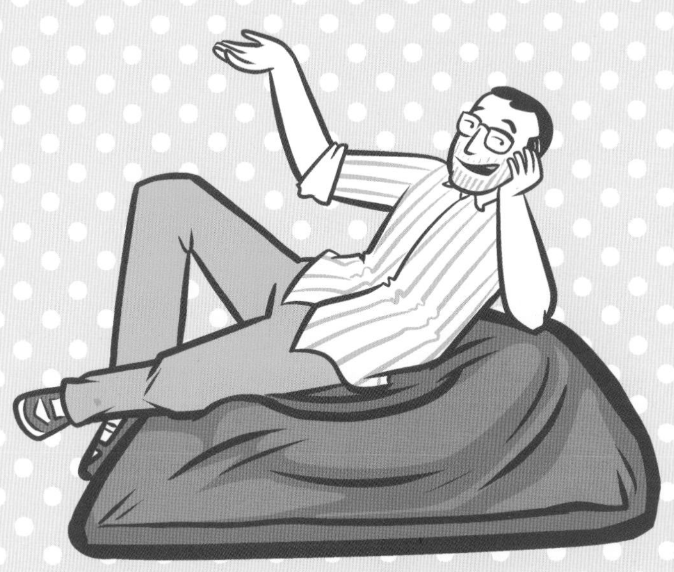

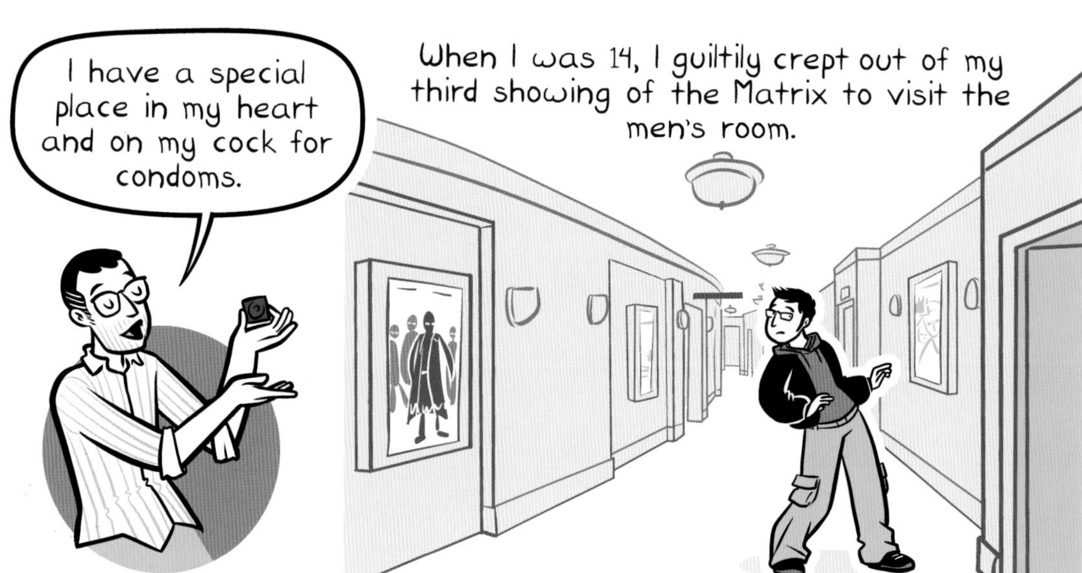
I have a special place in my heart and on my cock for condoms.
When I was 14, I guiltily crept out of my third showing of the Matrix to visit the men's room.

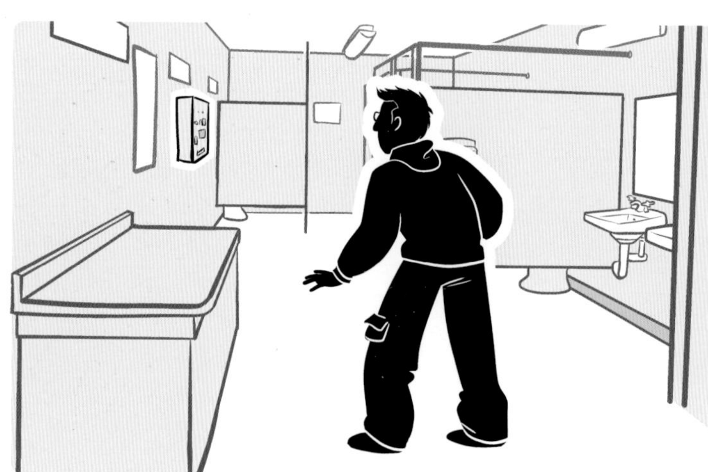
I didn't need the bathroom, but knew mid-movie I would get the room to myself.

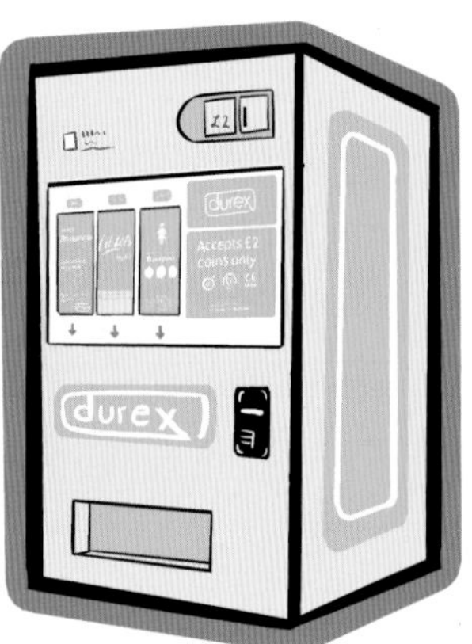
And this Odeon Theatre's men's room had a condom machine.
durex
durex

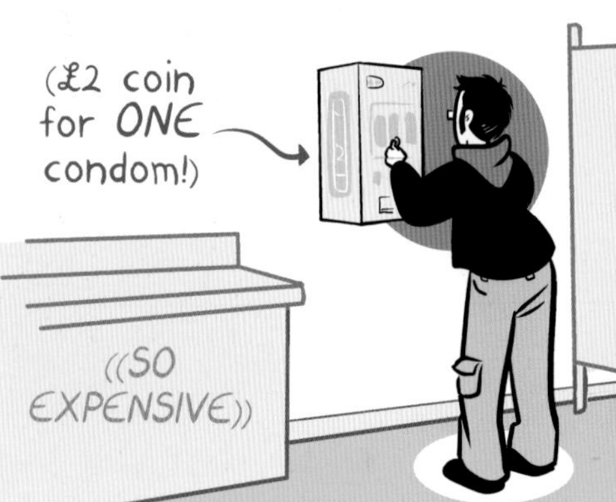
At the time I barely knew anybody of the opposite sex, let alone any I might eventually have sex with.
(£2 coin for ONE condom!)
((SO EXPENSIVE))

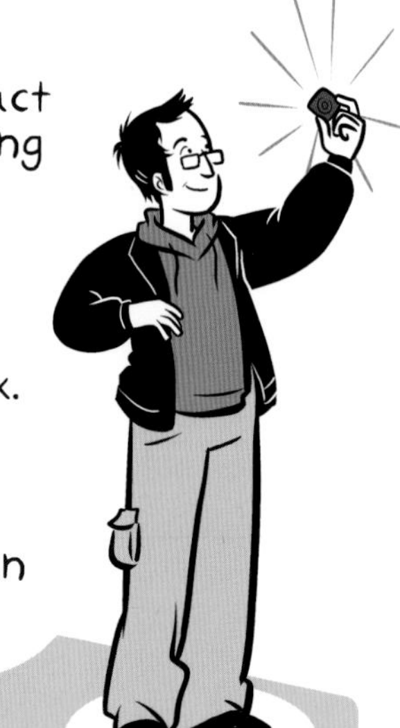
But the act of simply buying and HAVING a condom, becoming PREPARED, brought me one step closer to actual sex.
It turned a *maybe* into an eventually.

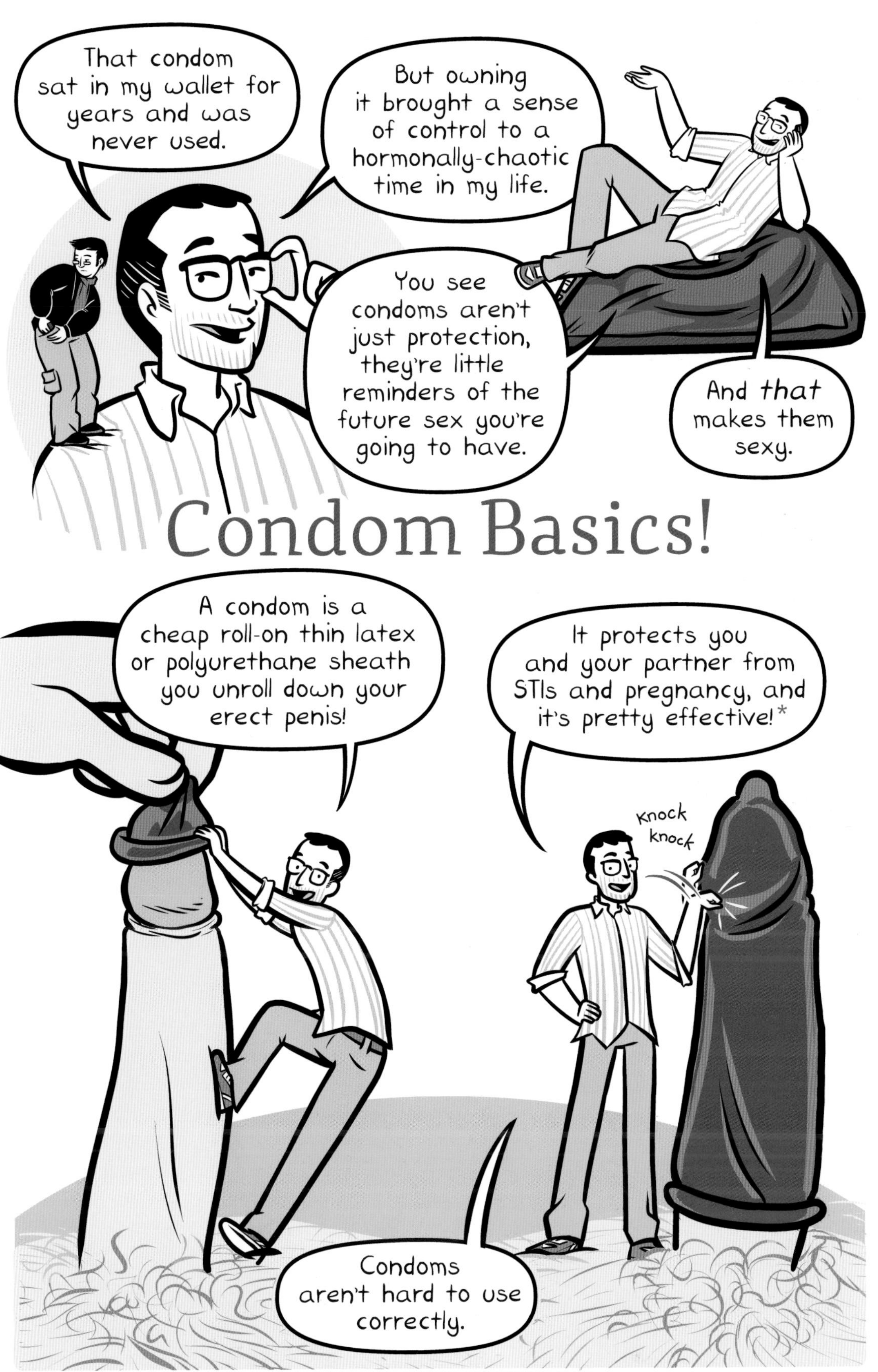
That condom sat in my wallet for years and was never used.
But owning it brought a sense of control to a hormonally-chaotic time in my life.
You see condoms aren't just protection, they're little reminders of the future sex you're going to have.
And *that* makes them sexy.
Condom Basics!
A condom is a cheap roll-on thin latex or polyurethane sheath you unroll down your erect penis!
It protects you and your partner from STIs and pregnancy, and it's pretty effective!*
Knock knock
Condoms aren't hard to use correctly.

*plannedparenthood.org/health-info/birth-control/condom

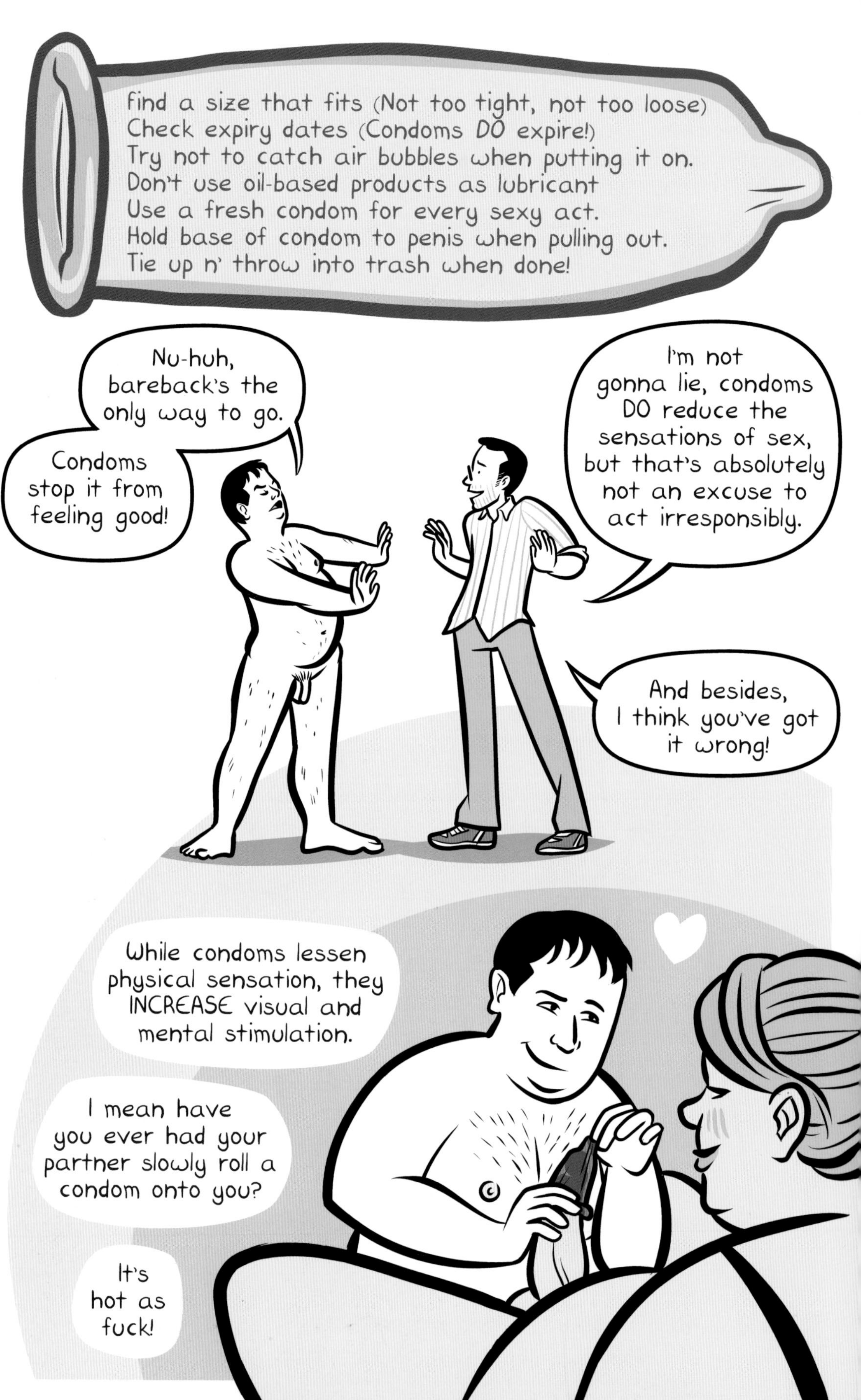
find a size that fits (Not too tight, not too loose)
Check expiry dates (Condoms DO expire!)
Try not to catch air bubbles when putting it on.
Don't use oil-based products as lubricant
Use a fresh condom for every sexy act.
Hold base of condom to penis when pulling out.
Tie up n' throw into trash when done!
Nu-huh, bareback's the only way to go.
Condoms stop it from feeling good!
I'm not gonna lie, condoms DO reduce the sensations of sex, but that's absolutely not an excuse to act irresponsibly.
And besides, I think you've got it wrong!
While condoms lessen physical sensation, they INCREASE visual and mental stimulation.
I mean have you ever had your partner slowly roll a condom onto you?
It's hot as fuck!

And there are ways to bring the sensation back!

Find a thin condom you like and before rolling it on add a few drops of a silicone lube to the inside.

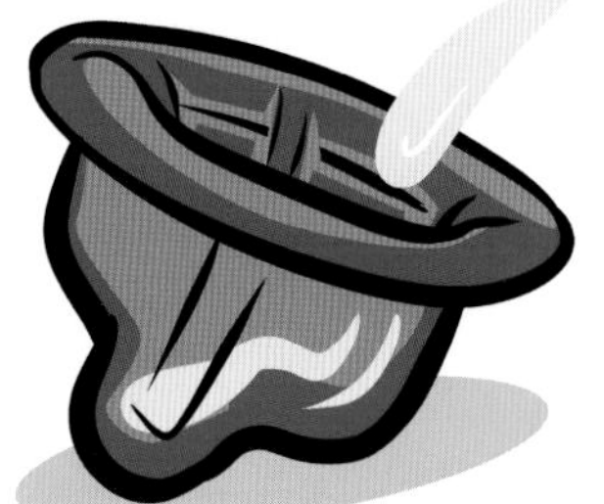

This non-drying lube will add a ton of smooth good-feeling friction.

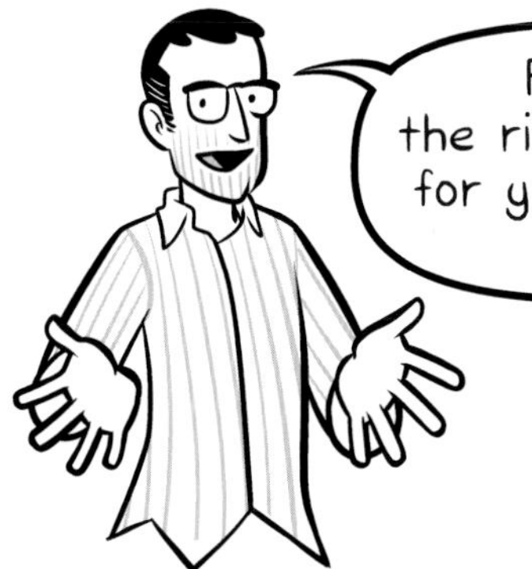

Finding the right condom for you will help too.
This past year I've gotten and tried TONS of different condoms.
And to give you somewhere to start, here are my current favorites*

*for the person with an averaged sized wang who has a preference for thin condoms.

Sir Richard's Ultra Thin

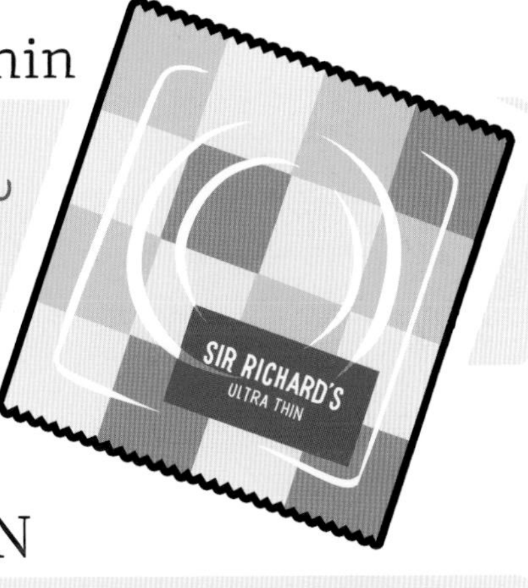

- Good looking wrapper!
- Low latex odor
- Ethical choice! For every condom you buy, one condom is sent to a developing country!
- Chemical-free

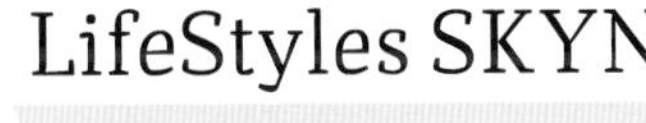

LifeStyles SKYN

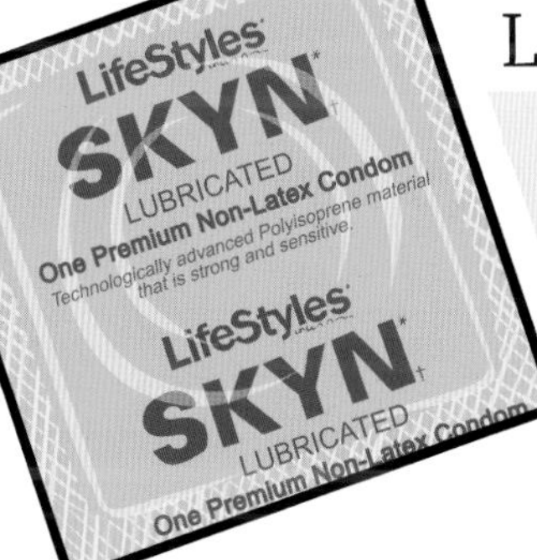

-Expensive

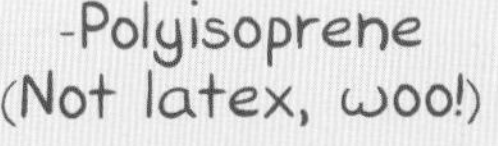

-Polyisoprene (Not latex, woo!)

-Strong and thin, well fitting!

Beyond Seven Ultra Thin

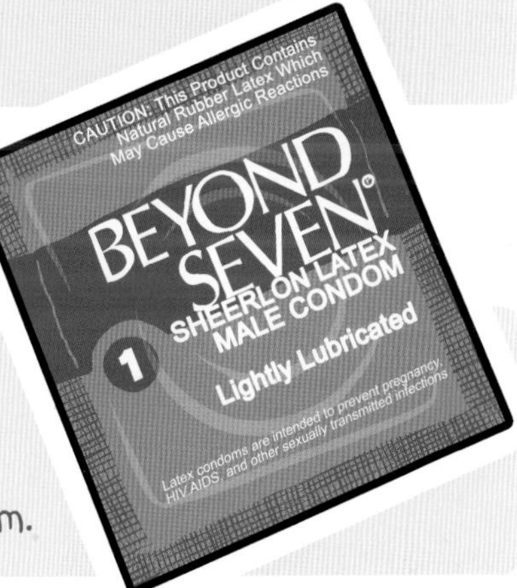

- Sheerlon latex (thinner than regular latex but still very durable)
- My current go to cheap condom.

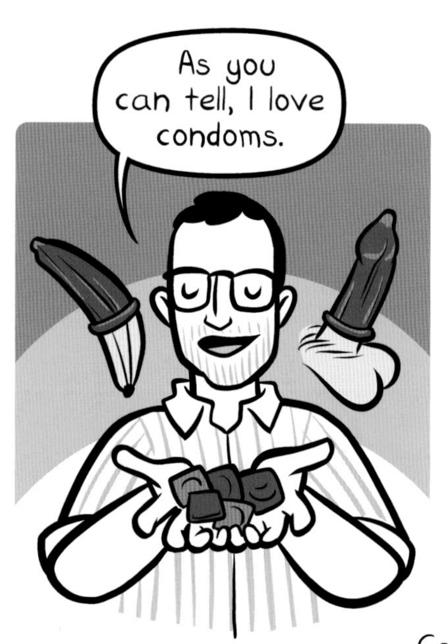

As you can tell, I love condoms.

Even though I don't need to use them with Erika*, we still often add them to our sex life.

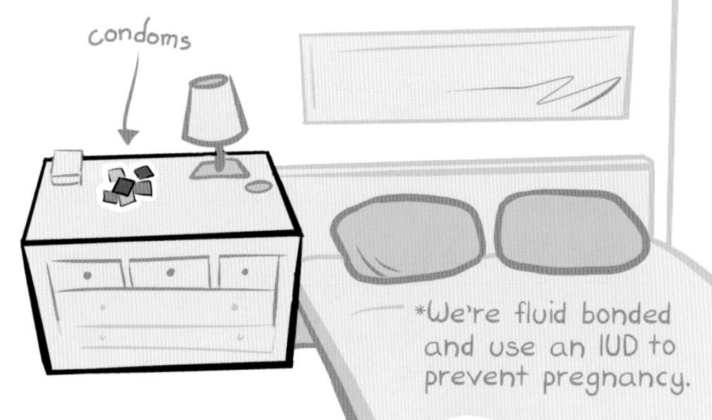

*We're fluid bonded and use an IUD to prevent pregnancy.

Condoms aren't a buzzkill, they're the starting gun of sexy times!

They're fun to use as role playing strangers,

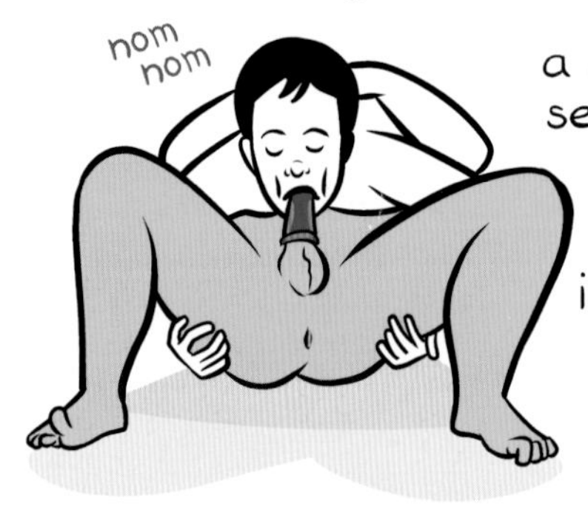

a switch in sensations,

a pause in our rolling around,

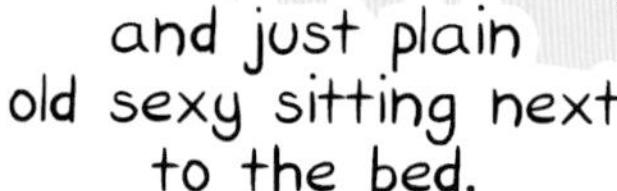

and just plain old sexy sitting next to the bed.

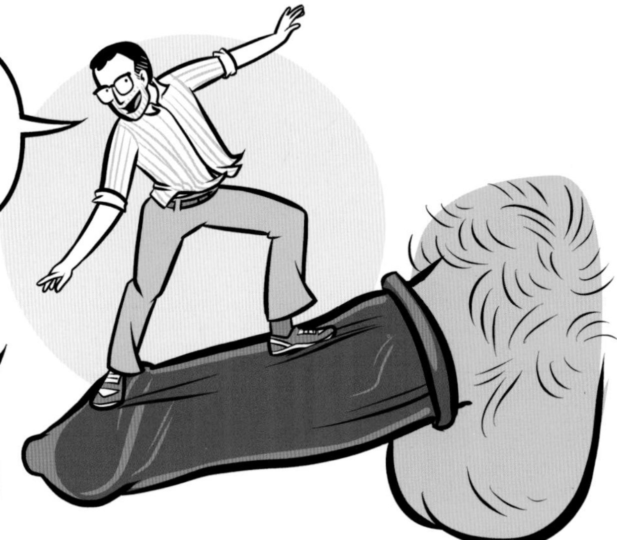

I'm gonna end this by saying that condoms are CHEAP and available everywhere.
If you're new to the world of sex, hunt some down and try them out solo.
I want you all to learn to love condoms!

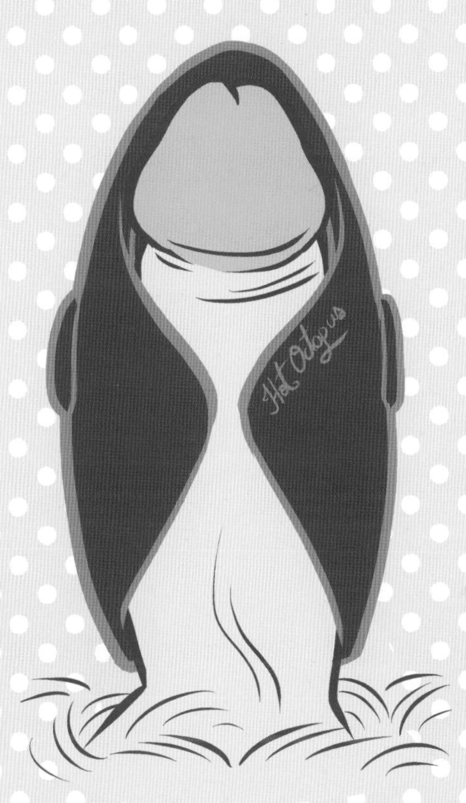
Hot Octopus

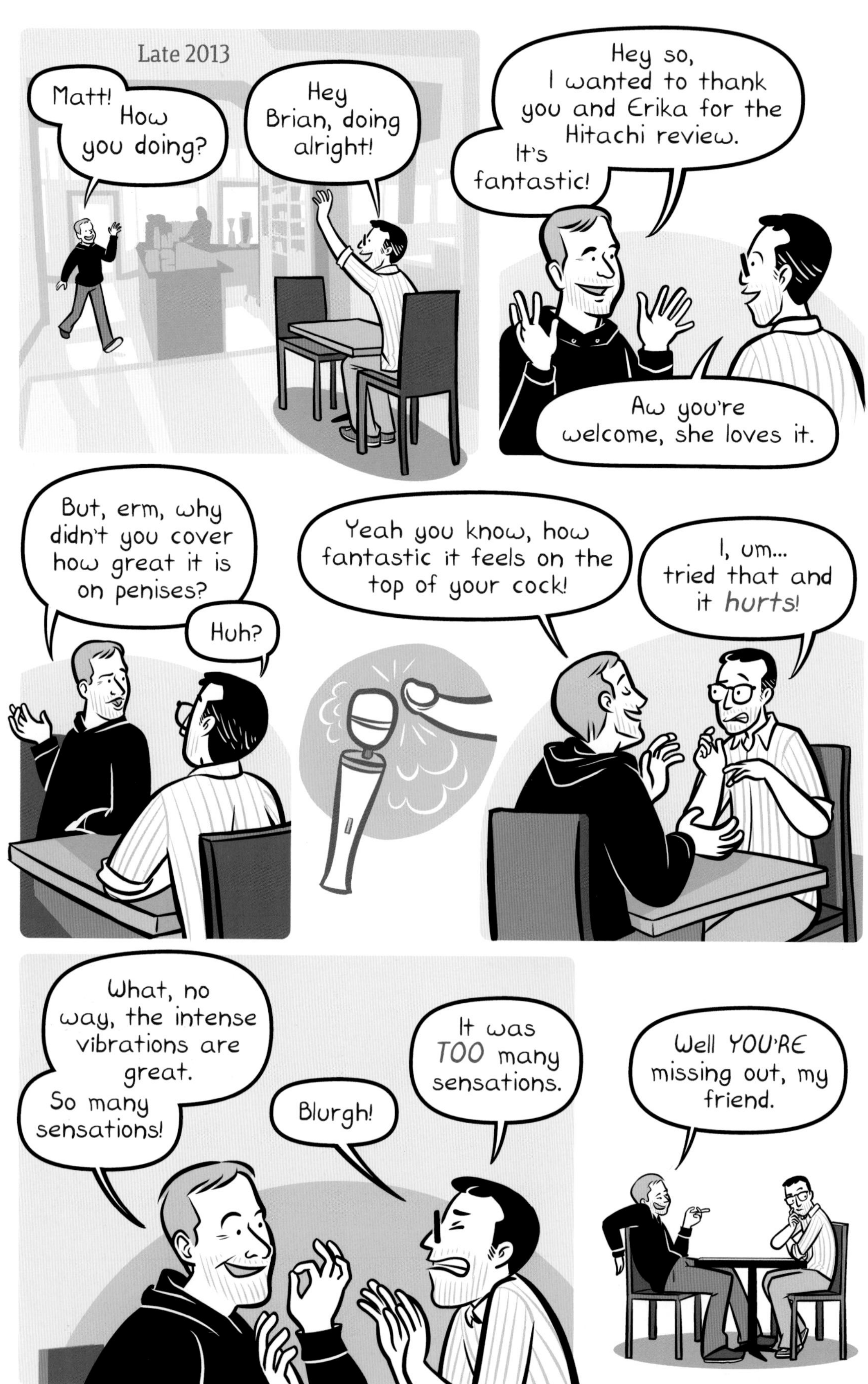
Late 2013
Matt! How you doing?
Hey Brian, doing alright!
Hey so, I wanted to thank you and Erika for the Hitachi review.
It's fantastic!
Aw you're welcome, she loves it.
But, erm, why didn't you cover how great it is on penises?
Huh?
Yeah you know, how fantastic it feels on the top of your cock!
I, um... tried that and it *hurts*!
What, no way, the intense vibrations are great.
So many sensations!
Blurgh!
It was *TOO* many sensations.
Well *YOU'RE* missing out, my friend.

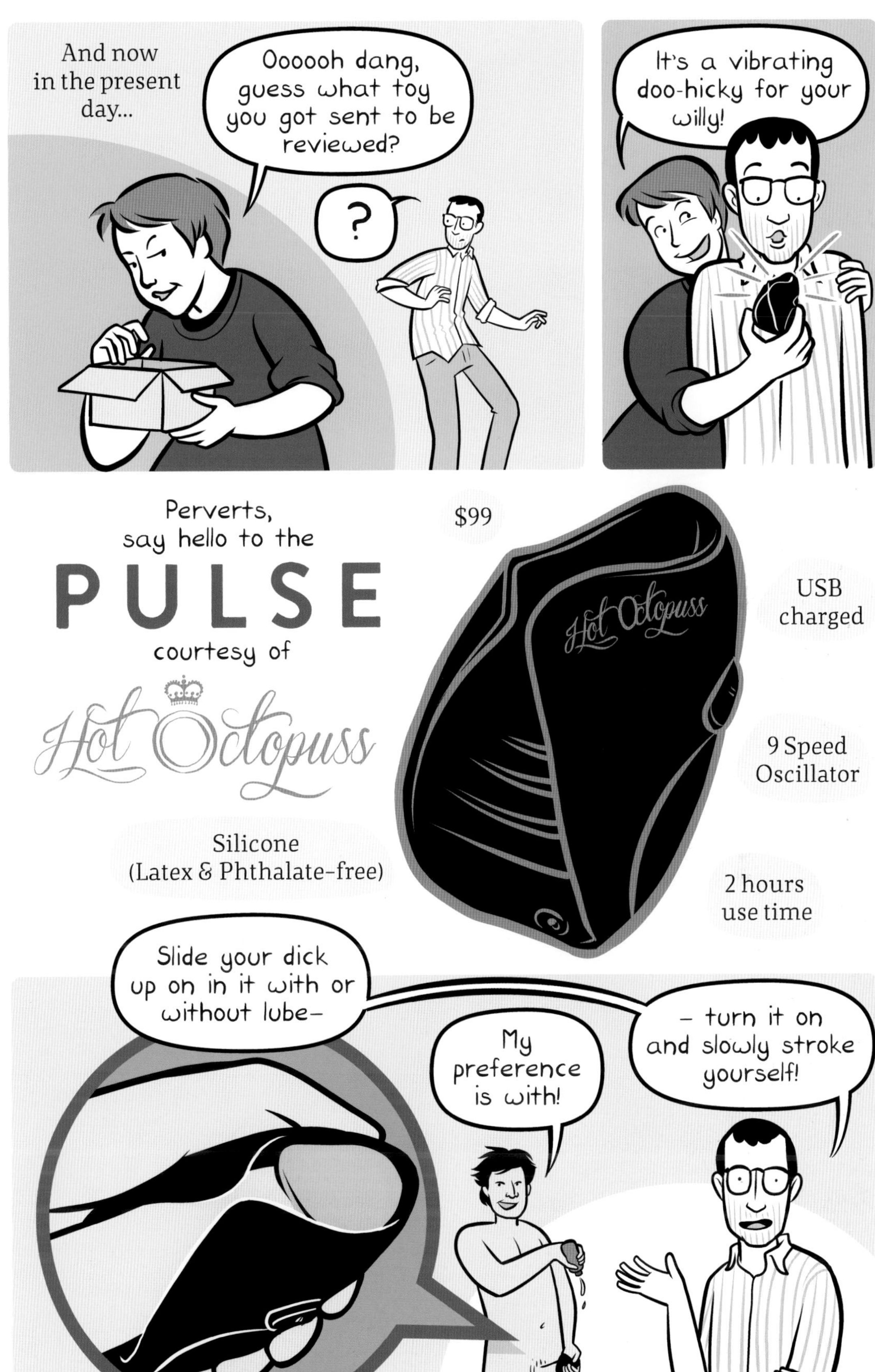
And now in the present day...
Oooooh dang, guess what toy you got sent to be reviewed?
?
It's a vibrating doo-hicky for your willy!
Perverts, say hello to the
PULSE
courtesy of
Hot Octopuss
$99
Hot Octopuss
USB charged
9 Speed Oscillator
Silicone (Latex & Phthalate-free)
2 hours use time
Slide your dick up on in it with or without lube–
– turn it on and slowly stroke yourself!
My preference is with!

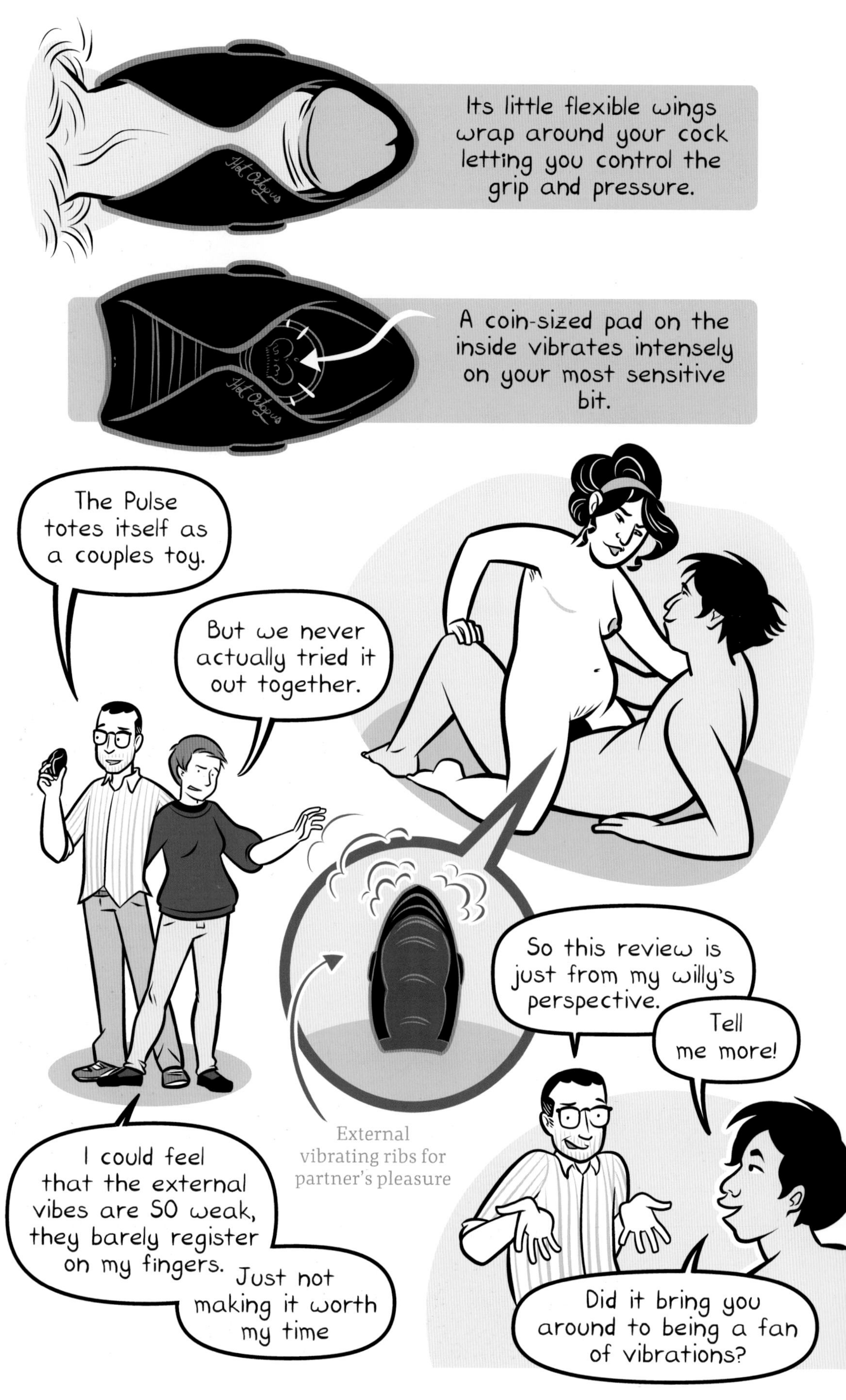
Its little flexible wings wrap around your cock letting you control the grip and pressure.
Hot Octopus
A coin-sized pad on the inside vibrates intensely on your most sensitive bit.
Hot Octopus
The Pulse totes itself as a couples toy.
But we never actually tried it out together.
External vibrating ribs for partner's pleasure
I could feel that the external vibes are SO weak, they barely register on my fingers.
Just not making it worth my time
So this review is just from my willy's perspective.
Tell me more!
Did it bring you around to being a fan of vibrations?

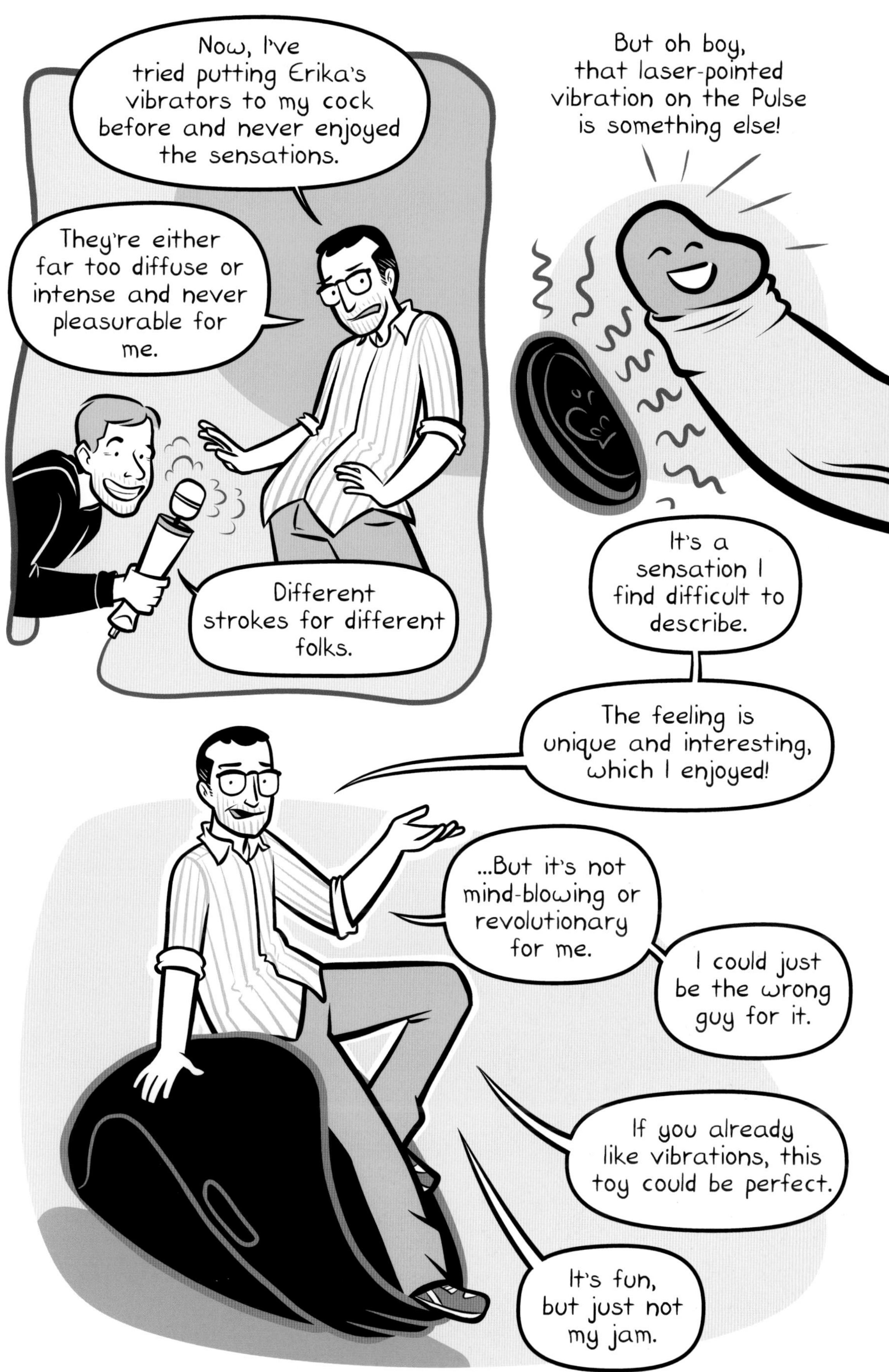
Now, I've tried putting Erika's vibrators to my cock before and never enjoyed the sensations.
They're either far too diffuse or intense and never pleasurable for me.
Different strokes for different folks.
But oh boy, that laser-pointed vibration on the Pulse is something else!
It's a sensation I find difficult to describe.
The feeling is unique and interesting, which I enjoyed!
...But it's not mind-blowing or revolutionary for me.
I could just be the wrong guy for it.
If you already like vibrations, this toy could be perfect.
It's fun, but just not my jam.

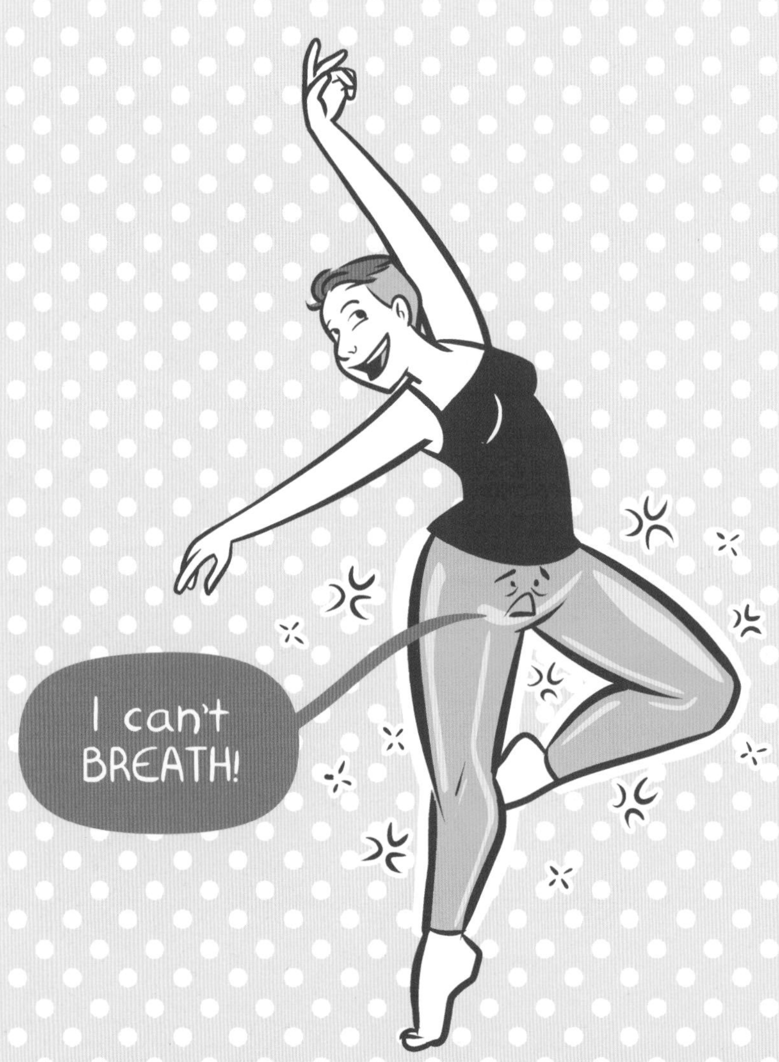
I can't
BREATH!

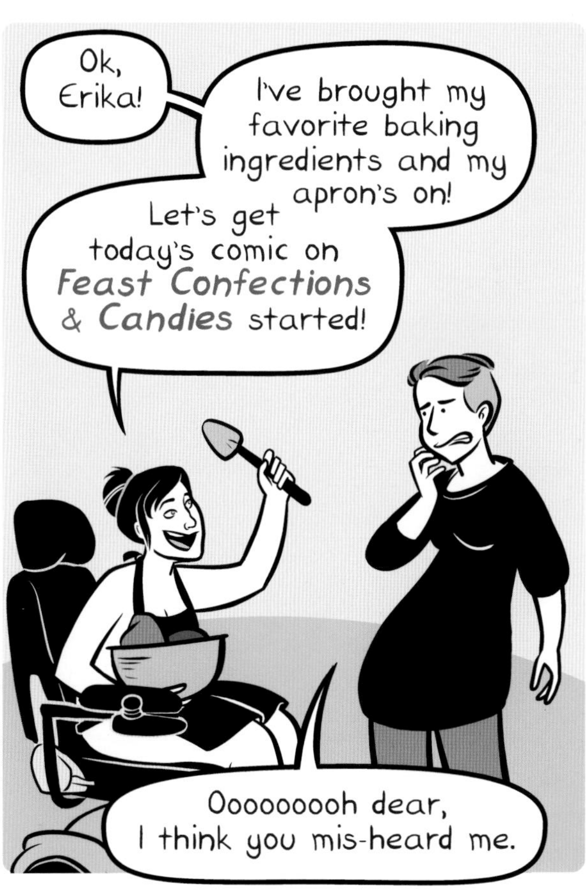
Ok, Erika!
I've brought my favorite baking ingredients and my apron's on!
Let's get today's comic on Feast Confections & Candies started!
Ooooooooh dear, I think you mis-heard me.

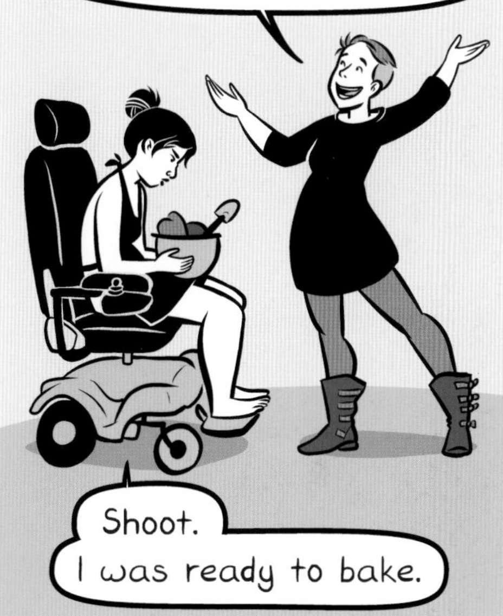
We're actually talking about the much less yummy Yeast Infections and Candidiasis
Shoot. I was ready to bake.

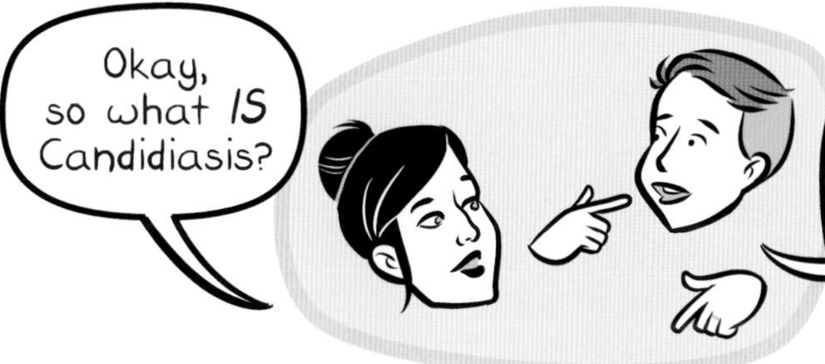
Okay, so what IS Candidiasis?
It is a super common & unpleasant fungal infection that can strike a variety of body parts, from mouths to toenails to genitals.

This comic is specifically about the vaginal kind, which is called a Yeast Infection.

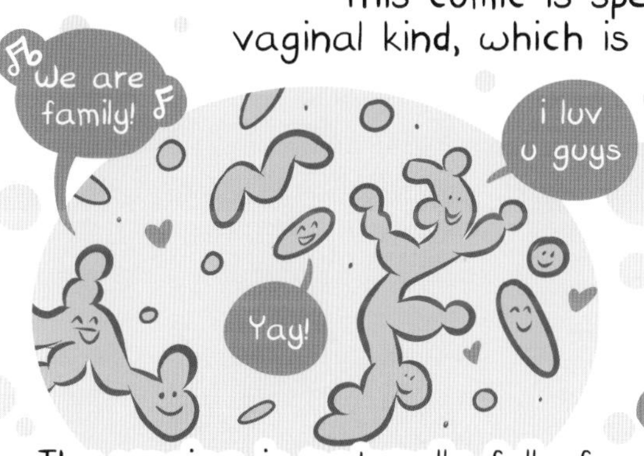

The vagina is naturally full of benign micro-organisms that live harmoniously inside that warm little ecosystem.

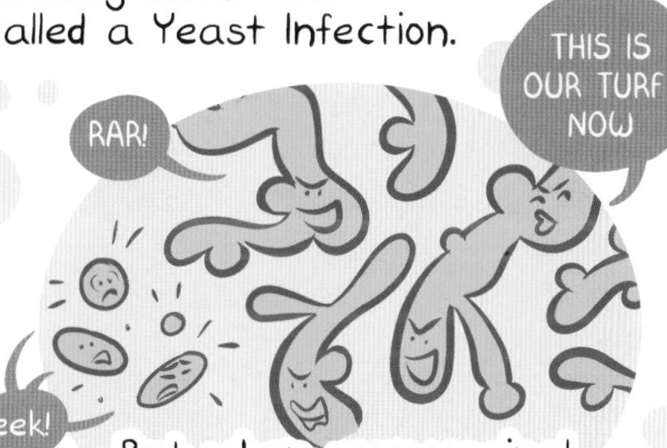

But when your vaginal acidity becomes unbalanced, the ever-present fungus candida albicans can grow out of control, resulting in a yeast infection.

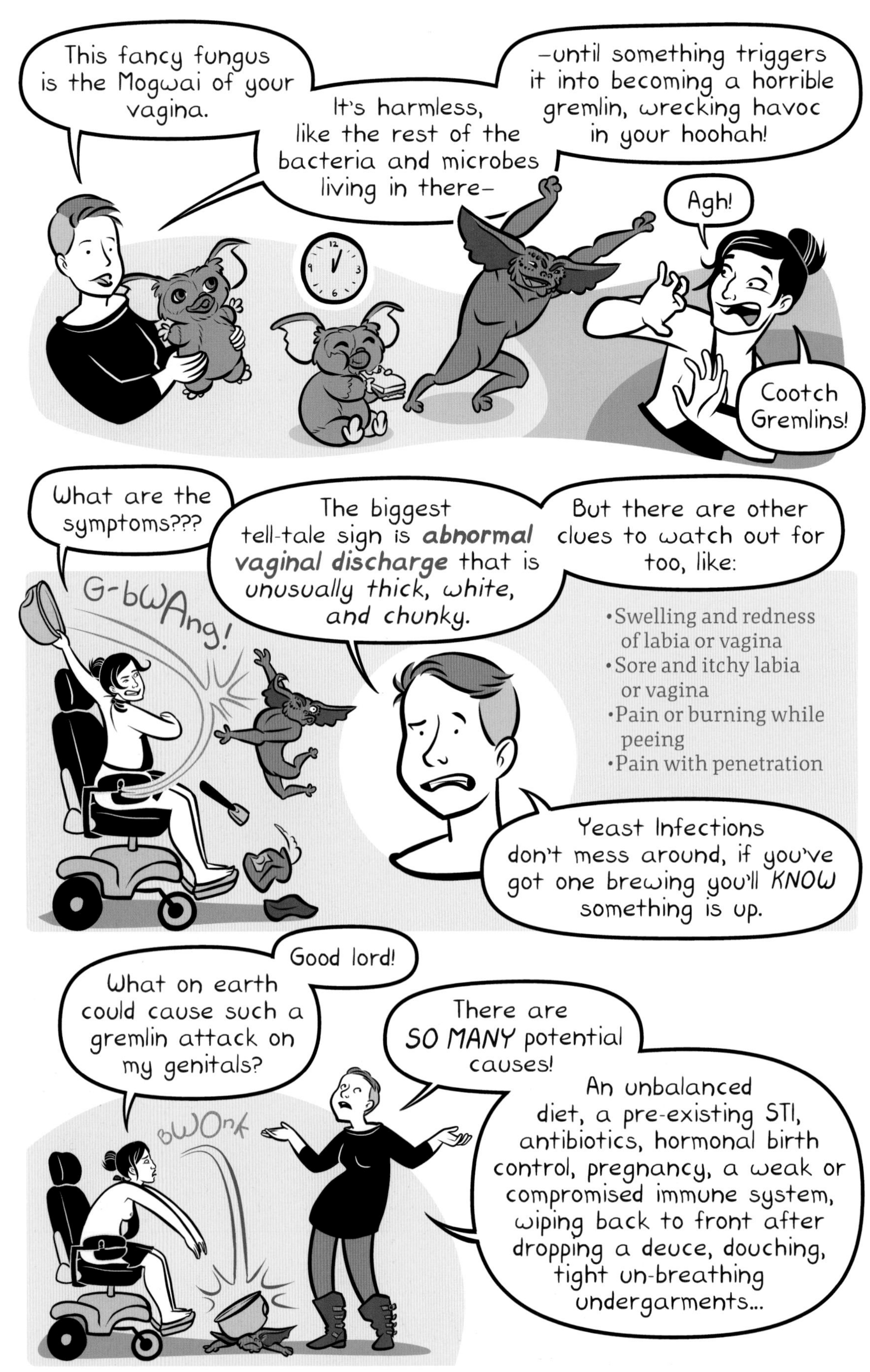
This fancy fungus is the Mogwai of your vagina.
It's harmless, like the rest of the bacteria and microbes living in there–
–until something triggers it into becoming a horrible gremlin, wrecking havoc in your hoohah!
Agh!
Cootch Gremlins!
What are the symptoms???
G-bWAng!
The biggest tell-tale sign is **abnormal vaginal discharge** that is *unusually thick, white, and chunky.*
But there are other clues to watch out for too, like:
• Swelling and redness of labia or vagina
• Sore and itchy labia or vagina
• Pain or burning while peeing
• Pain with penetration
Yeast Infections don't mess around, if you've got one brewing you'll *KNOW* something is up.
Good lord!
What on earth could cause such a gremlin attack on my genitals?
bWOnk
There are *SO MANY* potential causes!
An unbalanced diet, a pre-existing STI, antibiotics, hormonal birth control, pregnancy, a weak or compromised immune system, wiping back to front after dropping a deuce, douching, tight un-breathing undergarments...

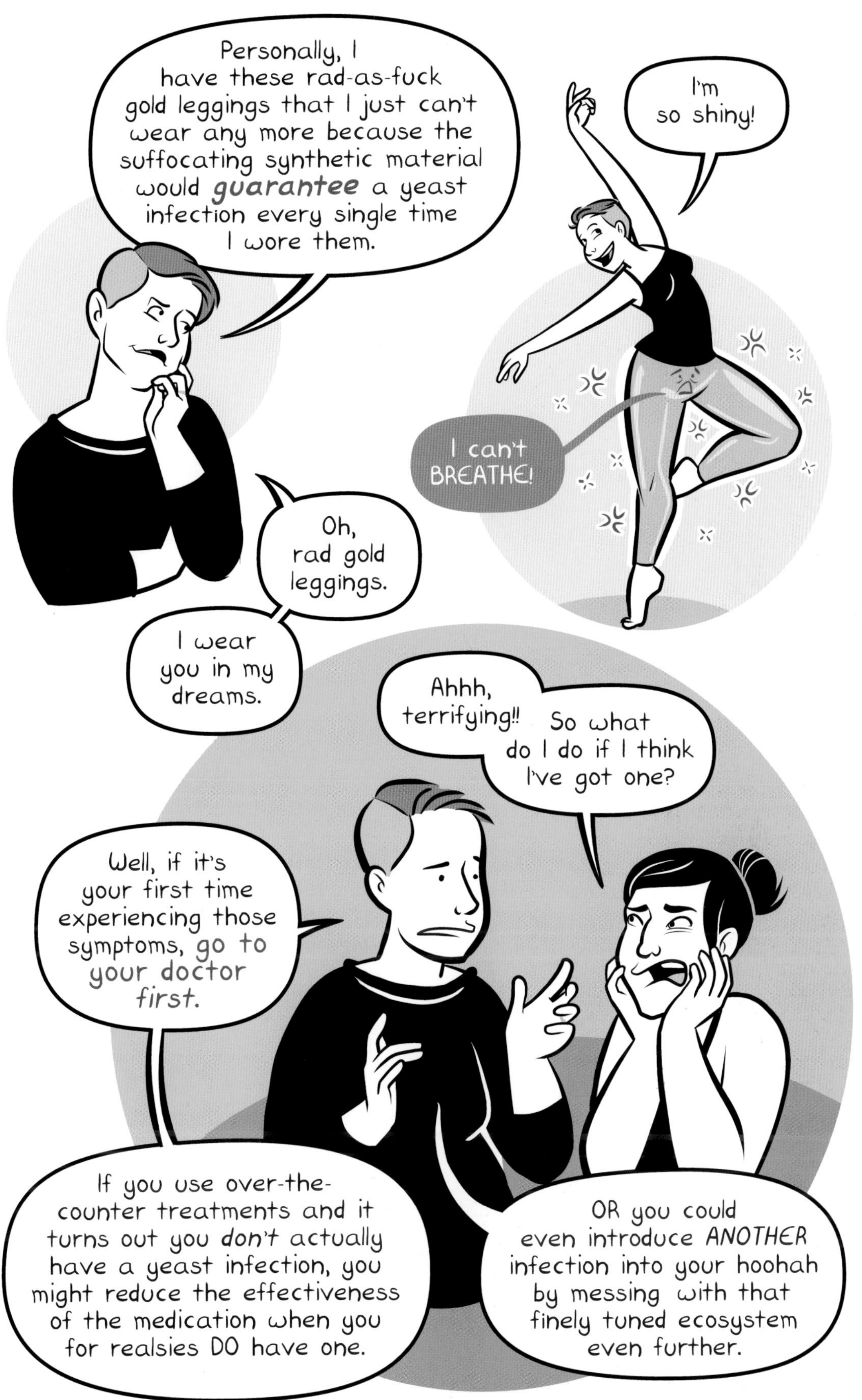

Personally, I have these rad-as-fuck gold leggings that I just can't wear any more because the suffocating synthetic material would guarantee a yeast infection every single time I wore them.
I'm so shiny!
I can't BREATHE!
Oh, rad gold leggings.
I wear you in my dreams.
Ahhh, terrifying!!
So what do I do if I think I've got one?
Well, if it's your first time experiencing those symptoms, go to your doctor first.
If you use over-the-counter treatments and it turns out you don't actually have a yeast infection, you might reduce the effectiveness of the medication when you for realsies DO have one.
OR you could even introduce ANOTHER infection into your hoohah by messing with that finely tuned ecosystem even further.

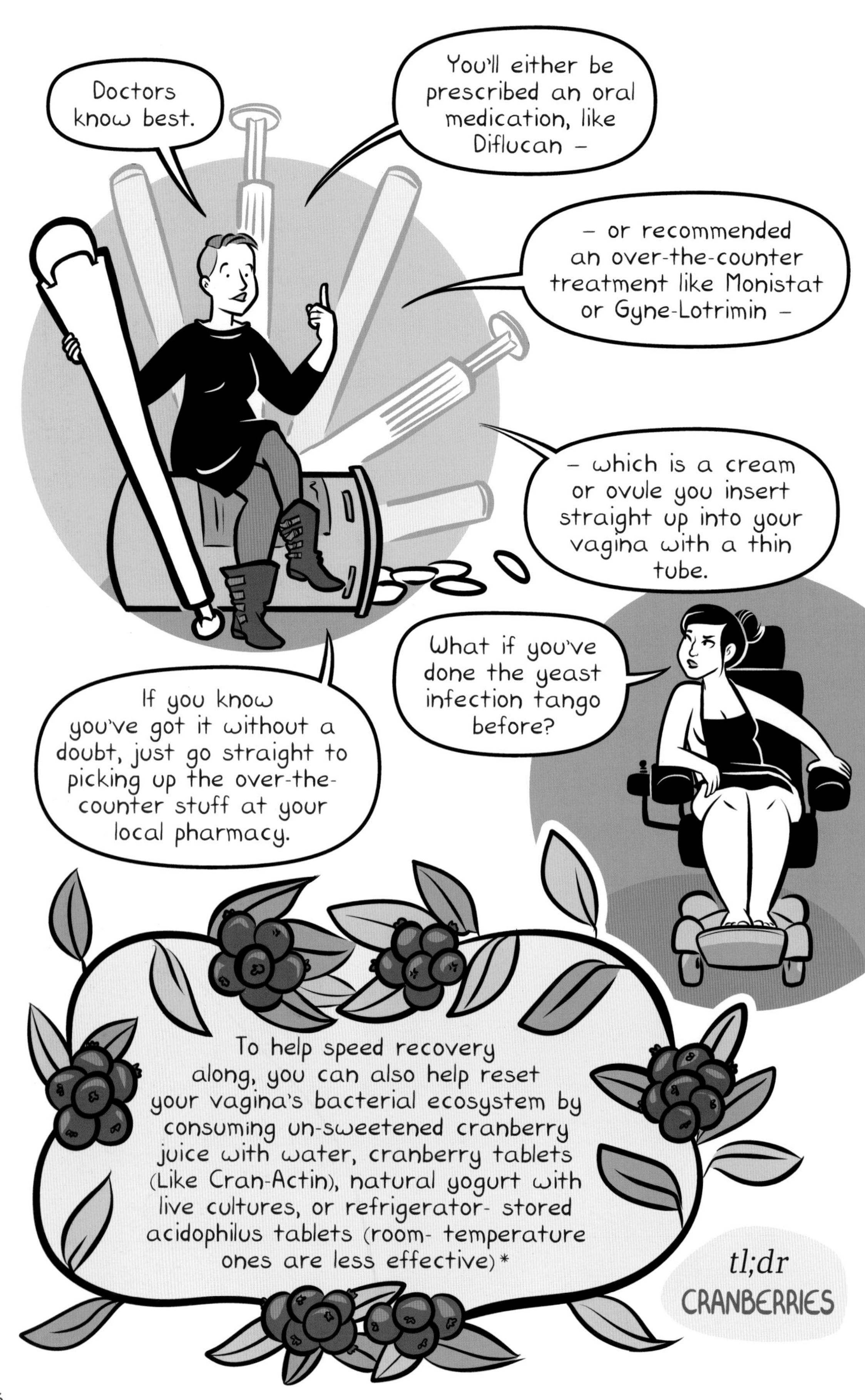
Doctors know best.
You'll either be prescribed an oral medication, like Diflucan –
– or recommended an over-the-counter treatment like Monistat or Gyne-Lotrimin –
– which is a cream or ovule you insert straight up into your vagina with a thin tube.
What if you've done the yeast infection tango before?
If you know you've got it without a doubt, just go straight to picking up the over-the-counter stuff at your local pharmacy.
To help speed recovery along, you can also help reset your vagina's bacterial ecosystem by consuming un-sweetened cranberry juice with water, cranberry tablets (Like Cran-Actin), natural yogurt with live cultures, or refrigerator- stored acidophilus tablets (room- temperature ones are less effective)*
tl;dr
CRANBERRIES

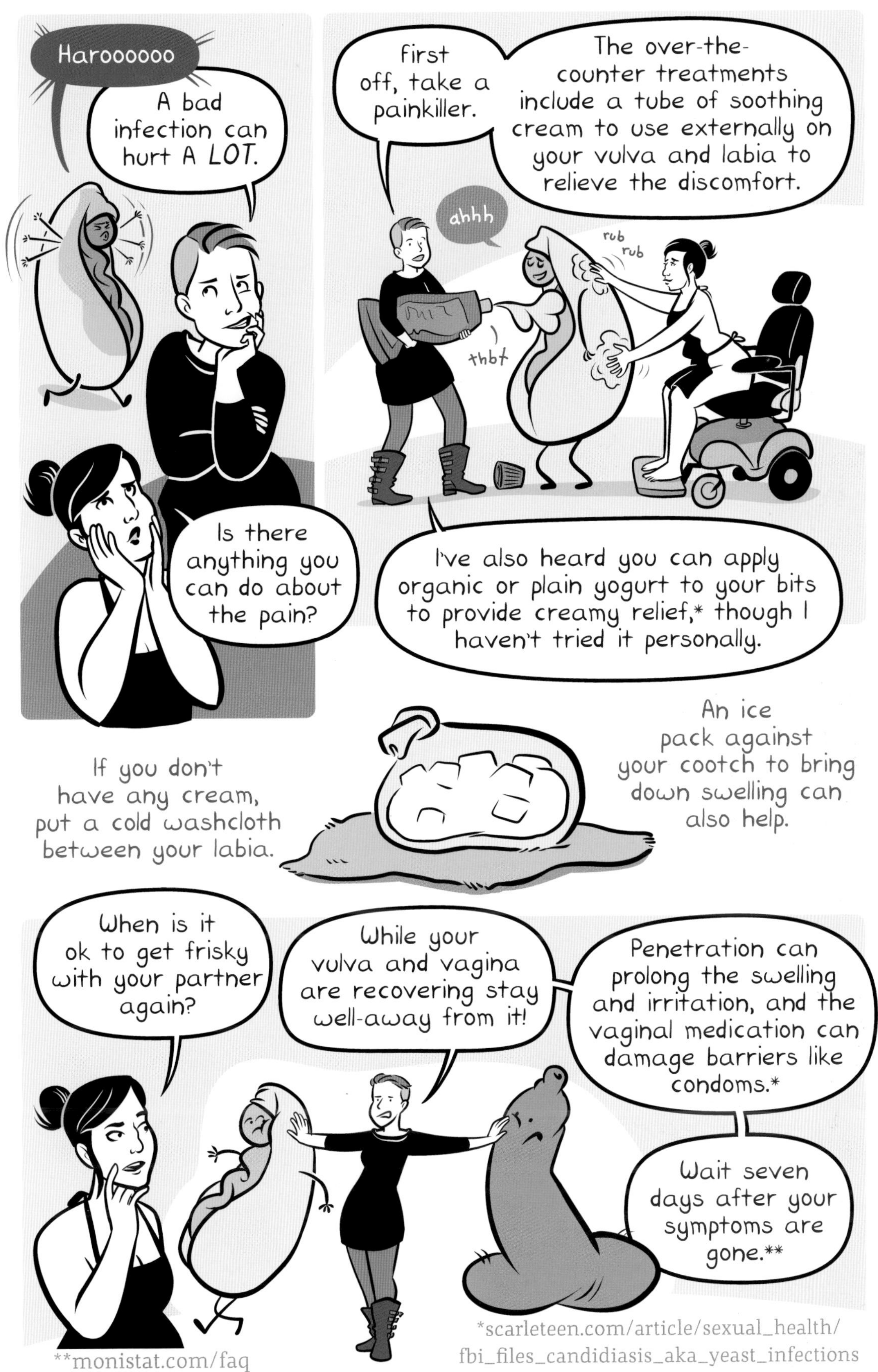
Haroooooo
A bad infection can hurt A LOT.
Is there anything you can do about the pain?
First off, take a painkiller.
The over-the-counter treatments include a tube of soothing cream to use externally on your vulva and labia to relieve the discomfort.
ahhh
rub rub
thbt
I've also heard you can apply organic or plain yogurt to your bits to provide creamy relief,* though I haven't tried it personally.
If you don't have any cream, put a cold washcloth between your labia.
An ice pack against your cootch to bring down swelling can also help.
When is it ok to get frisky with your partner again?
While your vulva and vagina are recovering stay well-away from it!
Penetration can prolong the swelling and irritation, and the vaginal medication can damage barriers like condoms.*
Wait seven days after your symptoms are gone.**

*scarleteen.com/article/sexual_health/fbi_files_candidiasis_aka_yeast_infections

**monistat.com/faq

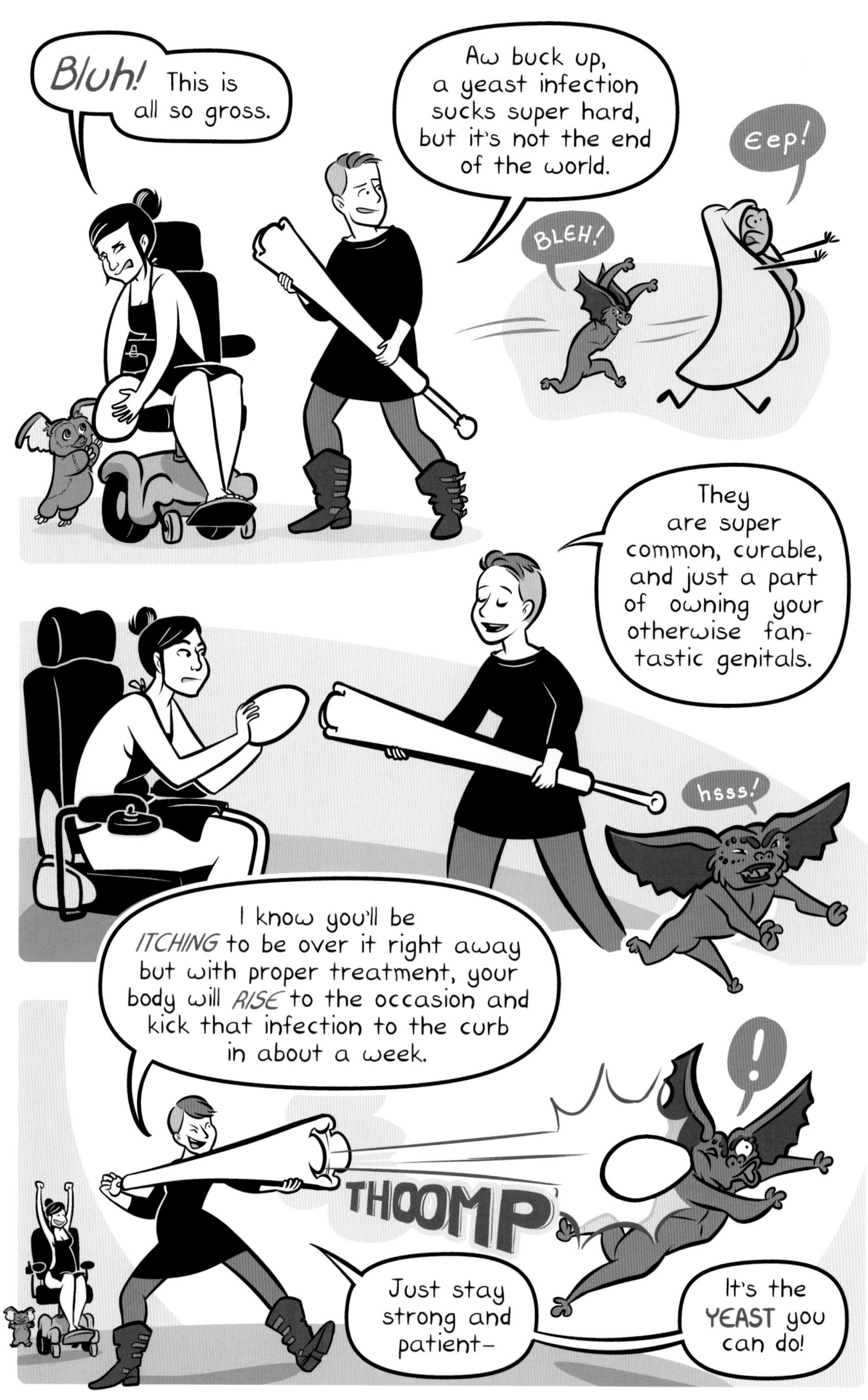
Bluh! This is all so gross.
Aw buck up, a yeast infection sucks super hard, but it's not the end of the world.
Eep!
BLEH!
They are super common, curable, and just a part of owning your otherwise fantastic genitals.
hsss!
I know you'll be ITCHING to be over it right away but with proper treatment, your body will RISE to the occasion and kick that infection to the curb in about a week.
!
THOOMP
Just stay strong and patient–
It's the YEAST you can do!

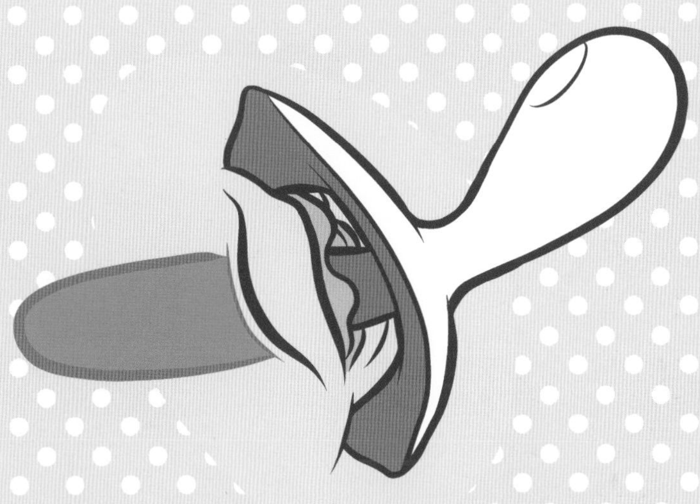

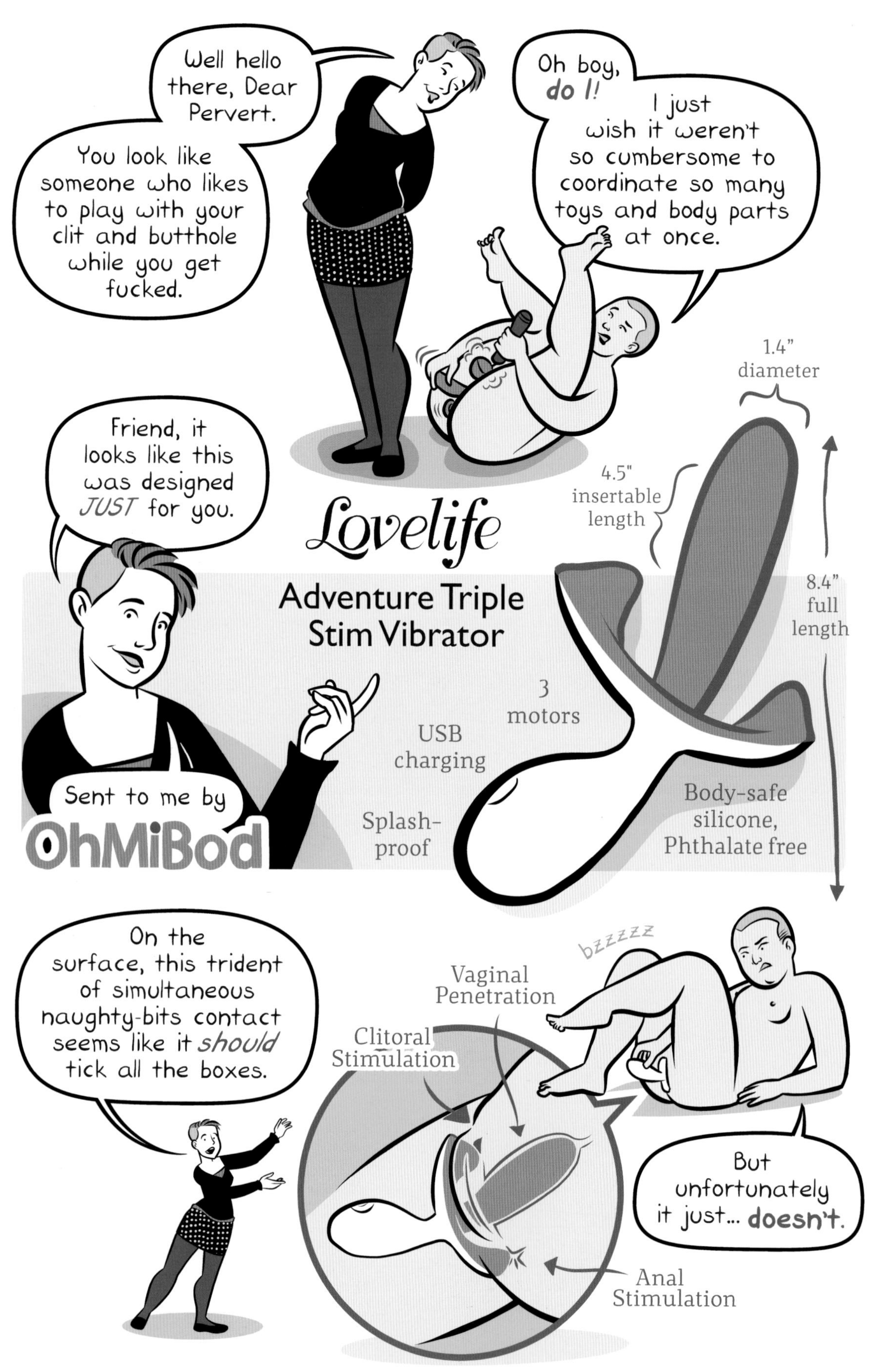
Well hello there, Dear Pervert.
You look like someone who likes to play with your clit and butthole while you get fucked.
Oh boy, do I!
I just wish it weren't so cumbersome to coordinate so many toys and body parts at once.
Friend, it looks like this was designed JUST for you.
Lovelife
Adventure Triple Stim Vibrator
1.4" diameter
4.5" insertable length
8.4" full length
3 motors
USB charging
Splash-proof
Body-safe silicone, Phthalate free
Sent to me by
OhMiBod
On the surface, this trident of simultaneous naughty-bits contact seems like it should tick all the boxes.
bzzzzz
Vaginal Penetration
Clitoral Stimulation
Anal Stimulation
But unfortunately it just... doesn't.

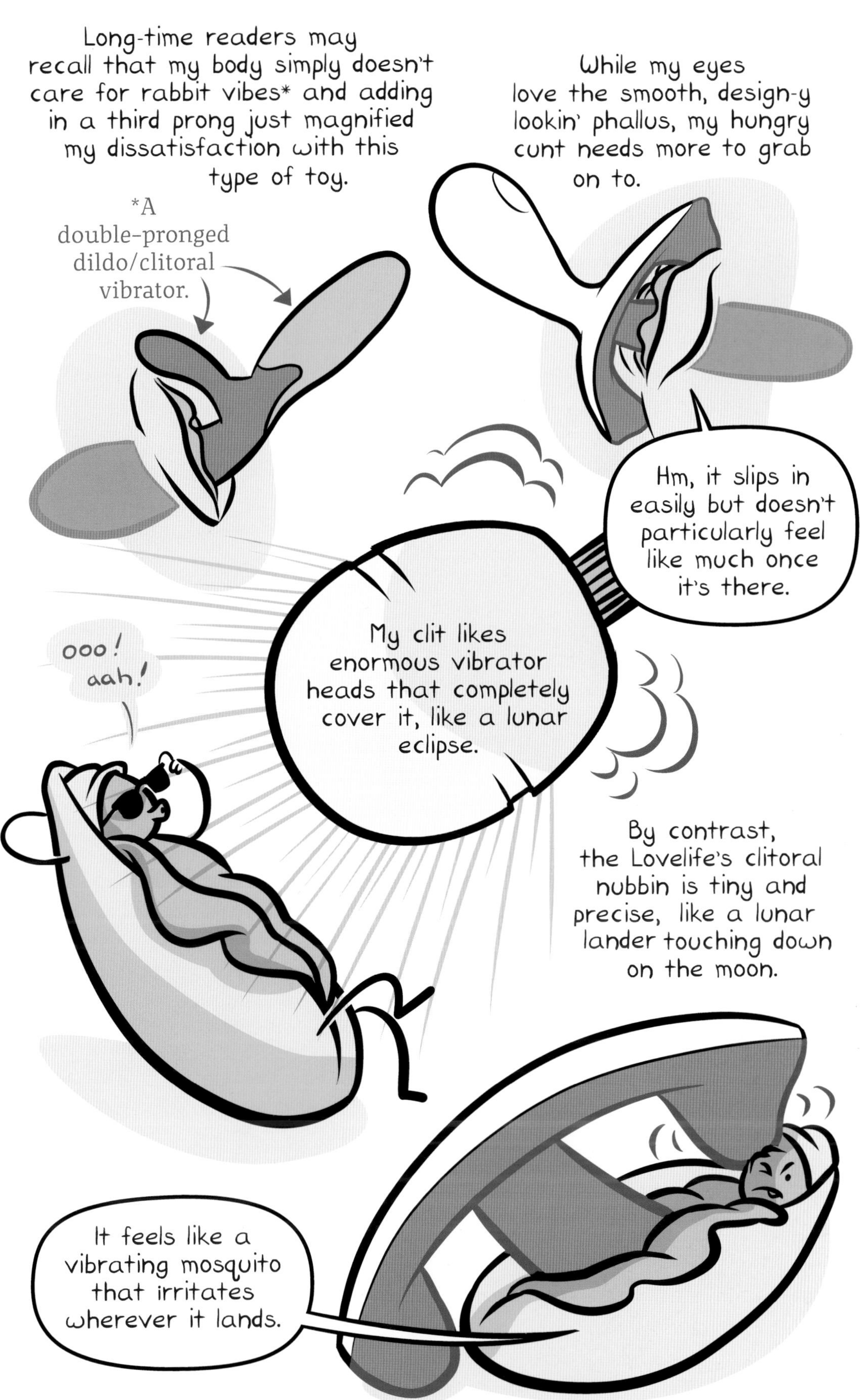
Long-time readers may recall that my body simply doesn't care for rabbit vibes* and adding in a third prong just magnified my dissatisfaction with this type of toy.
*A double-pronged dildo/clitoral vibrator.
While my eyes love the smooth, design-y lookin' phallus, my hungry cunt needs more to grab on to.
Hm, it slips in easily but doesn't particularly feel like much once it's there.
My clit likes enormous vibrator heads that completely cover it, like a lunar eclipse.
ooo! aah!
By contrast, the Lovelife's clitoral nubbin is tiny and precise, like a lunar lander touching down on the moon.
It feels like a vibrating mosquito that irritates wherever it lands.

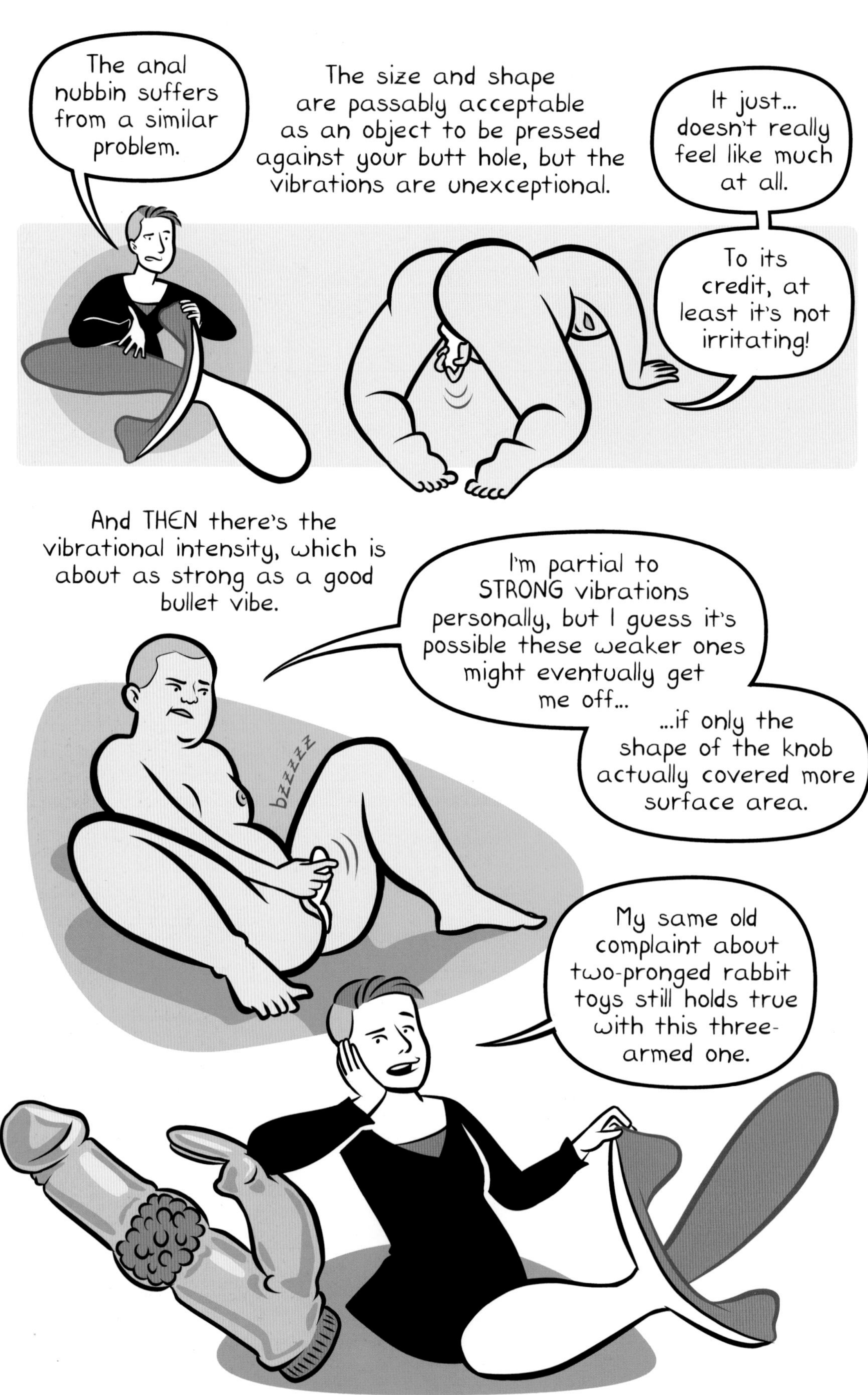
The anal nubbin suffers from a similar problem.
The size and shape are passably acceptable as an object to be pressed against your butt hole, but the vibrations are unexceptional.
It just... doesn't really feel like much at all.
To its credit, at least it's not irritating!
And THEN there's the vibrational intensity, which is about as strong as a good bullet vibe.
I'm partial to STRONG vibrations personally, but I guess it's possible these weaker ones might eventually get me off...
...if only the shape of the knob actually covered more surface area.
bzzzzz
My same old complaint about two-pronged rabbit toys still holds true with this three-armed one.

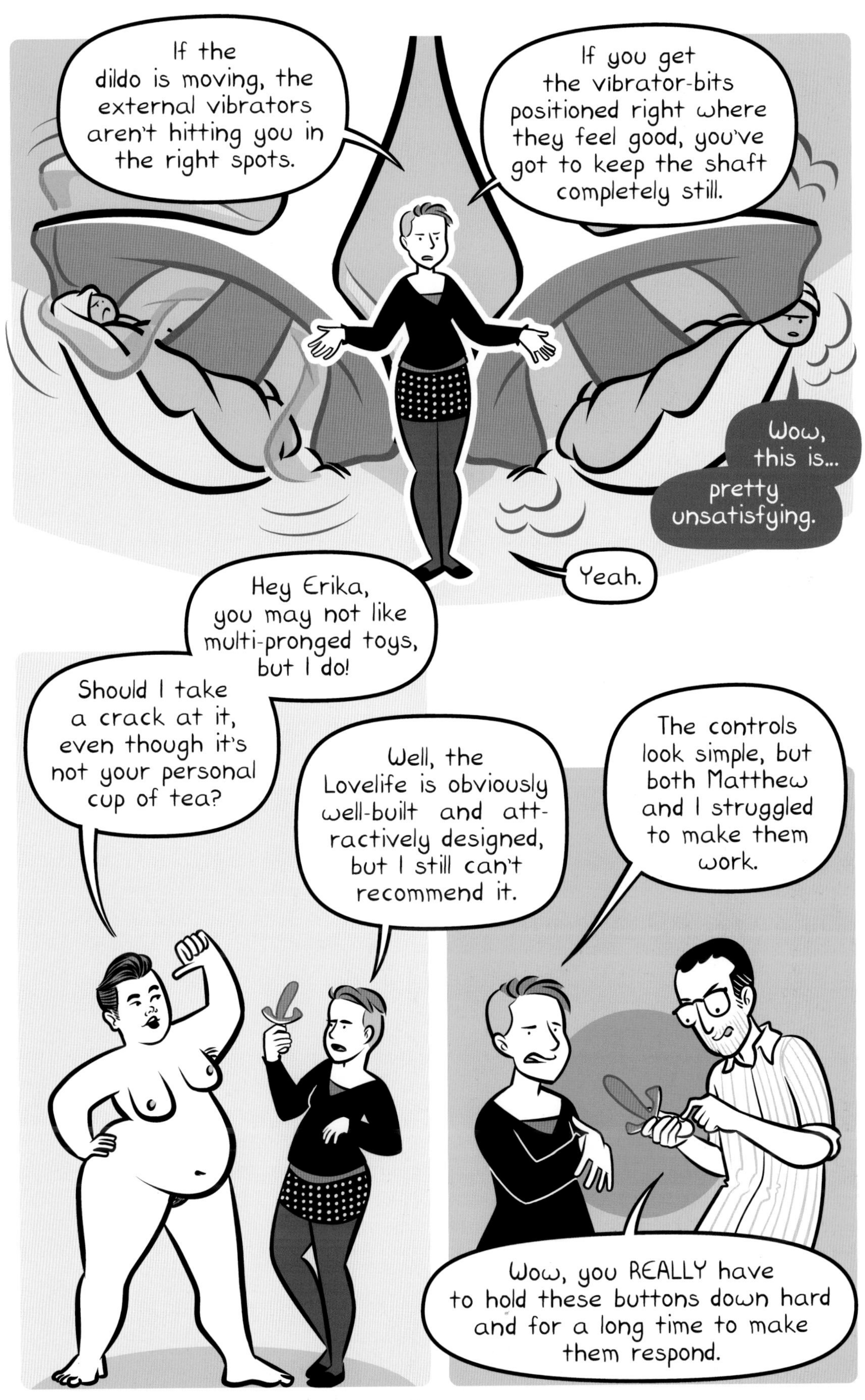
If the dildo is moving, the external vibrators aren't hitting you in the right spots.
If you get the vibrator-bits positioned right where they feel good, you've got to keep the shaft completely still.
Wow, this is...
pretty unsatisfying.
Yeah.
Hey Erika, you may not like multi-pronged toys, but I do!
Should I take a crack at it, even though it's not your personal cup of tea?
Well, the Lovelife is obviously well-built and attractively designed, but I still can't recommend it.
The controls look simple, but both Matthew and I struggled to make them work.
Wow, you REALLY have to hold these buttons down hard and for a long time to make them respond.

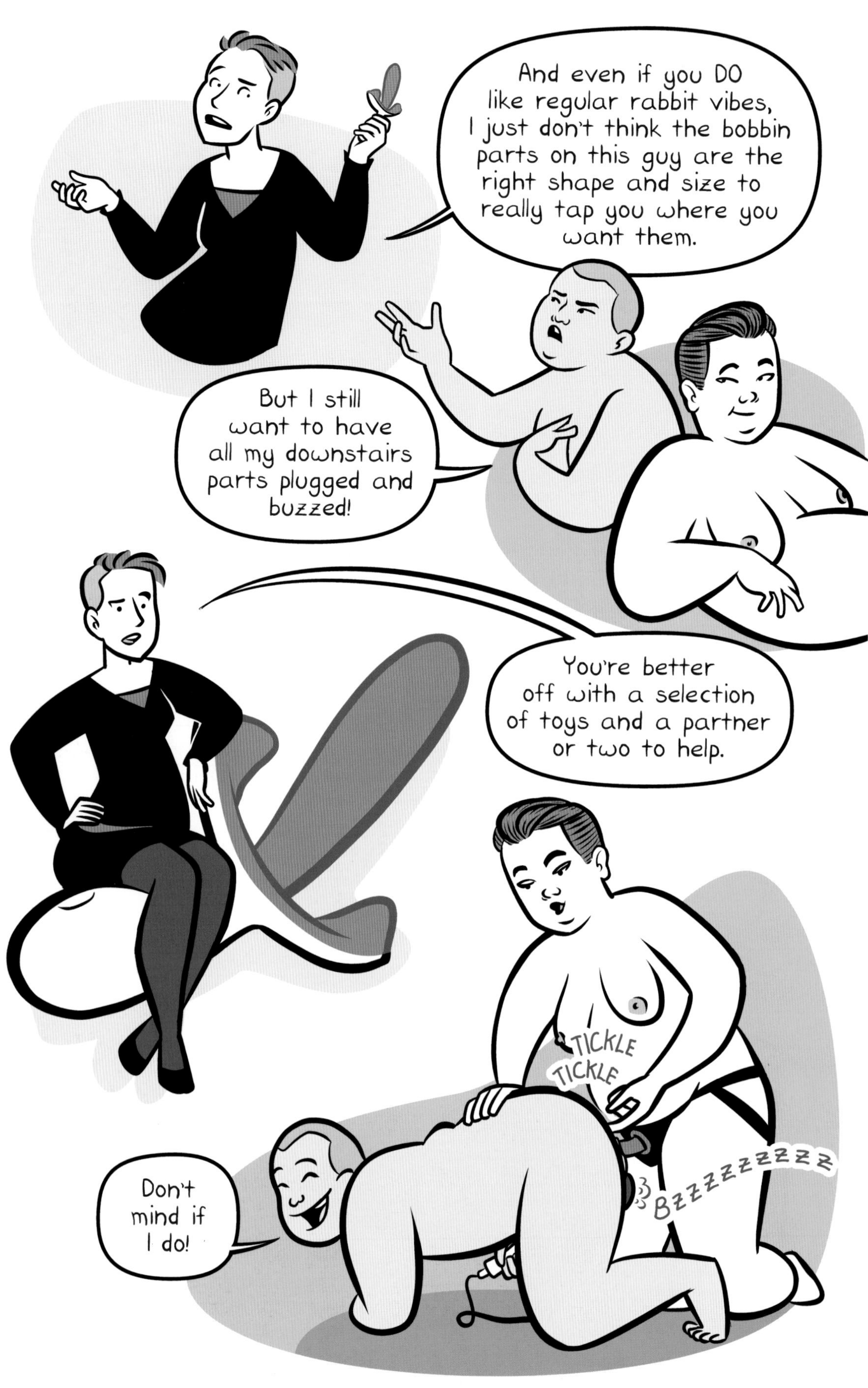
And even if you DO like regular rabbit vibes, I just don't think the bobbin parts on this guy are the right shape and size to really tap you where you want them.
But I still want to have all my downstairs parts plugged and buzzed!
You're better off with a selection of toys and a partner or two to help.
TICKLE
TICKLE
BZZZZZZZZZZ
Don't mind if I do!

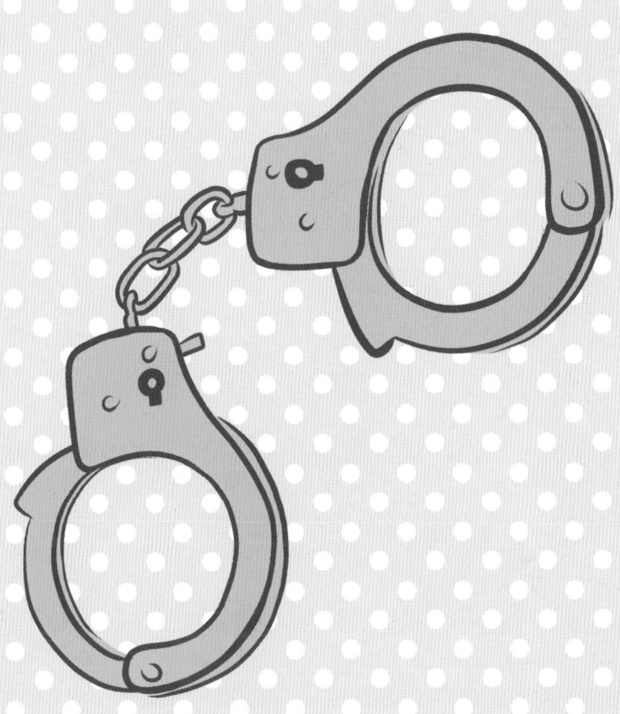

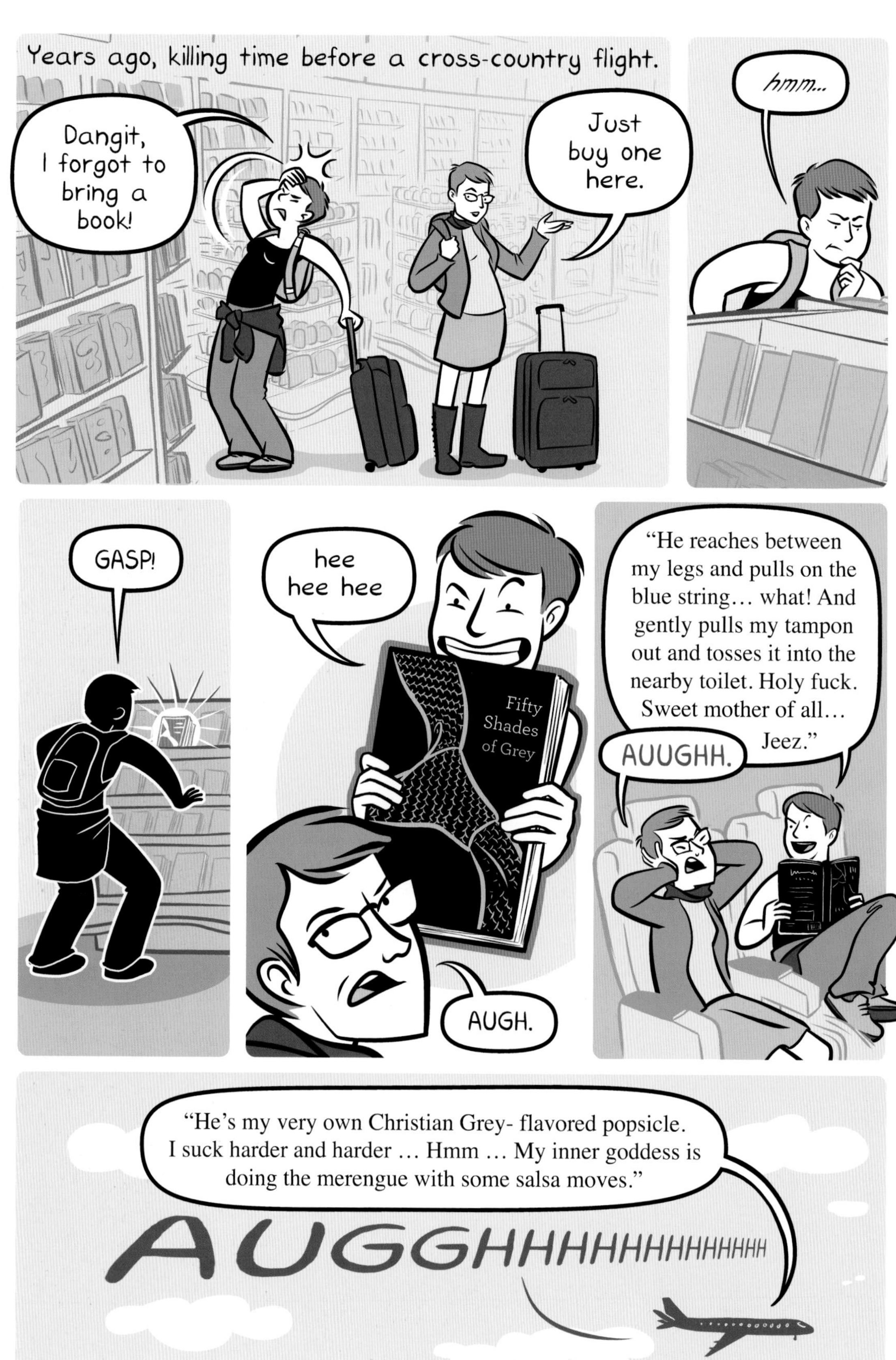

We all know the story by now.

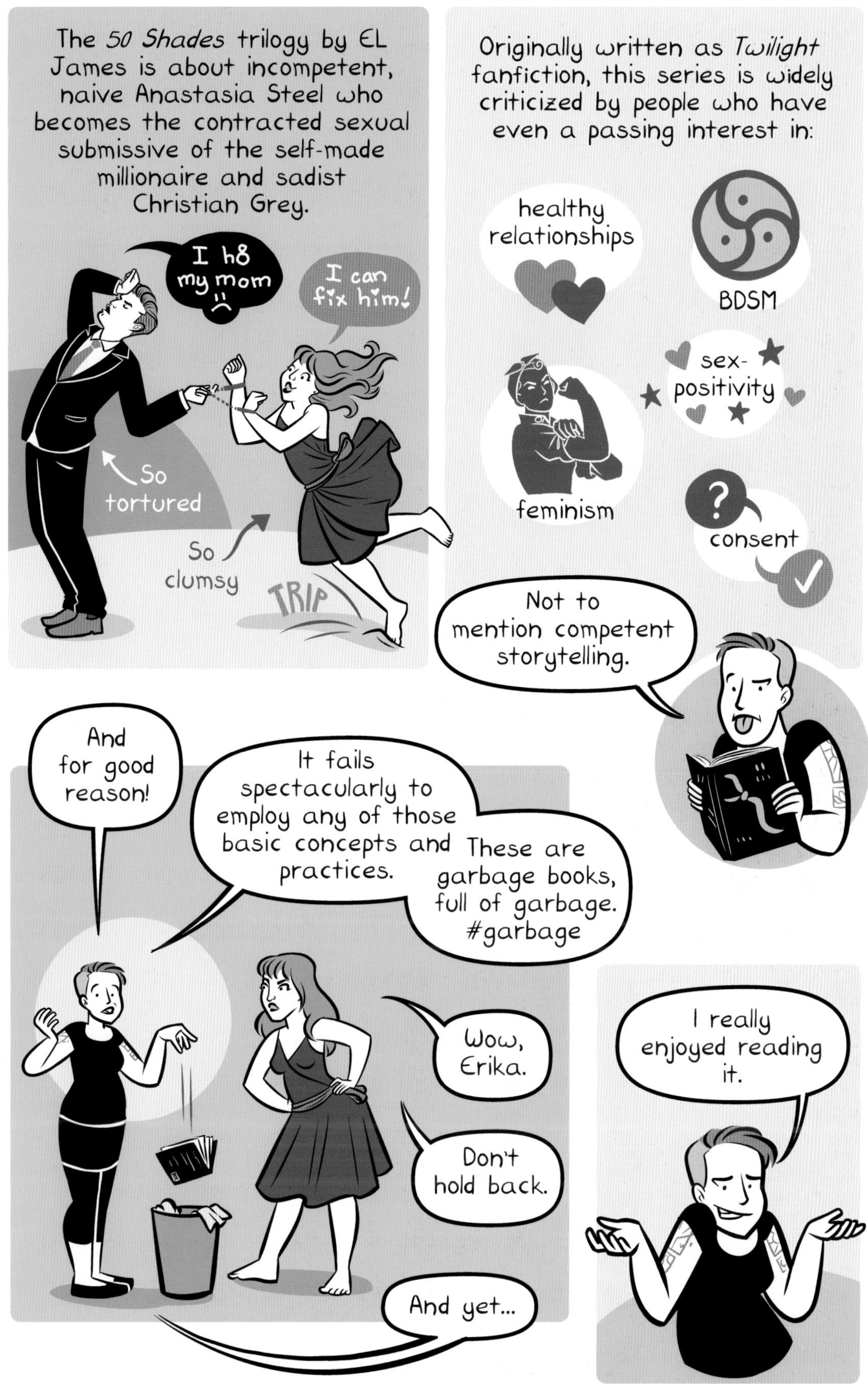
The *50 Shades* trilogy by EL James is about incompetent, naive Anastasia Steel who becomes the contracted sexual submissive of the self-made millionaire and sadist Christian Grey.
I h8 my mom :(
I can fix him!
So tortured
So clumsy
TRIP
Originally written as *Twilight* fanfiction, this series is widely criticized by people who have even a passing interest in:
healthy relationships
BDSM
sex-positivity
feminism
consent
Not to mention competent storytelling.
And for good reason!
It fails spectacularly to employ any of those basic concepts and practices.
These are garbage books, full of garbage. #garbage
Wow, Erika.
Don't hold back.
And yet...
I really enjoyed reading it.

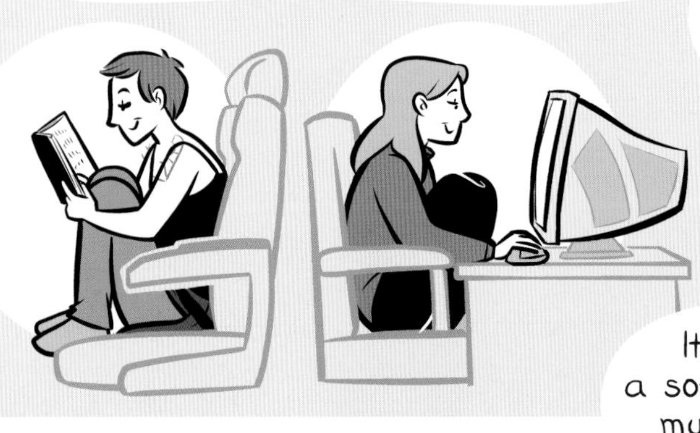
50 Shades unexpectedly tapped into my decades-old buried memories of reading terrible erotic Sonic the Hedgehog fanfiction as an adolescent in the '90s.
There's this certain unsophisticated style that's ever-present amongst juvenile fandom writers.
It's so earnest, so unvarnished, so devoid of real life experience and nuance.
It holds a soft spot in my heart.

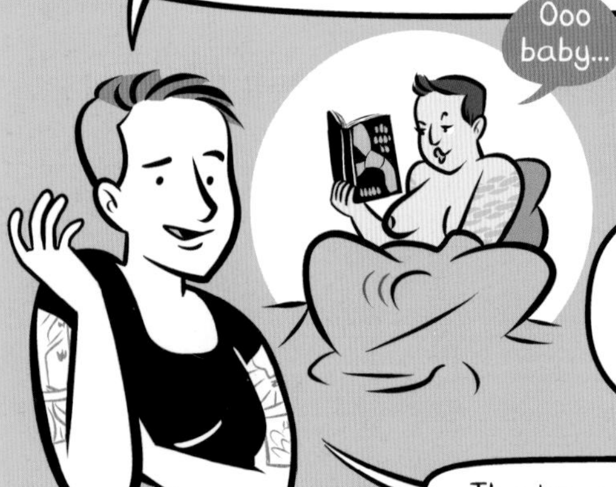
As a sex-positive feminist, I know I'm supposed to condemn this series for contradicting my agenda...
Ooo baby...
but I just can't.
This story is making a lot of readers happy and turning them on.
That's cool with me.
...Erika, *how **could** you?*

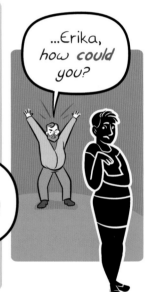

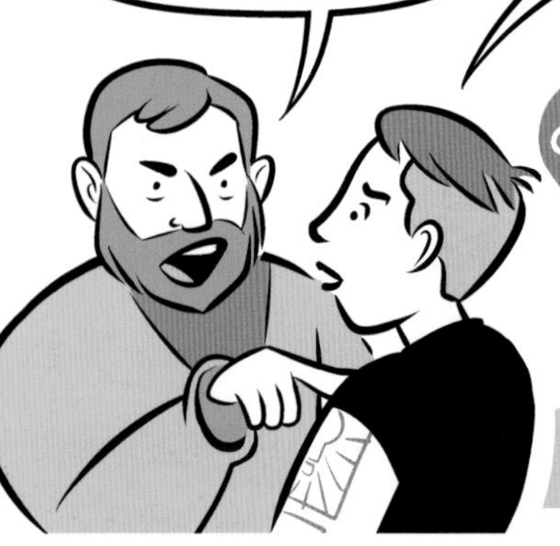
50 Shades is the antithesis of healthy sexual relationships and proper BDSM practices!!!
Well... I'm just not into policing what people are allowed to find arousing in their fantasy porn.

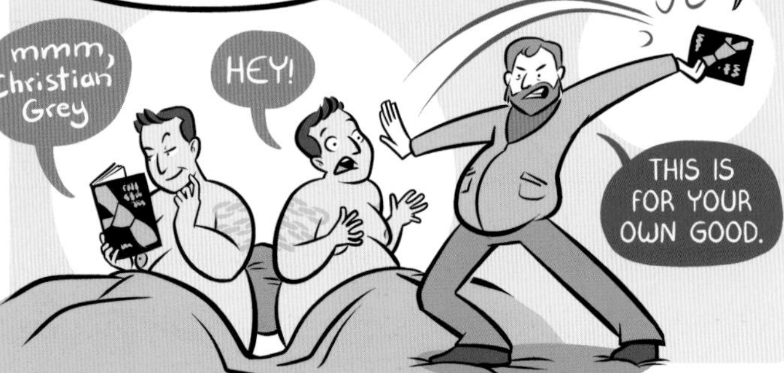
But what if easily impressionable people read this and use it in real life?
mmm, Christian Grey
HEY!
THIS IS FOR YOUR OWN GOOD.

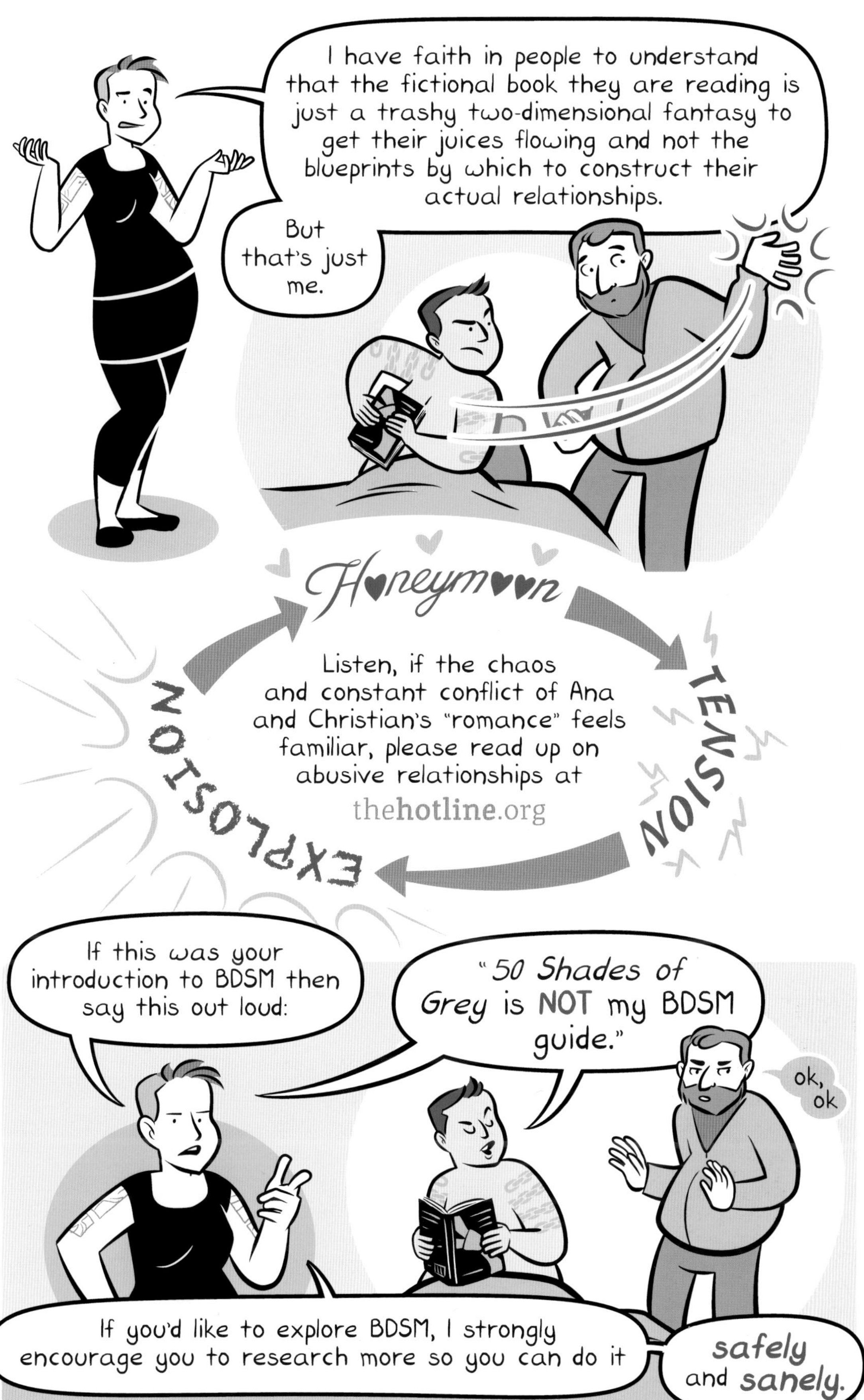
I have faith in people to understand that the fictional book they are reading is just a trashy two-dimensional fantasy to get their juices flowing and not the blueprints by which to construct their actual relationships.
But that's just me.
Honeymoon
Tension
Explosion
Listen, if the chaos and constant conflict of Ana and Christian's "romance" feels familiar, please read up on abusive relationships at
thehotline.org
If this was your introduction to BDSM then say this out loud:
"*50 Shades of Grey* is **NOT** my BDSM guide."
ok, ok
If you'd like to explore BDSM, I strongly encourage you to research more so you can do it
safely and sanely.

Unlike this work of fiction, you're a real person who can be hurt physically and emotionally, so make sure you don't unintentionally damage yourself or your partner.

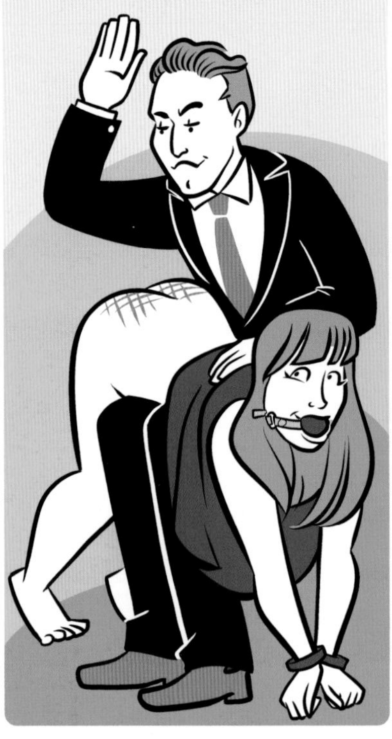

You deserve to have the best, most fulfilling BDSM experience, so do it right!

I've heard seasoned kinksters recommend Tristan Taormino's "*50 Shades of Kink*", give that a try.

TRISTAN TAORMINO
50 shades of kink
AN INTRODUCTION TO BDSM

The *50 Shades* series is junk food.

Fifty Shades Freed
E L James

Fifty Shades Darker
E L James

It's fun to eat every now and then, but don't believe for a second that it's got any nutritional value.

If you can consume fiction without basing your life on it, then there's no harm in giving it a read to see what all the fuss is about.

It's bad in a fun way, and I certainly don't regret reading it...

...just like I don't regret consuming the occasional Big Mac.

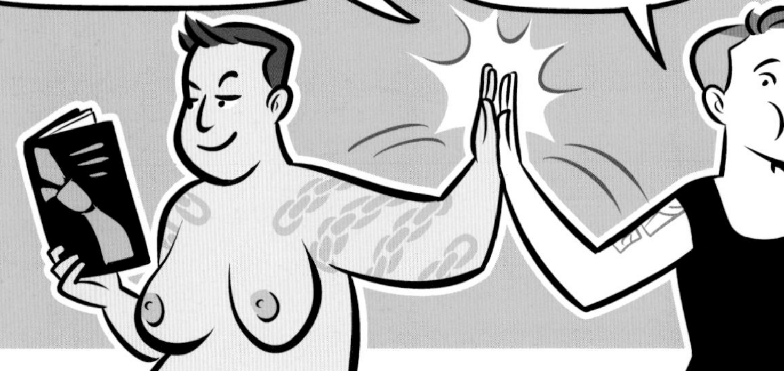

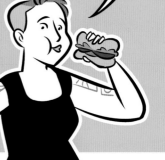

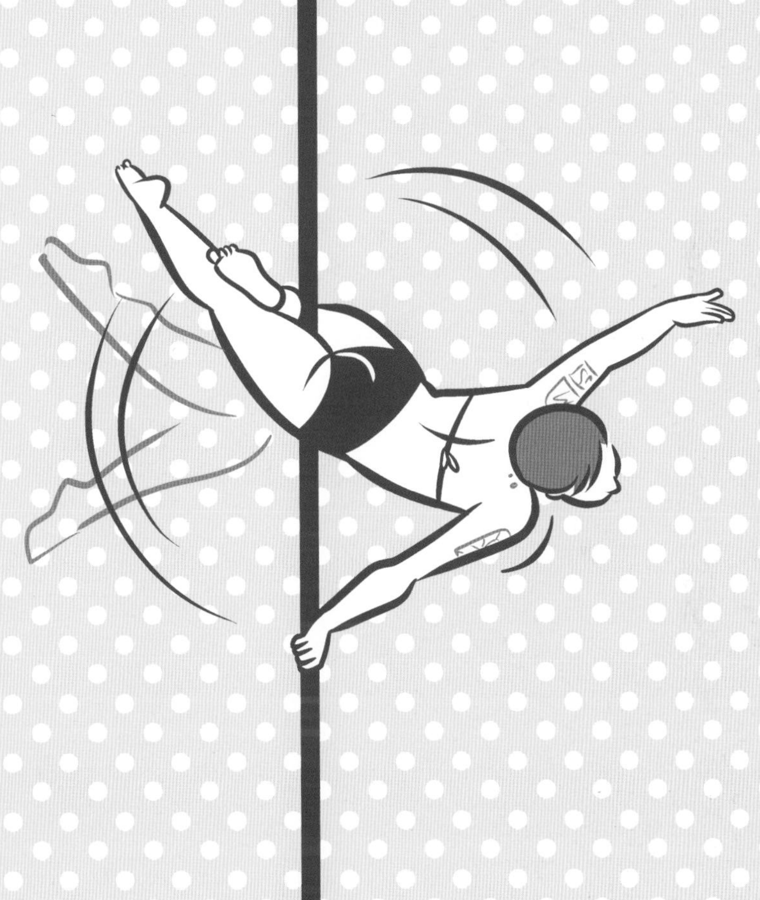

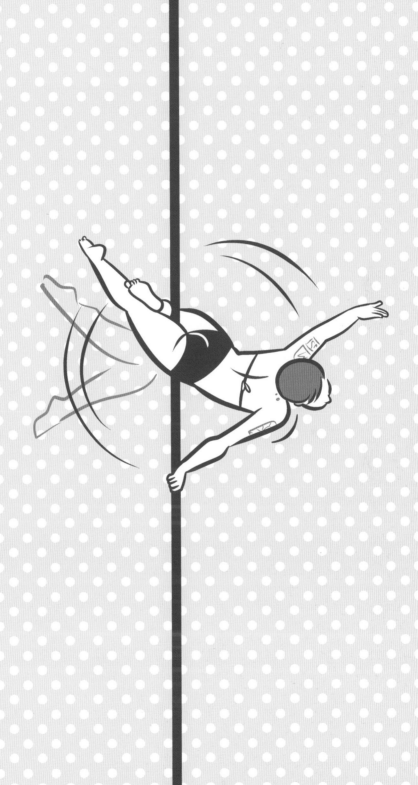

I have never been athletic.

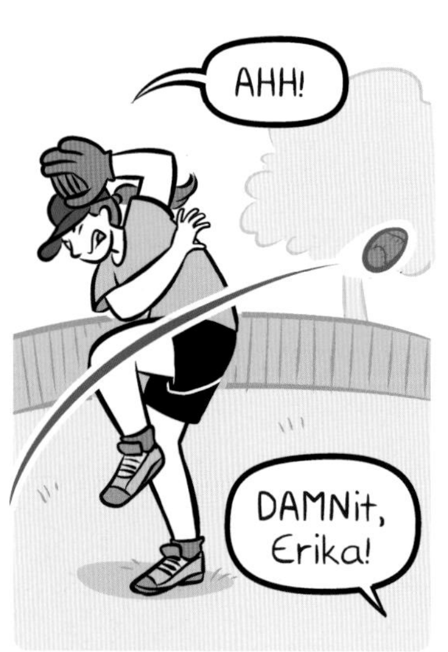
AHH!
DAMNit, Erika!

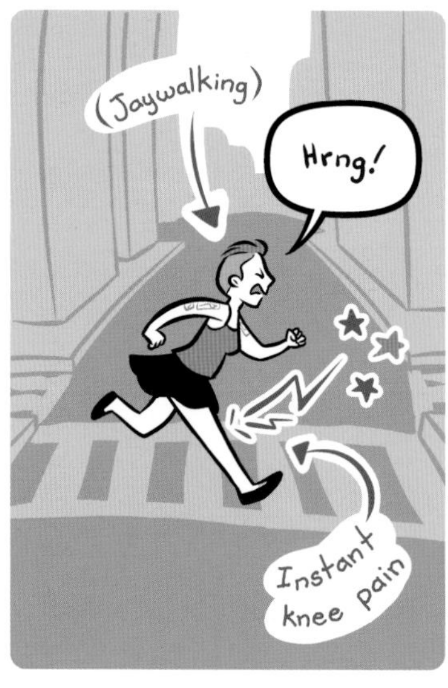
(Jaywalking)
Hrng!
Instant knee pain

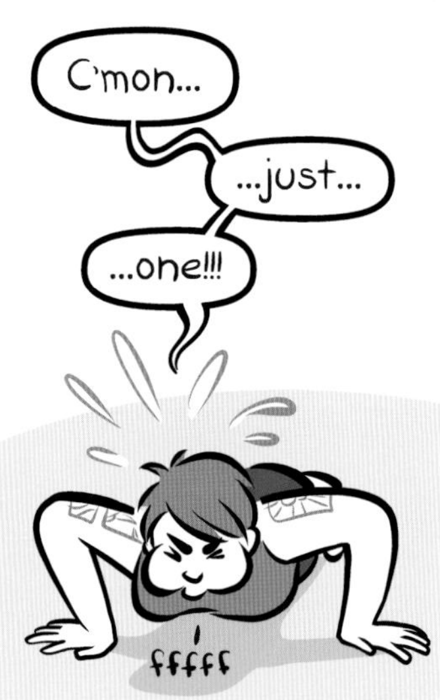
C'mon...
...just...
...one!!!
fffff

But like many people, I NEED exercise to help manage my depression and anxiety, not to mention keep my body healthy.

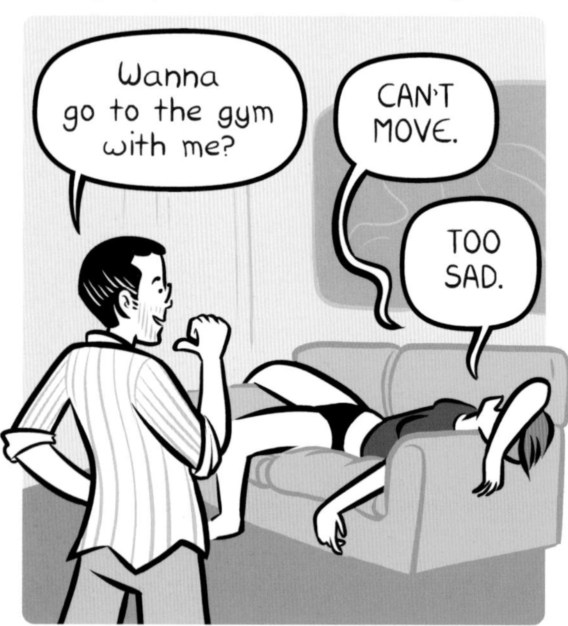
Wanna go to the gym with me?
CAN'T MOVE.
TOO SAD.

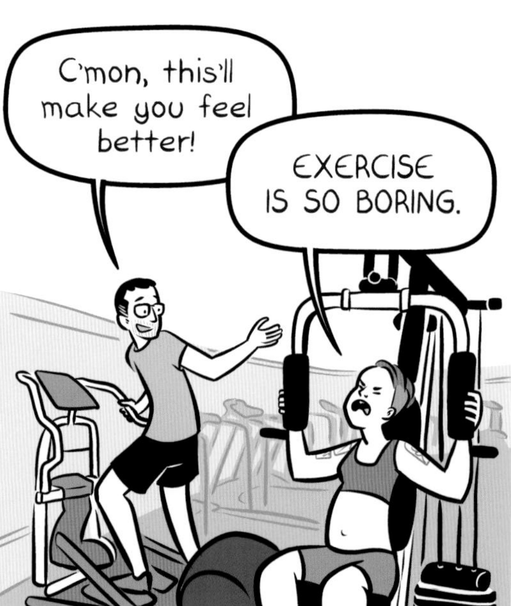
C'mon, this'll make you feel better!
EXERCISE IS SO BORING.

And then one day I found this ad in the *Portland Mercury*.

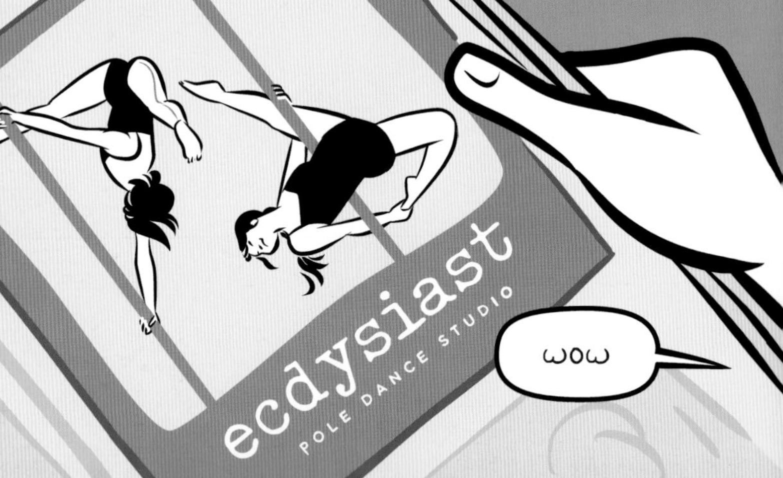
ecdysiast
POLE DANCE STUDIO
wow

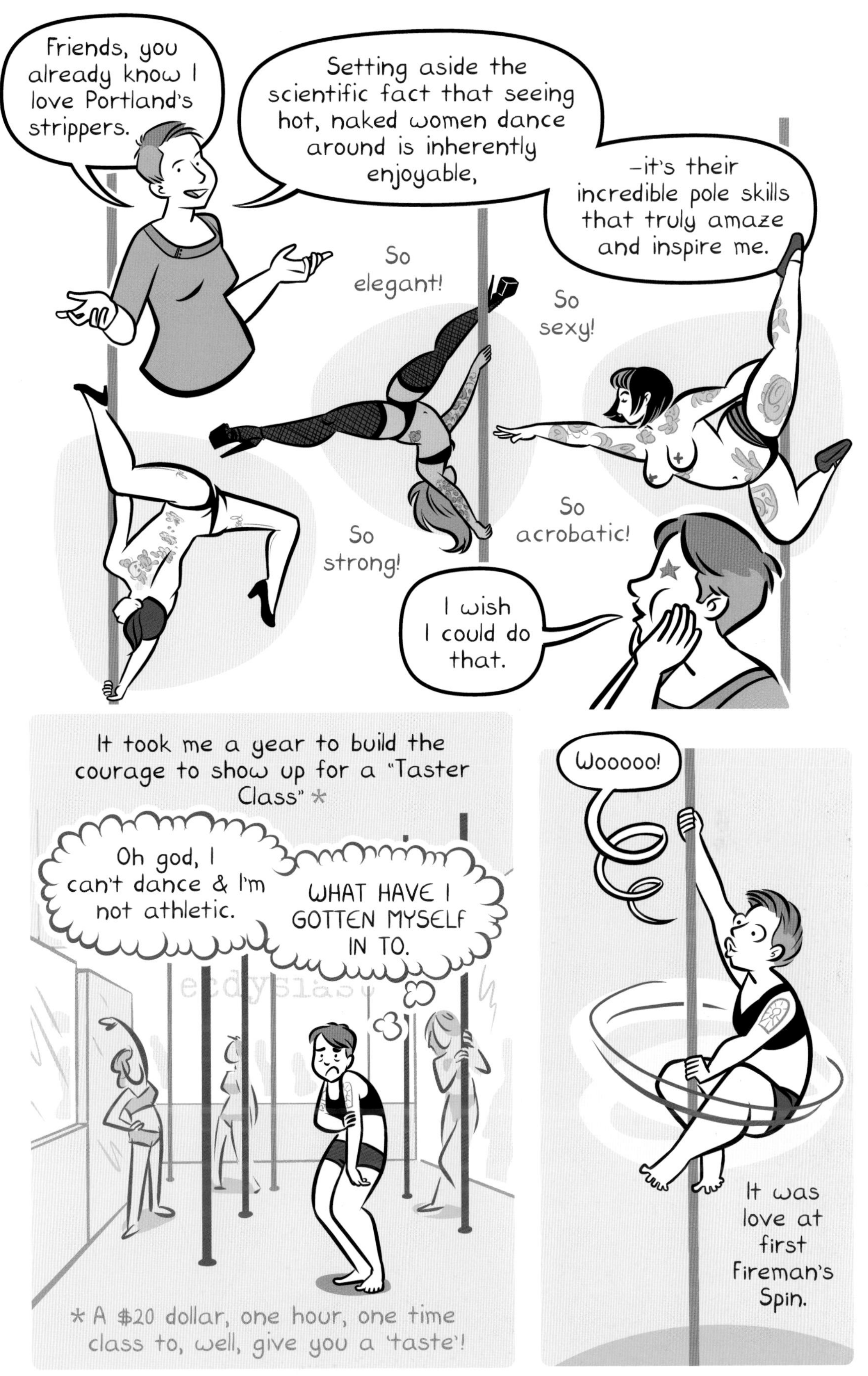
Friends, you already know I love Portland's strippers.
Setting aside the scientific fact that seeing hot, naked women dance around is inherently enjoyable,
–it's their incredible pole skills that truly amaze and inspire me.
So elegant!
So sexy!
So strong!
So acrobatic!
I wish I could do that.
It took me a year to build the courage to show up for a "Taster Class" *
Oh god, I can't dance & I'm not athletic.
WHAT HAVE I GOTTEN MYSELF IN TO.
* A $20 dollar, one hour, one time class to, well, give you a 'taste'!
Wooooo!
It was love at first Fireman's Spin.

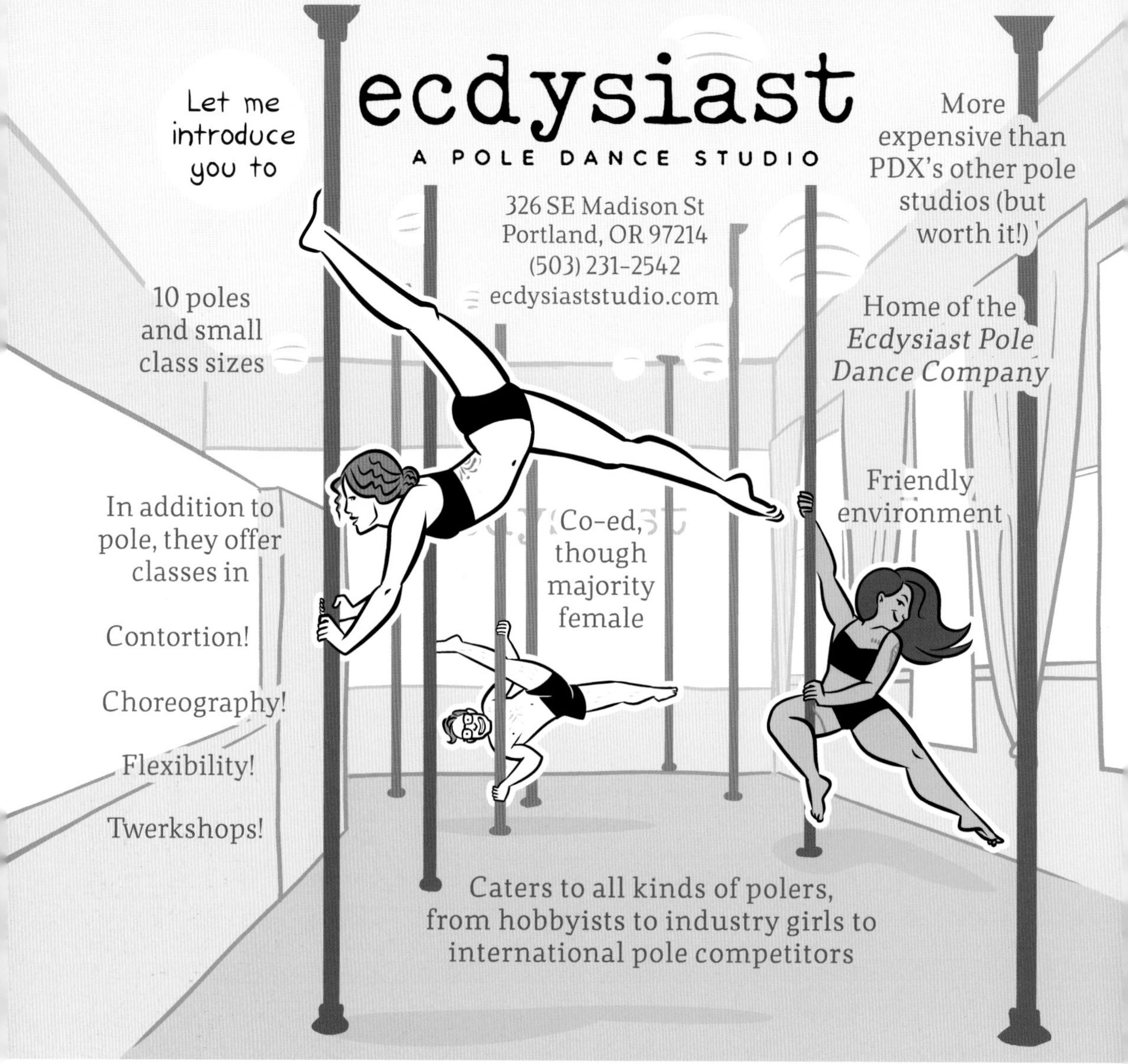

Let me introduce you to

ecdysiast

A POLE DANCE STUDIO

326 SE Madison St
Portland, OR 97214
(503) 231-2542
ecdysiaststudio.com

More expensive than PDX's other pole studios (but worth it!)

10 poles and small class sizes

Home of the *Ecdysiast Pole Dance Company*

In addition to pole, they offer classes in

Contortion!

Choreography!

Flexibility!

Twerkshops!

Co-ed, though majority female

Friendly environment

Caters to all kinds of polers, from hobbyists to industry girls to international pole competitors

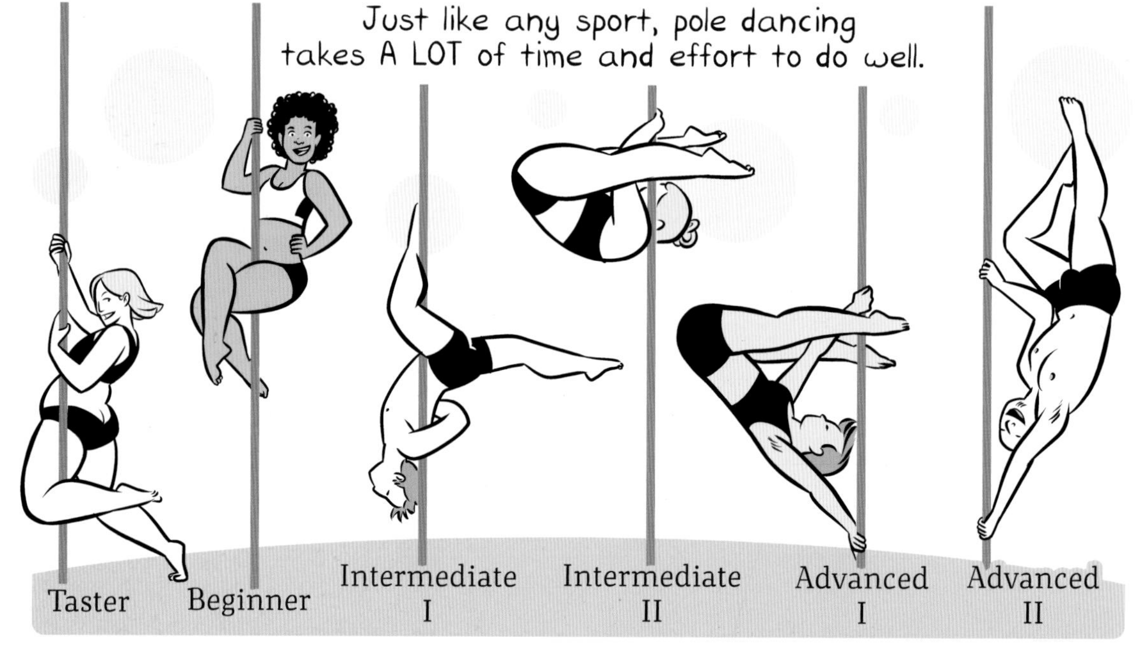

Just like any sport, pole dancing takes A LOT of time and effort to do well.
Taster
Beginner
Intermediate I
Intermediate II
Advanced I
Advanced II

Though it wasn't my goal, by the time I finished Advanced II, two years after my first class–

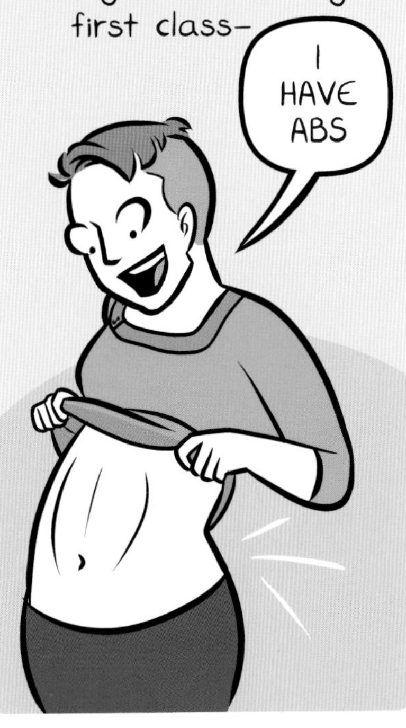

I'm not going to suggest that pole dance is for everyone.

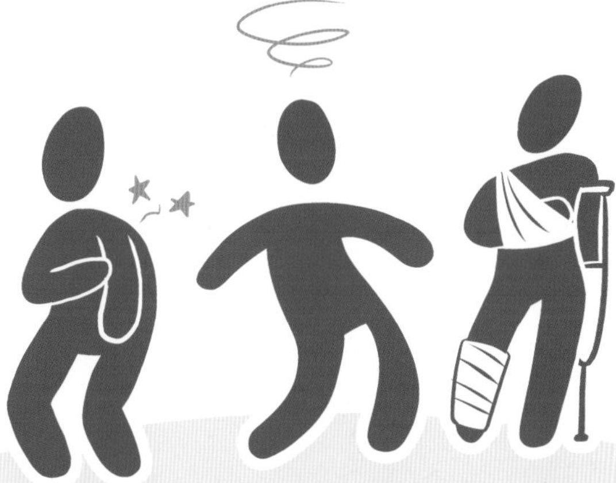

You'll walk away from classes bruised, dizzy, sore, and occasionally injured.

And students are *strongly* encouraged to dance in a public recital.

ecdysiast

Which I did once, but for an introvert like me, that just isn't my jam.

But those moments, after months of hard work when I finally pull off a difficult move, it's incredibly empowering and anything that makes me feel strong and sexy is totally worth the effort.

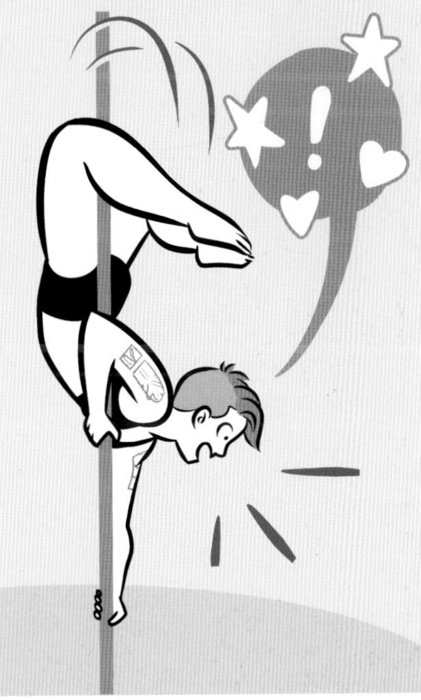

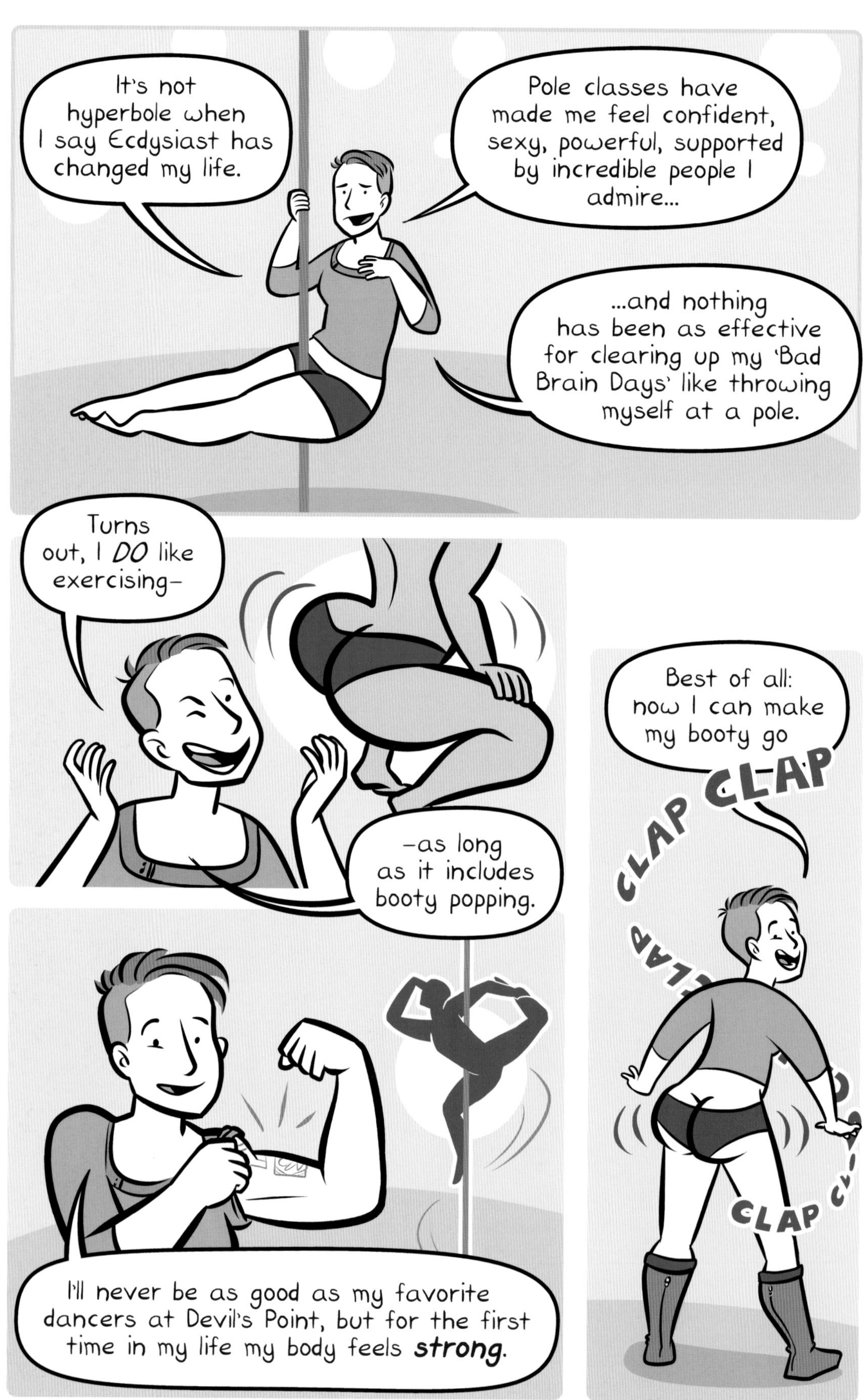
It's not hyperbole when I say Ecdysiast has changed my life.
Pole classes have made me feel confident, sexy, powerful, supported by incredible people I admire...
...and nothing has been as effective for clearing up my 'Bad Brain Days' like throwing myself at a pole.
Turns out, I *DO* like exercising–
–as long as it includes booty popping.
I'll never be as good as my favorite dancers at Devil's Point, but for the first time in my life my body feels **strong**.
Best of all: now I can make my booty go
CLAP CLAP
CLAP
CLAP
CLAP

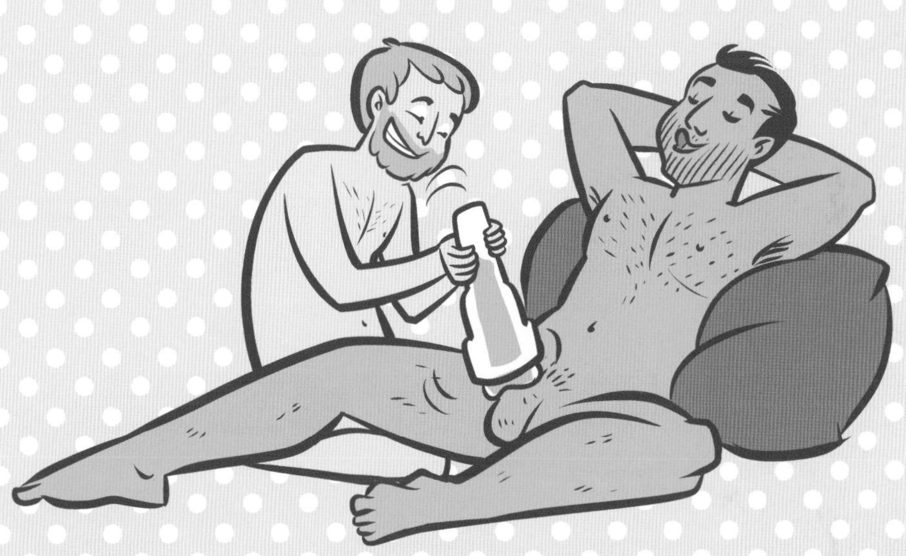

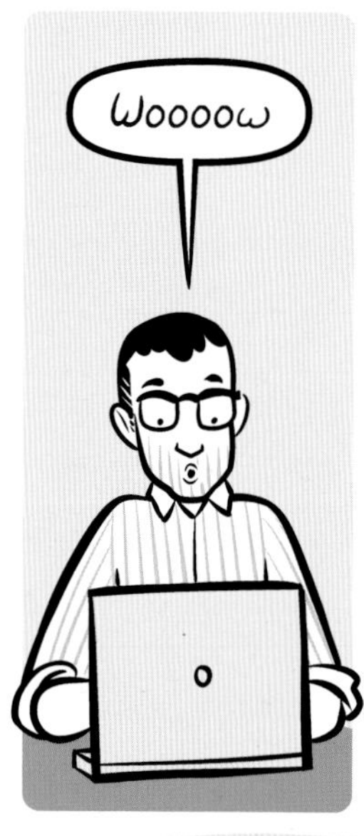

Woooow

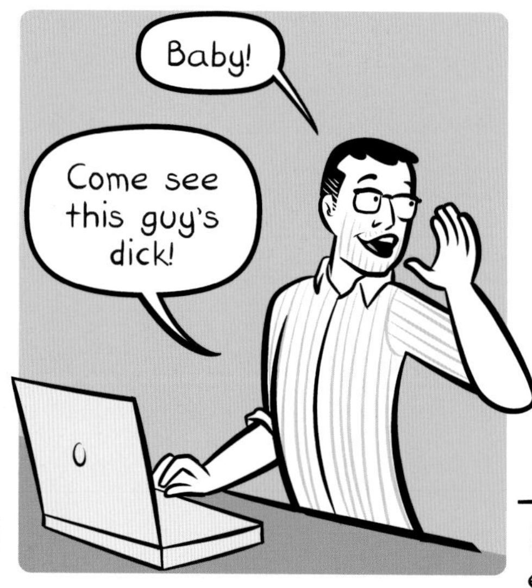

Baby!
Come see this guy's dick!

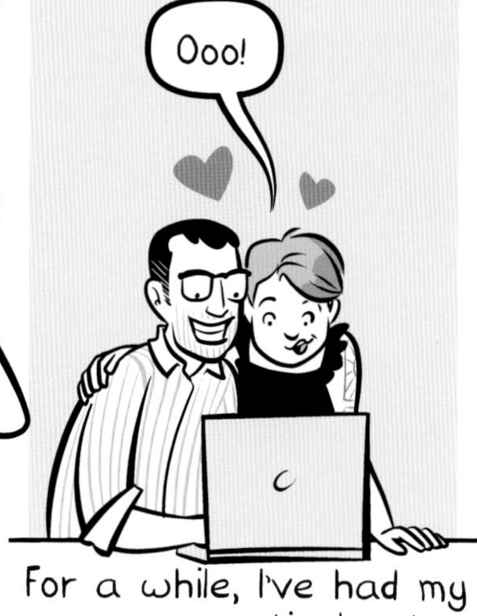

Ooo!

For a while, I've had my eye on a particular toy.

After seeing many a hunk using fleshlight's see-through Ice masturbation sleeve in tumblr gifs, I've been keen to get one myself.

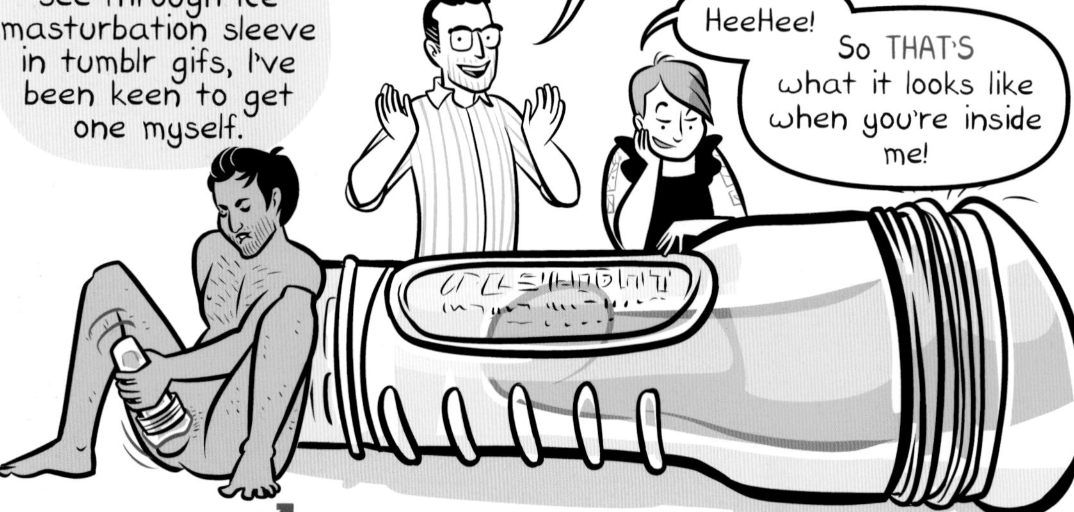

Paired with a well-hung guy it's quite the visual treat, giving you that x-ray component you never realized you wanted.
HeeHee!
So THAT'S what it looks like when you're inside me!

FLESHLIGHT kindly stepped up and supplied me with the "Lady" sleeve and I'm now the proud owner of this fancy do-daddy!

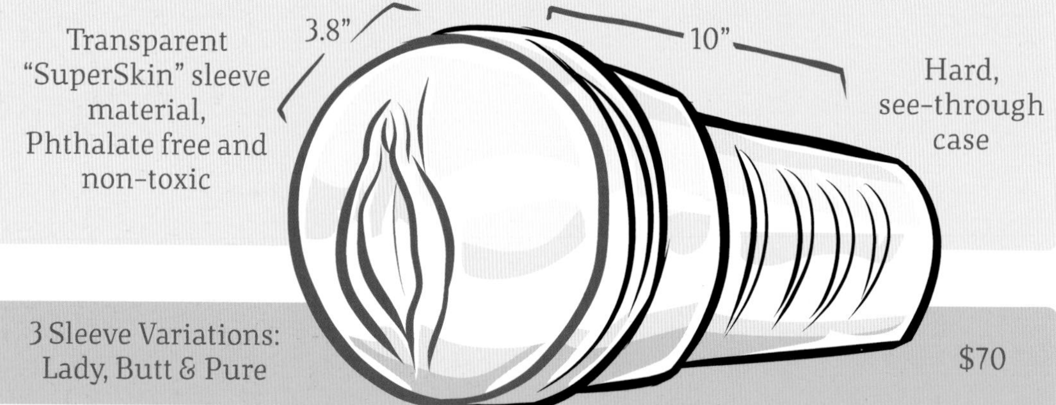

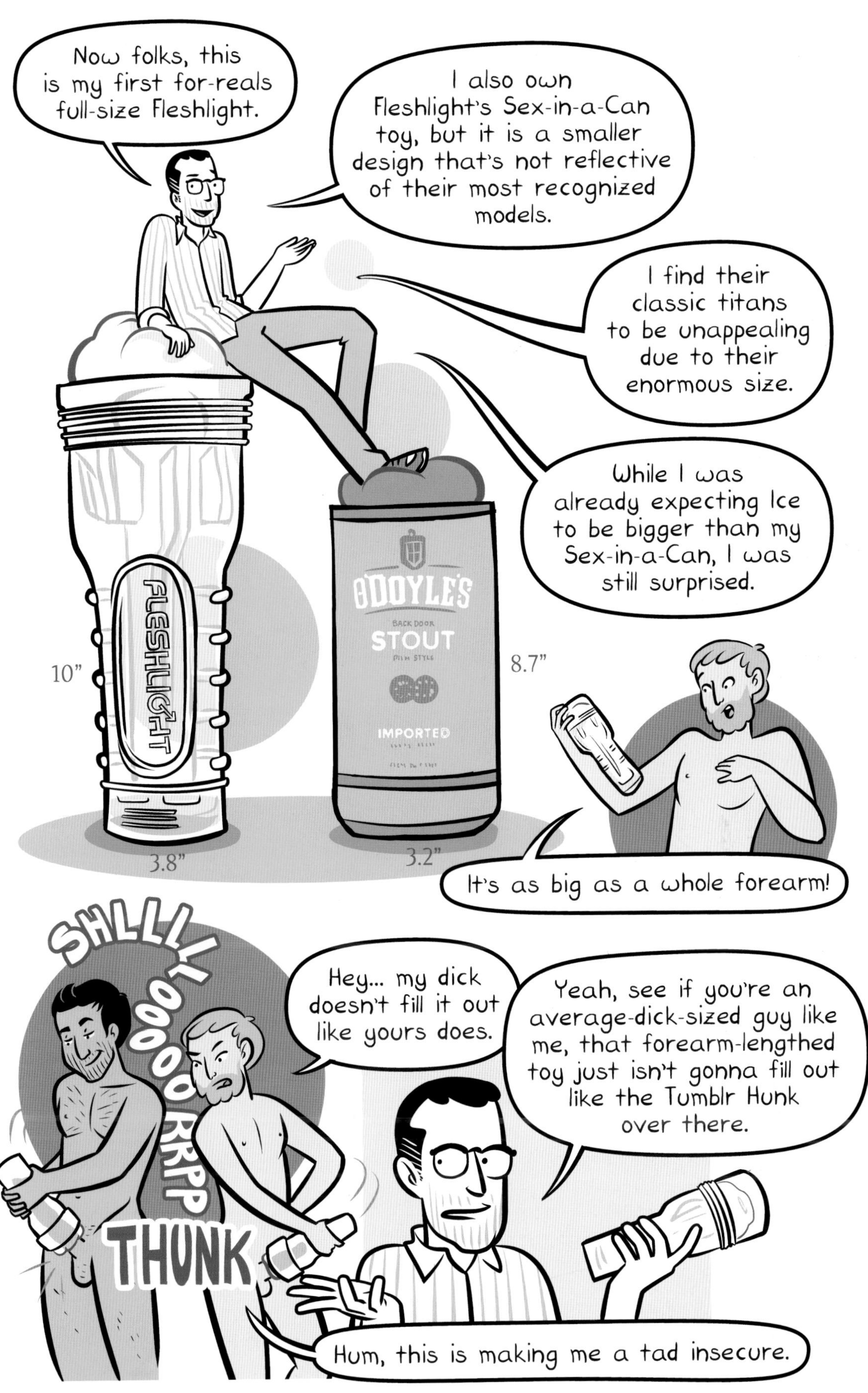
Now folks, this is my first for-reals full-size Fleshlight.
I also own Fleshlight's Sex-in-a-Can toy, but it is a smaller design that's not reflective of their most recognized models.
I find their classic titans to be unappealing due to their enormous size.
While I was already expecting Ice to be bigger than my Sex-in-a-Can, I was still surprised.
FLESHLIGHT
O'DOYLE'S
BACK DOOR
STOUT
IMPORTED
10"
3.8"
8.7"
3.2"
It's as big as a whole forearm!
SHLLLLOOOOORRPP
THUNK
Hey... my dick doesn't fill it out like yours does.
Yeah, see if you're an average-dick-sized guy like me, that forearm-lengthed toy just isn't gonna fill out like the Tumblr Hunk over there.
Hum, this is making me a tad insecure.

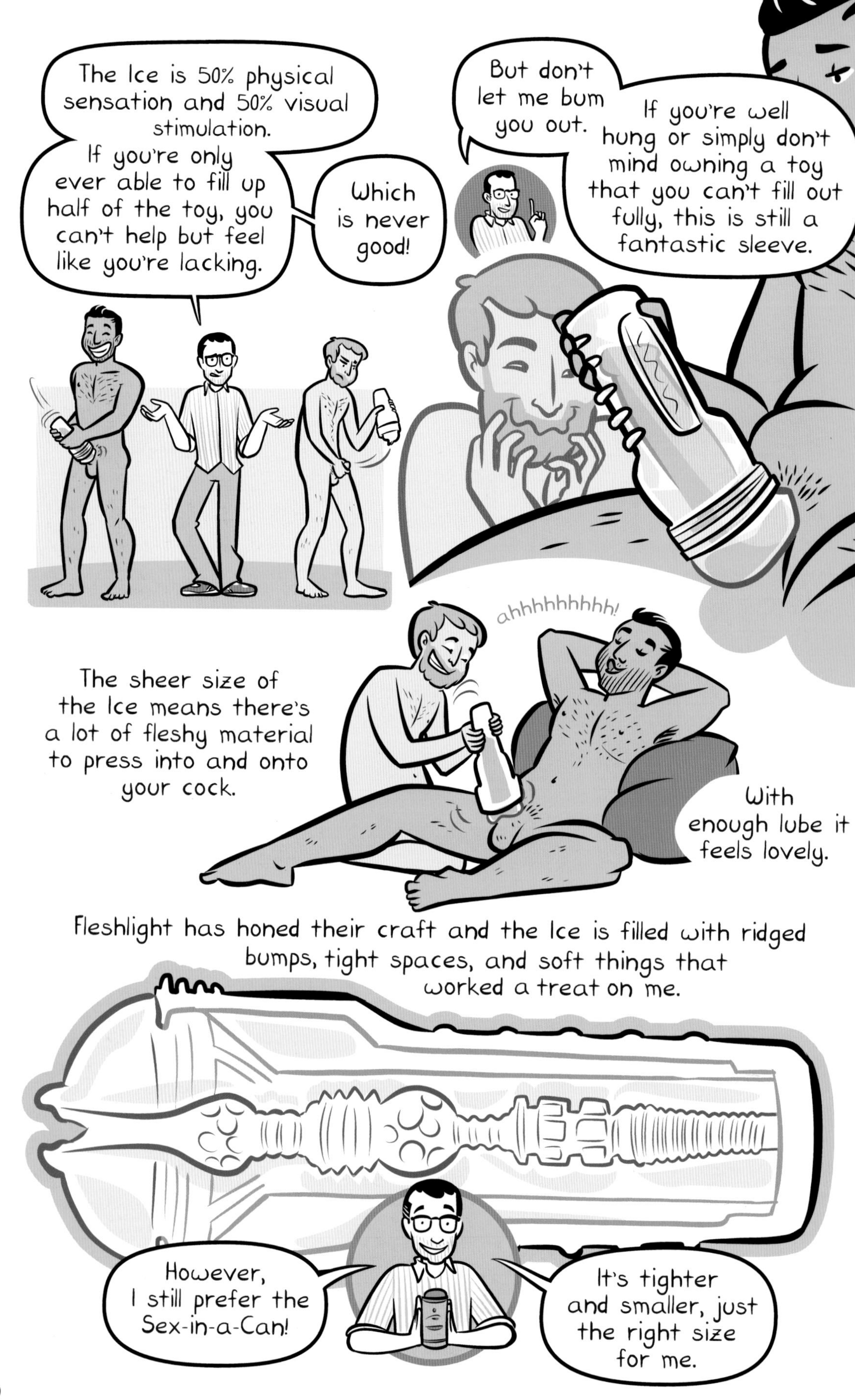
The Ice is 50% physical sensation and 50% visual stimulation.
If you're only ever able to fill up half of the toy, you can't help but feel like you're lacking.
Which is never good!
But don't let me bum you out.
If you're well hung or simply don't mind owning a toy that you can't fill out fully, this is still a fantastic sleeve.
ahhhhhhhhh!
The sheer size of the Ice means there's a lot of fleshy material to press into and onto your cock.
With enough lube it feels lovely.
Fleshlight has honed their craft and the Ice is filled with ridged bumps, tight spaces, and soft things that worked a treat on me.
However, I still prefer the Sex-in-a-Can!
It's tighter and smaller, just the right size for me.

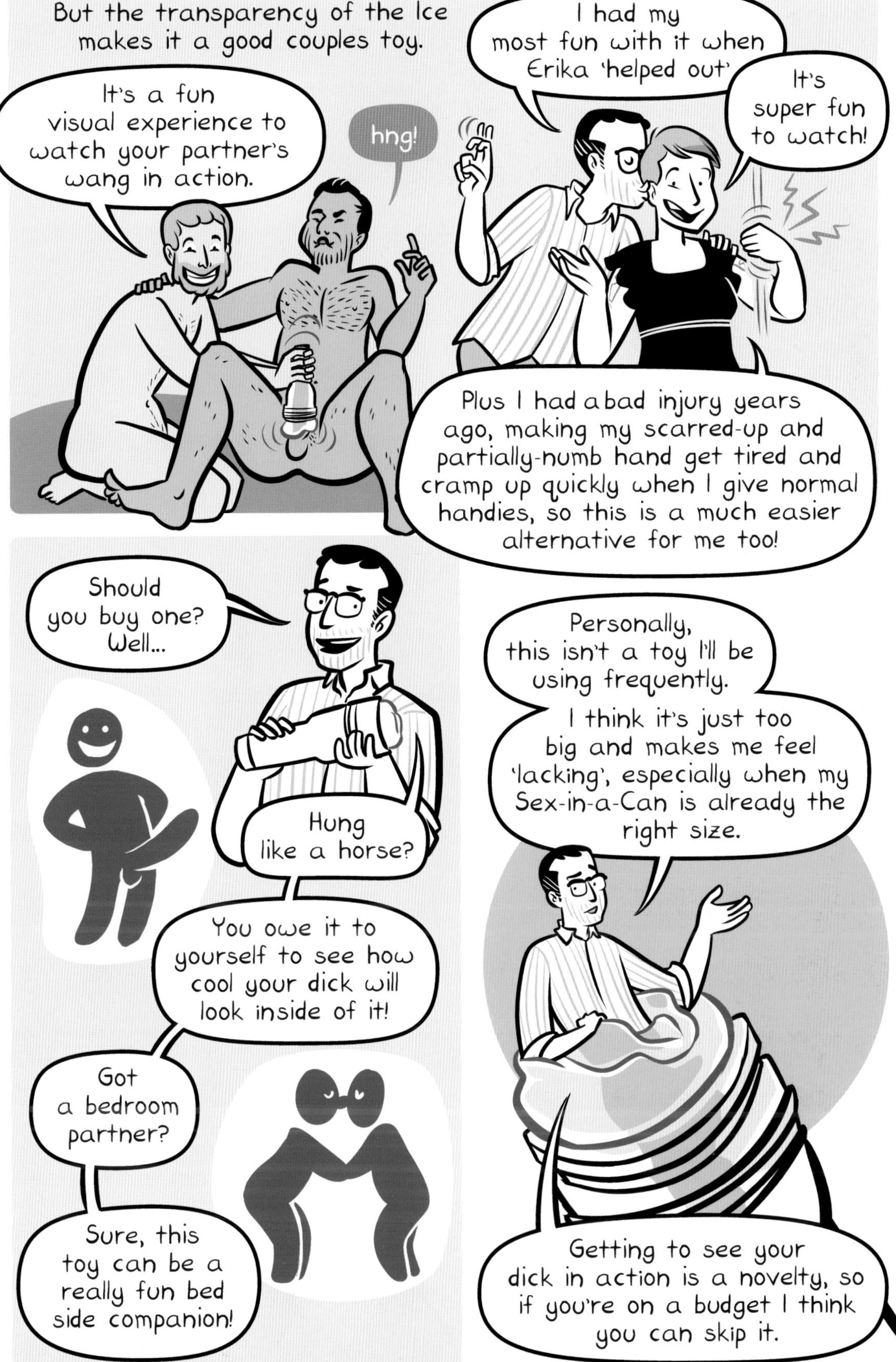
But the transparency of the Ice makes it a good couples toy.
It's a fun visual experience to watch your partner's wang in action.
hng!
I had my most fun with it when Erika 'helped out'
It's super fun to watch!
Plus I had a bad injury years ago, making my scarred-up and partially-numb hand get tired and cramp up quickly when I give normal handies, so this is a much easier alternative for me too!
Should you buy one? Well...
Hung like a horse?
You owe it to yourself to see how cool your dick will look inside of it!
Got a bedroom partner?
Sure, this toy can be a really fun bed side companion!
Personally, this isn't a toy I'll be using frequently.
I think it's just too big and makes me feel 'lacking', especially when my Sex-in-a-Can is already the right size.
Getting to see your dick in action is a novelty, so if you're on a budget I think you can skip it.

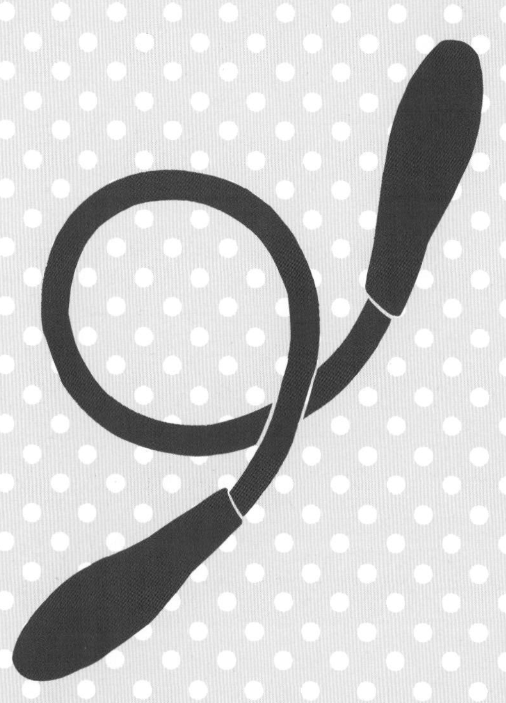

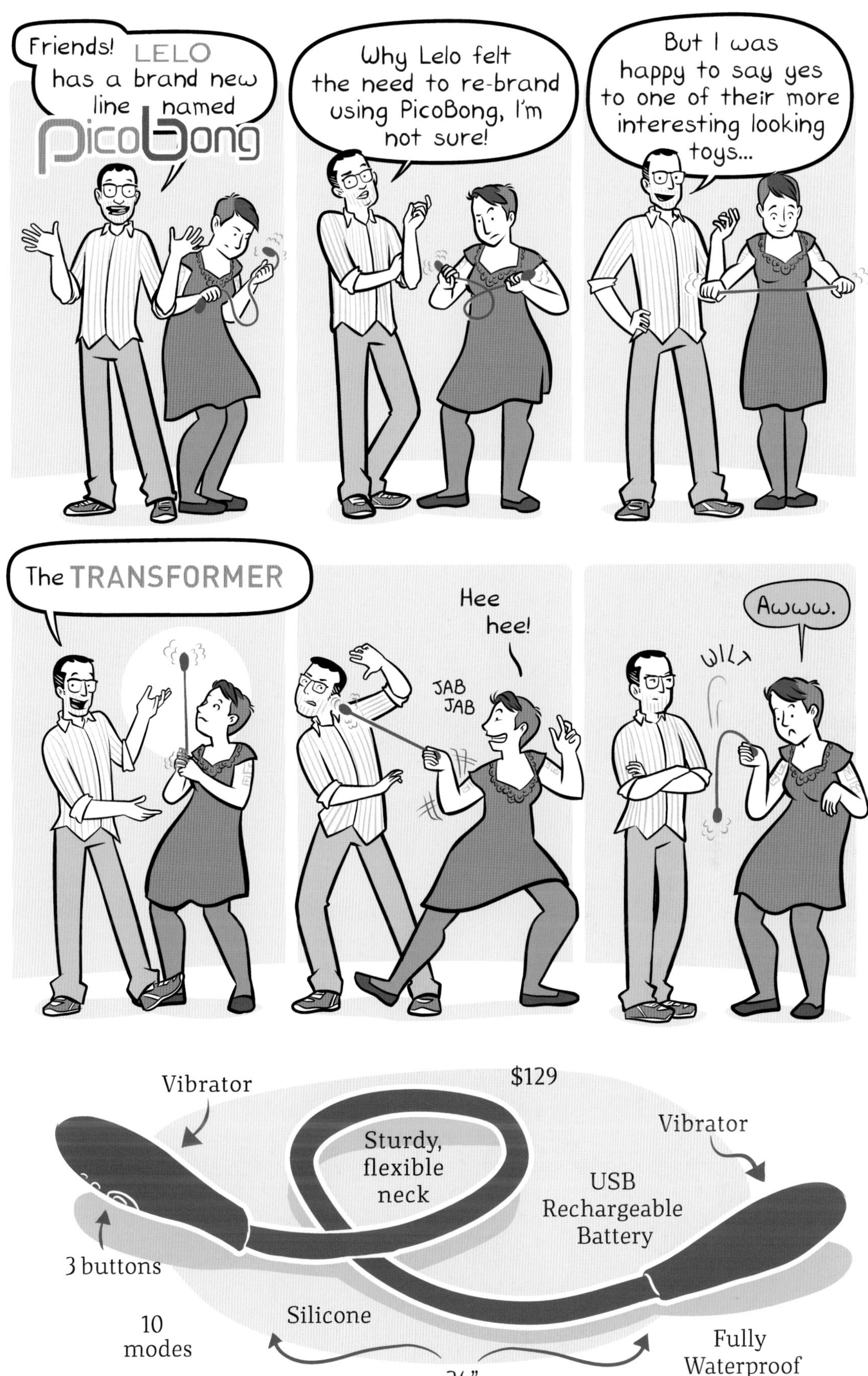
Friends! LELO has a brand new line named PicoBong
Why Lelo felt the need to re-brand using PicoBong, I'm not sure!
But I was happy to say yes to one of their more interesting looking toys...
The TRANSFORMER
Hee hee!
JAB JAB
WILT
Awww.
Vibrator
$129
Sturdy, flexible neck
Vibrator
USB Rechargeable Battery
3 buttons
10 modes
Silicone
24"
Fully Waterproof

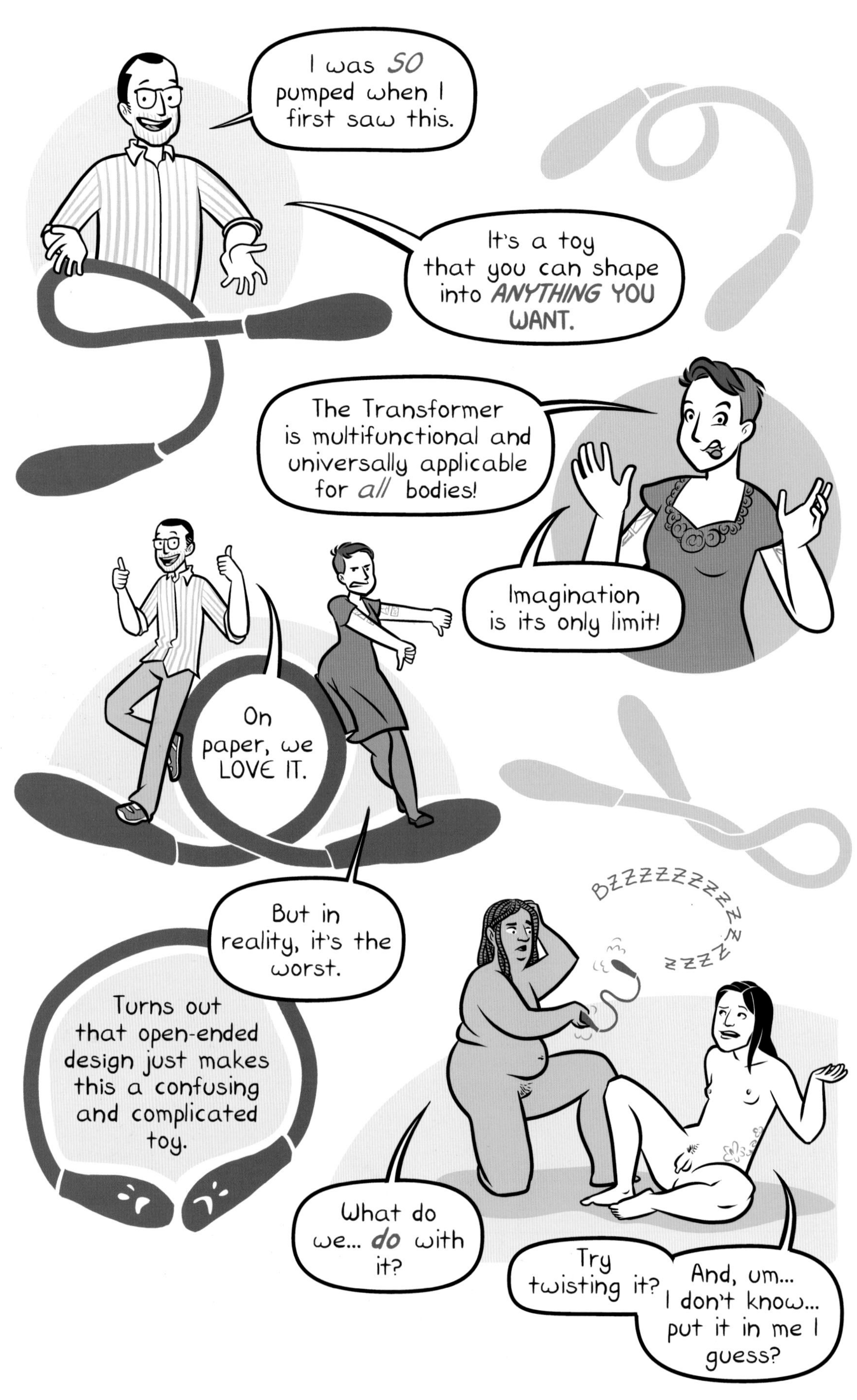
I was SO pumped when I first saw this.
It's a toy that you can shape into ANYTHING YOU WANT.
The Transformer is multifunctional and universally applicable for all bodies!
Imagination is its only limit!
On paper, we LOVE IT.
But in reality, it's the worst.
Turns out that open-ended design just makes this a confusing and complicated toy.
BZZZZZZZZZZZZZZZ
What do we... do with it?
Try twisting it?
And, um... I don't know... put it in me I guess?

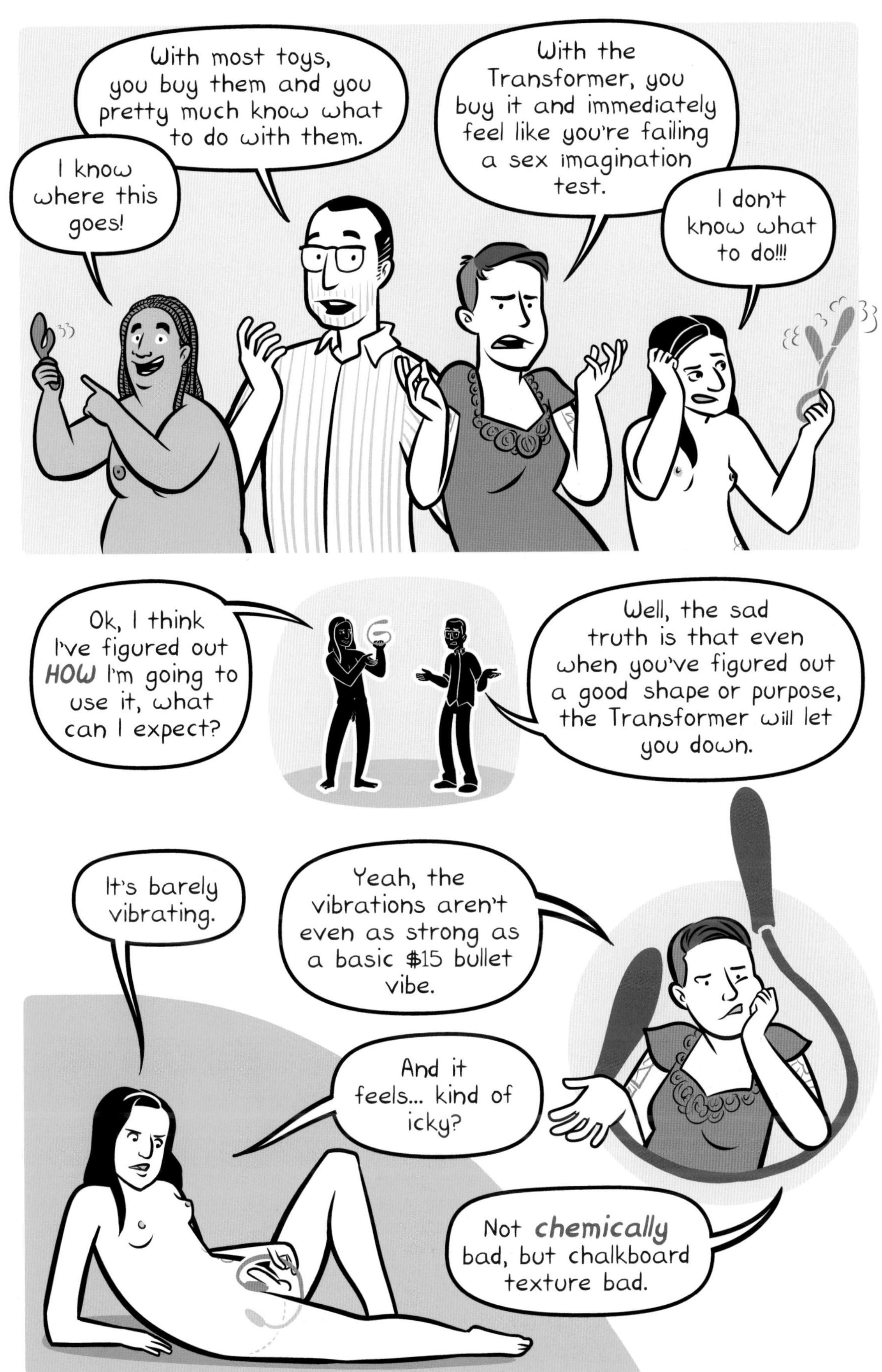
With most toys, you buy them and you pretty much know what to do with them.
I know where this goes!
With the Transformer, you buy it and immediately feel like you're failing a sex imagination test.
I don't know what to do!!!
Ok, I think I've figured out HOW I'm going to use it, what can I expect?
Well, the sad truth is that even when you've figured out a good shape or purpose, the Transformer will let you down.
It's barely vibrating.
Yeah, the vibrations aren't even as strong as a basic $15 bullet vibe.
And it feels... kind of icky?
Not chemically bad, but chalkboard texture bad.

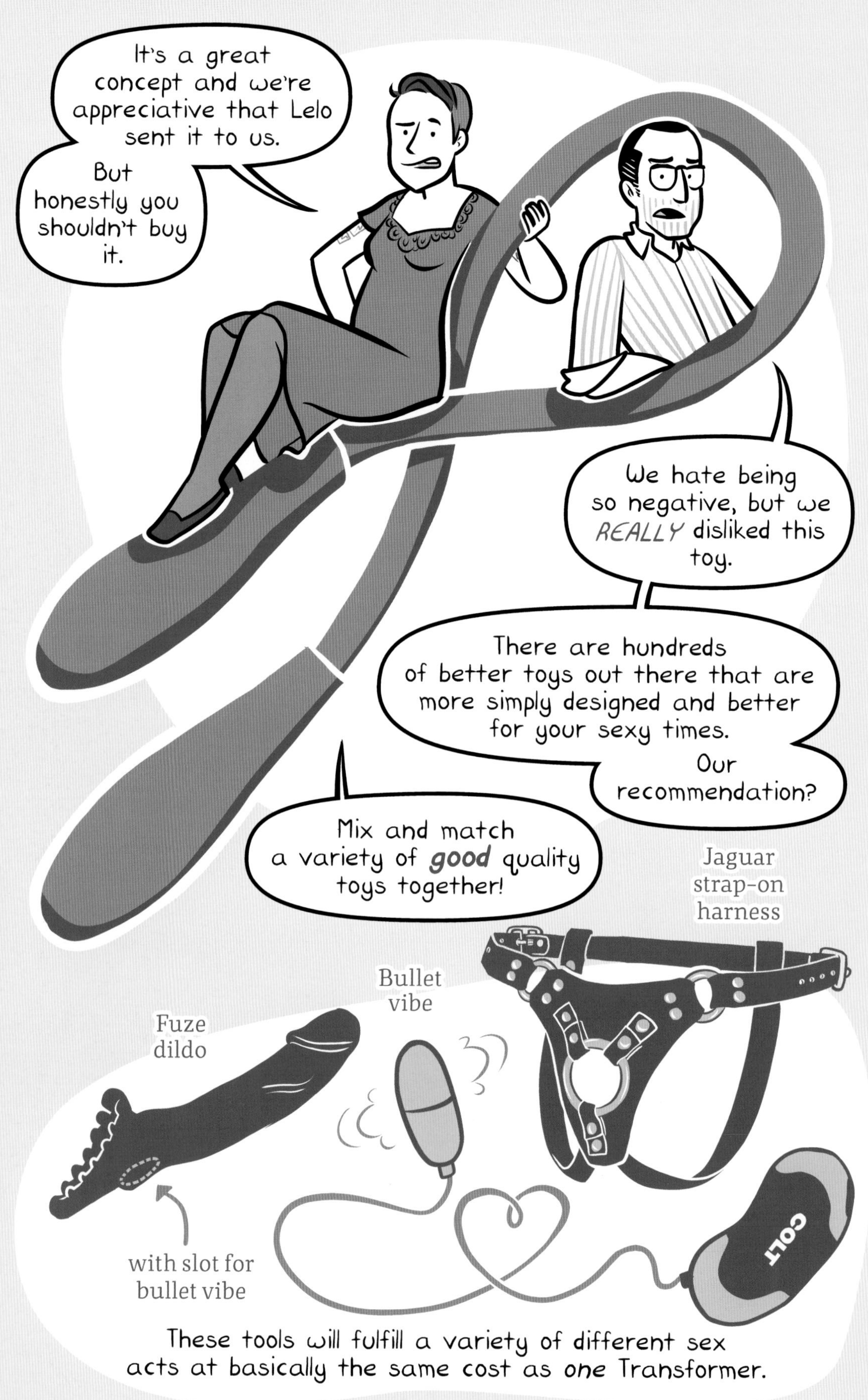
It's a great concept and we're appreciative that Lelo sent it to us.
But honestly you shouldn't buy it.
We hate being so negative, but we REALLY disliked this toy.
There are hundreds of better toys out there that are more simply designed and better for your sexy times.
Our recommendation?
Mix and match a variety of good quality toys together!
Jaguar strap-on harness
Bullet vibe
Fuze dildo
with slot for bullet vibe
COLT
These tools will fulfill a variety of different sex acts at basically the same cost as one Transformer.

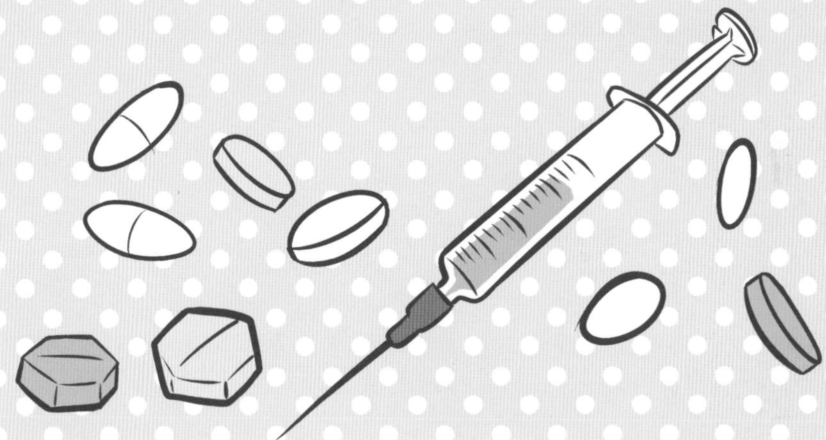

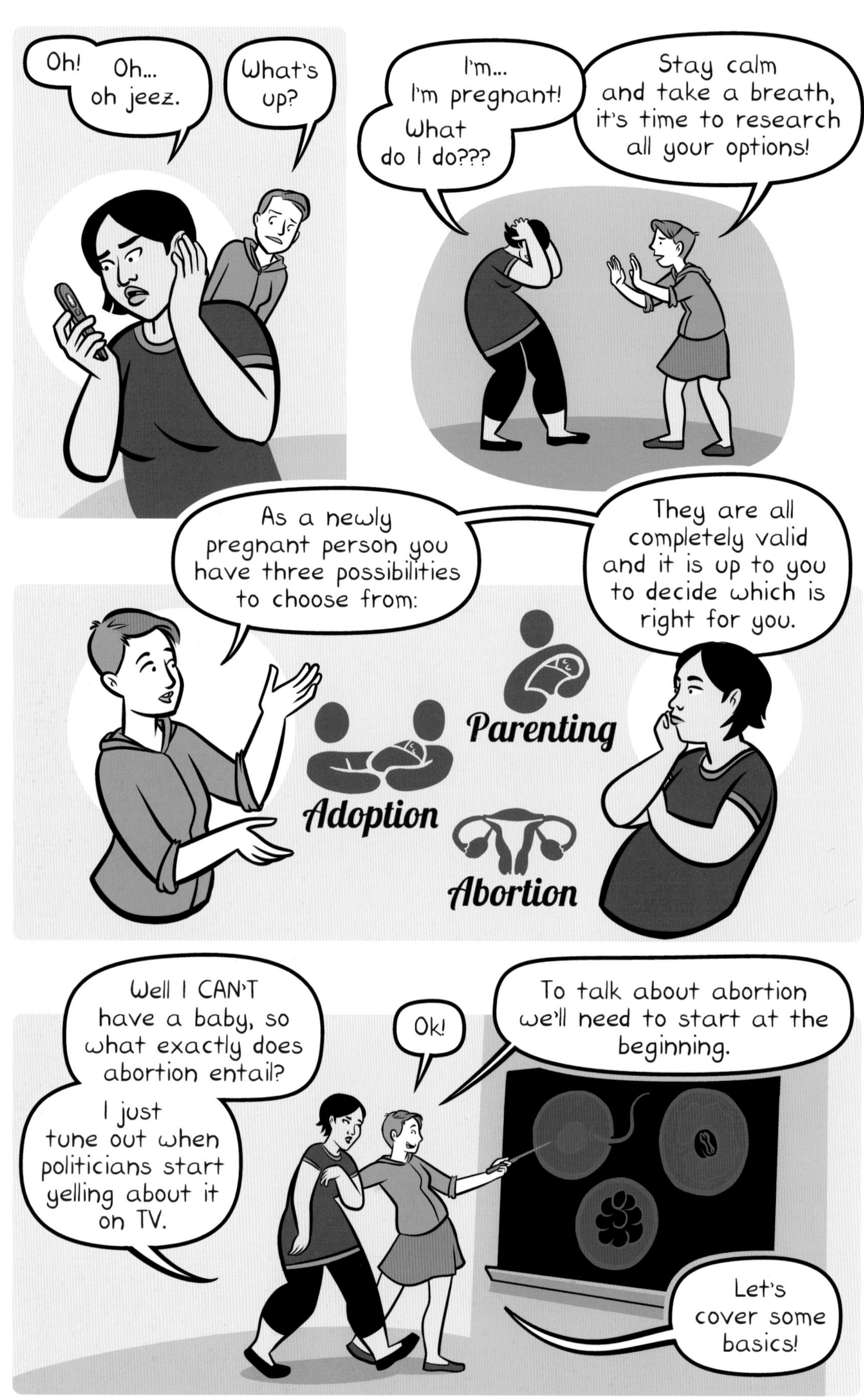
Oh!
Oh... oh jeez.
What's up?
I'm... I'm pregnant!
What do I do???
Stay calm and take a breath, it's time to research all your options!
As a newly pregnant person you have three possibilities to choose from:
They are all completely valid and it is up to you to decide which is right for you.
Parenting
Adoption
Abortion
Well I CAN'T have a baby, so what exactly does abortion entail?
I just tune out when politicians start yelling about it on TV.
Ok!
To talk about abortion we'll need to start at the beginning.
Let's cover some basics!

Stages of Pregnancy

Conception

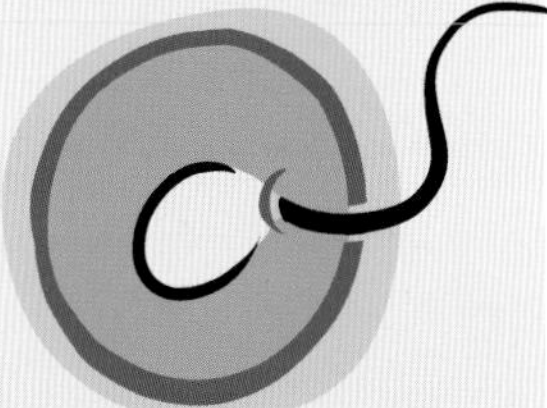

When your egg meets sperm in one of your fallopian tubes, we have conception!

Implantation & Embryo Development (1–5 weeks)

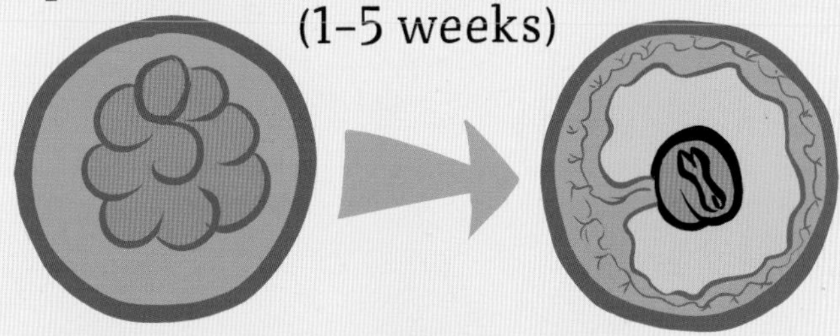

That fertilized egg (the *blastocyst*) will slowly travel to your uterus and implant itself, becoming an *embryo* and making you officially pregnant!

Around the 5 - 7 weeks mark, there's enough there for the embryo to have a detectable heartbeat, tiny buds (future hands and legs), and the beginning of a neural tube (future brain and spinal cord)

Fetus (8 weeks – 40 ish weeks)

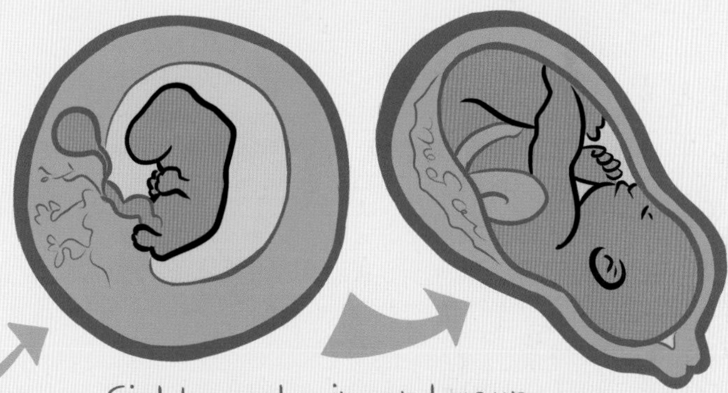

Eight weeks in and your embryo will develop into a fetus with organs, fingers, toes, and genitalia that will continue to grow through all the next stages until birth.

The timeline of a pregnancy is tracked through 'Trimesters'

First Trimester

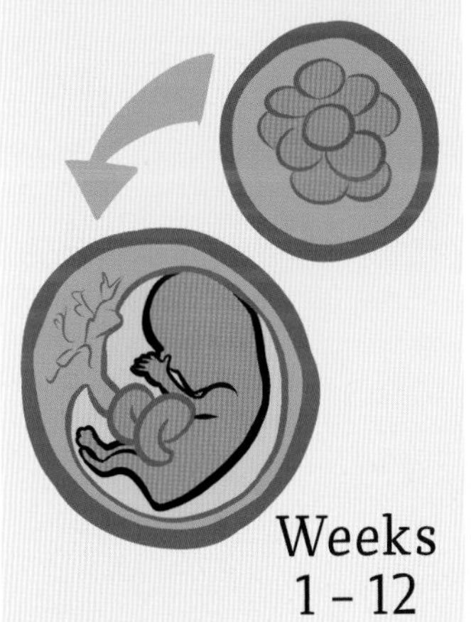

Second Trimester

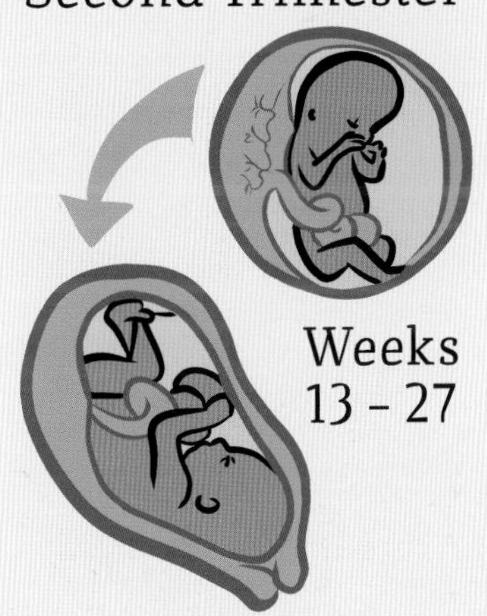

Third Trimester

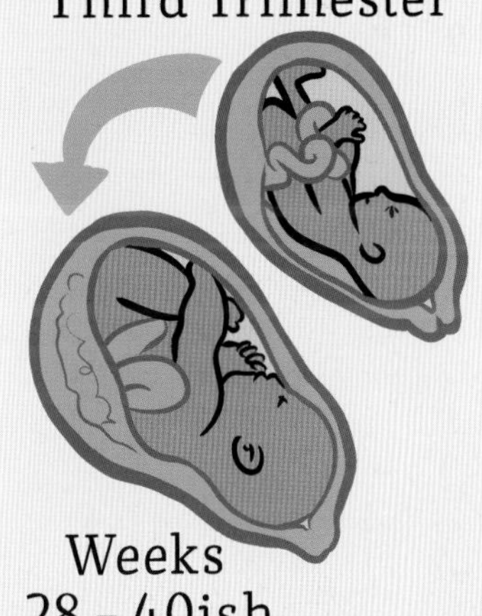

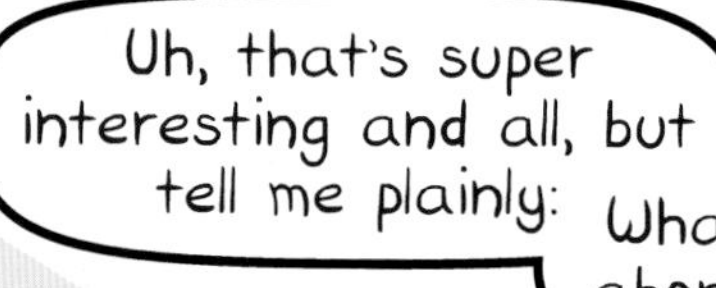
Uh, that's super interesting and all, but tell me plainly:
What *is* abortion?

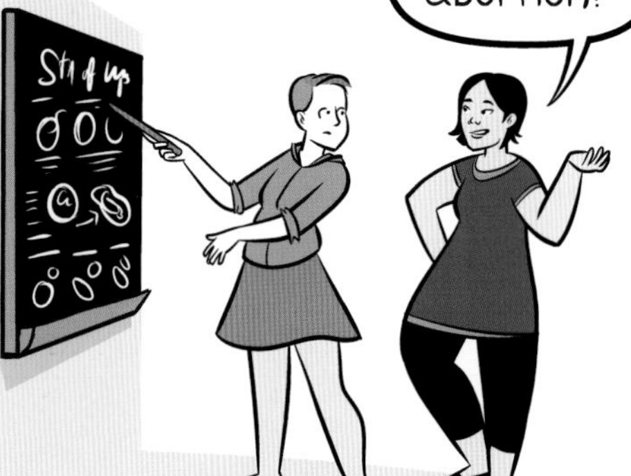
Stages of ...

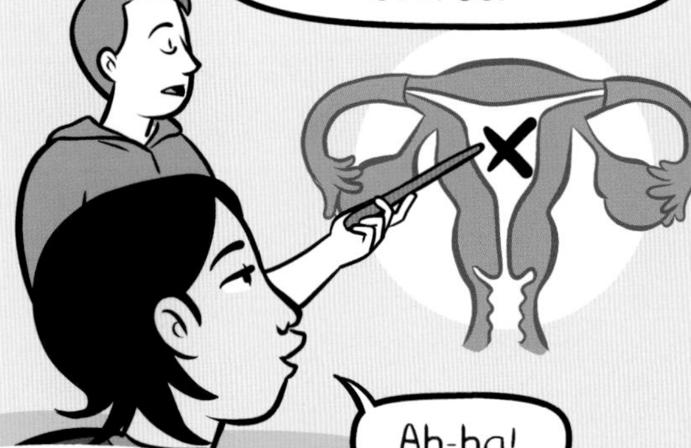
Nice and simple,
Abortion is the removal of an embryo or fetus before it can survive outside of the uterus.
Ah-ha!

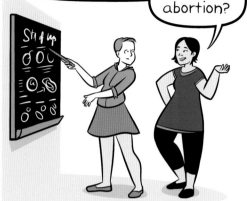

As someone considering abortion, you've got two options!

Surgical or ***medical***, which are both administered by a trained doctor or clinician.

Since I only have room to cover one of these today, I'm going to go over medical abortion

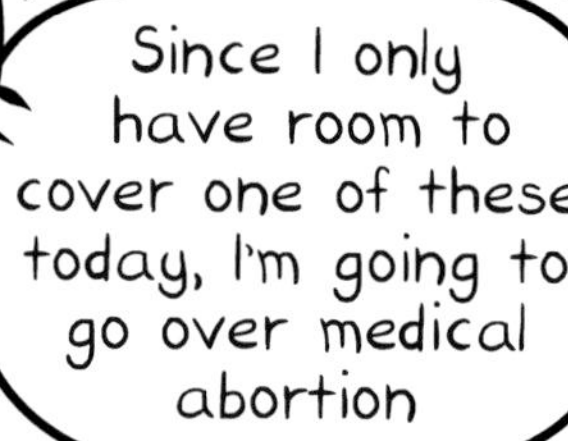

But you should definitely research surgical abortion on your own at:

Scarleteen.com
or
PlannedParenthood.com

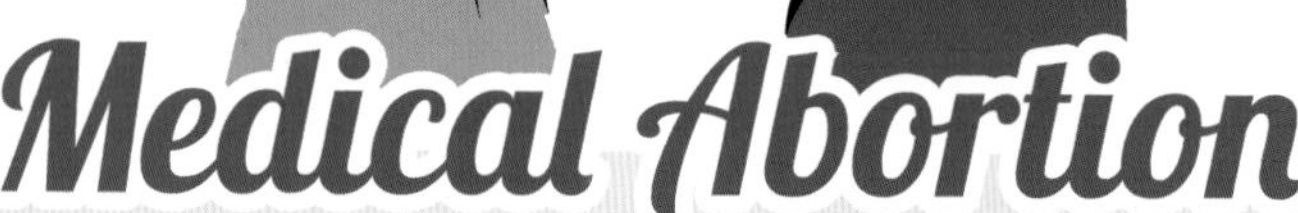

Medical Abortion

AKA: RU486, M&M, The Abortion Pill

(It is ***NOT*** Emergency Contraception)

Taken **before** 9 weeks of pregnancy.

95 – 98% effective

It's a combination of medications (typically mifepristone & misoprostol) that creates a reaction that is indistinguishable from a miscarriage.

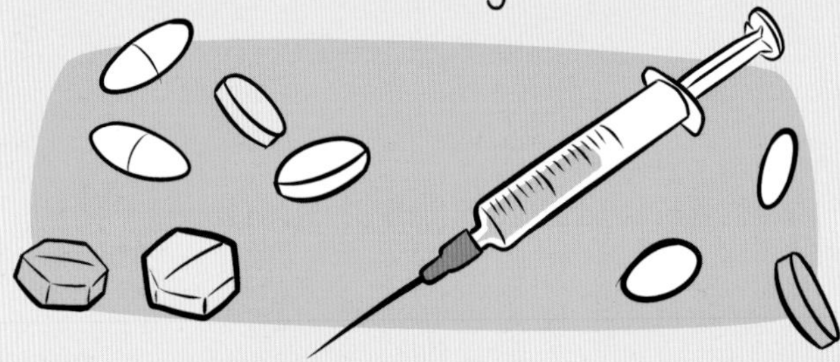

One dose is administered at the clinic (injection or orally) and a few days later another dose is taken orally or vaginally at home.

After the treatments you have a follow-up appointment with your abortion provider to make sure the procedure completed and that you're healthy.

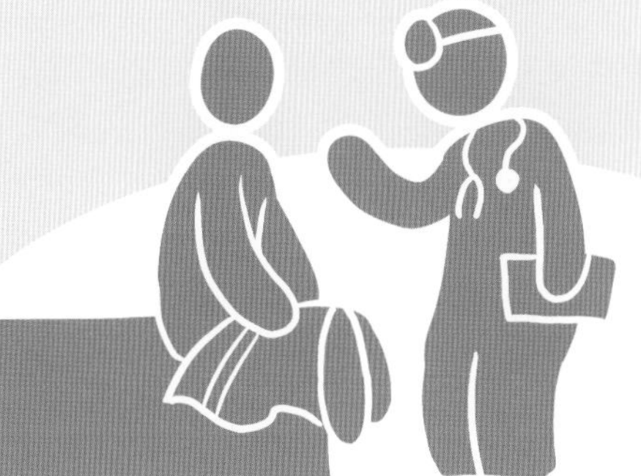

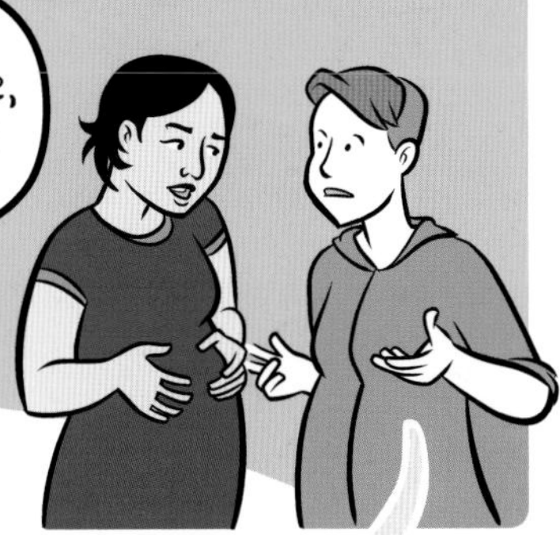
Indistinguishable from a miscarriage?
Geez I've never had one, what'll it feel like?

Well, there will be heavy cramping and bleeding.

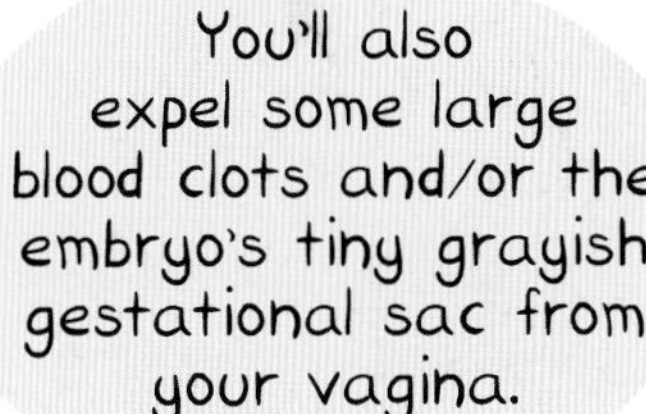

You *might* suffer some side effects like: nausea, headaches, barfing or bowel troubles, along with a week or two of spotting.

You'll also expel some large blood clots and/or the embryo's tiny grayish gestational sac from your vagina.

But it shouldn't be more horribly painful than a bad period and your provider will most likely supply you with some pain medication to keep it manageable.

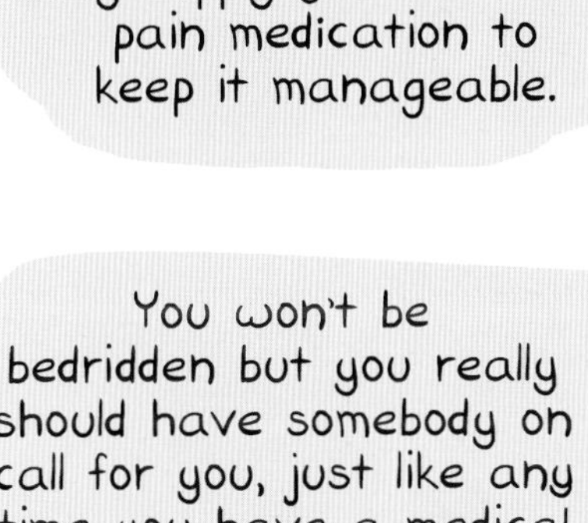

At nine weeks the embryo is still so small that it is unlikely to be seen when it passes out of you

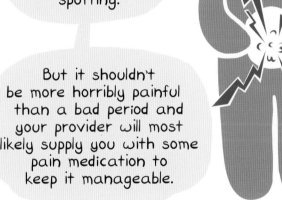

You won't be bedridden but you really should have somebody on call for you, just like any time you have a medical procedure done.

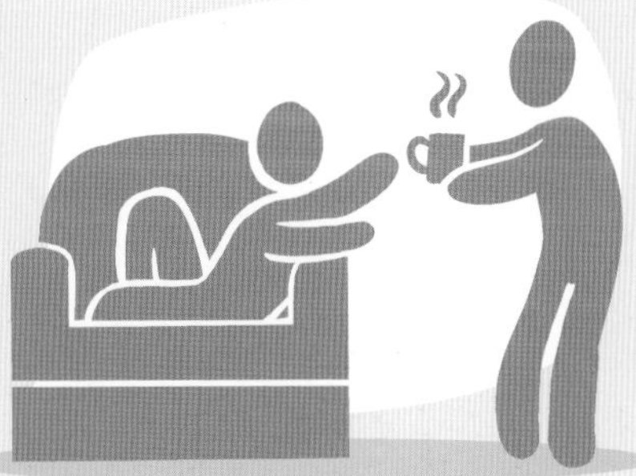

Whether it's for emotional support or to be your aid for anything you may need, it's nice to have someone around.

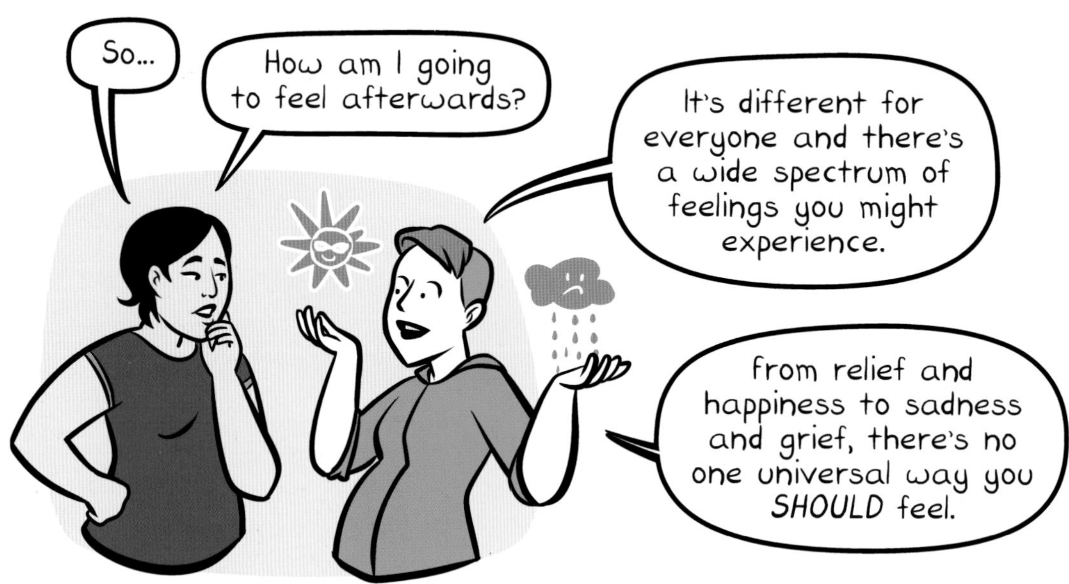

Pregnancy hormones not only cause big changes in your body but can also create **giant mood swings**, and it's normal to feel some depression or intense emotions when you're no longer pregnant–

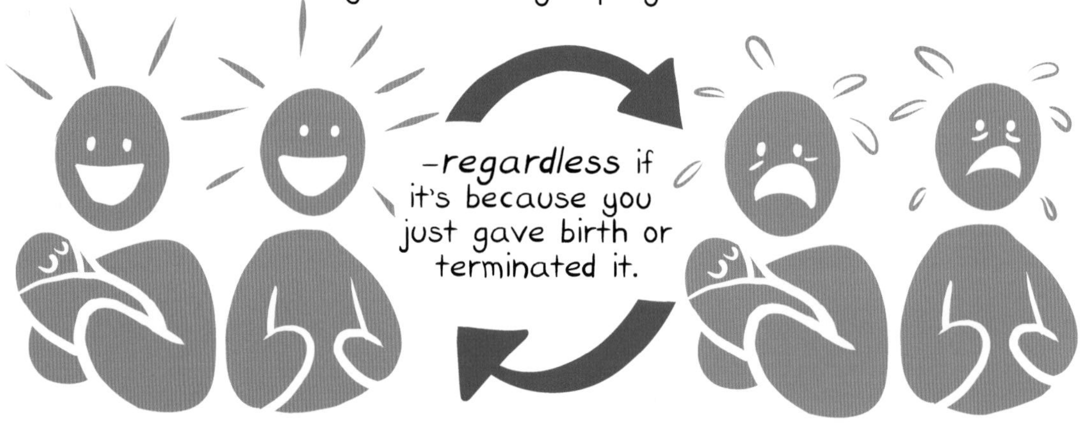
–*regardless* if it's because you just gave birth or terminated it.

Going through a life event is always better when you have supportive, loving, nonjudgmental people in your life that you can share your feelings with.

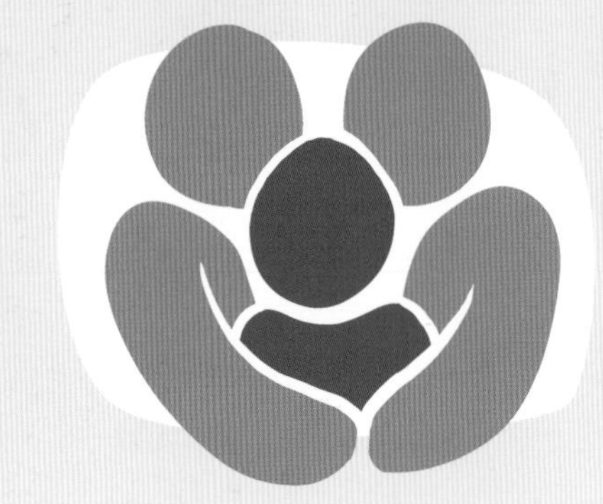

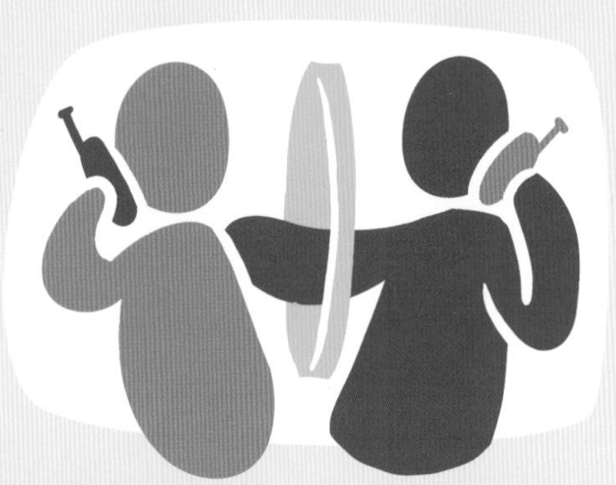

If you don't have someone like that near you, you can also turn to exhaleprovoice.org for some after-abortion support.

Take care of yourself physically and emotionally by doing things you enjoy afterwards, like spending time with friends, sleeping, eating, going to the movies, or whatever!

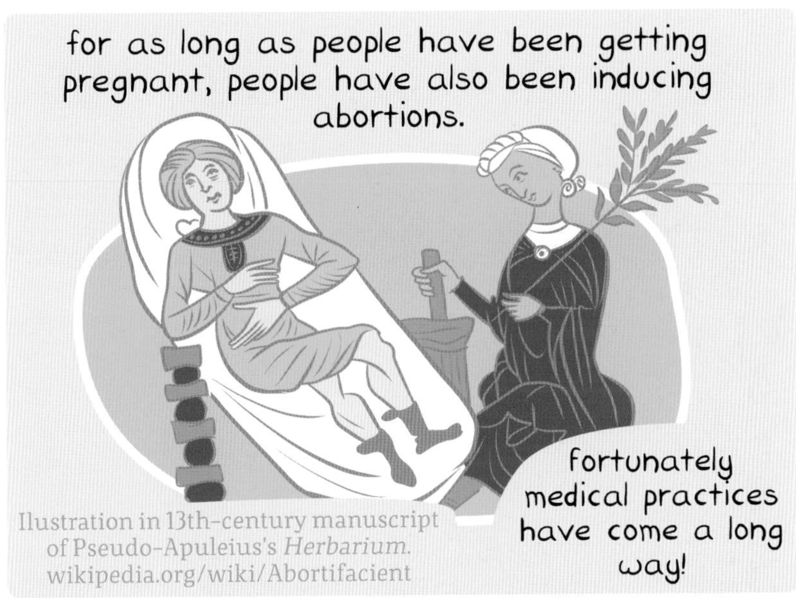

for as long as people have been getting pregnant, people have also been inducing abortions.
fortunately medical practices have come a long way!

Illustration in 13th-century manuscript of Pseudo-Apuleius's *Herbarium*. wikipedia.org/wiki/Abortifacient

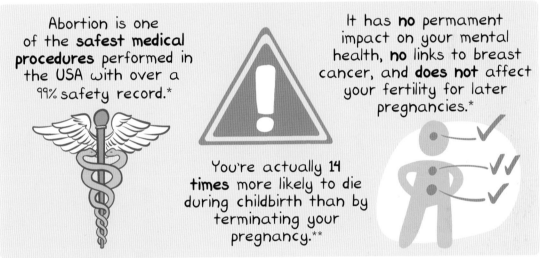

Abortion is one of the **safest medical procedures** performed in the USA with over a 99% safety record.*
It has **no** permament impact on your mental health, **no** links to breast cancer, and **does not** affect your fertility for later pregnancies.*
You're actually **14 times** more likely to die during childbirth than by terminating your pregnancy.**

*plannedparenthood.org/files/6014/2194/2001/Protect_Safe_and_Legal_Abortion.pdf

**http://www.ncbi.nlm.nih.gov/pubmed/22270271

Today in the USA...
50% of pregnancies are unplanned.

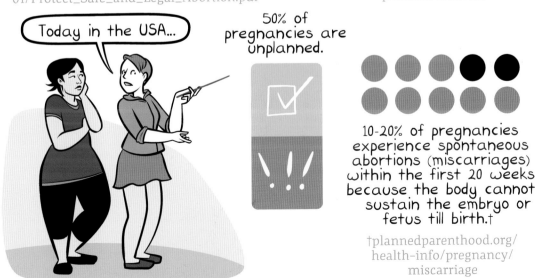

10-20% of pregnancies experience spontaneous abortions (miscarriages) within the first 20 weeks because the body cannot sustain the embryo or fetus till birth.†

†plannedparenthood.org/health-info/pregnancy/miscarriage

21% of all pregnancies (excluding miscarriages) end in abortion.‡

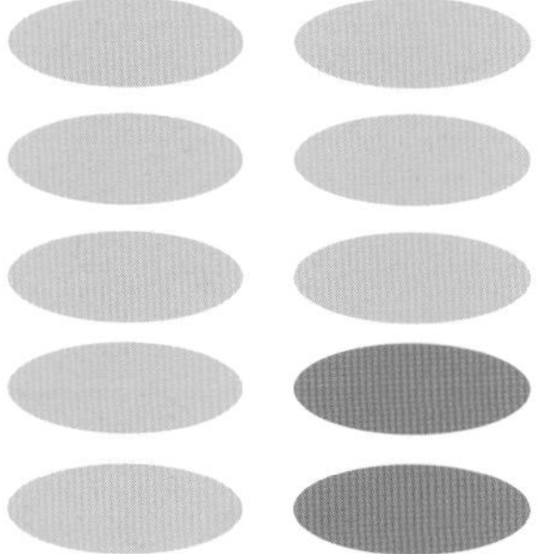

30% of abortions take place before six weeks of pregnancy.‡

‡guttmacher.org/pubs/fb_induced_abortion.html

30% of people with uteruses will have had an abortion by the time they're 45 years old.§

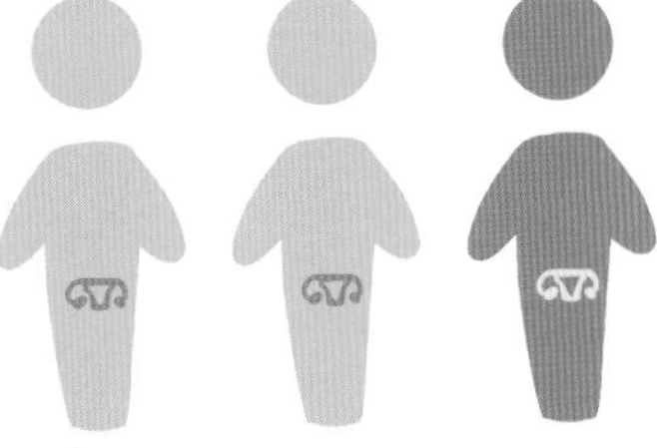

§plannedparenthood.org/health-info/pregnancy/pregnant-now-what/thinking-about-abortion

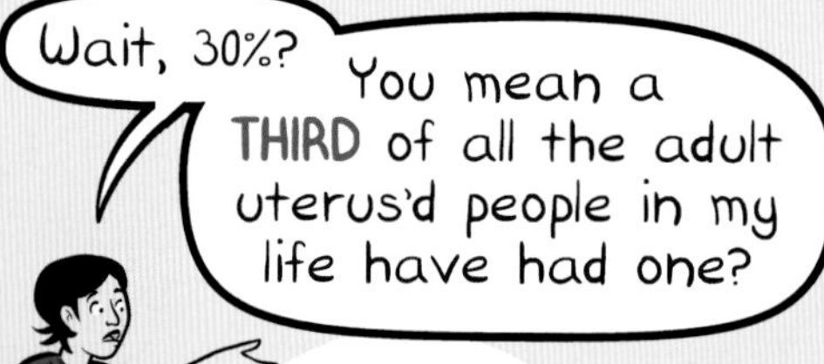

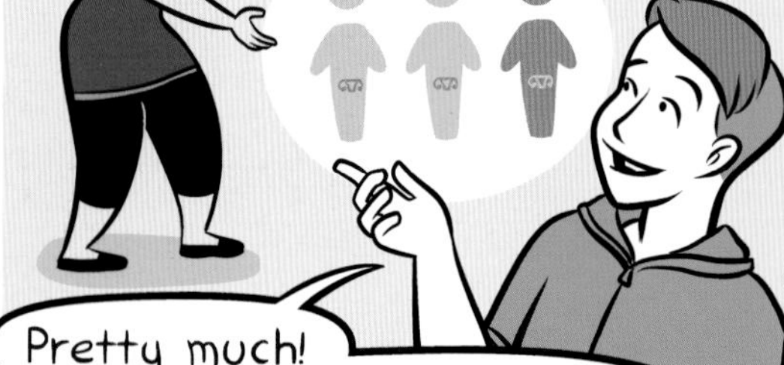
Pretty much!
People may not feel like bringing it up at dinner, but yes, everyone definitely knows at least a few people who have done it, even if they don't *know* they know them.

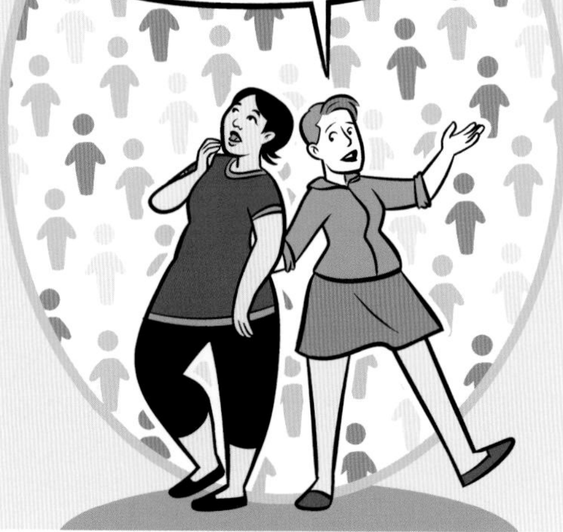
If you decide to have an abortion, remember ***YOU ARE NOT ALONE.***
Abortion is safe, legal, and each year over a million people in the USA have one performed.

For comprehensive information on abortion, please check out:

scarleteen.com/article/bodies/all_about_abortion

exhaleprovoice.org

plannedparenthood.org/health-info/pregnancy/pregnant-now-what/thinking-about-abortion

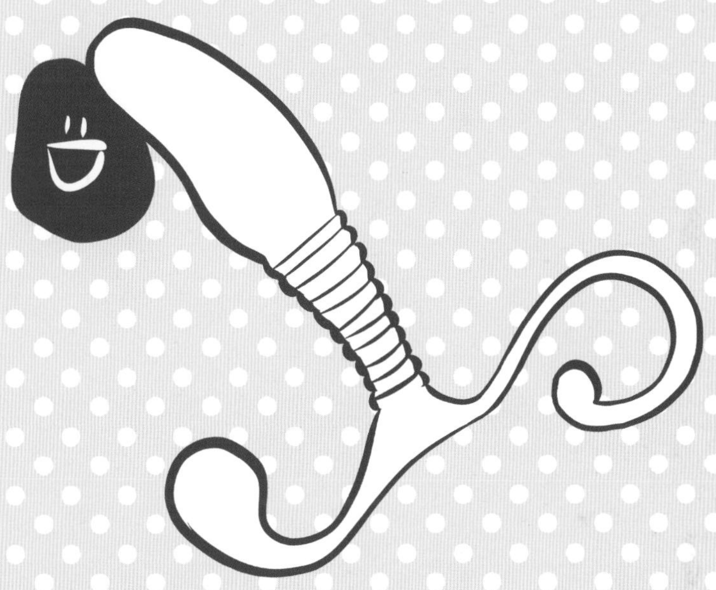

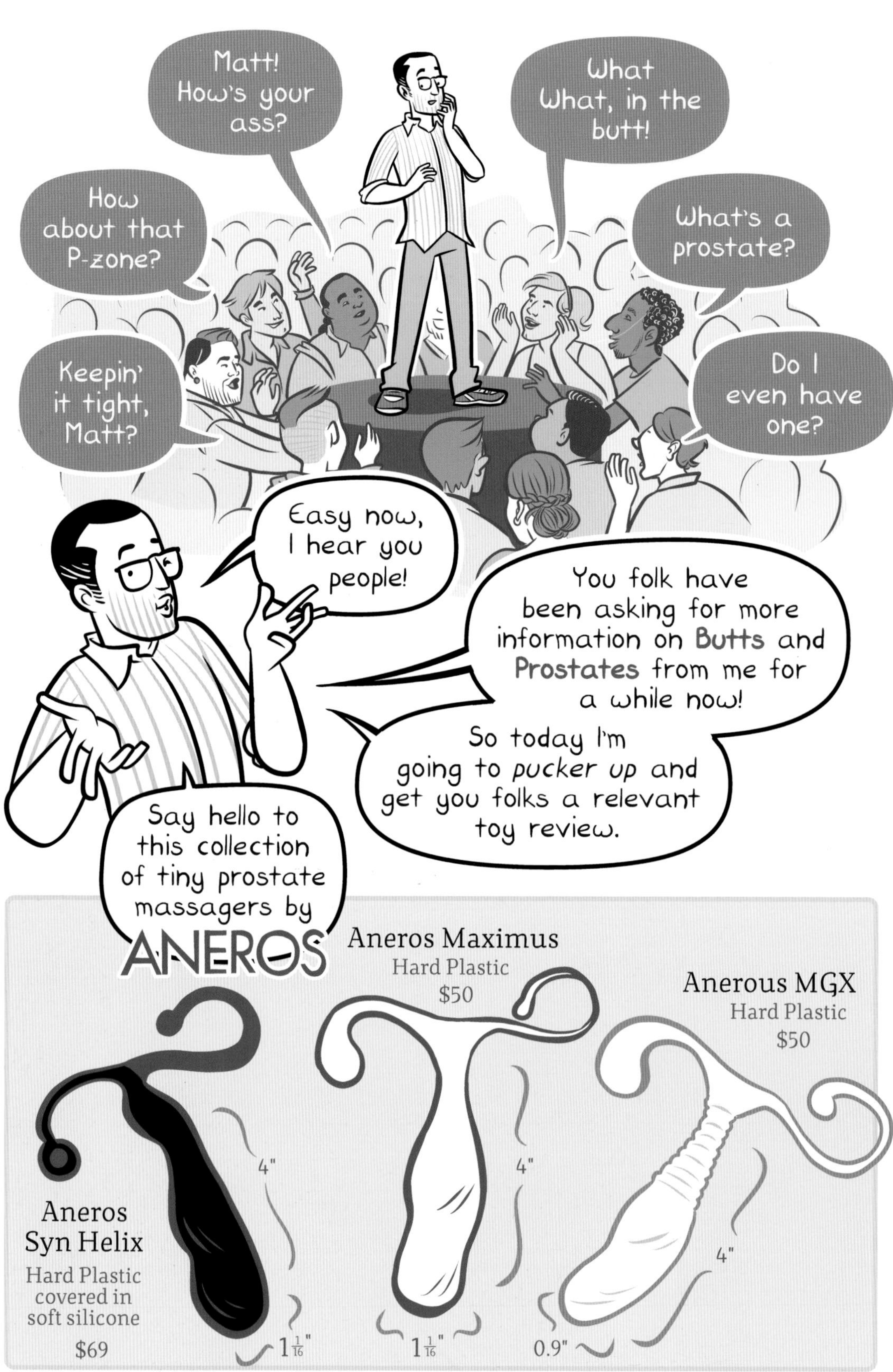

Matt! How's your ass?
What What, in the butt!
How about that P-zone?
What's a prostate?
Keepin' it tight, Matt?
Do I even have one?
Easy now, I hear you people!
You folk have been asking for more information on **Butts** and **Prostates** from me for a while now!
So today I'm going to *pucker up* and get you folks a relevant toy review.
Say hello to this collection of tiny prostate massagers by
ANEROS
Aneros Maximus
Hard Plastic
$50
Anerous MGX
Hard Plastic
$50
Aneros Syn Helix
Hard Plastic covered in soft silicone
$69
4"
4"
4"
1 1/16"
1 1/16"
0.9"

And these are just the ones I own! Aneros has a *LARGE* collection on offer with different sizes and shapes to suit your body.

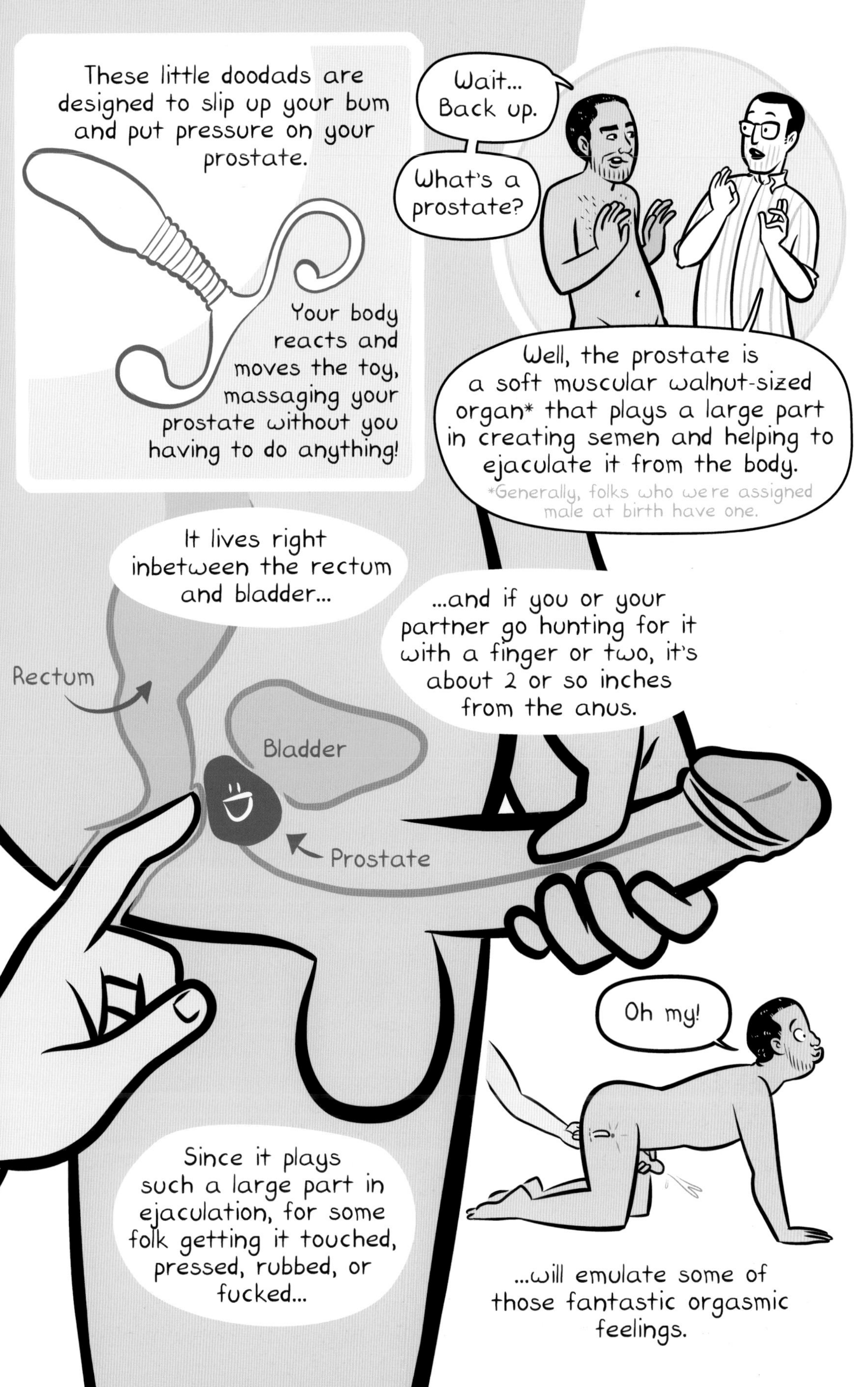
These little doodads are designed to slip up your bum and put pressure on your prostate.
Your body reacts and moves the toy, massaging your prostate without you having to do anything!
Wait... Back up.
What's a prostate?
Well, the prostate is a soft muscular walnut-sized organ* that plays a large part in creating semen and helping to ejaculate it from the body.
*Generally, folks who were assigned male at birth have one.
It lives right inbetween the rectum and bladder...
...and if you or your partner go hunting for it with a finger or two, it's about 2 or so inches from the anus.
Rectum
Bladder
Prostate
Since it plays such a large part in ejaculation, for some folk getting it touched, pressed, rubbed, or fucked...
Oh my!
...will emulate some of those fantastic orgasmic feelings.

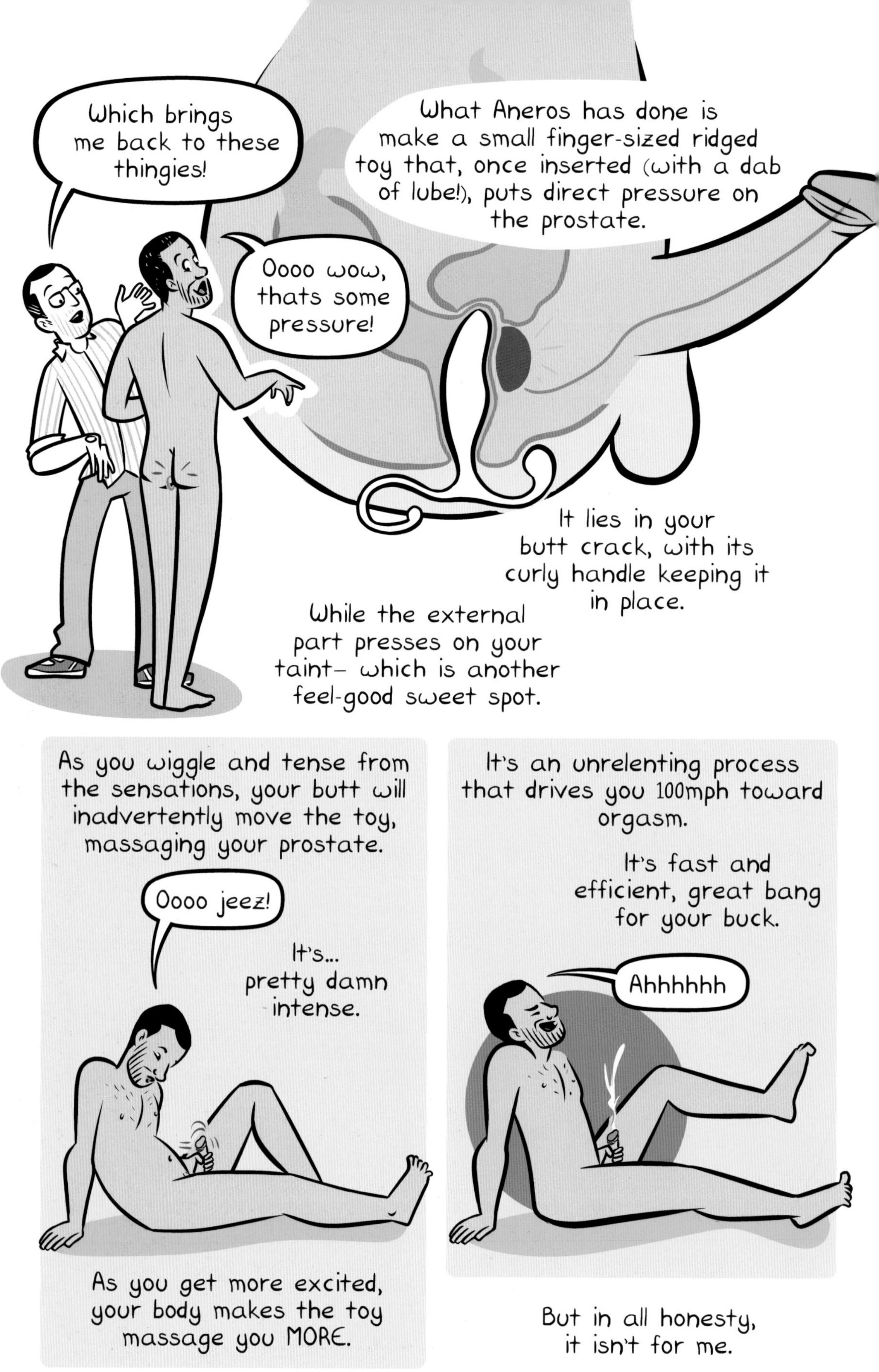

Which brings me back to these thingies!

What Aneros has done is make a small finger-sized ridged toy that, once inserted (with a dab of lube!), puts direct pressure on the prostate.

Oooo wow, thats some pressure!

It lies in your butt crack, with its curly handle keeping it in place.

While the external part presses on your taint– which is another feel-good sweet spot.

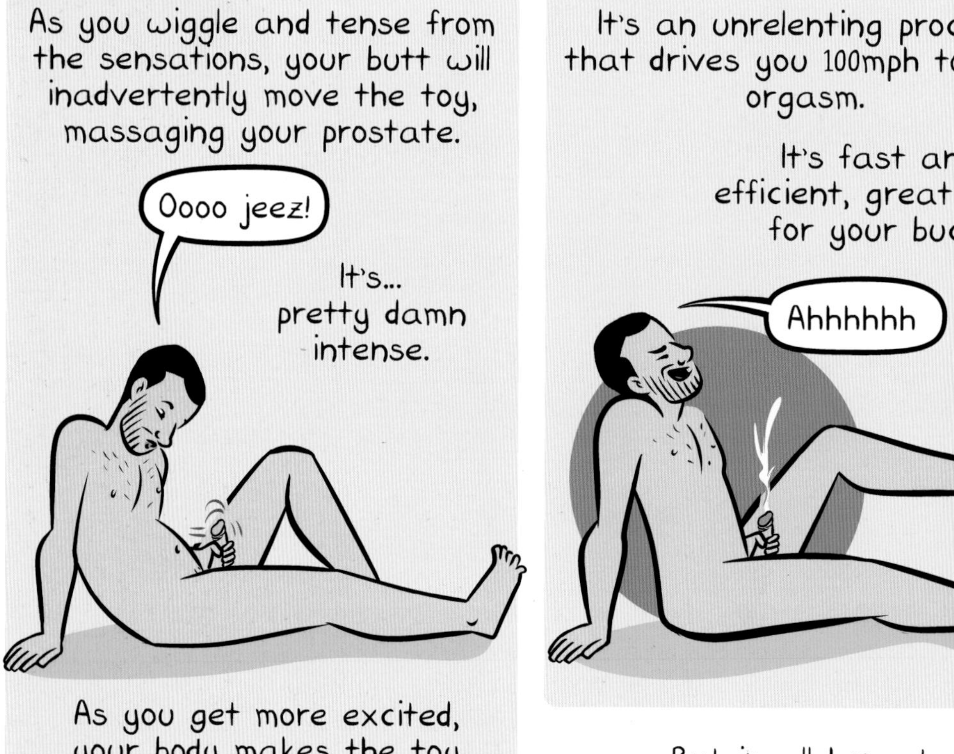

As you wiggle and tense from the sensations, your butt will inadvertently move the toy, massaging your prostate.
Oooo jeez!
It's... pretty damn intense.
As you get more excited, your body makes the toy massage you MORE.
It's an unrelenting process that drives you 100mph toward orgasm.
It's fast and efficient, great bang for your buck.
Ahhhhhh

But in all honesty, it isn't for me.

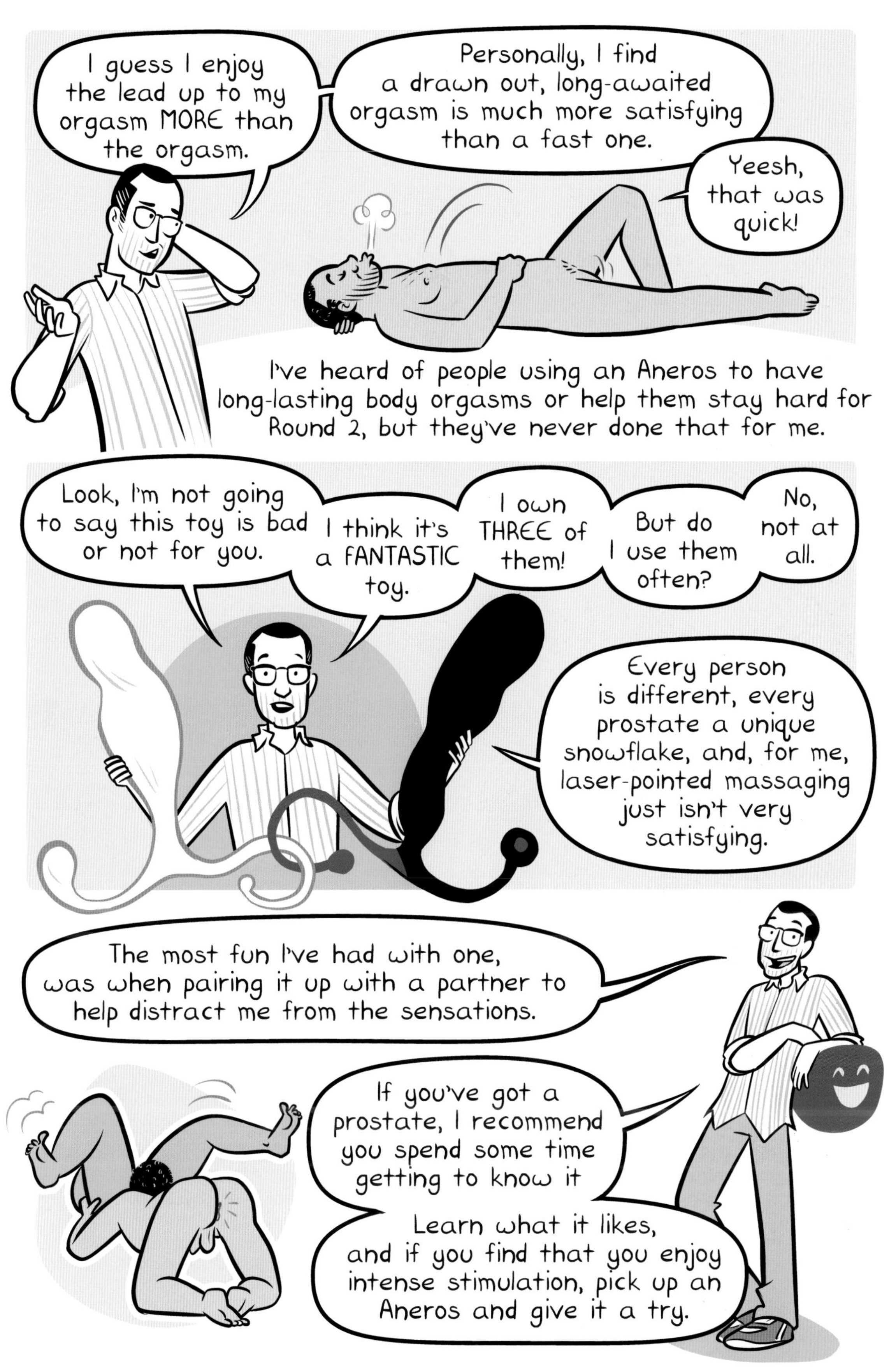
I guess I enjoy the lead up to my orgasm MORE than the orgasm.
Personally, I find a drawn out, long-awaited orgasm is much more satisfying than a fast one.
Yeesh, that was quick!
I've heard of people using an Aneros to have long-lasting body orgasms or help them stay hard for Round 2, but they've never done that for me.
Look, I'm not going to say this toy is bad or not for you.
I think it's a FANTASTIC toy.
I own THREE of them!
But do I use them often?
No, not at all.
Every person is different, every prostate a unique snowflake, and, for me, laser-pointed massaging just isn't very satisfying.
The most fun I've had with one, was when pairing it up with a partner to help distract me from the sensations.
If you've got a prostate, I recommend you spend some time getting to know it
Learn what it likes, and if you find that you enjoy intense stimulation, pick up an Aneros and give it a try.

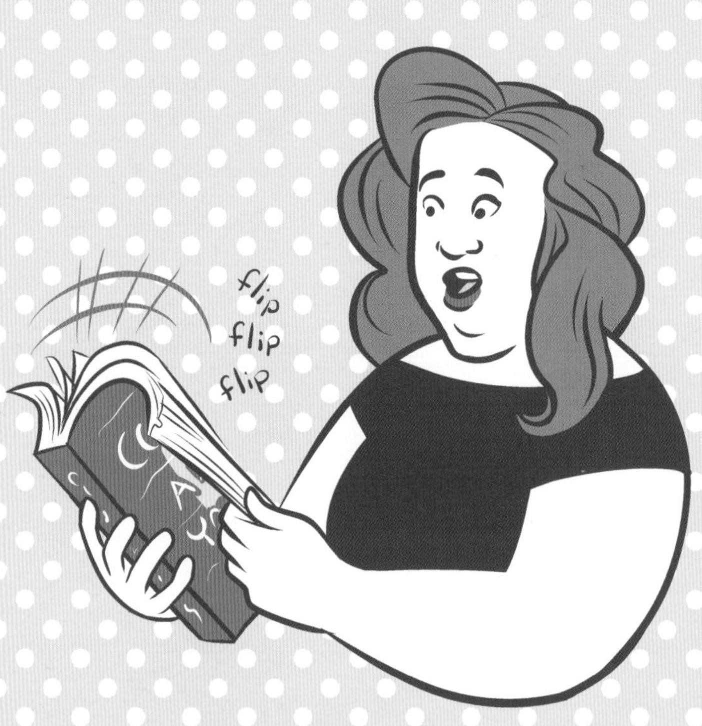
flip
flip
flip

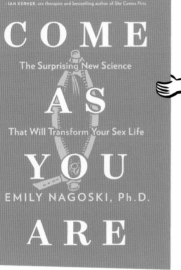

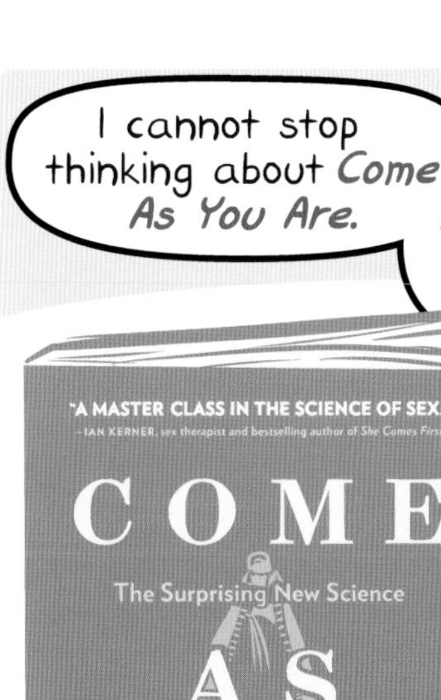
I cannot stop thinking about *Come As You Are.*
This book has absolutely blown my mind and I'm still reeling from it.
"A MASTER CLASS IN THE SCIENCE OF SEX."
–IAN KERNER, sex therapist and bestselling author of *She Comes First*
COME
The Surprising New Science
AS
That Will Transform Your Sex Life
YOU
EMILY NAGOSKI, Ph.D.
ARE

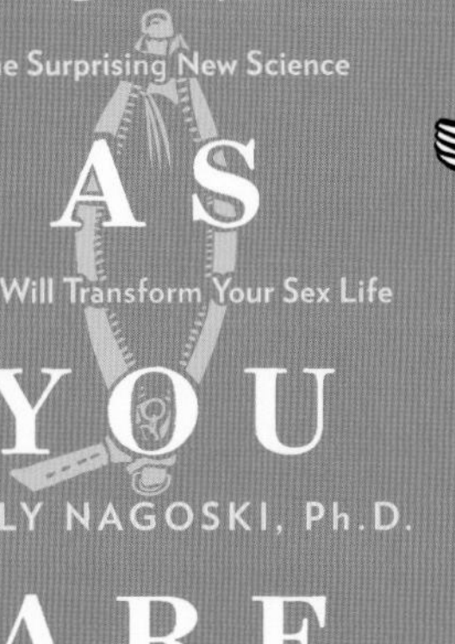

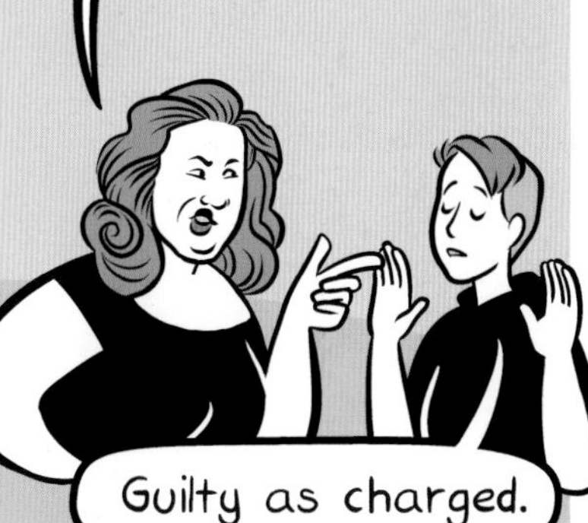
Waaaait a minute, didn't you draw the illustrations for this book?
And didn't Nagoski write the introduction to YOUR book?
And aren't you guys friends in real life?
Guilty as charged.

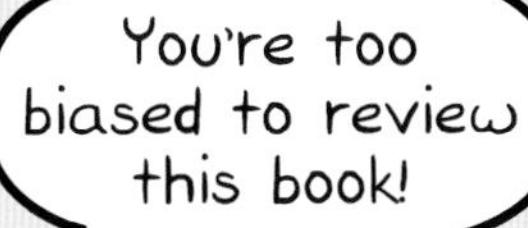

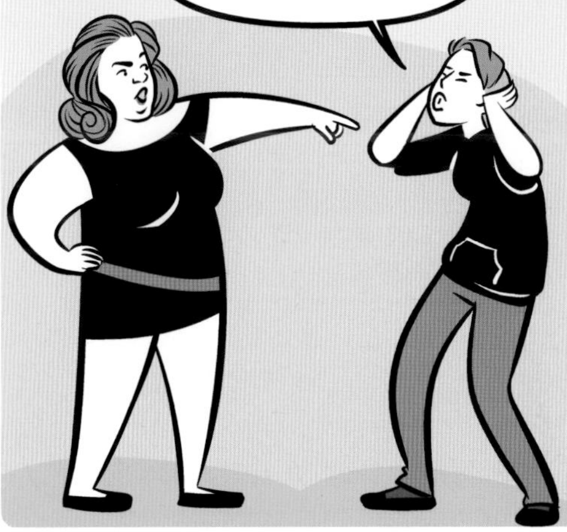
You're too biased to review this book!
I knoooooooo-oooow!
Nobody asked me to and I wasn't planning on it...

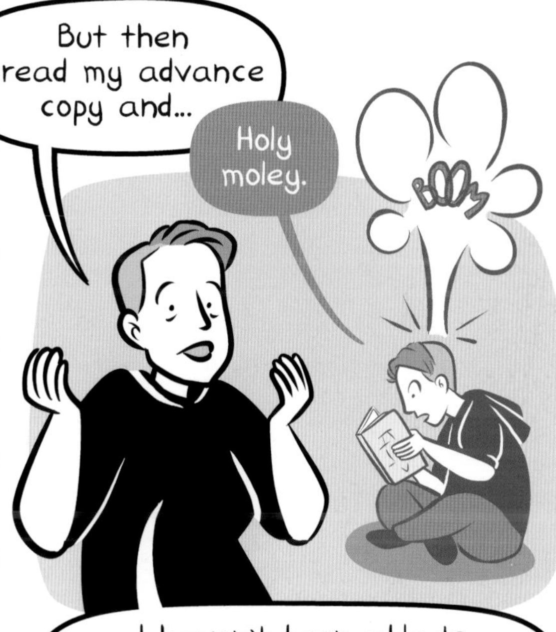
But then I read my advance copy and...
Holy moley.
BOOM
I haven't been able to shut up about it in real life and I honestly think I'd be doing a bigger disservice to you folks if I *DIDN'T* tell you all about it.

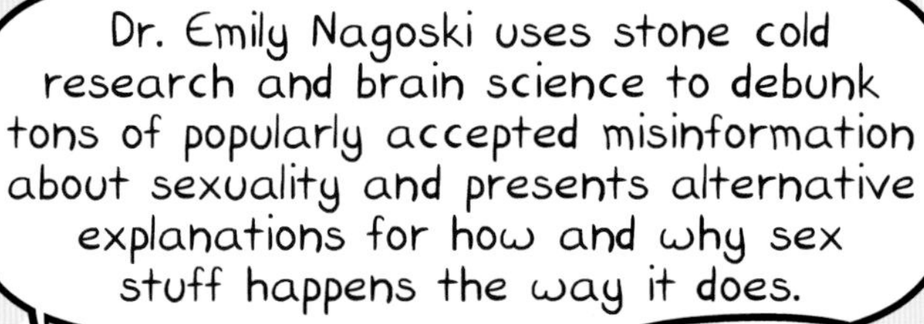

Dr. Emily Nagoski uses stone cold research and brain science to debunk tons of popularly accepted misinformation about sexuality and presents alternative explanations for how and why sex stuff happens the way it does.

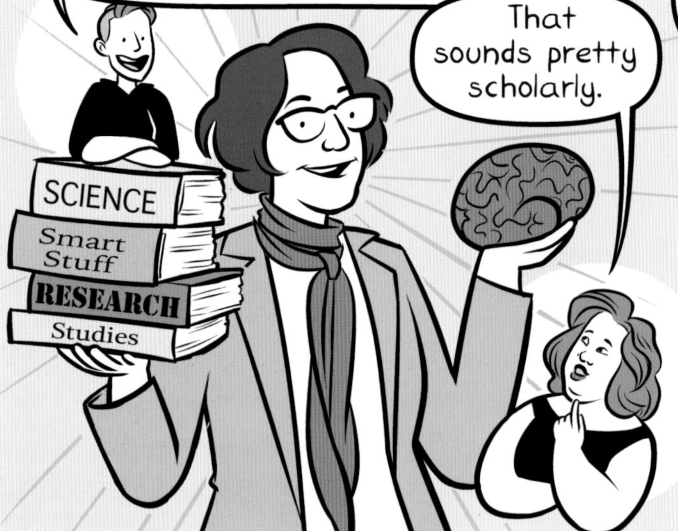

That sounds pretty scholarly.
SCIENCE
Smart Stuff
RESEARCH
Studies

It's more than just intellectual, though!

She's got real, practical solutions to help people resolve their sexual frustrations and woes.

Oo, worksheets!

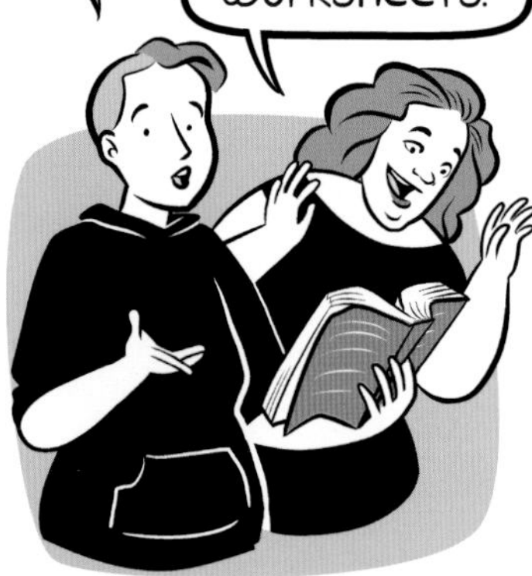

At first I tried to just make a mental note every time she introduced a new concept to me or said something thought-provoking.

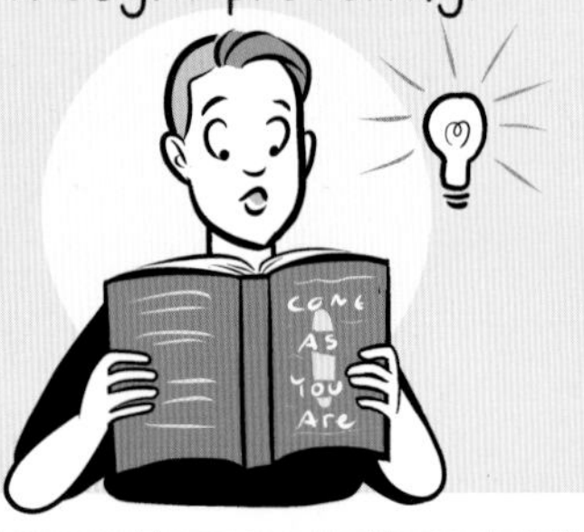

Pretty quickly I realized my brain couldn't realistically keep track of everything.

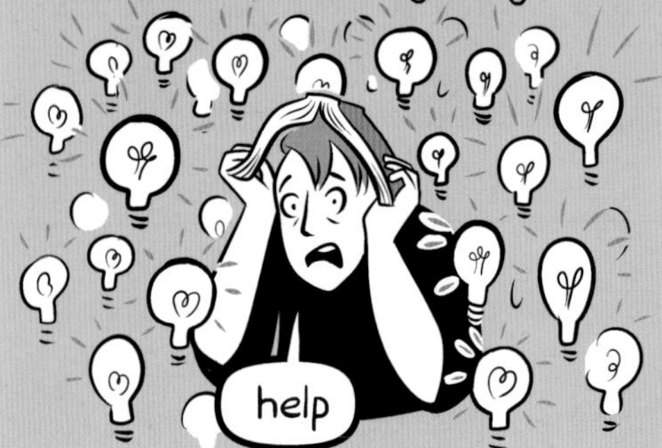

So then I started underlining passages with a red pencil!

Jesus, you underlined the whole flippin' book!

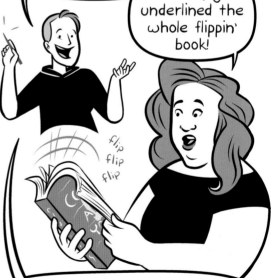

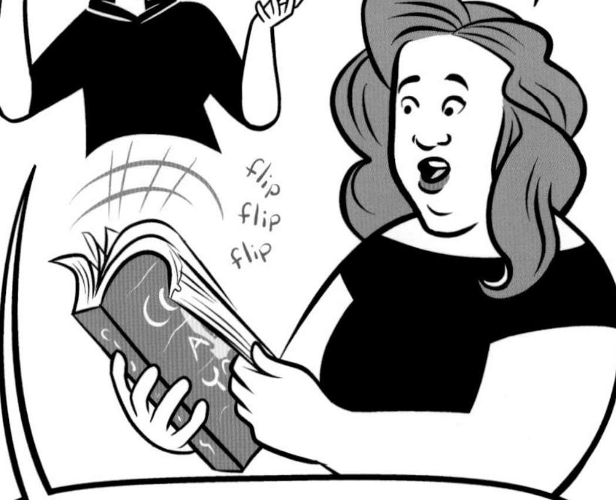

Just for you, my dearest perverts, I present to you the top three mind-blowing concepts I learned from *Come As You Are.*

The Dual Control Model of Sexual Desire

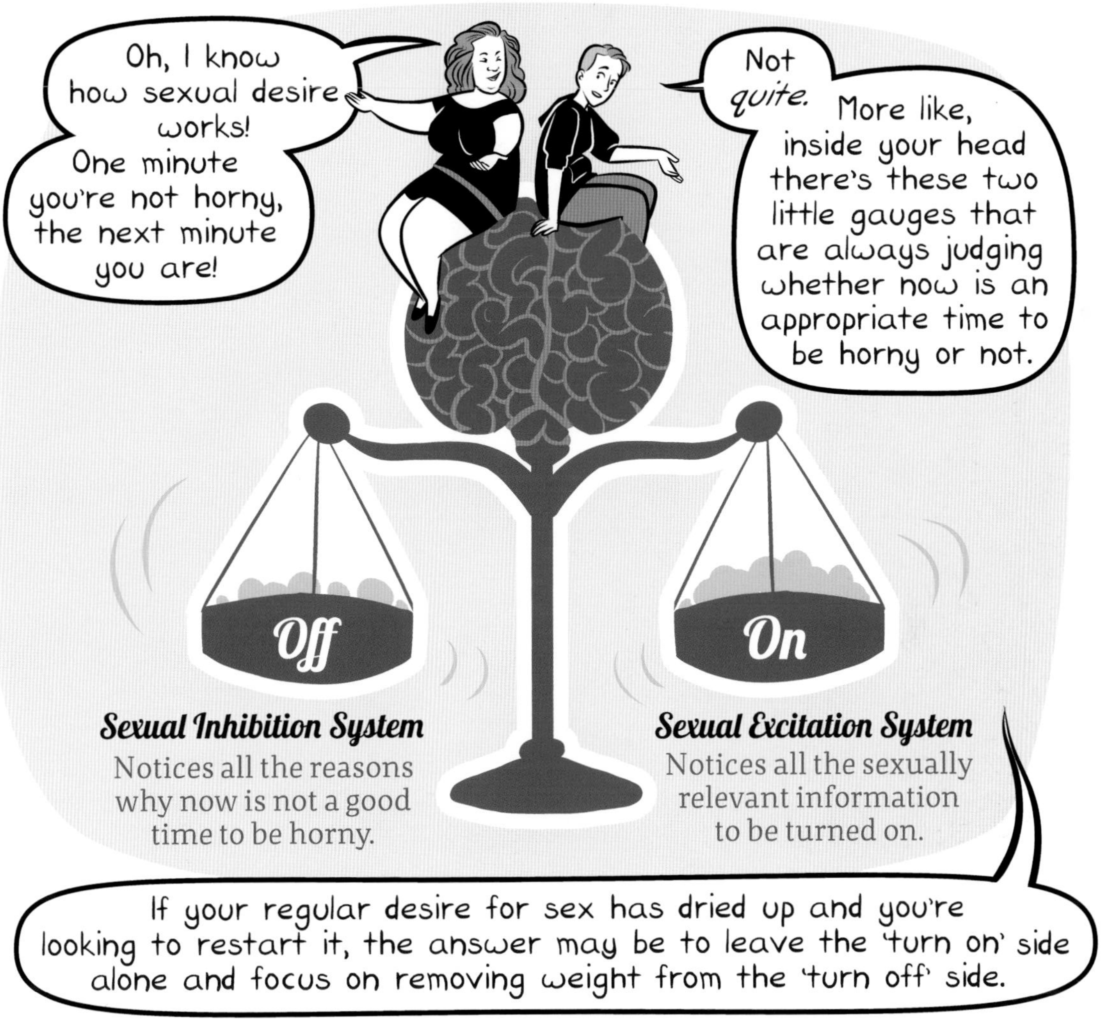

Oh, I know how sexual desire works! One minute you're not horny, the next minute you are!

Not *quite.* More like, inside your head there's these two little gauges that are always judging whether now is an appropriate time to be horny or not.

Off

On

Sexual Inhibition System

Notices all the reasons why now is not a good time to be horny.

Sexual Excitation System

Notices all the sexually relevant information to be turned on.

If your regular desire for sex has dried up and you're looking to restart it, the answer may be to leave the 'turn on' side alone and focus on removing weight from the 'turn off' side.

Spontaneous Desire and Responsive Desire

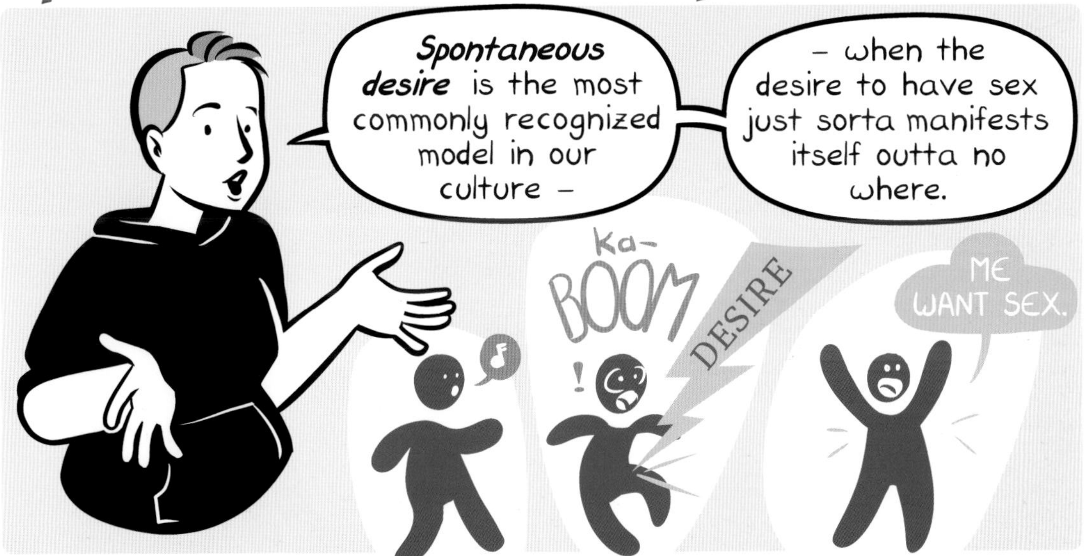

Spontaneous desire is the most commonly recognized model in our culture –
– when the desire to have sex just sorta manifests itself outta no where.
Ka-BOOM
!
DESIRE
ME WANT SEX.

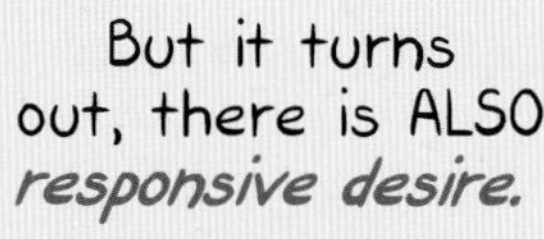
But it turns out, there is ALSO *responsive desire.*

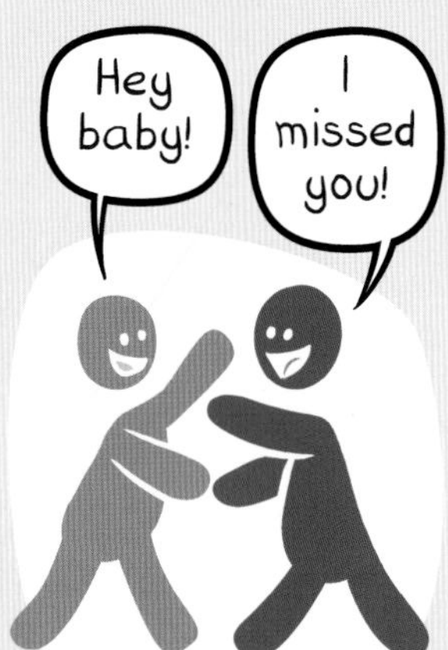
Hey baby!
I missed you!

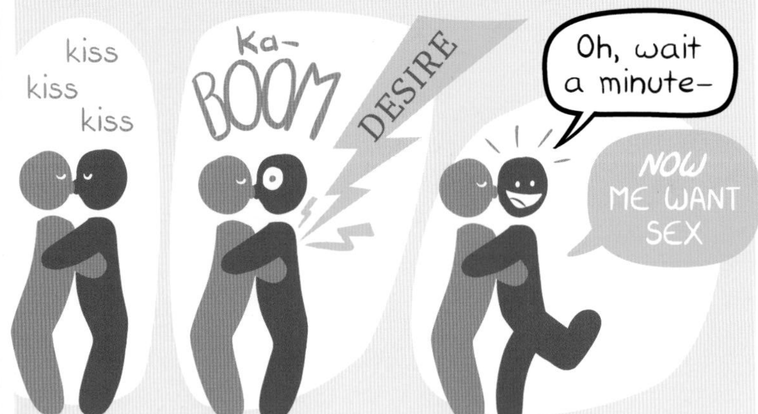
Which is when folks only want sex **after** consensually sexy things are already happening, and then their mind and body turns on ***in response to*** that sexy context.
kiss kiss kiss
Ka-BOOM
DESIRE
Oh, wait a minute–
NOW ME WANT SEX

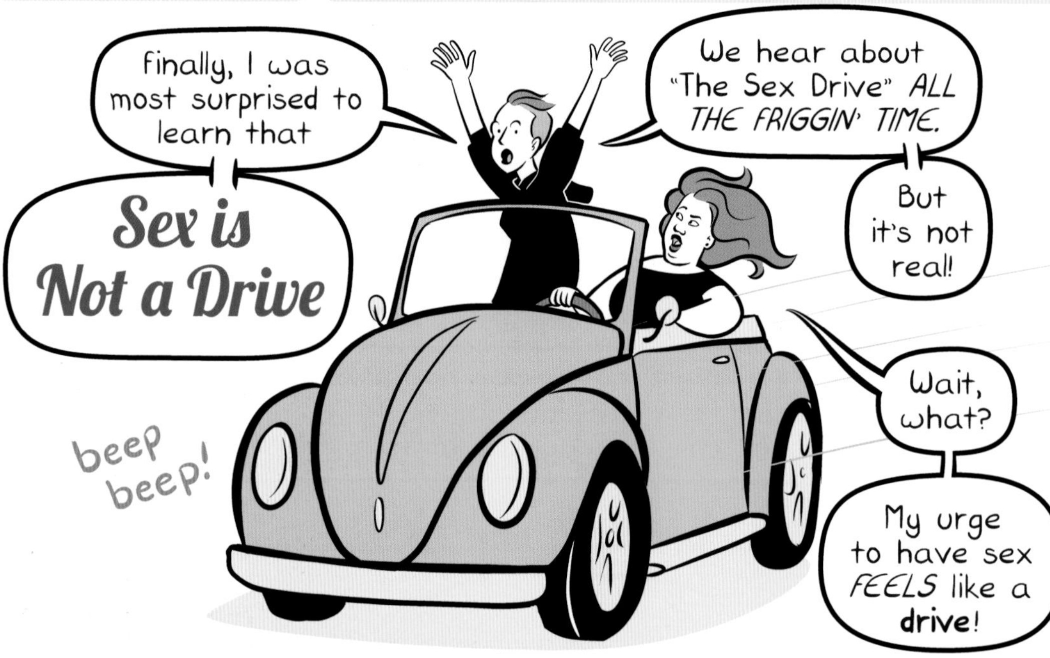
Finally, I was most surprised to learn that
Sex is Not a Drive
We hear about "The Sex Drive" *ALL THE FRIGGIN' TIME.*
But it's not real!
beep beep!
Wait, what?
My urge to have sex *FEELS* like a **drive**!

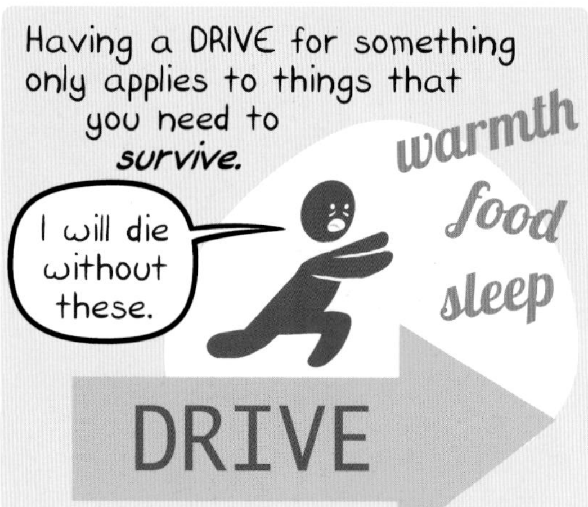
Having a DRIVE for something only applies to things that you need to ***survive.***
I will die without these.
warmth
food
sleep
DRIVE

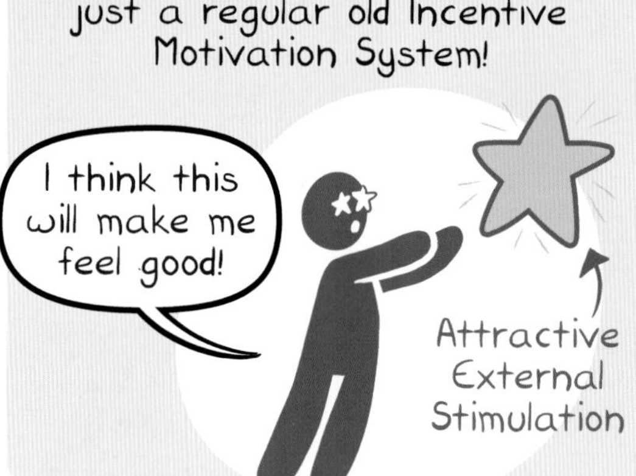
Instead of a drive, sex is just a regular old Incentive Motivation System!
I think this will make me feel good!
Attractive External Stimulation

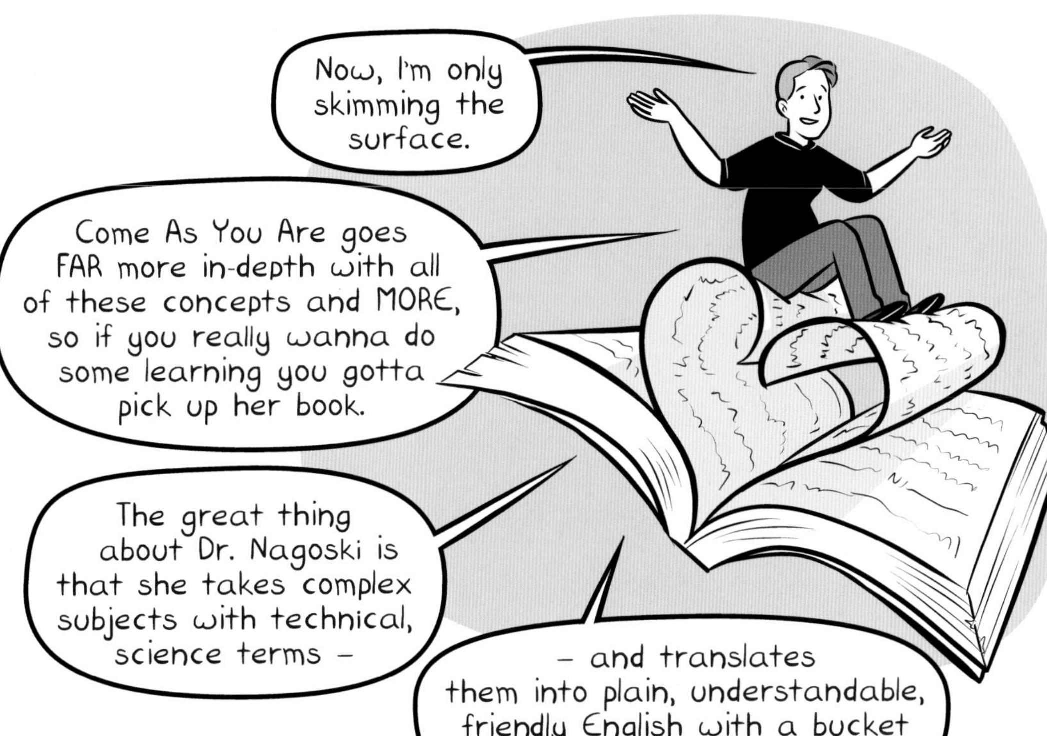

Now, I'm only skimming the surface.
Come As You Are goes FAR more in-depth with all of these concepts and MORE, so if you really wanna do some learning you gotta pick up her book.
The great thing about Dr. Nagoski is that she takes complex subjects with technical, science terms –
– and translates them into plain, understandable, friendly English with a bucket fulla real compassion.

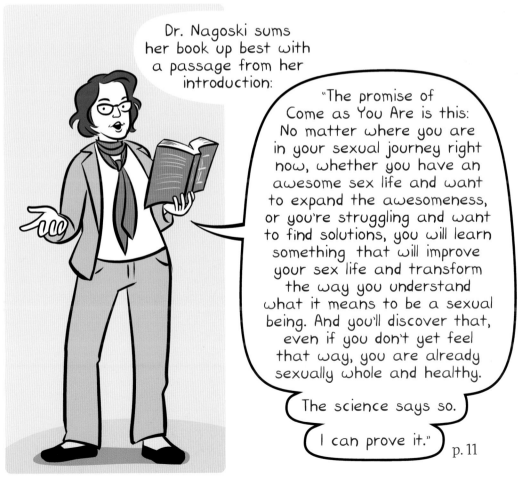

Dr. Nagoski sums her book up best with a passage from her introduction:

"The promise of Come as You Are is this: No matter where you are in your sexual journey right now, whether you have an awesome sex life and want to expand the awesomeness, or you're struggling and want to find solutions, you will learn something that will improve your sex life and transform the way you understand what it means to be a sexual being. And you'll discover that, even if you don't yet feel that way, you are already sexually whole and healthy.

The science says so.

I can prove it." p. 11

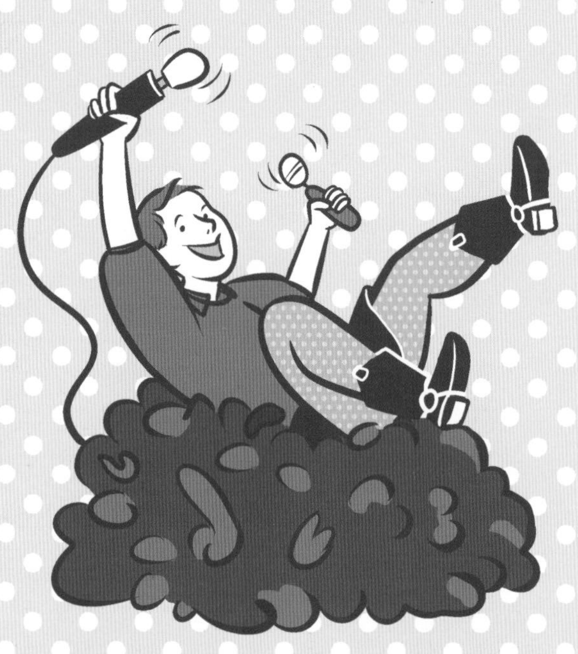

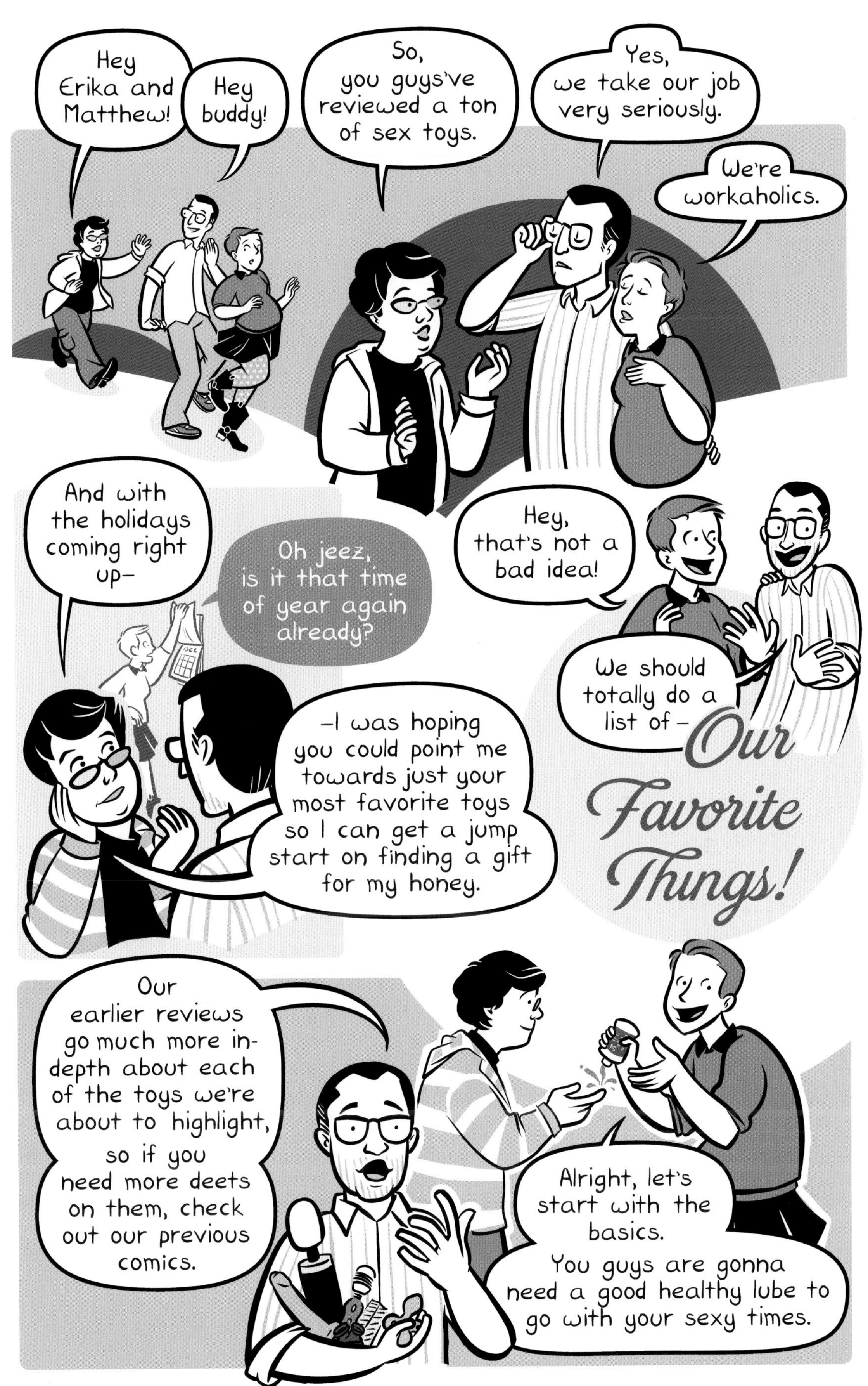
Hey Erika and Matthew!
Hey buddy!
So, you guys've reviewed a ton of sex toys.
Yes, we take our job very seriously.
We're workaholics.
And with the holidays coming right up–
Oh jeez, is it that time of year again already?
DEC
–I was hoping you could point me towards just your most favorite toys so I can get a jump start on finding a gift for my honey.
Hey, that's not a bad idea!
We should totally do a list of–
Our Favorite Things!
Our earlier reviews go much more in-depth about each of the toys we're about to highlight,
so if you need more deets on them, check out our previous comics.
Alright, let's start with the basics.
You guys are gonna need a good healthy lube to go with your sexy times.

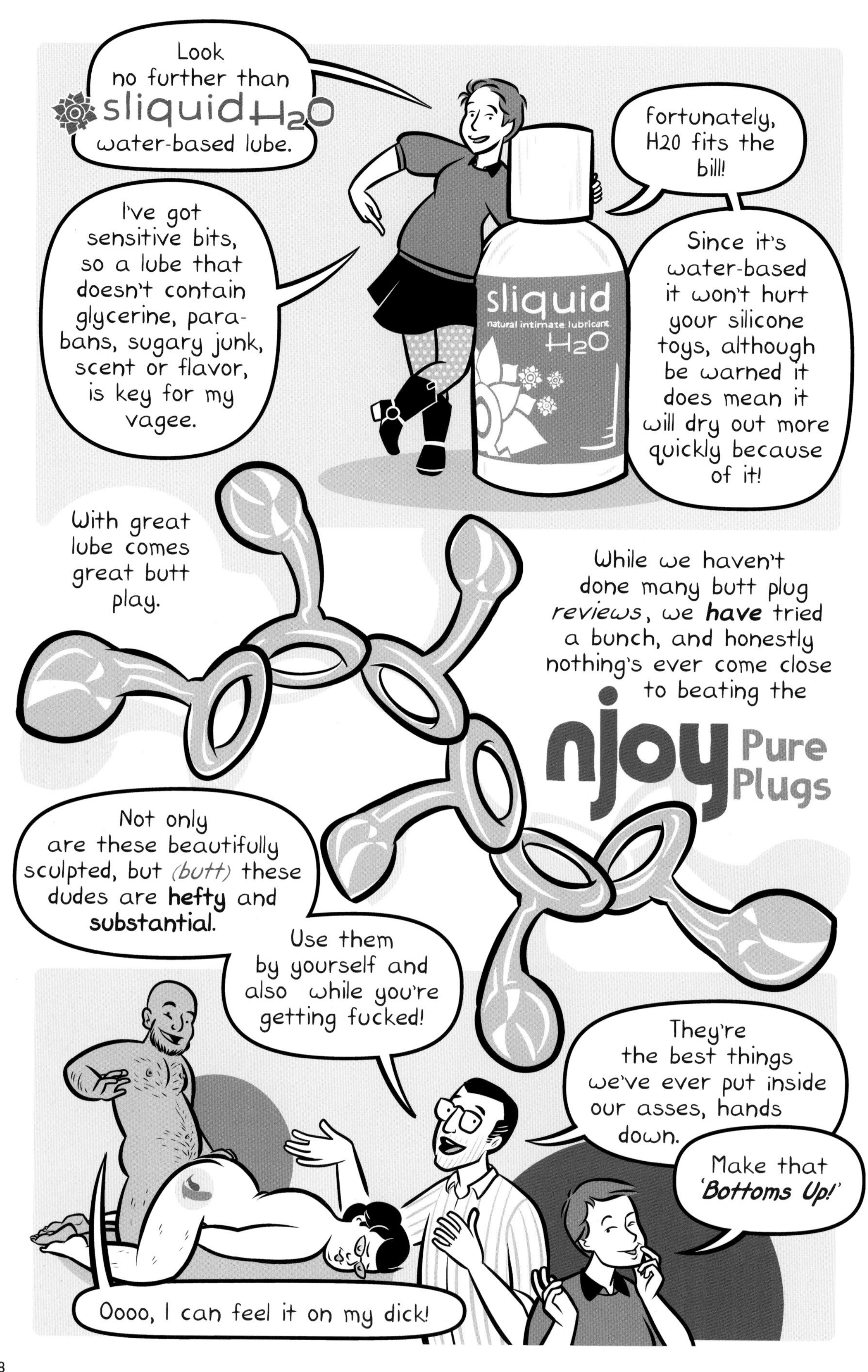
Look no further than sliquid H2O water-based lube.
I've got sensitive bits, so a lube that doesn't contain glycerine, parabans, sugary junk, scent or flavor, is key for my vagee.
Fortunately, H20 fits the bill!
Since it's water-based it won't hurt your silicone toys, although be warned it does mean it will dry out more quickly because of it!
sliquid
natural intimate lubricant
H2O
With great lube comes great butt play.
While we haven't done many butt plug *reviews*, we **have** tried a bunch, and honestly nothing's ever come close to beating the
njoy Pure Plugs
Not only are these beautifully sculpted, but *(butt)* these dudes are **hefty** and **substantial**.
Use them by yourself and also while you're getting fucked!
They're the best things we've ever put inside our asses, hands down.
Make that *'Bottoms Up!'*
Oooo, I can feel it on my dick!

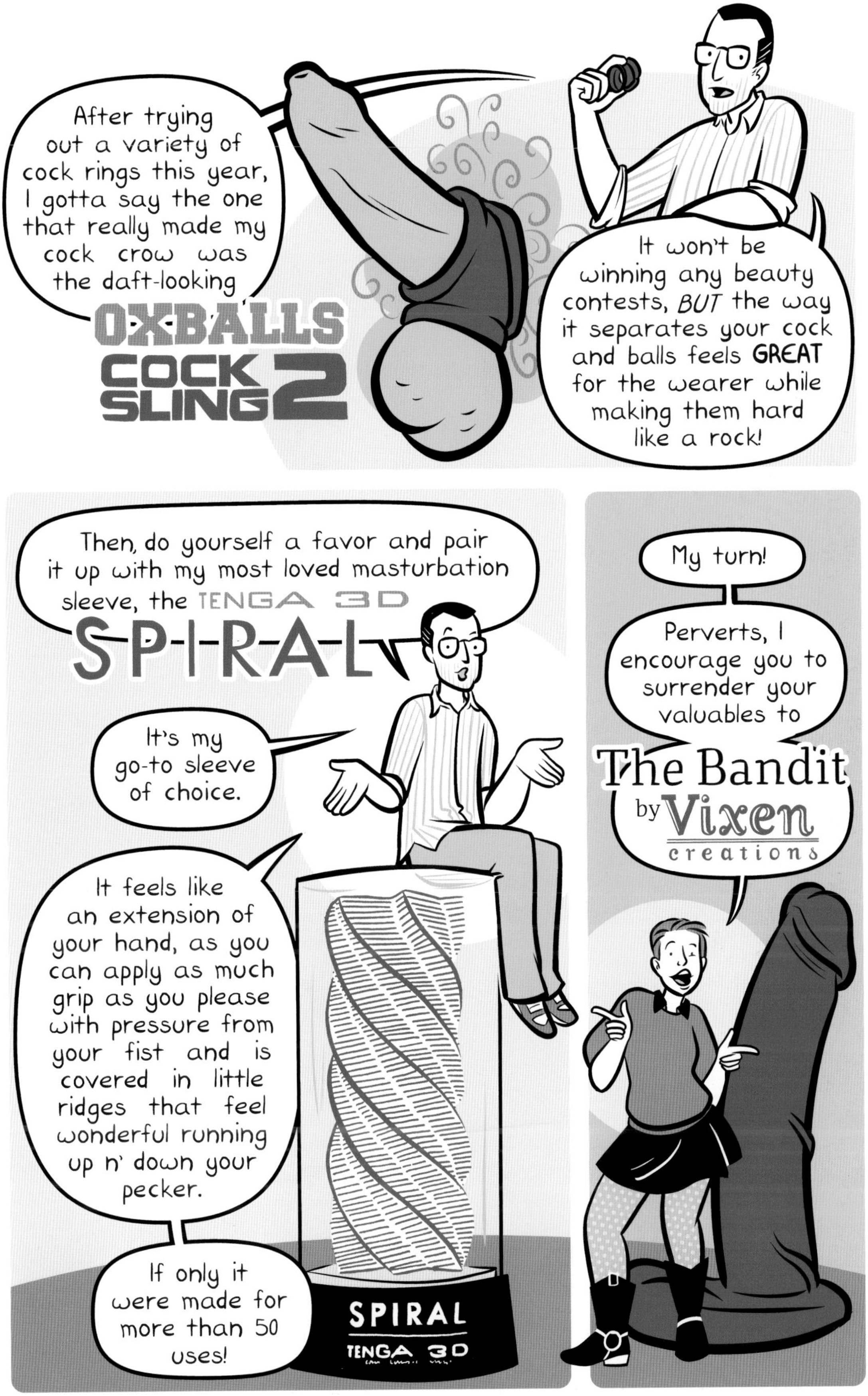

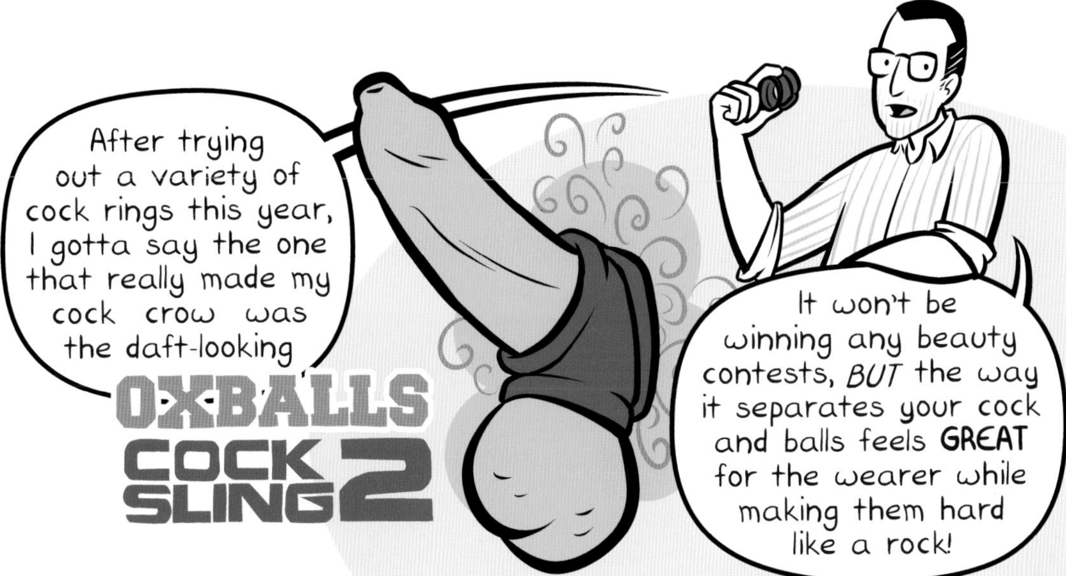
After trying out a variety of cock rings this year, I gotta say the one that really made my cock crow was the daft-looking
OXBALLS
COCK SLING 2
It won't be winning any beauty contests, *BUT* the way it separates your cock and balls feels **GREAT** for the wearer while making them hard like a rock!

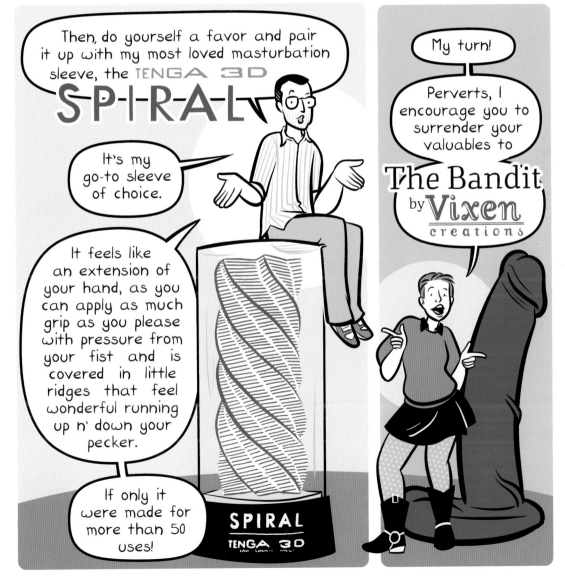

Then, do yourself a favor and pair it up with my most loved masturbation sleeve, the TENGA 3D SPIRAL

It's my go-to sleeve of choice.

It feels like an extension of your hand, as you can apply as much grip as you please with pressure from your fist and is covered in little ridges that feel wonderful running up n' down your pecker.

If only it were made for more than 50 uses!

SPIRAL

TENGA 3D

My turn!

Perverts, I encourage you to surrender your valuables to

The Bandit by Vixen creations

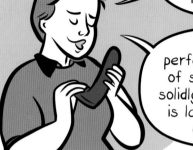

Ho-o-o-o-ly *MOLEY*, do I love this toy.

This is the most luxurious-feeling dildo that has ever graced my vagina with its presence.

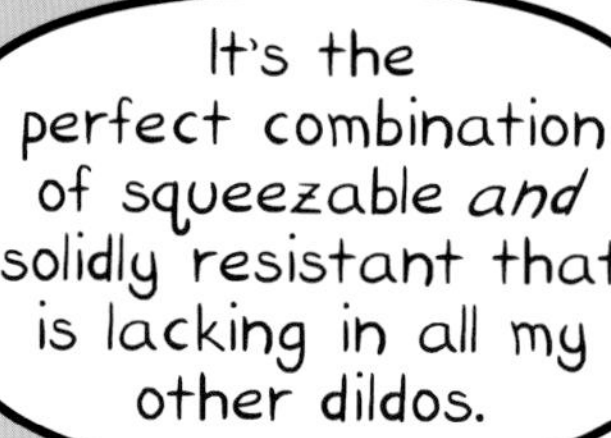

It's the perfect combination of squeezable *and* solidly resistant that is lacking in all my other dildos.

I love a good dong, but vibrators are my bread and butter and I can't just pick one as my favsies.

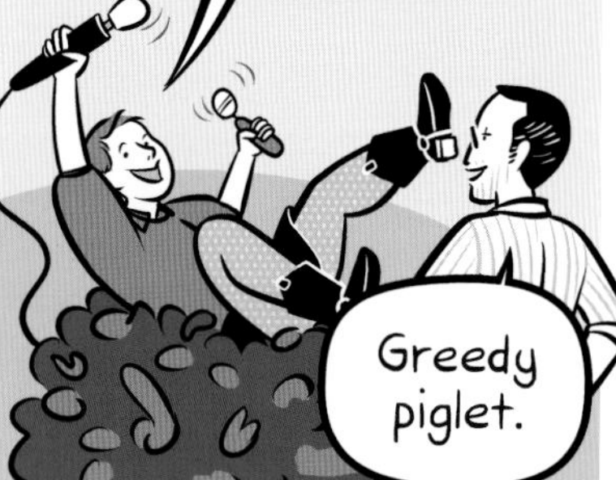

The standard Bullet Vibe puts the **fun** in ***fun**damental* as the beginner toy everyone should have in their tool chest.

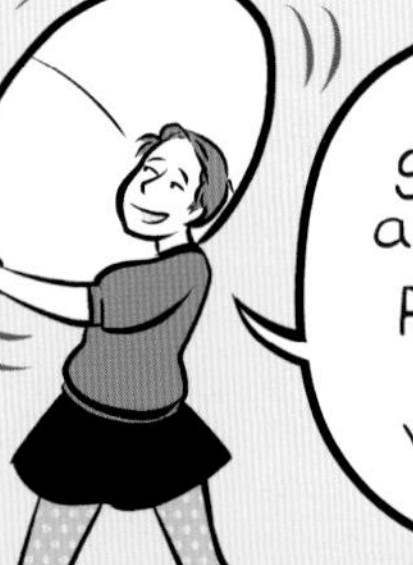

It's a great, gentle starter toy and forever holds a place in my heart for giving me my very first orgasm ever.

(Bonus points if you recognized it in our logo)

My cunt has come a long way since my bullet vibe days and now I need a toy that can really rumble my jungle.

The Mystic Wand by Vibratex is the strongest battery-powered vibrator I've ever found and a super convenient size for travel or partnered fucking.

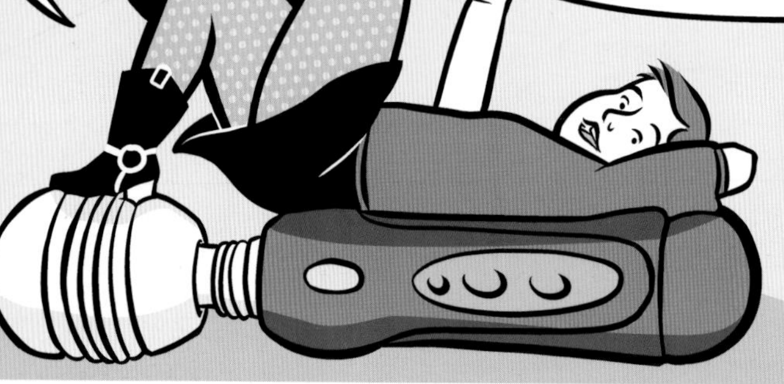

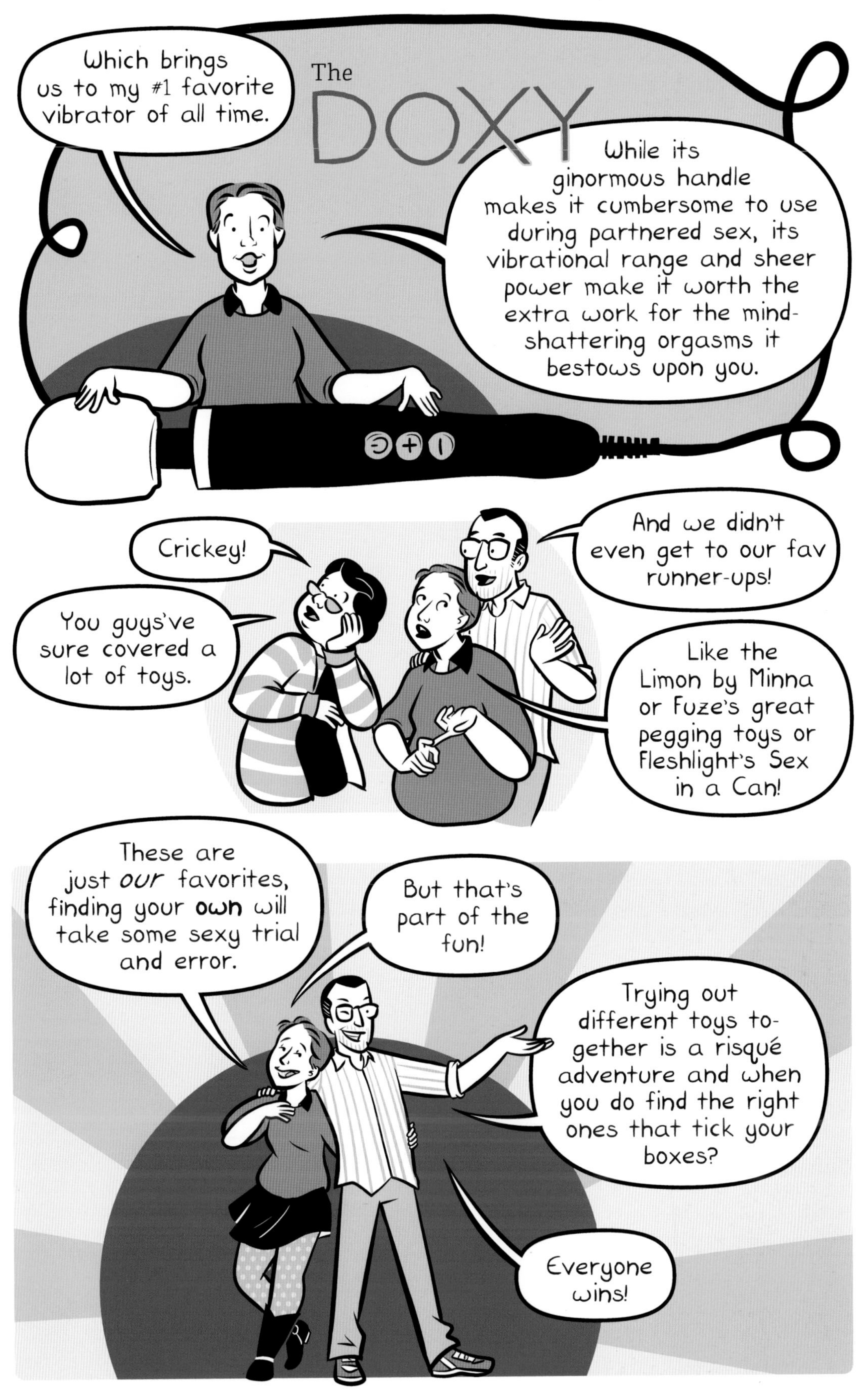
Which brings us to my #1 favorite vibrator of all time.
The DOXY
While its ginormous handle makes it cumbersome to use during partnered sex, its vibrational range and sheer power make it worth the extra work for the mind-shattering orgasms it bestows upon you.
Crickey!
You guys've sure covered a lot of toys.
And we didn't even get to our fav runner-ups!
Like the Limon by Minna or Fuze's great pegging toys or Fleshlight's Sex in a Can!
These are just *our* favorites, finding your **own** will take some sexy trial and error.
But that's part of the fun!
Trying out different toys together is a risqué adventure and when you do find the right ones that tick your boxes?
Everyone wins!

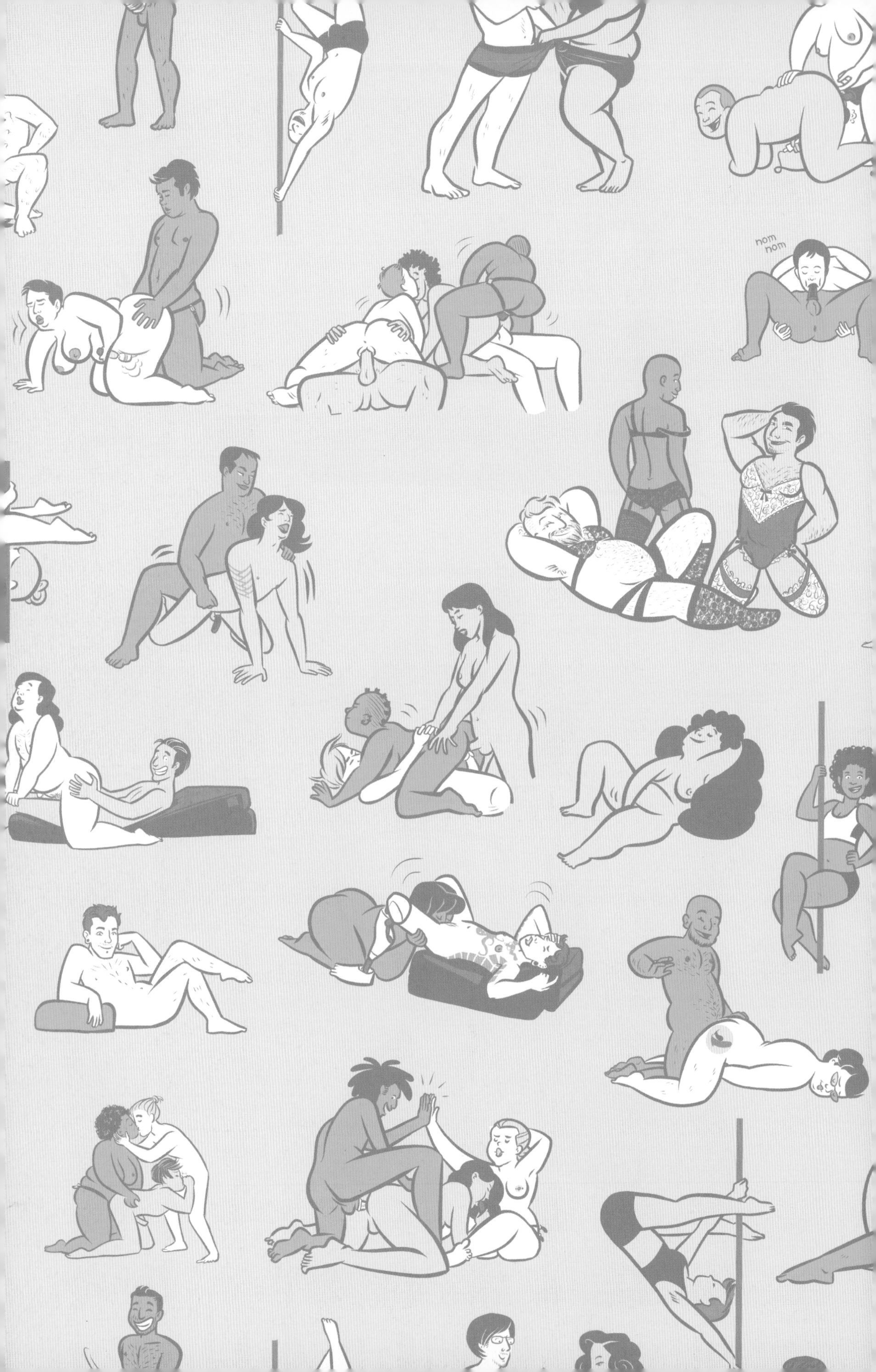
nom
nom

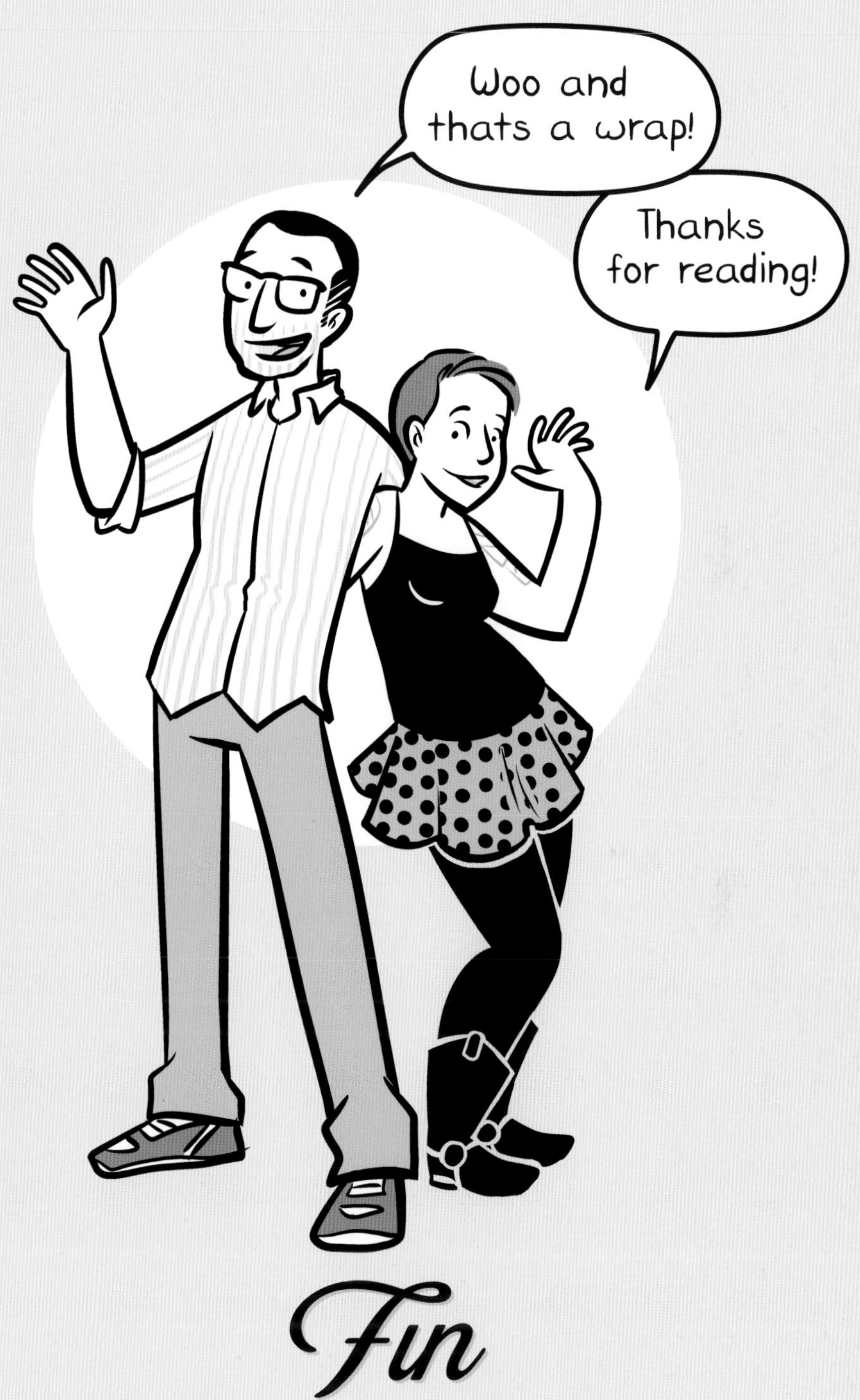

Fin

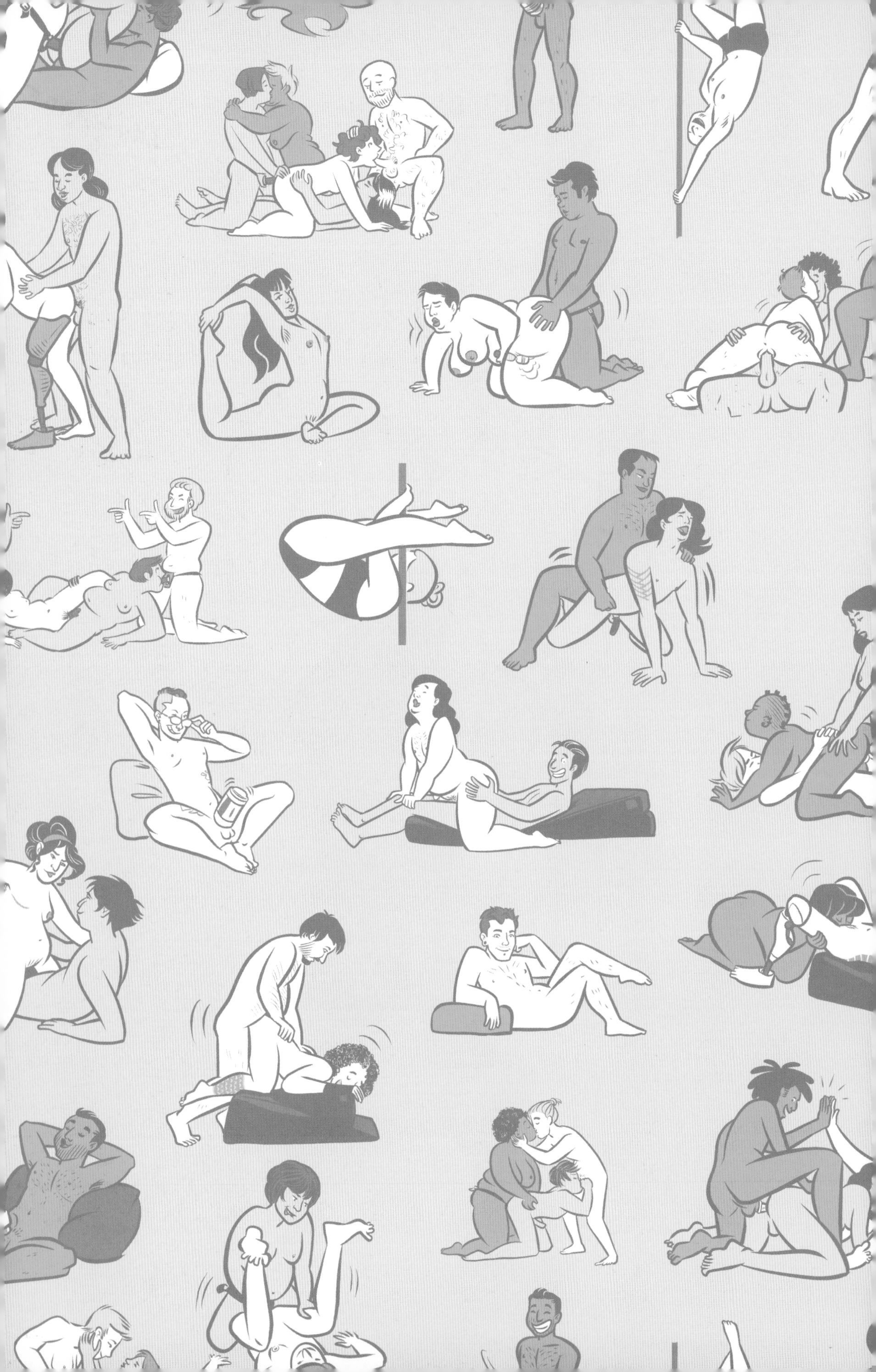

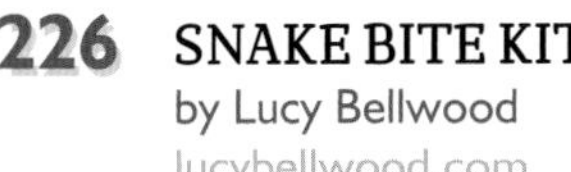

Guest Strips

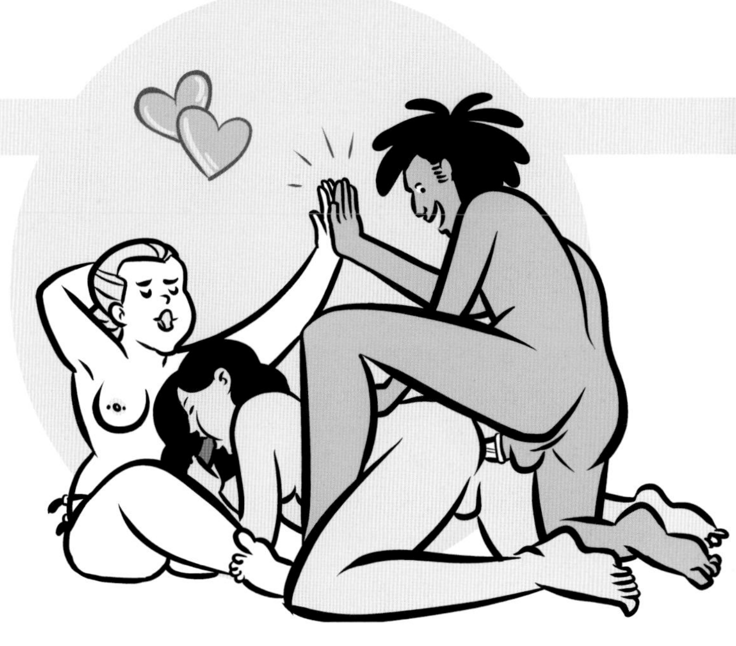

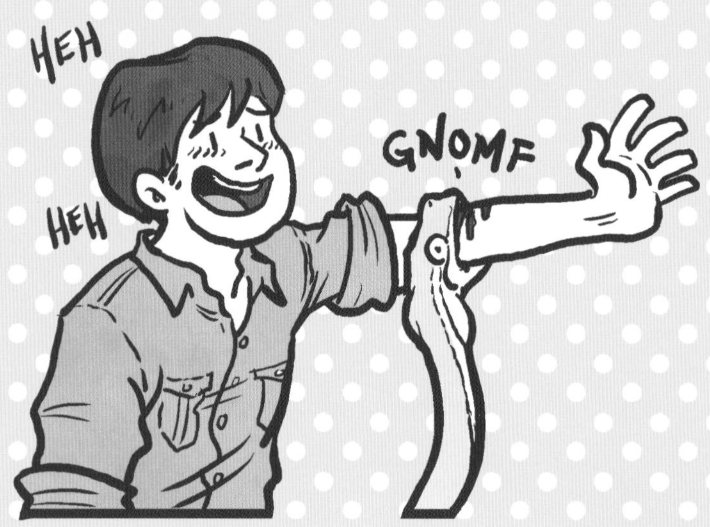

SNAKE BITE KIT

by Lucy Bellwood

lucybellwood.com

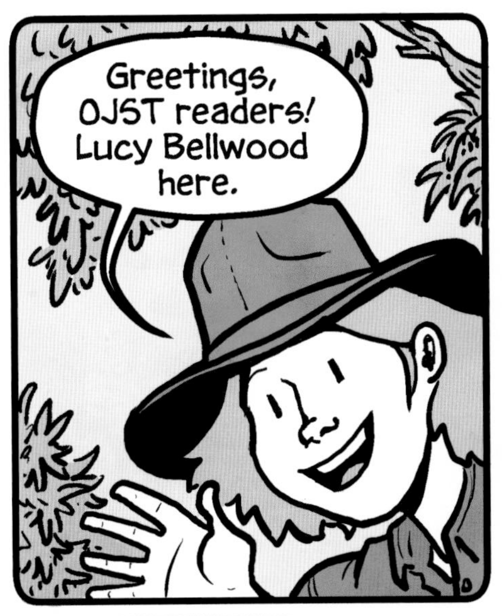
Greetings, OJST readers! Lucy Bellwood here.

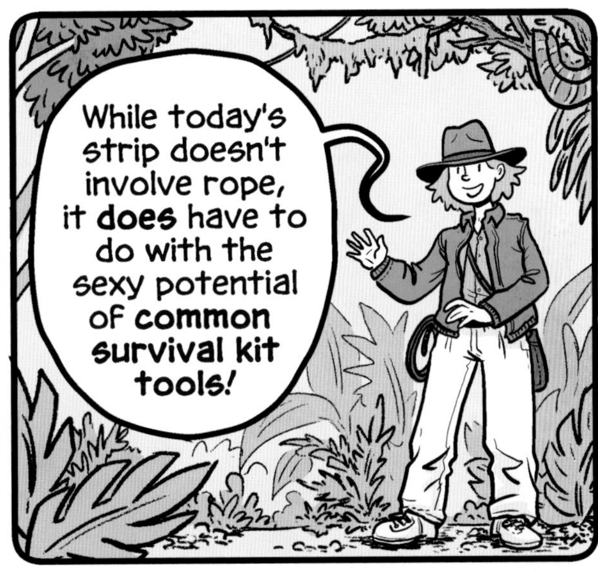
While today's strip doesn't involve rope, it **does** have to do with the sexy potential of **common survival kit tools!**

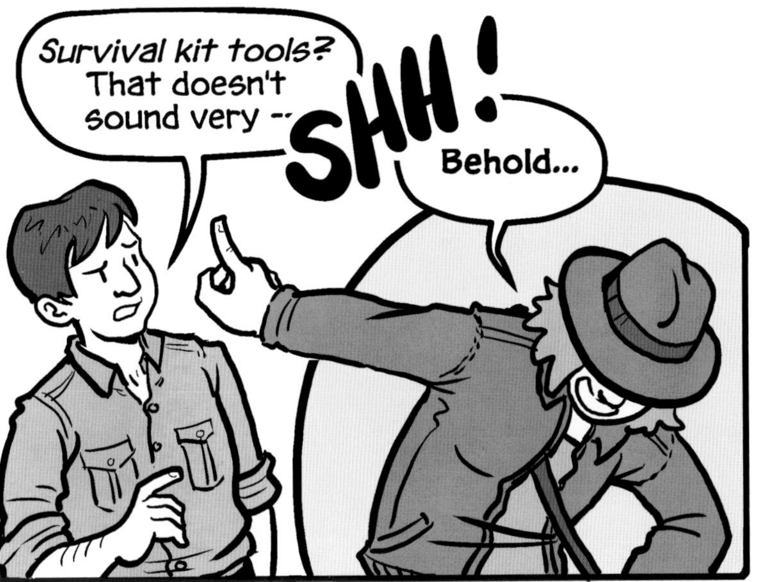
Survival kit tools? That doesn't sound very --
SHH!
Behold...

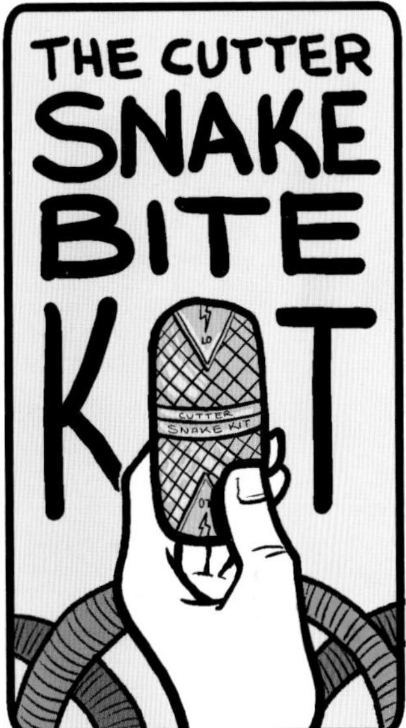
THE CUTTER SNAKE BITE KIT
CUTTER SNAKE KIT

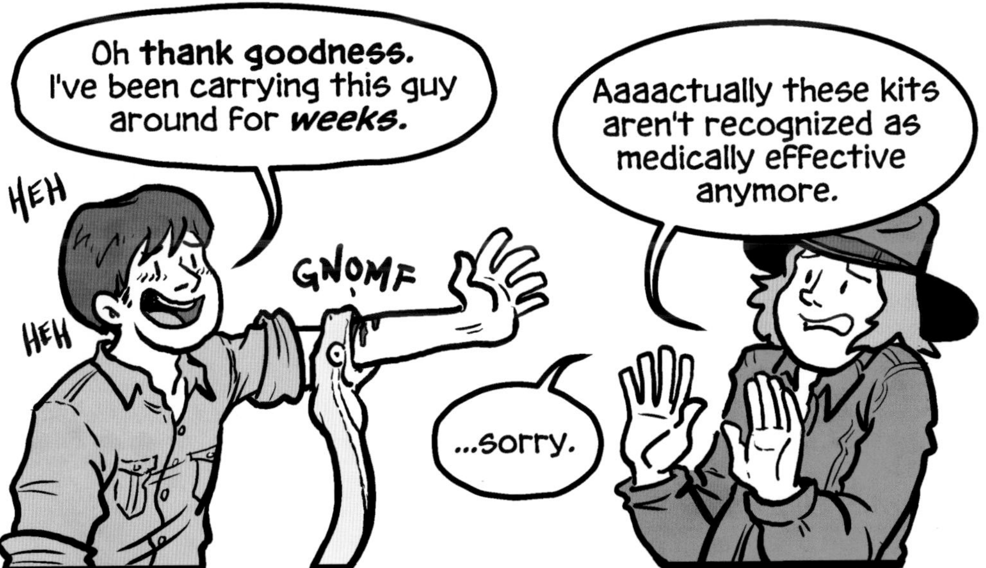
Oh **thank goodness.** I've been carrying this guy around for ***weeks.***
HEH
HEH
GNOMF
Aaaactually these kits aren't recognized as medically effective anymore.
...sorry.

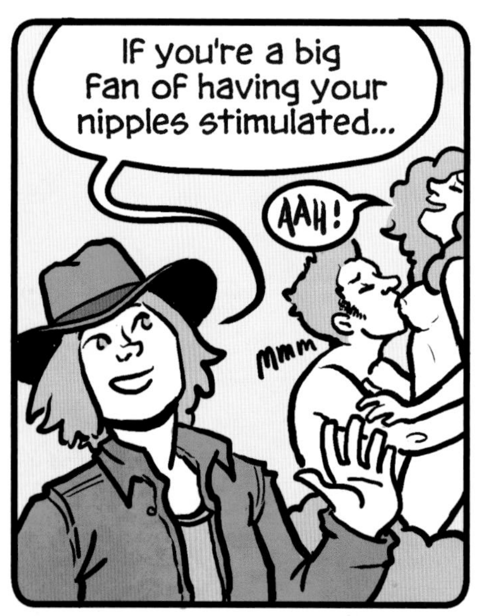

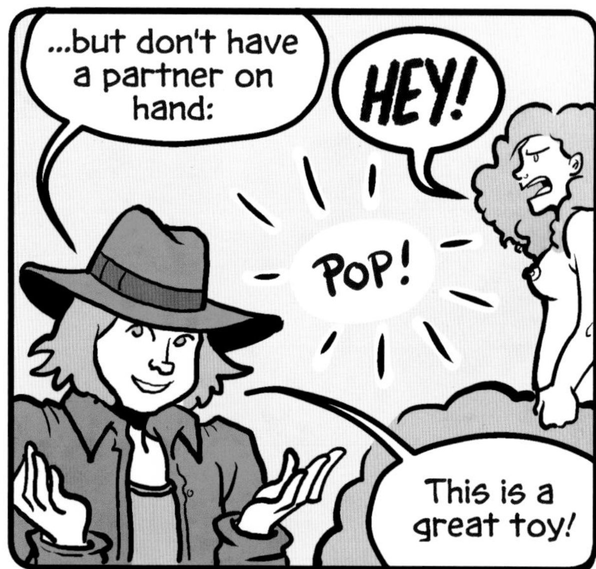

HERE'S THE SCOOP

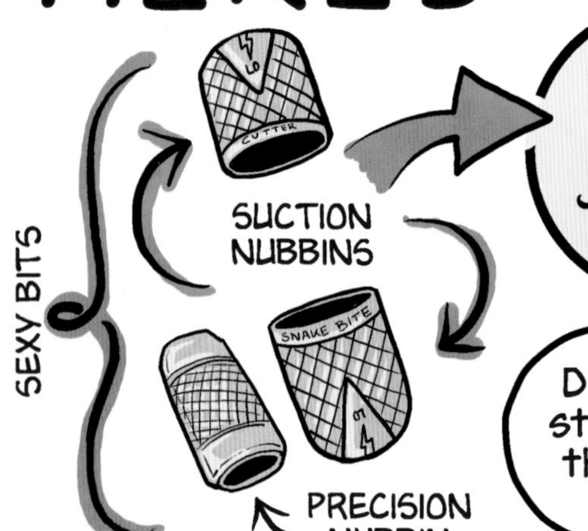

NOT-SEXY BITS
- BIT OF STRING
- RAZOR BLADE
- ANTISEPTIC SOLUTION

Ditch this stuff, keep the other stuff.

Due to being obsolete for its intended purpose, the kit is really cheap compared to similar, sex-specific toys.

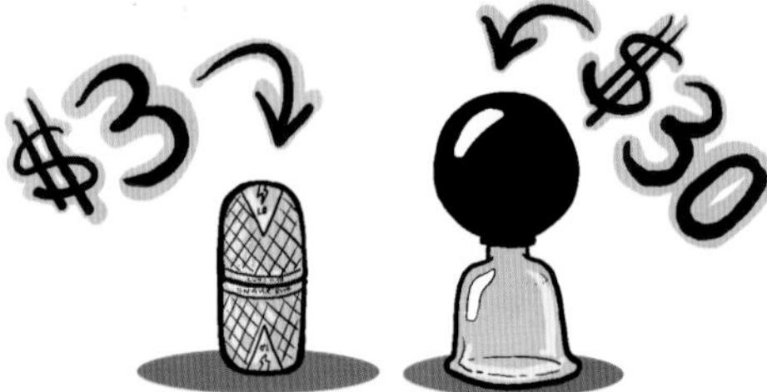

Also why use something called a "NIPPLE HONKER" when you can casually reach for your ***SNAKE BITE KIT?***

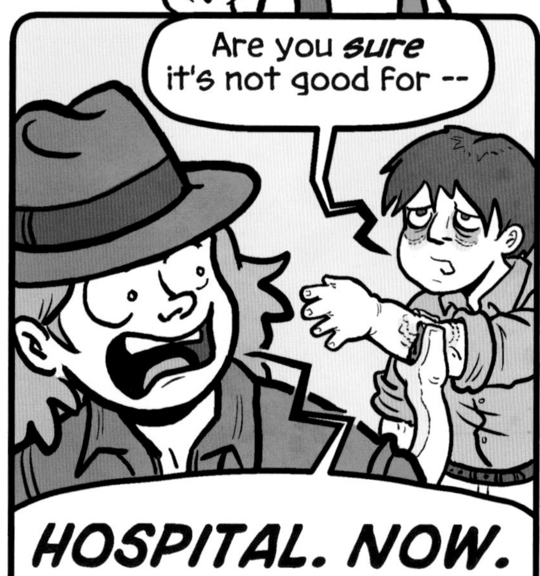

Are you *sure* it's not good for --
HOSPITAL. NOW.

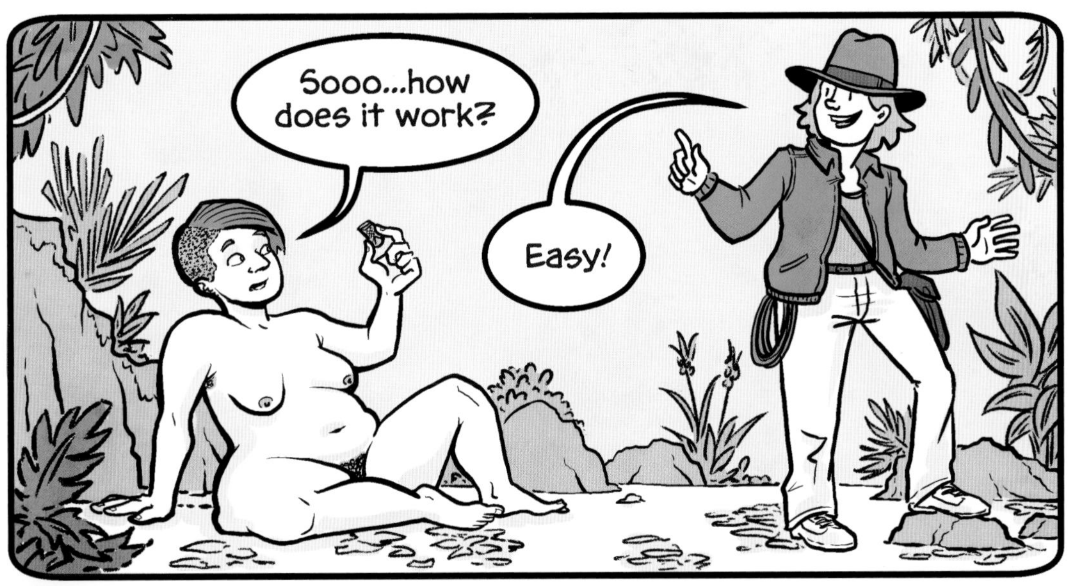
Sooo...how does it work?
Easy!

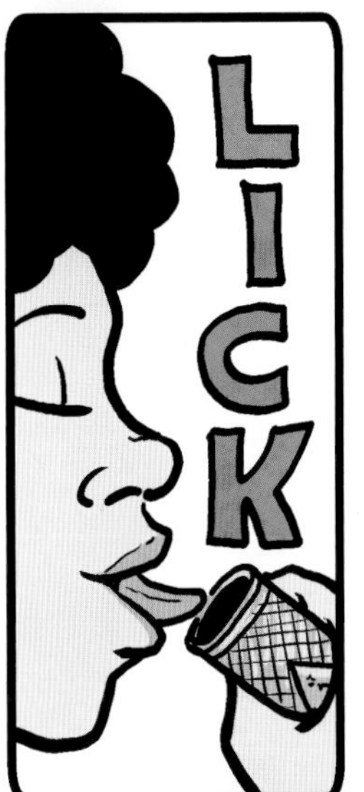
LICK

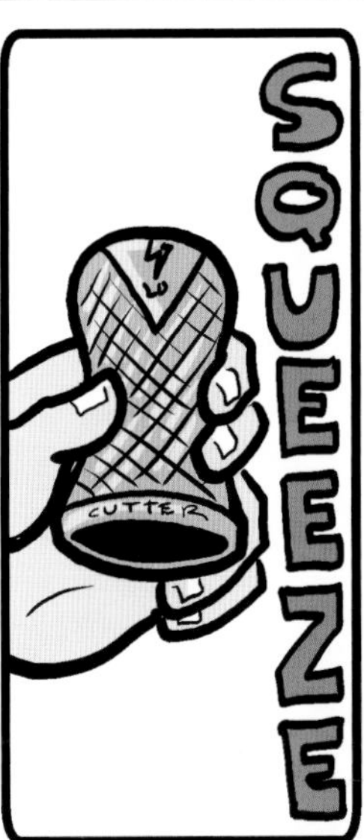
SQUEEZE
CUTTER

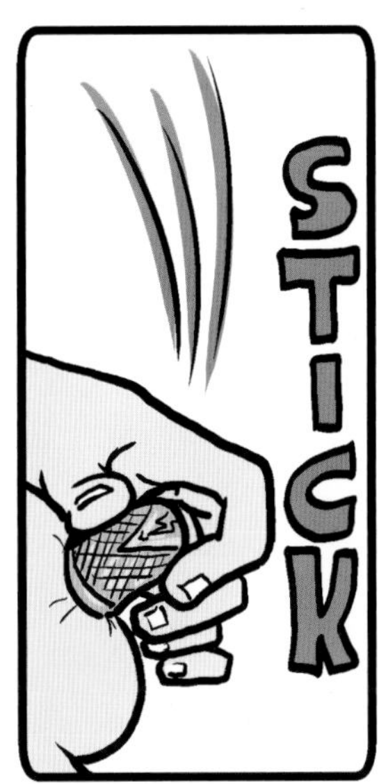
STICK

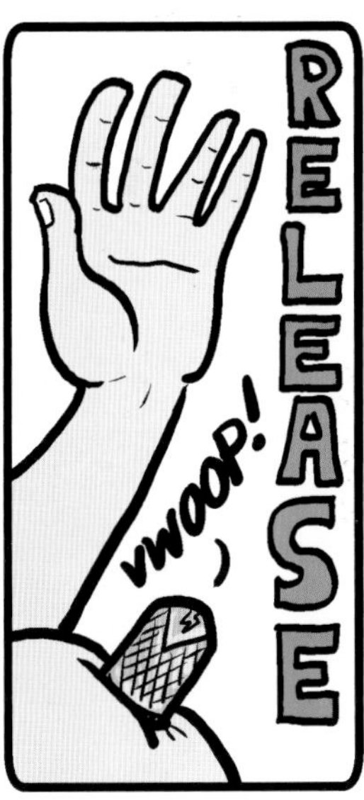
RELEASE
VWOOP!

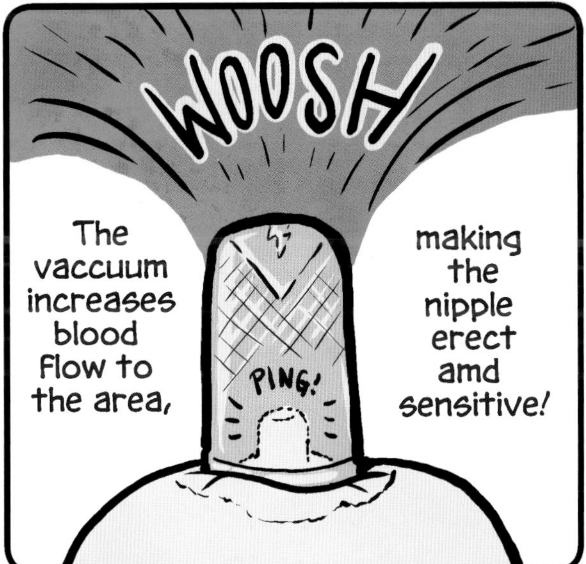
WOOSH
The vaccuum increases blood flow to the area,
PING!
making the nipple erect amd sensitive!

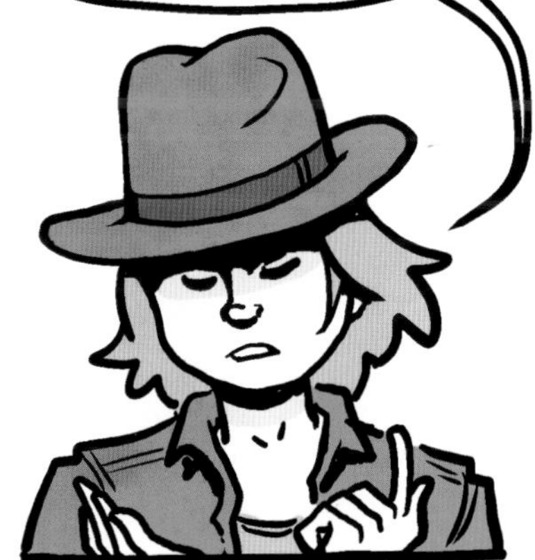
Now, before we go any further, I need to level with you:

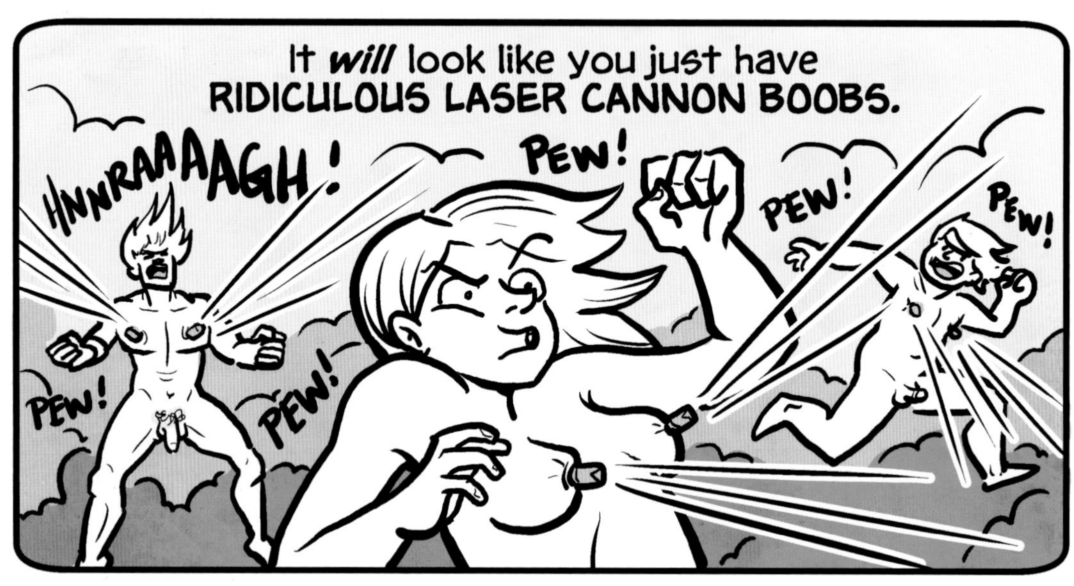
It *will* look like you just have
RIDICULOUS LASER CANNON BOOBS.
HNNRAAAAAGH!
PEW!
PEW!
PEW!
PEW!
PEW!

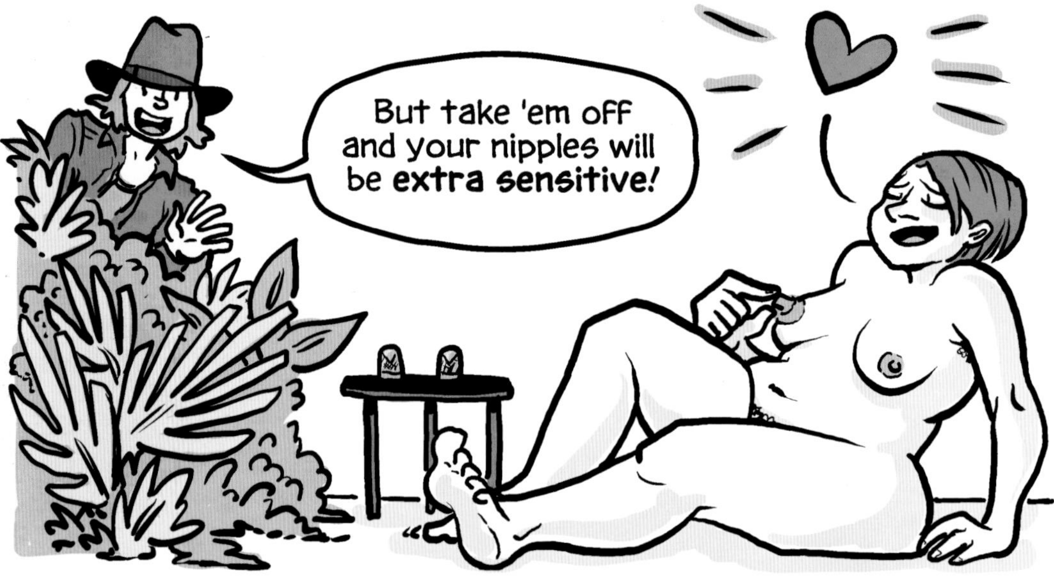
But take 'em off and your nipples will be **extra sensitive!**

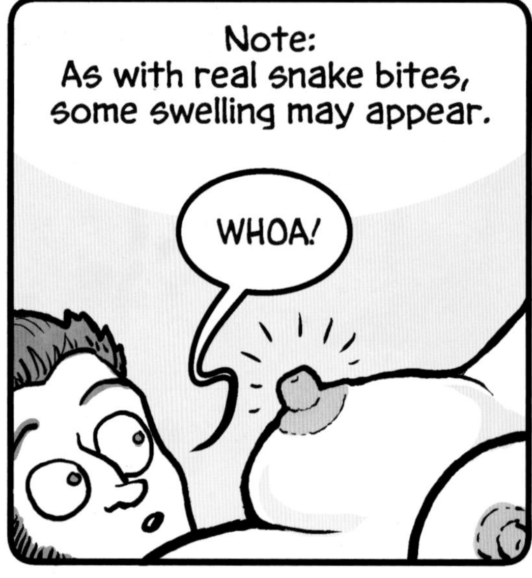
Note:
As with real snake bites, some swelling may appear.
WHOA!

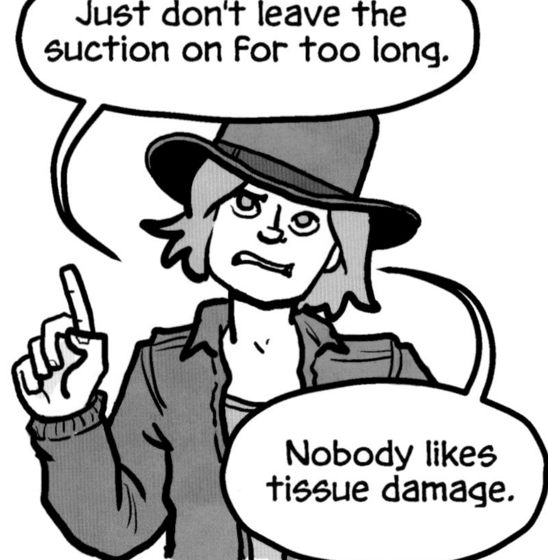
Just don't leave the suction on for too long.
Nobody likes tissue damage.

If you have sensivitve nipples, I wouldn't recommend this toy.

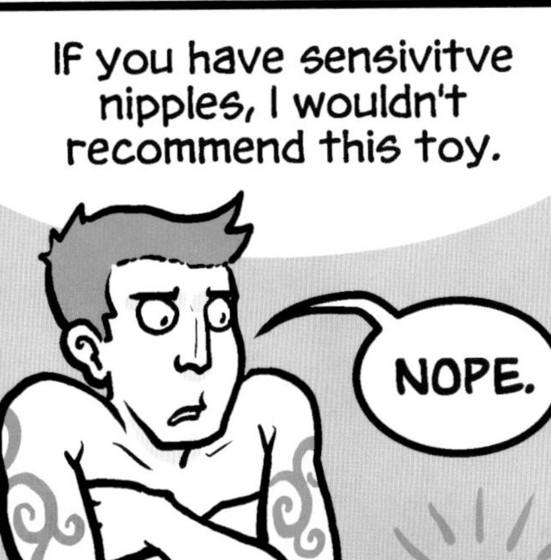

But if you like nipple stimulation and want to branch out, they're small and affordable...

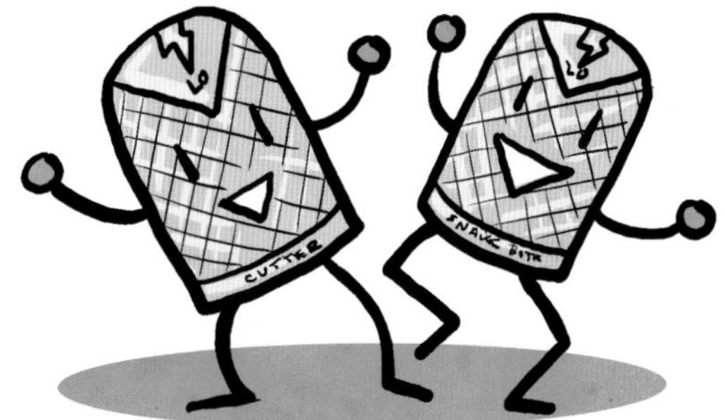

...and no one will suspect you're gonna use 'em on your titties!

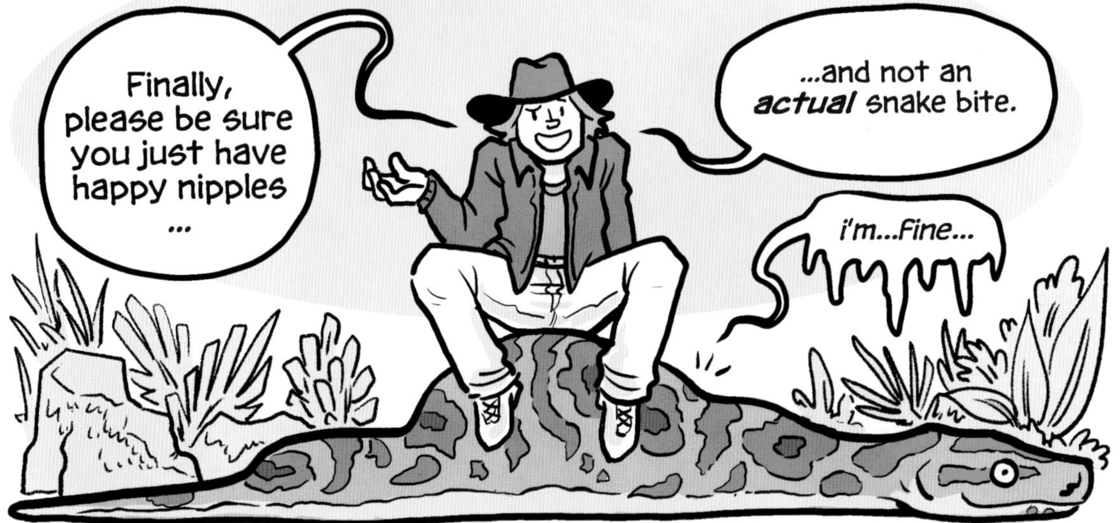

Finally, please be sure you just have happy nipples ...
...and not an *actual* snake bite.
i'm...fine...

TUNE IN NEXT TIME

TO LEARN HOW YOU CAN NEUTRALIZE AN ***ENRAGED GRIZZLY BEAR***
ARMED ONLY WITH A ***SMALL WARTENBURG WHEEL***
AND A ***HITCHAI MAGIC WAND!***

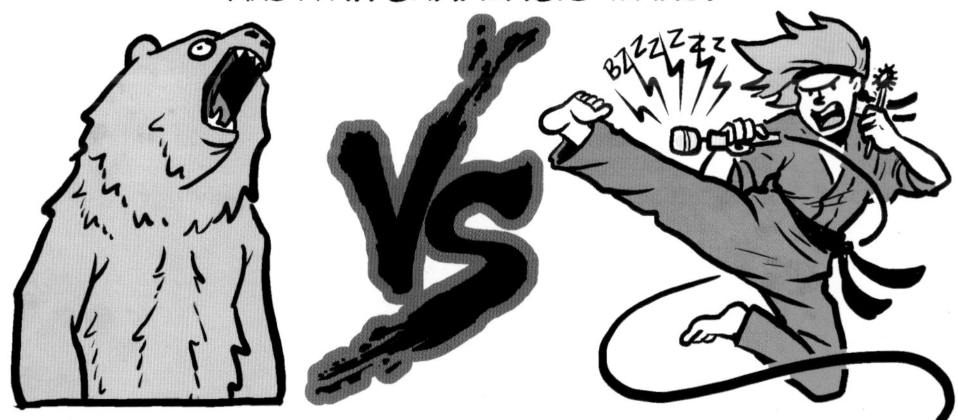

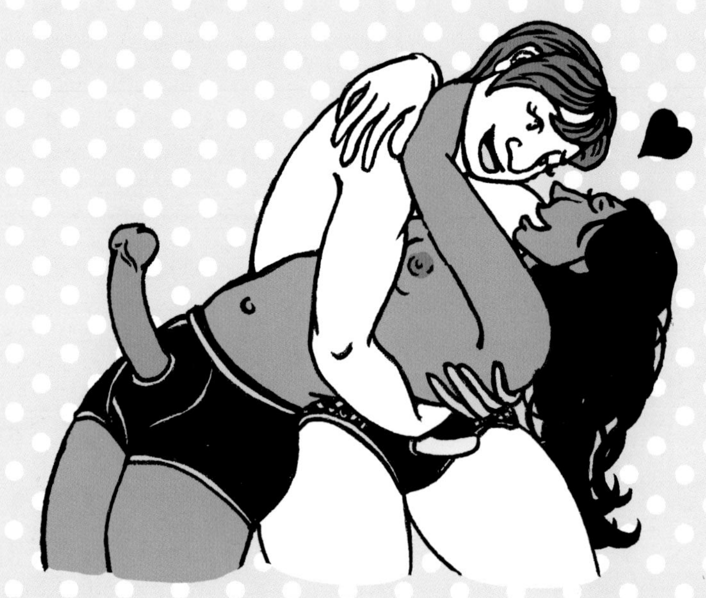

HARNESSING SAVINGS

by Isabella Rotman

isabellarotman.com

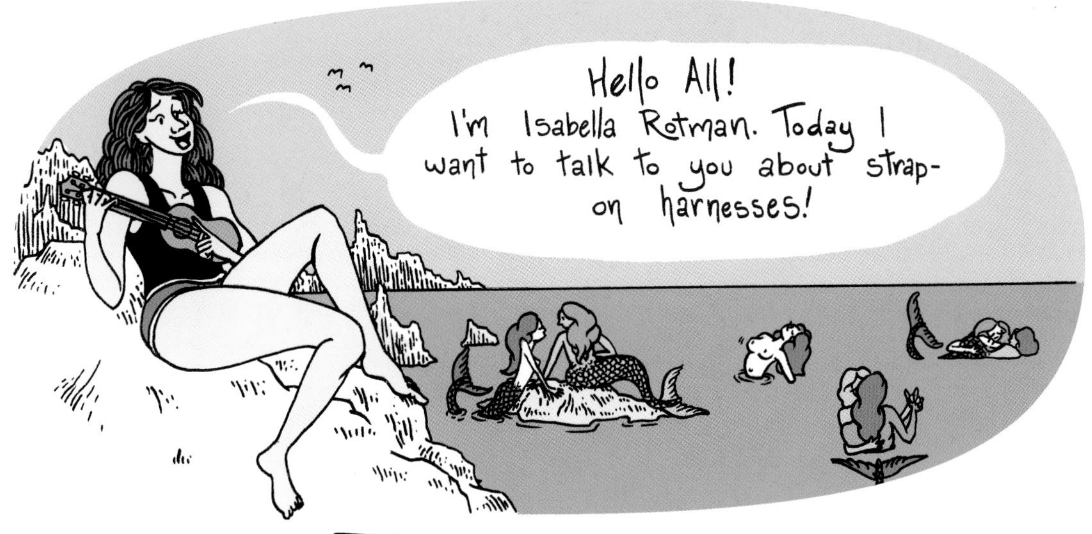
Hello All!
I'm Isabella Rotman. Today I want to talk to you about strap-on harnesses!

THERE ARE 3 Major Types

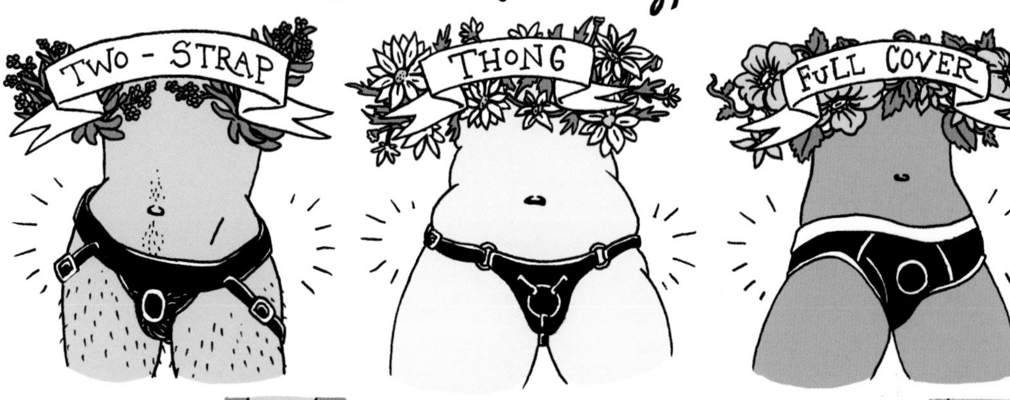
TWO - STRAP
THONG
FULL COVER

STRAP AROUND MID-SECTION AND TWO STRAPS AROUND LEGS, LEAVING GENITALS AVAILABLE FOR "PLAY".

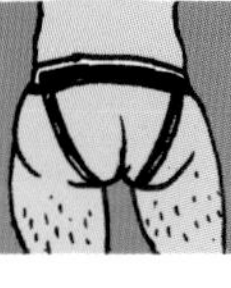

SINGLE STRAP BETWEEN LEGS. SOME FIND IT ALL SORTS OF AWESOME ON THEIR CLIT.

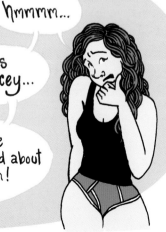

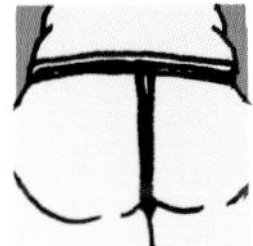

OFTEN LOOK LIKE A PAIR OF BRIEFS OR TIGHT SHORTS.

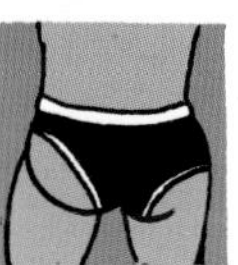

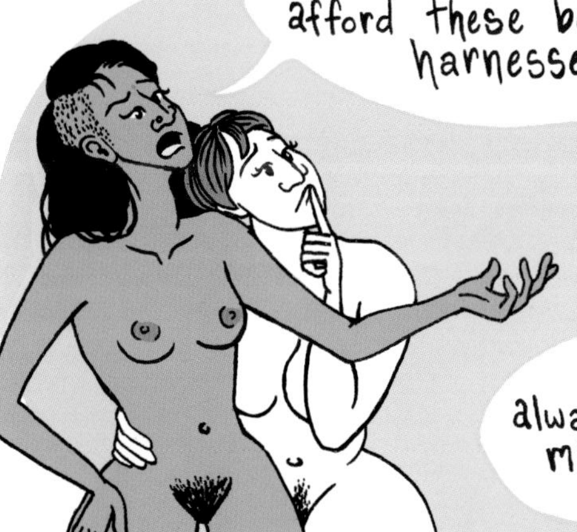
but wait, I can't afford these beautiful harnesses!

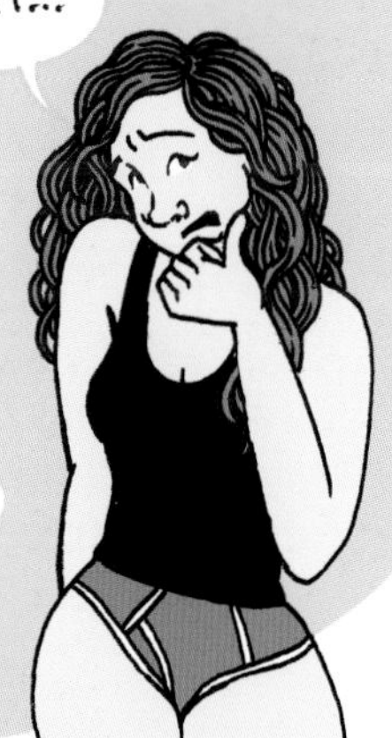
hmmmm...
it does get pricey...
and I have always fantasized about making my own!

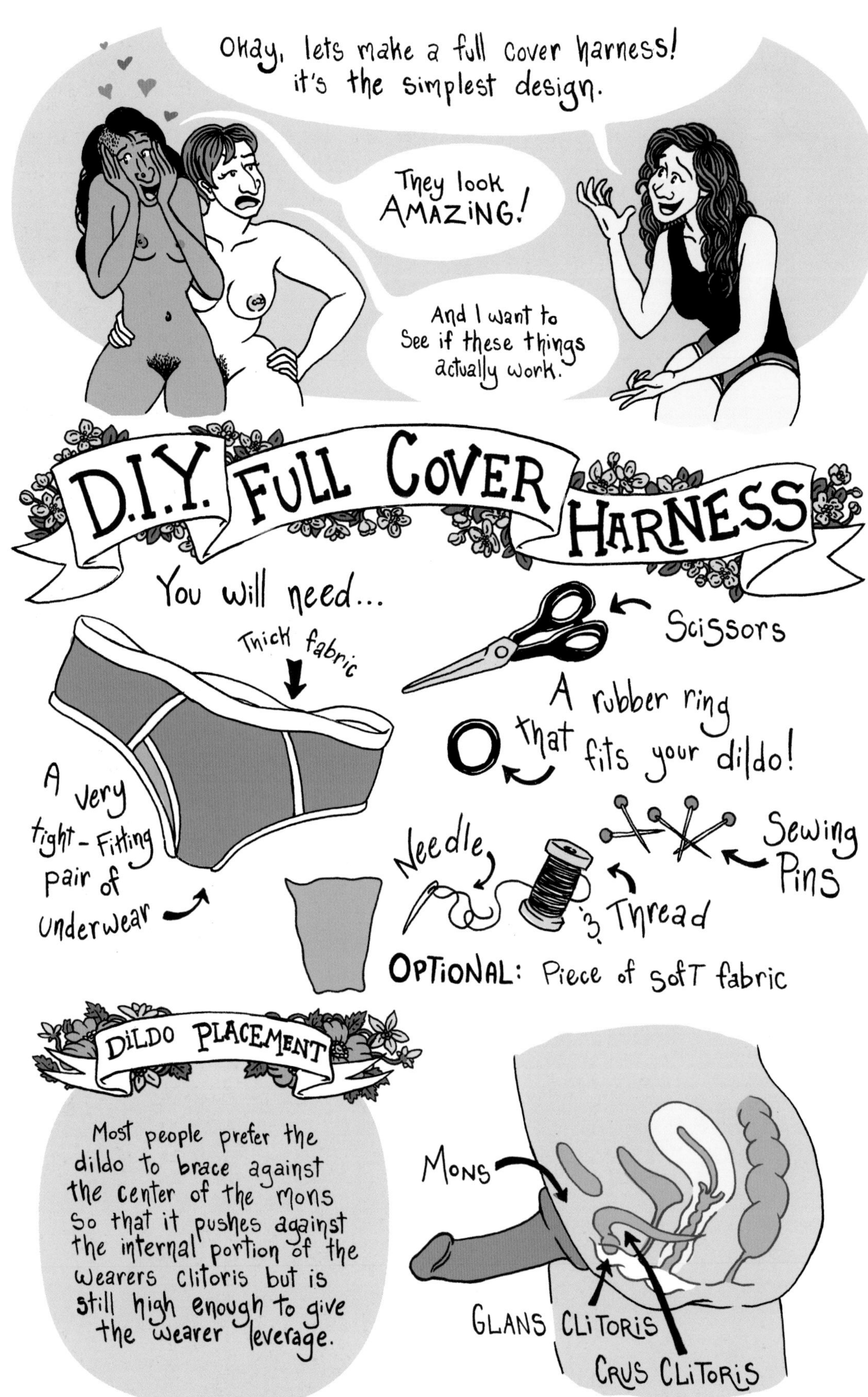
Okay, lets make a full cover harness! it's the simplest design.
They look AMAZING!
And I want to see if these things actually work.
D.I.Y. FULL COVER HARNESS
You will need...
Thick fabric
A very tight-fitting pair of underwear
Scissors
A rubber ring that fits your dildo!
Needle
Sewing Pins
Thread
OPTIONAL: Piece of soft fabric
DILDO PLACEMENT
Most people prefer the dildo to brace against the center of the mons so that it pushes against the internal portion of the wearers clitoris but is still high enough to give the wearer leverage.
Mons
GLANS CLITORIS
CRUS CLITORIS

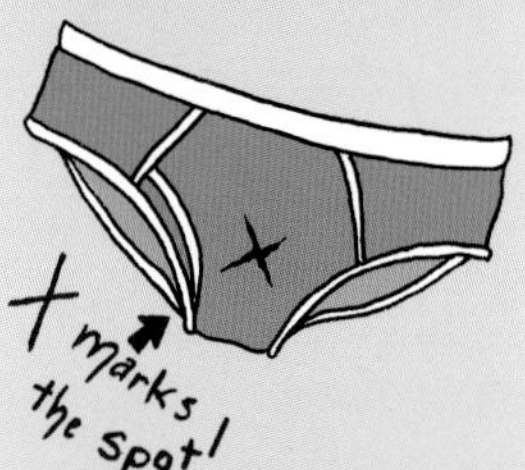
CUT AN X WHERE THE DILDO WILL GO.
X marks the spot!
THE X SHOULD BE SLIGHTLY SMALLER THAN THE RING.

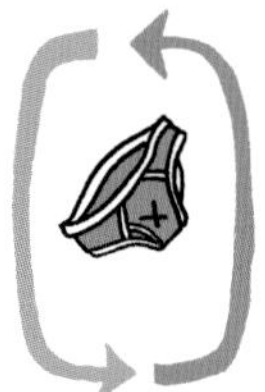
TURN THE UNDERWEAR
INSIDE-OUT!

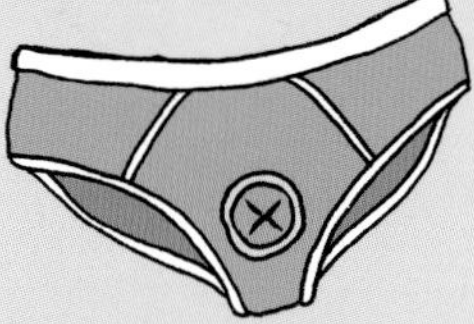

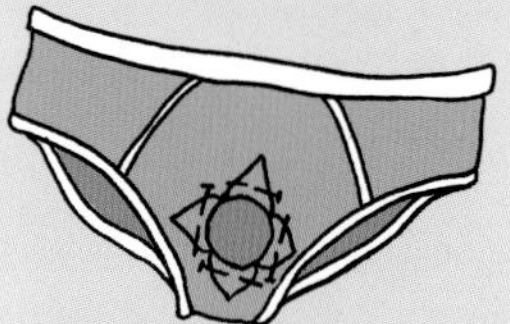

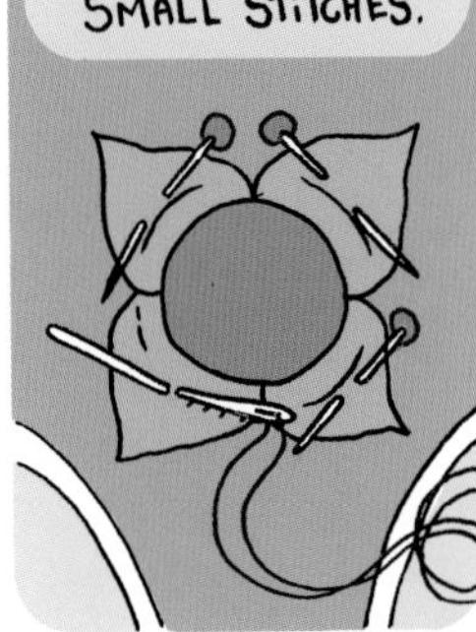

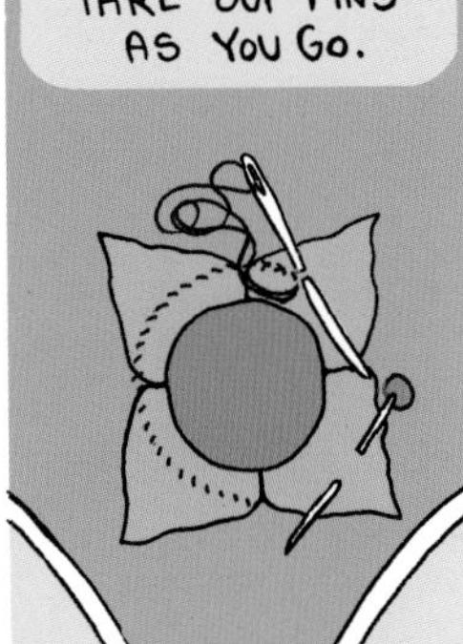

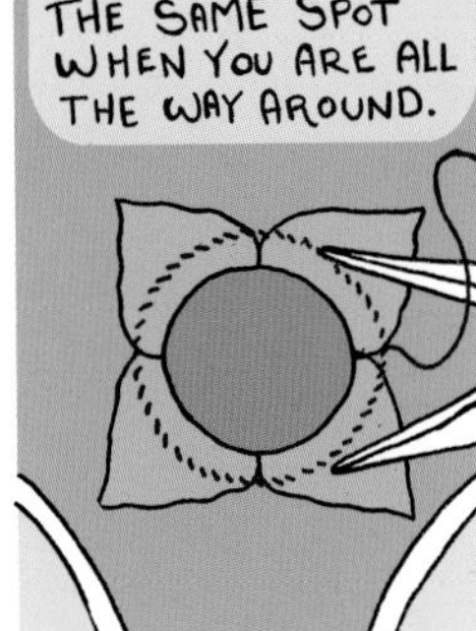

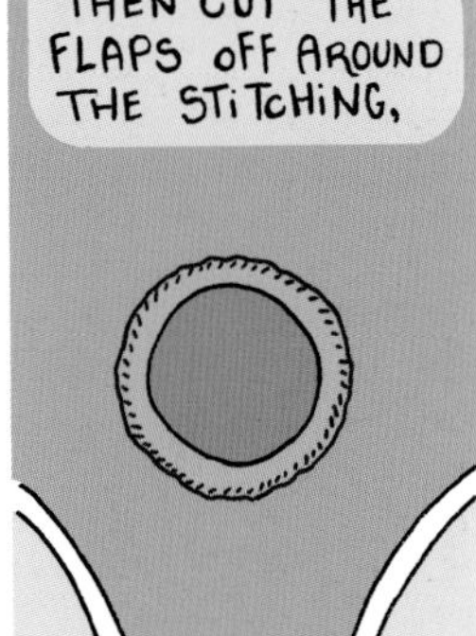

PLACE THE RING AROUND THE X,
AND STRETCH THE FABRIC FLAPS AROUND THE RING.

PIN THE FLAPS DOWN AROUND THE RING.
THE RING SHOULD BE COMPLELY COVERED BY THE FLAPS.

SEW THE RING IN TIGHTLY WITH SMALL STITCHES.

TAKE OUT PINS AS YOU GO.

SEW EXTRA LOOPS IN THE SAME SPOT WHEN YOU ARE ALL THE WAY AROUND.

THEN CUT THE FLAPS OFF AROUND THE STITCHING,

OPTIONAL STEP:

Some people like the base of the dildo directly on their skin and some don't. If you would prefer a barrier, sew a piece of fabric behind the ring, leaving an opening large enough to slide a dildo in the back.

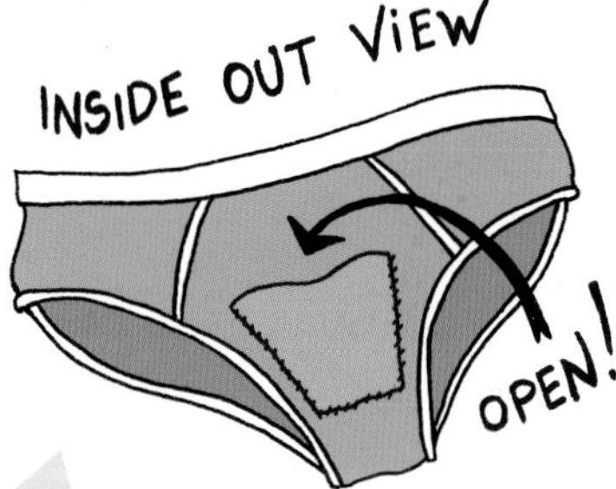

TA-DA!

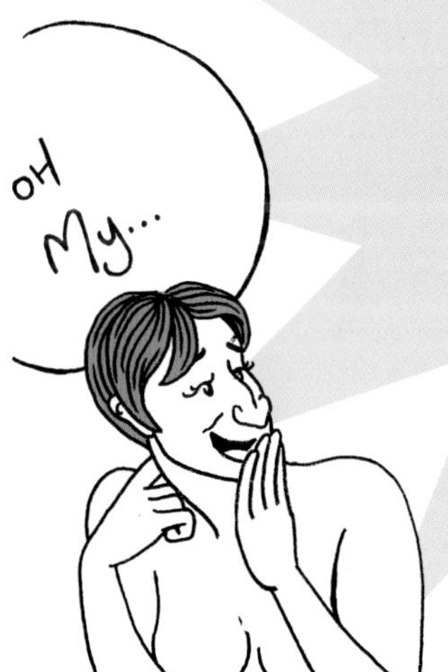
OH My...

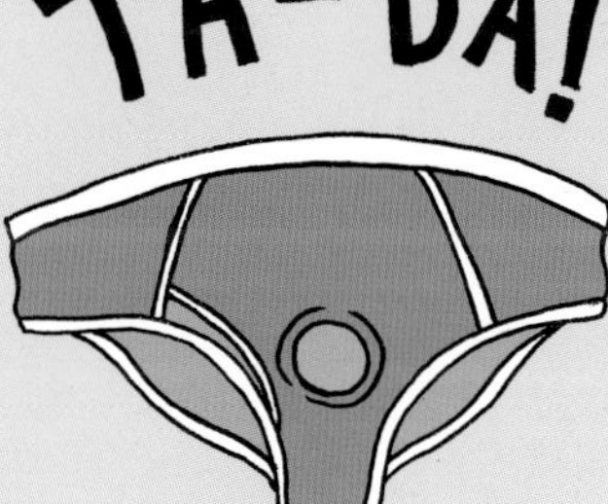

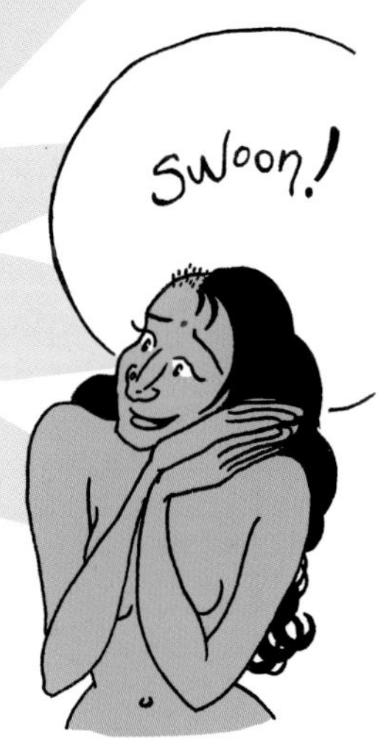
Swoon!

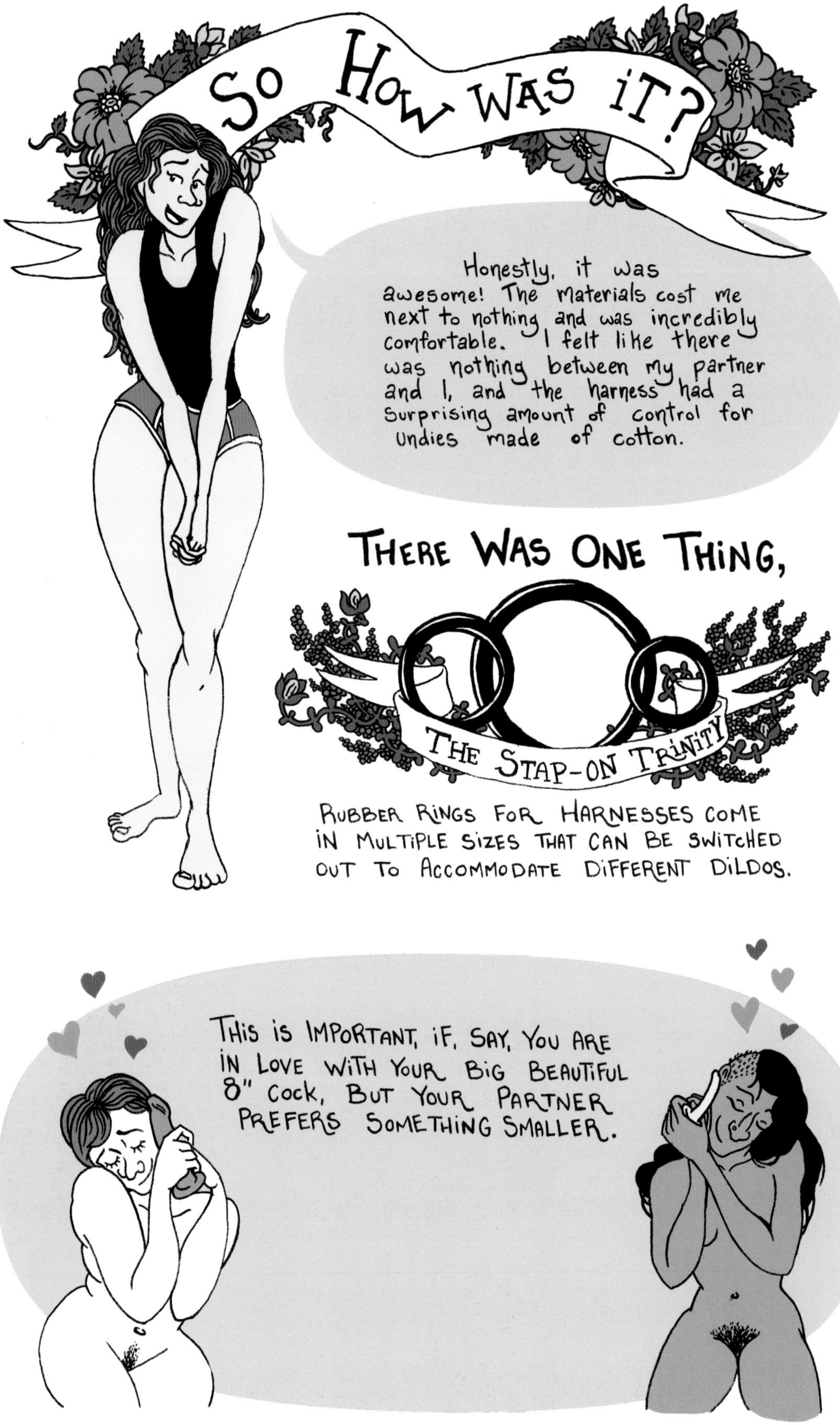

So How Was iT?

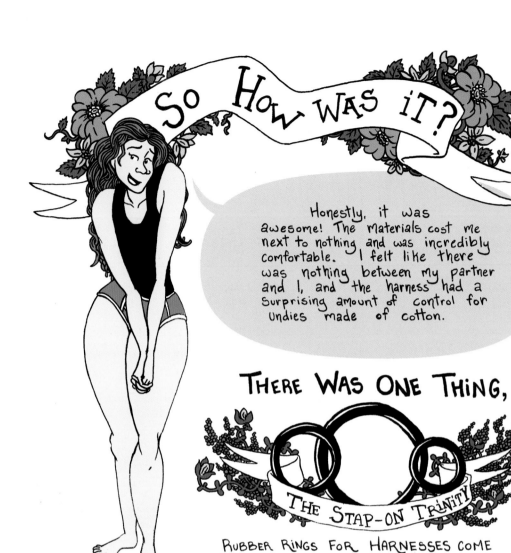

Honestly, it was awesome! The materials cost me next to nothing and was incredibly comfortable. I felt like there was nothing between my partner and I, and the harness had a surprising amount of control for undies made of cotton.

THERE WAS ONE THING,

THE STAP-ON TRINITY

RUBBER RINGS FOR HARNESSES COME IN MULTIPLE SIZES THAT CAN BE SWITCHED OUT TO ACCOMMODATE DIFFERENT DILDOS.

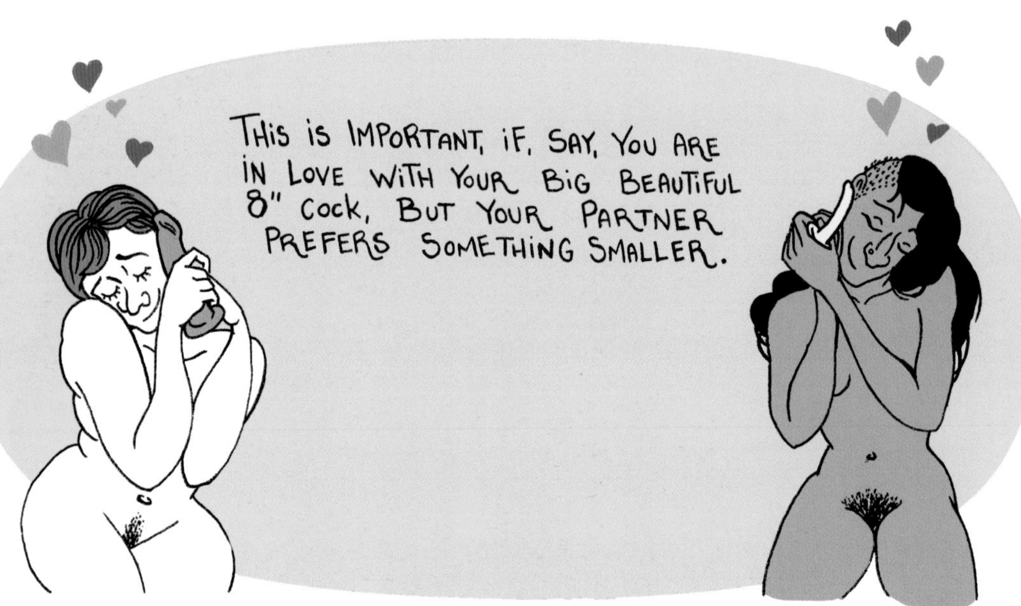

THIS IS IMPORTANT, IF, SAY, YOU ARE IN LOVE WITH YOUR BIG BEAUTIFUL 8" COCK, BUT YOUR PARTNER PREFERS SOMETHING SMALLER.

UNFORTUNATELY, SINCE I SECURELY SEWED THE RUBBER RING INTO THE UNDERWEAR I COULDN'T SWITCH IT OUT FOR A DIFFERENT SIZE.

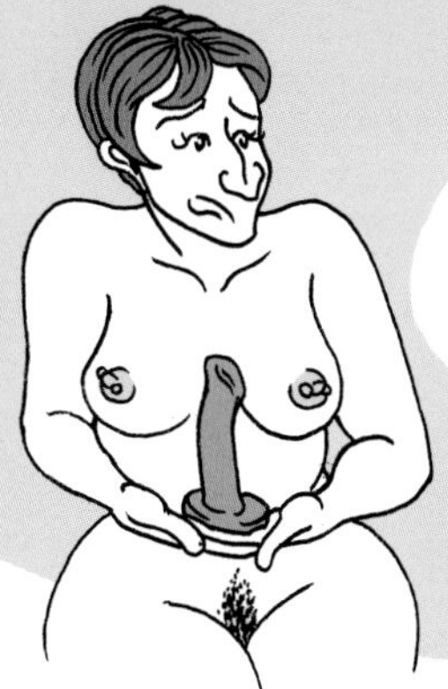

Hmmmm... I'm not sure I want that inside of me.

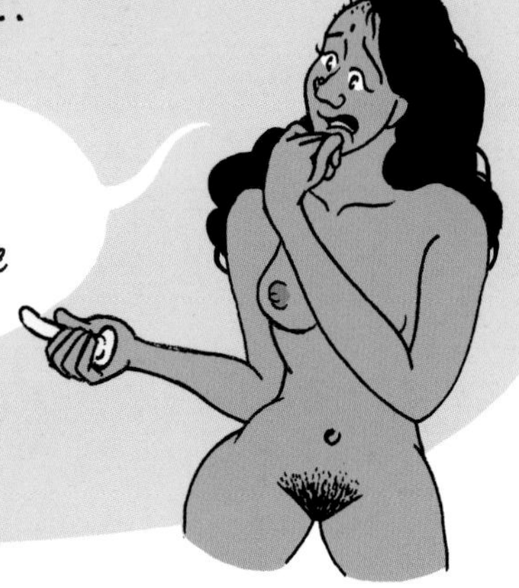

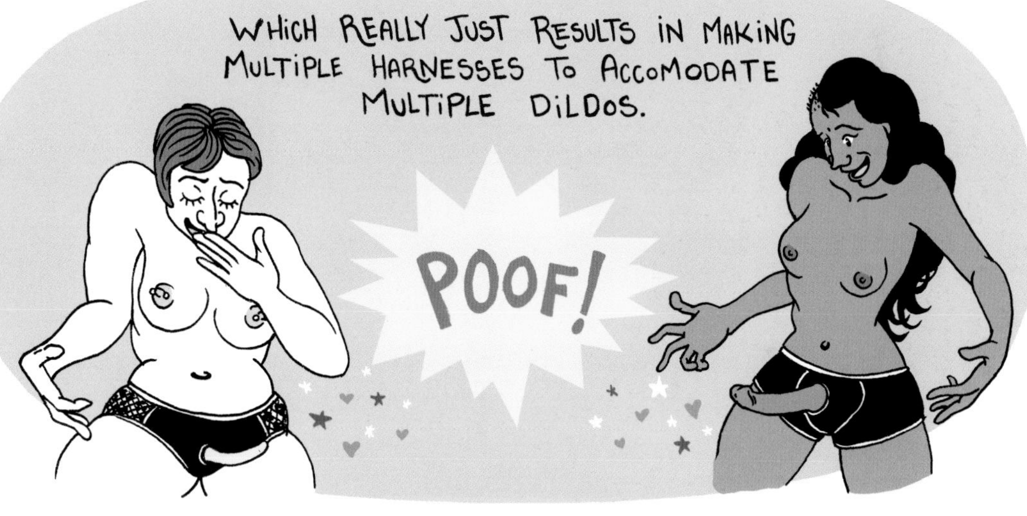

WHICH REALLY JUST RESULTS IN MAKING MULTIPLE HARNESSES TO ACCOMODATE MULTIPLE DILDOS.
POOF!

AND IS THAT REALLY SUCH A BAD THING?

And it's machine washable!

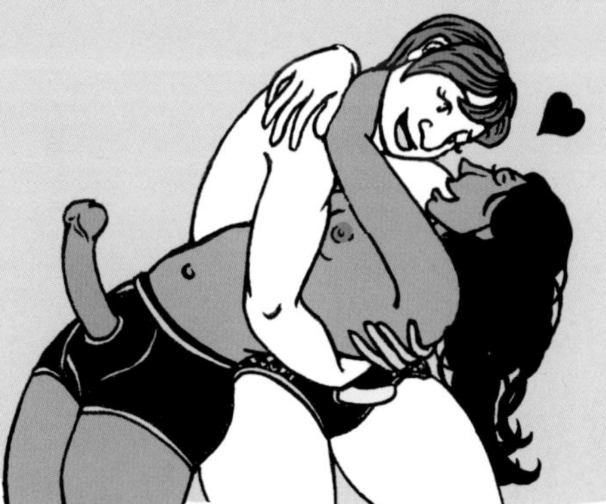

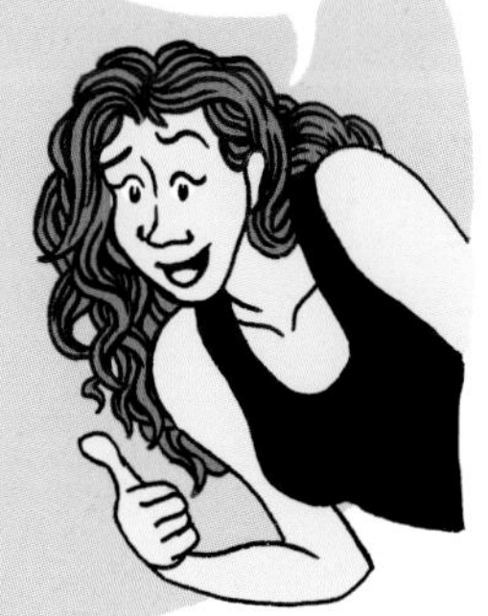

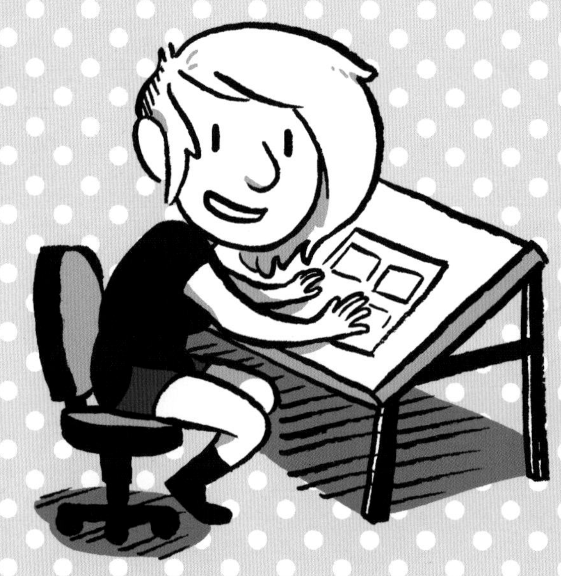

EROTIC COMICS

by Jess Fink

jessfink.com

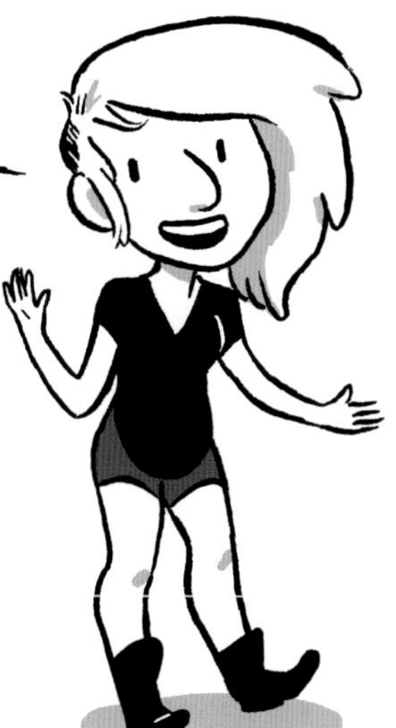

Hi I'm Jess! I'm an illustator/cartoonist and my work is equal parts "clean" stuff and sexy stuff. I've never felt the need to use a pseudonym to hide my identity.
I've worked in kid's games, illustrated all ages books, and making erotica hasn't hindered me because I am able to seperate the two.
However, it has changed how some people treat me!

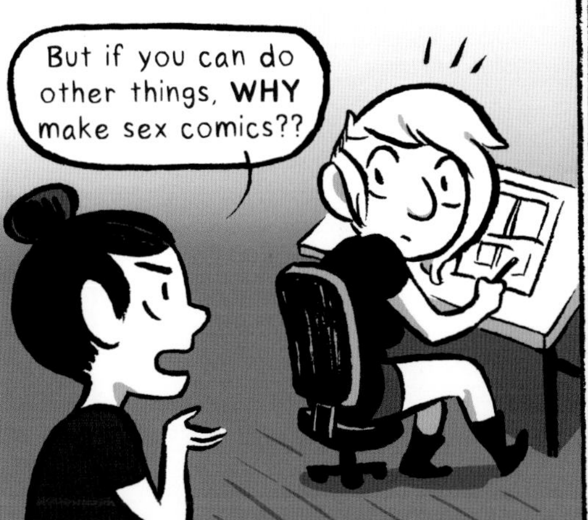

I've been working professionally for about 12 years and sometimes people ask me:
But if you can do other things, **WHY** make sex comics??

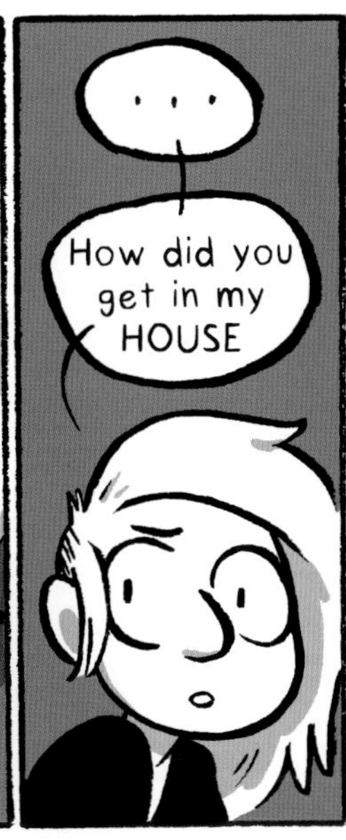

. . .
How did you get in my HOUSE

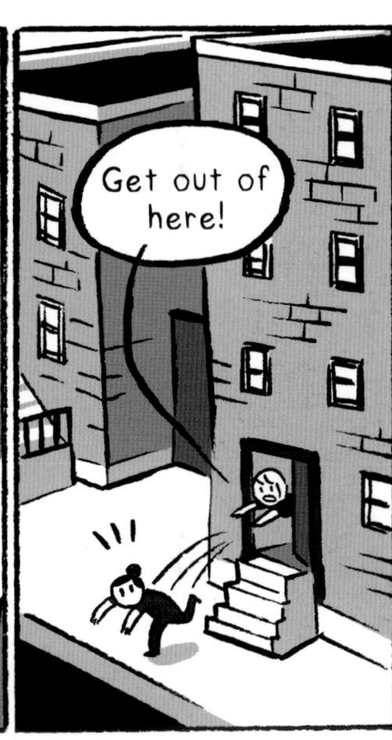

Get out of here!

LOCK

The truth is I make sex comics because ...why not?? And because most of the time I like sexy drawings and stories better than the alternatives!

CURVY

ARTIFICE

It's not that I don't look at or like photos and videos, but erotic stories and characters are FAR more preferable to me. I'm not alone either, people have been getting off to drawings for a long time!

SMUT PEDDLER

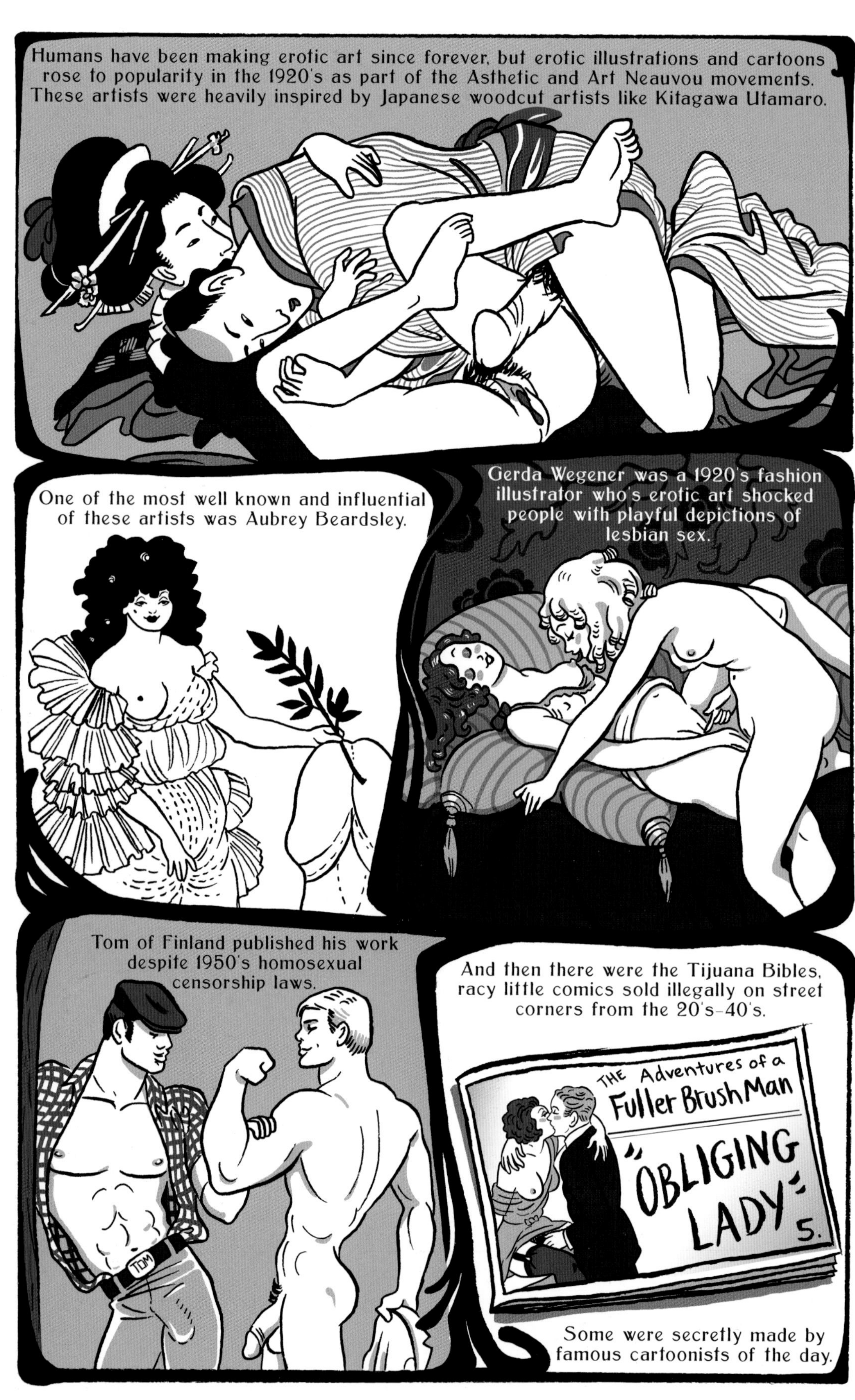
Humans have been making erotic art since forever, but erotic illustrations and cartoons rose to popularity in the 1920's as part of the Asthetic and Art Neauvou movements. These artists were heavily inspired by Japanese woodcut artists like Kitagawa Utamaro.
One of the most well known and influential of these artists was Aubrey Beardsley.
Gerda Wegener was a 1920's fashion illustrator who's erotic art shocked people with playful depictions of lesbian sex.
Tom of Finland published his work despite 1950's homosexual censorship laws.
TOM
And then there were the Tijuana Bibles, racy little comics sold illegally on street corners from the 20's-40's.
THE Adventures of a
Fuller Brush Man
"OBLIGING LADY"
5.
Some were secretly made by famous cartoonists of the day.

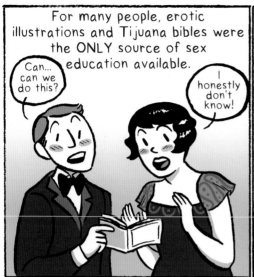
For many people, erotic illustrations and Tijuana bibles were the ONLY source of sex education available.
Can... can we do this?
I honestly don't know!

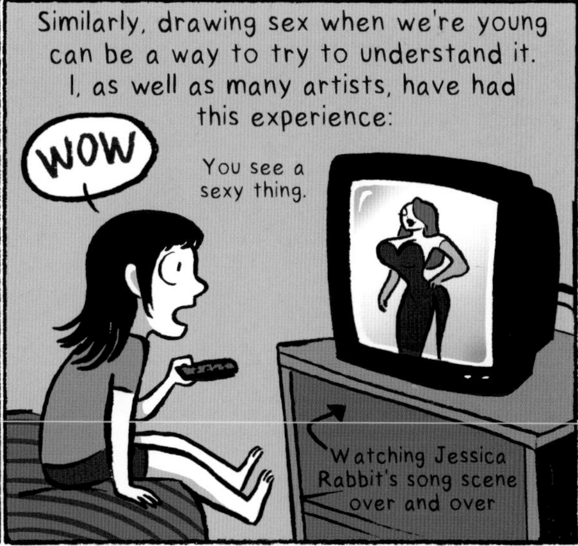
Similarly, drawing sex when we're young can be a way to try to understand it. I, as well as many artists, have had this experience:
WOW
You see a sexy thing.
Watching Jessica Rabbit's song scene over and over

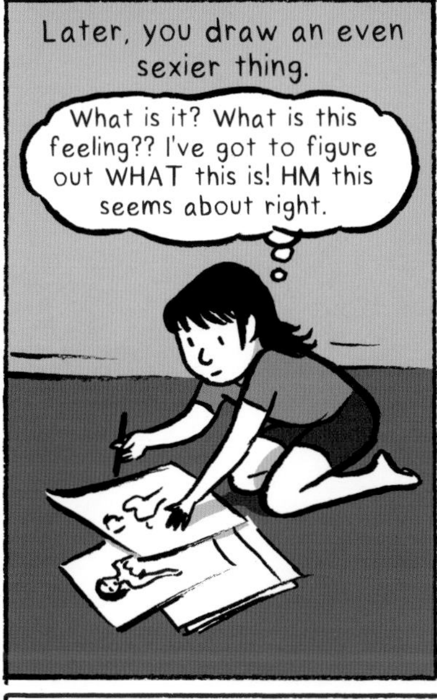
Later, you draw an even sexier thing.
What is it? What is this feeling?? I've got to figure out WHAT this is! HM this seems about right.

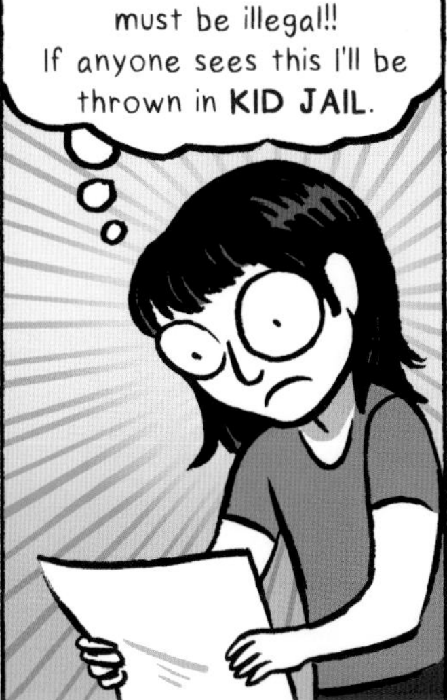
OH NOOOO, what have I DONE? This is so sexy it must be illegal!! If anyone sees this I'll be thrown in **KID JAIL**.

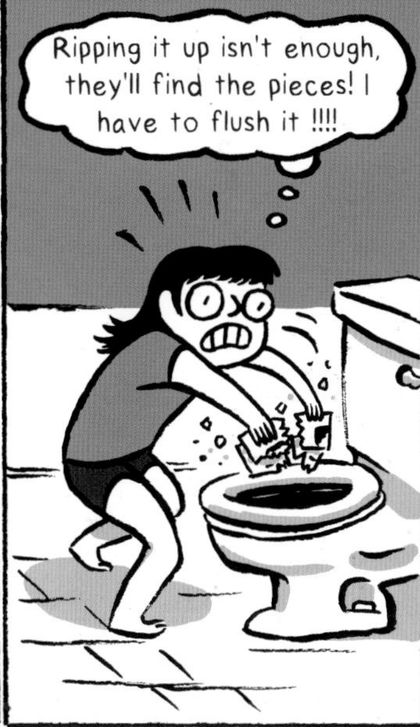
Ripping it up isn't enough, they'll find the pieces! I have to flush it !!!!

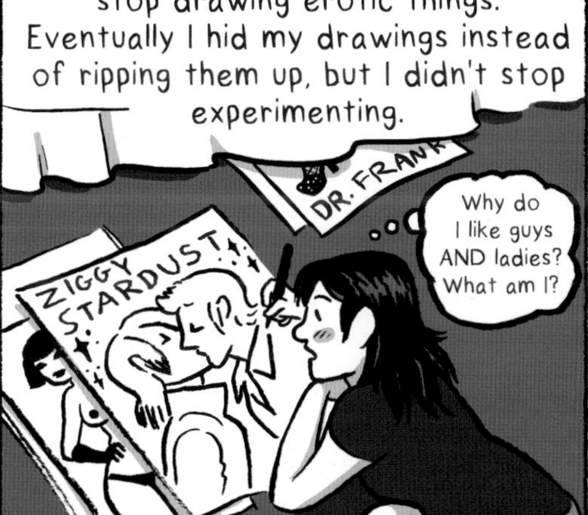
That guilt causes many artists to stop drawing erotic things. Eventually I hid my drawings instead of ripping them up, but I didn't stop experimenting.
DR. FRANK
ZIGGY STARDUST
Why do I like guys AND ladies? What am I?

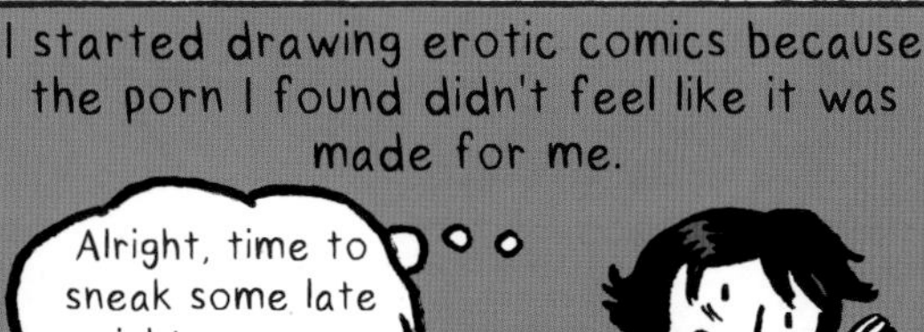
I started drawing erotic comics because the porn I found didn't feel like it was made for me.
Alright, time to sneak some late night porn on the living room tv!!

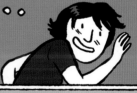

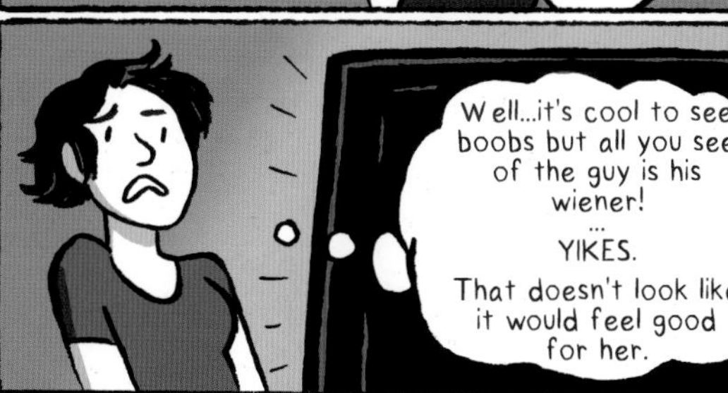
Well...it's cool to see boobs but all you see of the guy is his wiener!
...
YIKES.
That doesn't look like it would feel good for her.

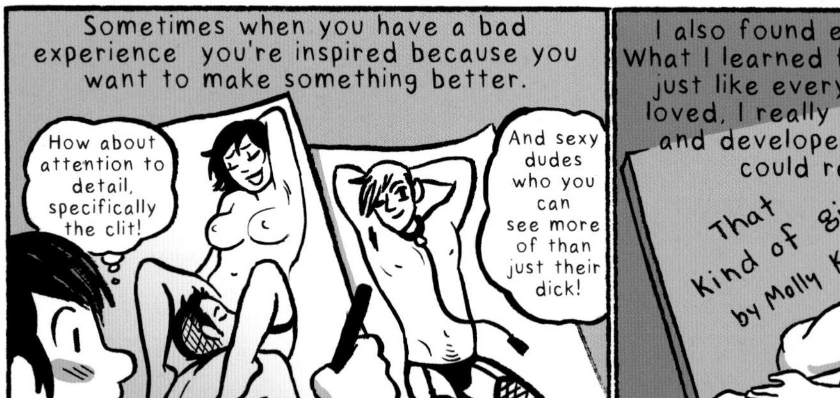
Sometimes when you have a bad experience you're inspired because you want to make something better.
How about attention to detail, specifically the clit!
And sexy dudes who you can see more of than just their dick!
I also found erotica I loved! What I learned from it was that, just like every other comic I loved, I really wanted stories and developed characters I could relate to.
That Kind of girl
by Molly Kiely

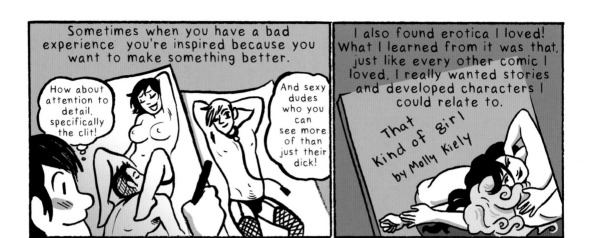

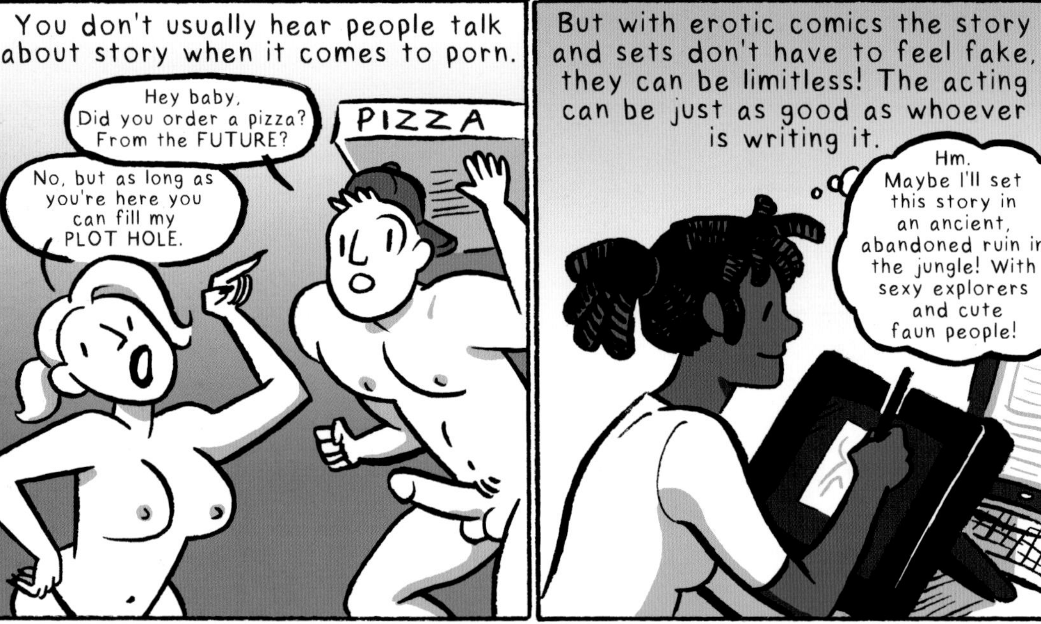
You don't usually hear people talk about story when it comes to porn.
Hey baby, Did you order a pizza? From the FUTURE?
No, but as long as you're here you can fill my PLOT HOLE.
PIZZA
But with erotic comics the story and sets don't have to feel fake, they can be limitless! The acting can be just as good as whoever is writing it.
Hm. Maybe I'll set this story in an ancient, abandoned ruin in the jungle! With sexy explorers and cute faun people!

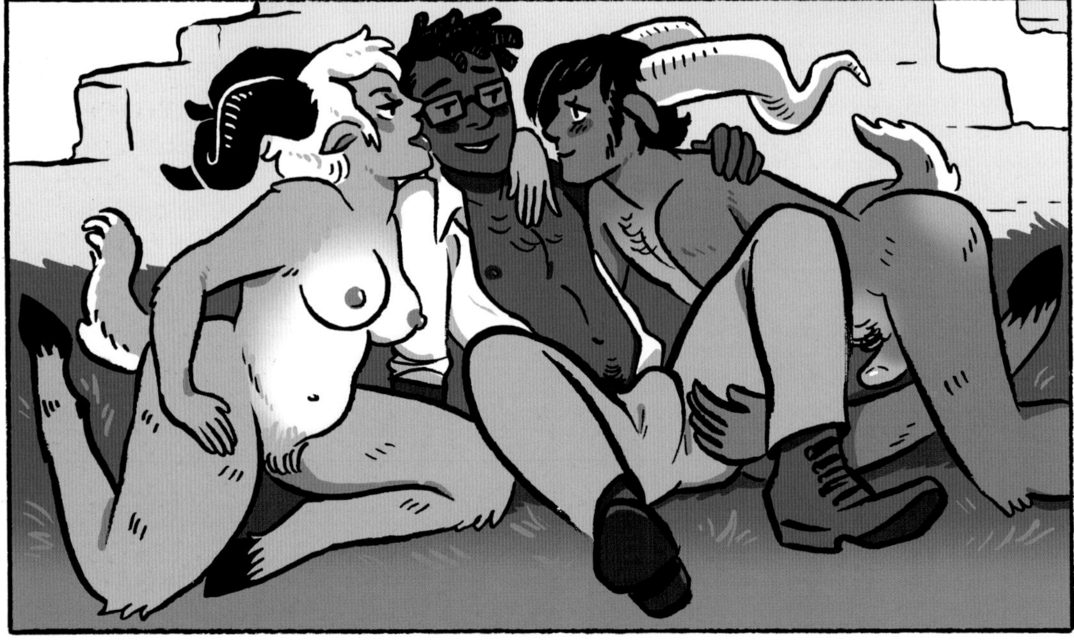

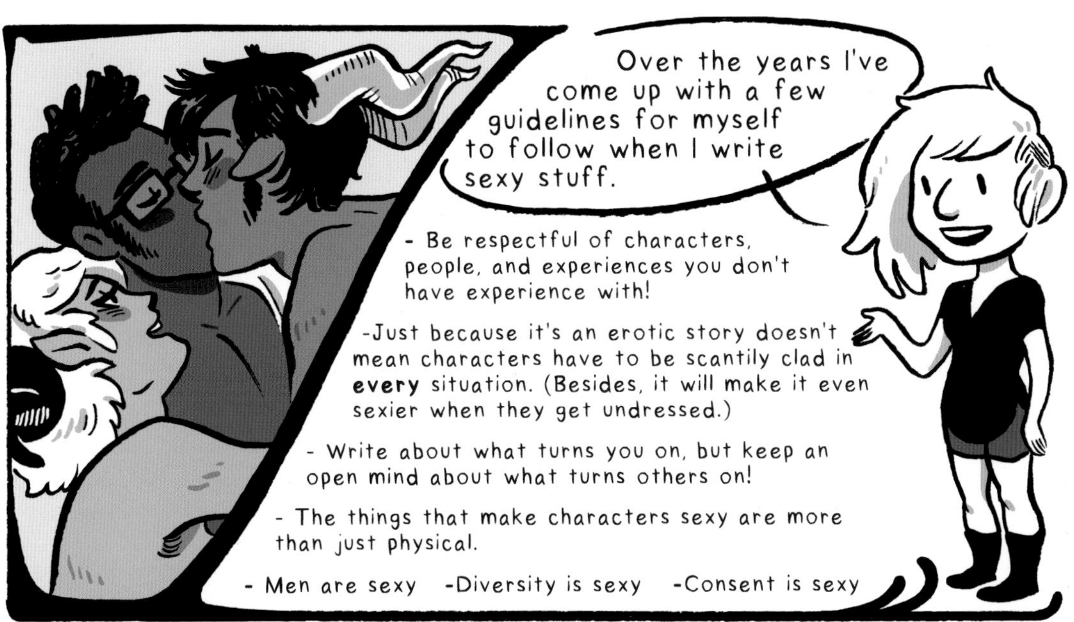
Over the years I've come up with a few guidelines for myself to follow when I write sexy stuff.
- Be respectful of characters, people, and experiences you don't have experience with!
-Just because it's an erotic story doesn't mean characters have to be scantily clad in **every** situation. (Besides, it will make it even sexier when they get undressed.)
- Write about what turns you on, but keep an open mind about what turns others on!
- The things that make characters sexy are more than just physical.
- Men are sexy -Diversity is sexy -Consent is sexy

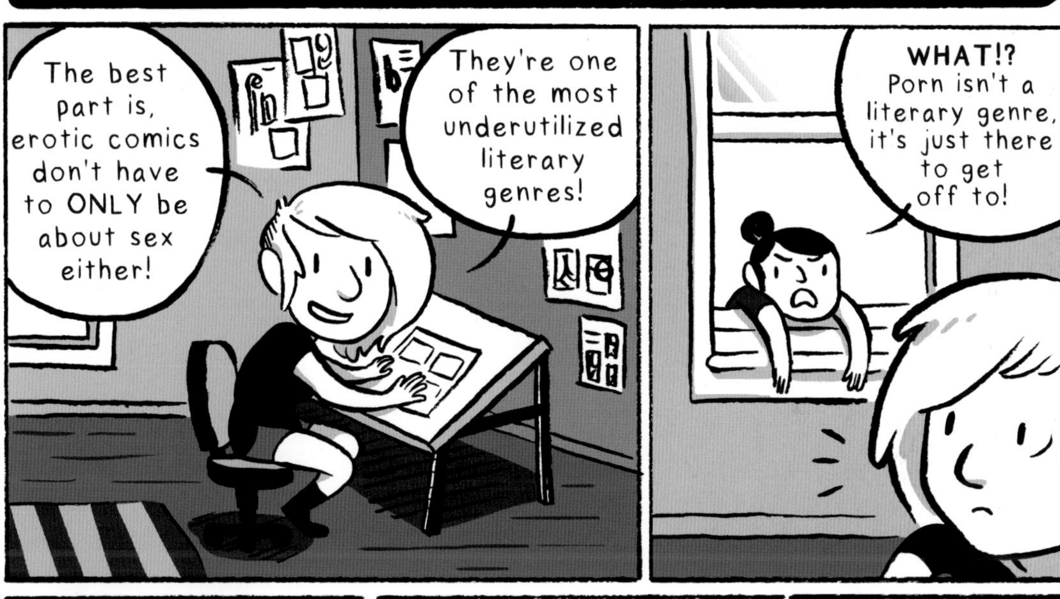
The best part is, erotic comics don't have to ONLY be about sex either!
They're one of the most underutilized literary genres!
WHAT!? Porn isn't a literary genre, it's just there to get off to!

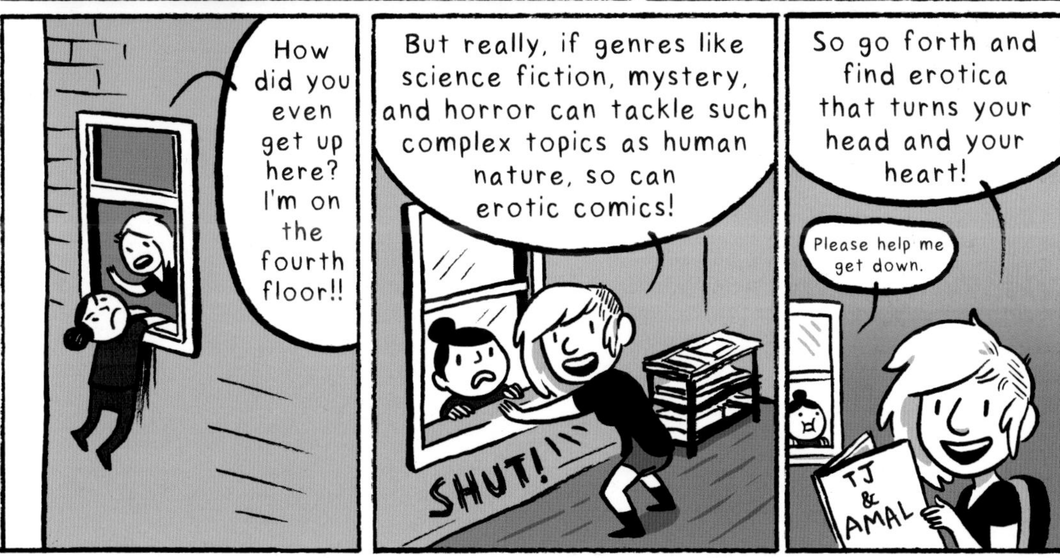
How did you even get up here? I'm on the fourth floor!!
But really, if genres like science fiction, mystery, and horror can tackle such complex topics as human nature, so can erotic comics!
SHUT!
So go forth and find erotica that turns your head and your heart!
Please help me get down.
TJ & AMAL

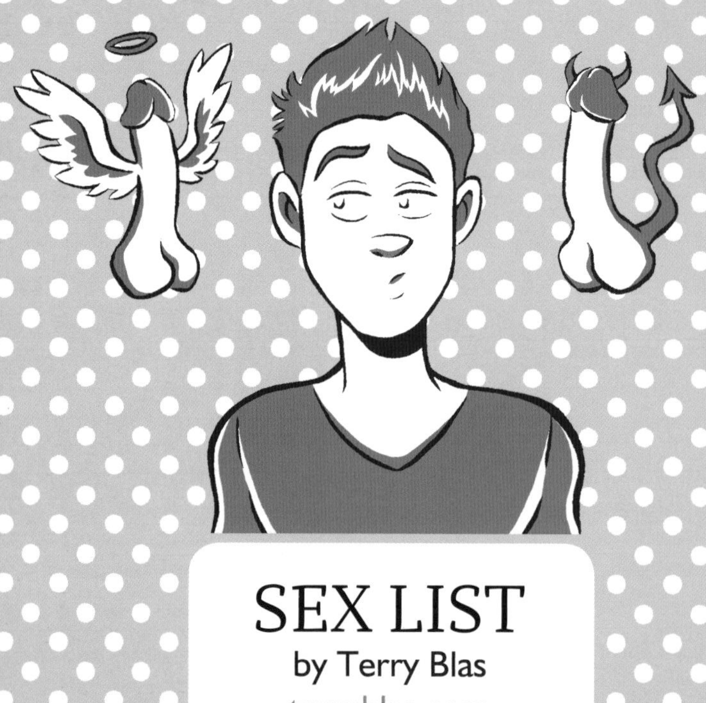

SEX LIST

by Terry Blas

terryblas.com

YES, NO, MAYBE SO!

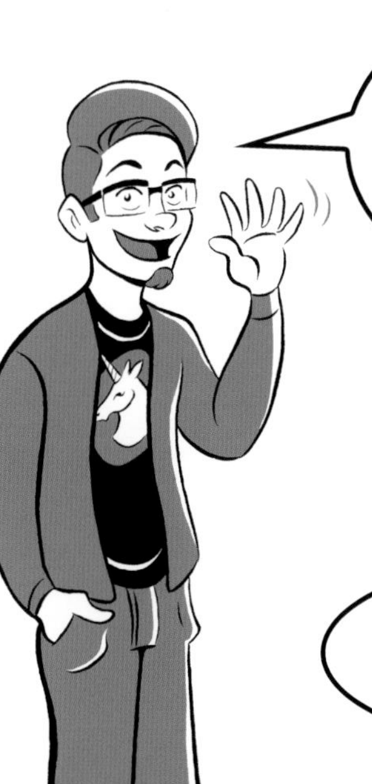

HI THERE! FOR THOSE OF YOU WHO DON'T KNOW ME, I'M TERRY BLAS.
I'M NOT SURE BUT I THINK I MIGHT BE PORTLAND'S ONLY GAY, EX-MORMON, LATIN, COMIC BOOK DRAWING NERD.
IF NOT, HEY, LET ME KNOW!

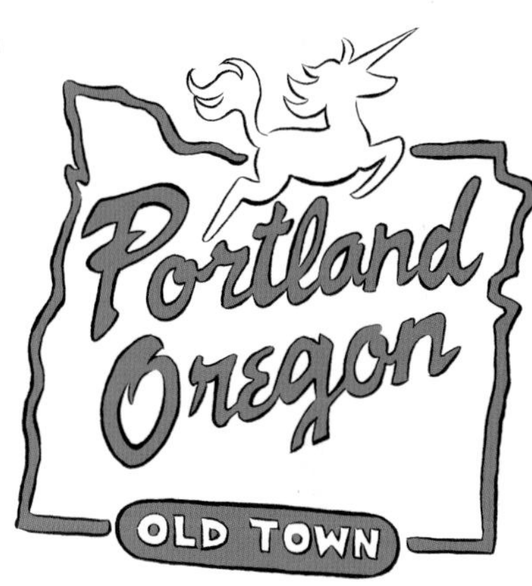

Portland Oregon
OLD TOWN
BUT SOMEONE ONCE TOLD ME THAT IF YOU TAKE A LOOK AT MY BACKGROUND, IT'S CLEAR TO SEE WHY I ENJOY...
ORGANIZING AND MAKING LISTS!

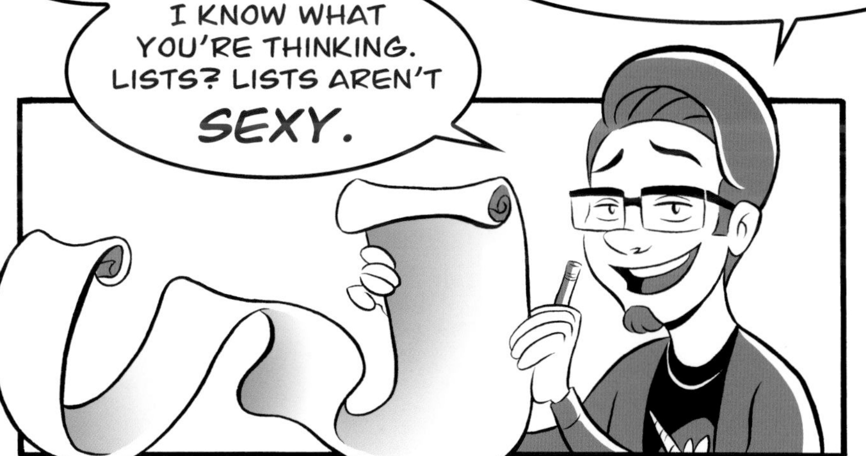

I KNOW WHAT YOU'RE THINKING. LISTS? LISTS AREN'T SEXY.
AU CONTRAIRE!

A GREAT WAY TO **SPICE THINGS UP** IN YOUR RELATIONSHIP IS TO TAKE A STAB AT FILLING OUT A...

SEX LIST!

EVERYONE KNOWS THAT ONE OF THE MOST IMPORTANT THINGS IN A RELATIONSHIP IS:

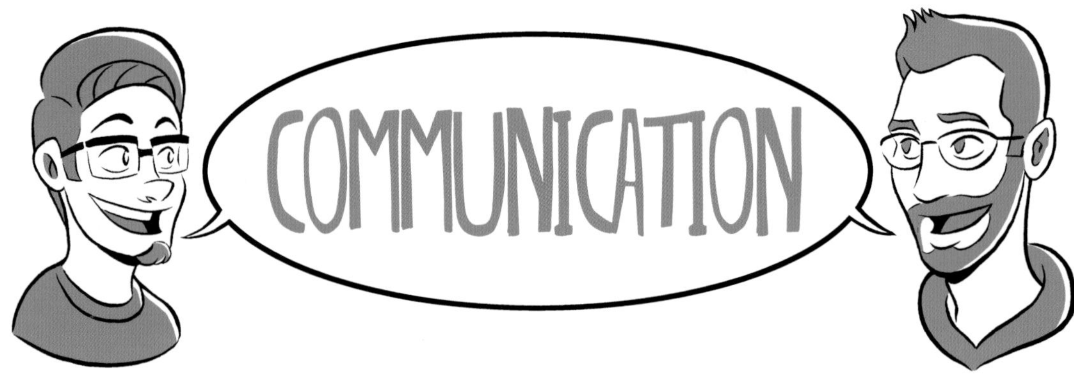

IF YOU AREN'T FAMILIAR,
A ***SEX LIST*** IS A LIST OF SEXUAL ACTIVITIES
WITH COLUMNS FOR ***YES, NO AND MAYBE.***
YOU FILL IT OUT AND SEE WHAT YOU
ARE OR MIGHT BE INTO!

AND OF COURSE WHAT YOU
DEFINITELY AREN'T INTO!

GIVE IT A TRY!

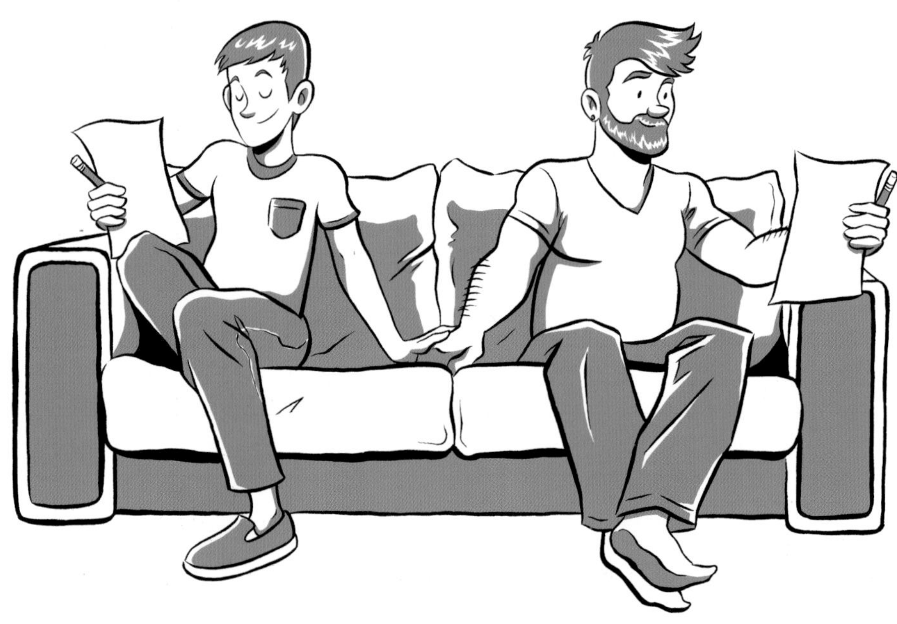

YOU CAN FIND ONE ONLINE OR BEGIN WITH THIS ADMITTEDLY LIMITED ONE. LET'S JUST CALL IT A BEGINNER'S LIST!

ACTIVITY	YES	NO	MAYBE
69			
ANALINGUS			
BONDAGE			
COCK RINGS			
DIRTY TALK			
DOMINATION & SUBMISSION			
EROTIC MASSAGE			
FELLATIO			
FETISH PLAY			
FINGERING			
FISTING			
GENDER PLAY			
GLORY HOLES			
GOLDEN SHOWERS			
GROUP SEX			
INTERCOURSE			
LAP DANCE			
MASTURBATION			
NIPPLE PLAY			
PHONE SEX			
PORNOGRAPHY			
PROSTATE MASSAGE			
QUICKIES			
RAINBOW SHOWERS			
ROLE PLAY			
ROUGH PLAY			
SCAT PLAY			
SENSORY DEPRIVATION			
SEX CLUBS			
SEX PARTIES			
SHRIMPING			
S & M			
SPANKING			
STRIP TEASE			
THREESOMES			
TOYS			
VIBRATORS			
VOYEURISM			

STEP ONE

GRAB A PEN. GET COMFORTABLE AND ***FILL OUT THE LIST ALONE.***

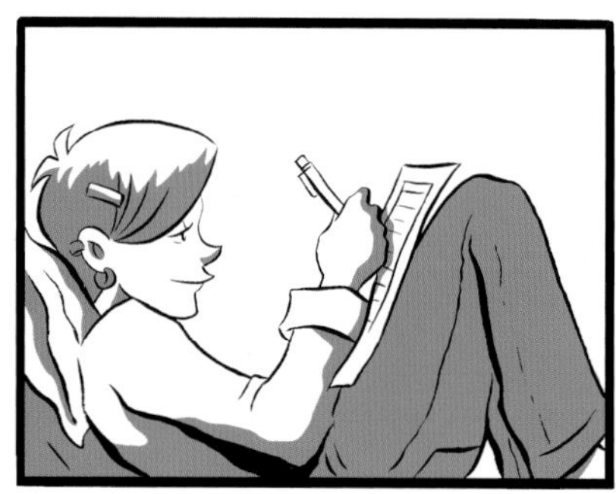

STEP TWO

BE HONEST. DON'T LISTEN TO THAT LITTLE SHOULDER DEVIL. IT'S ALL ABOUT COMMUNICATING YOUR INTERESTS AND NEEDS.

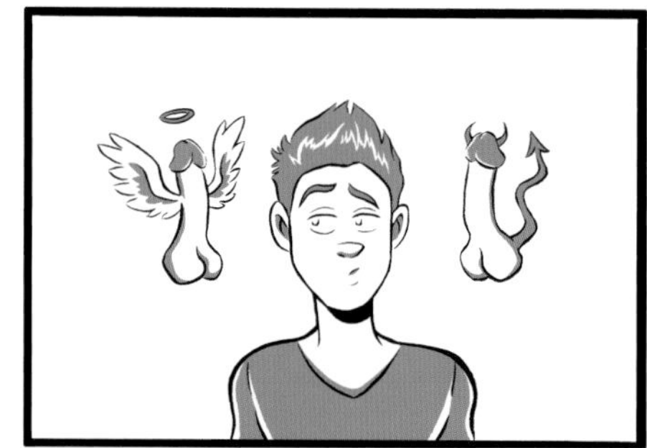

STEP THREE

EDIT YOUR LIST. TAKE THINGS OUT THAT DON'T APPLY TO YOU.

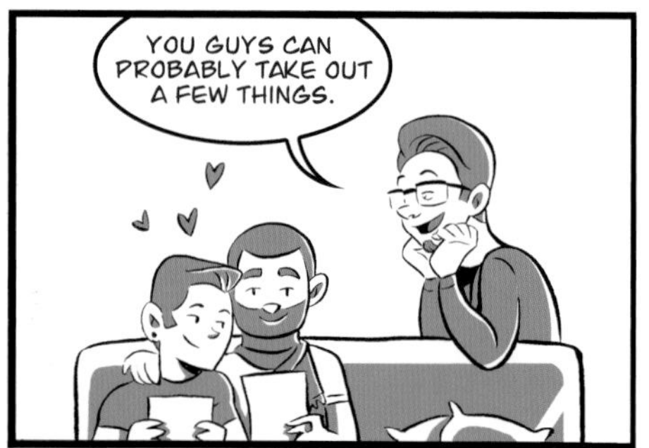
YOU GUYS CAN PROBABLY TAKE OUT A FEW THINGS.

STEP FOUR

GET TOGETHER AND DISCUSS! NO JUDGEMENT! LISTEN AND COMPARE YOUR LISTS!

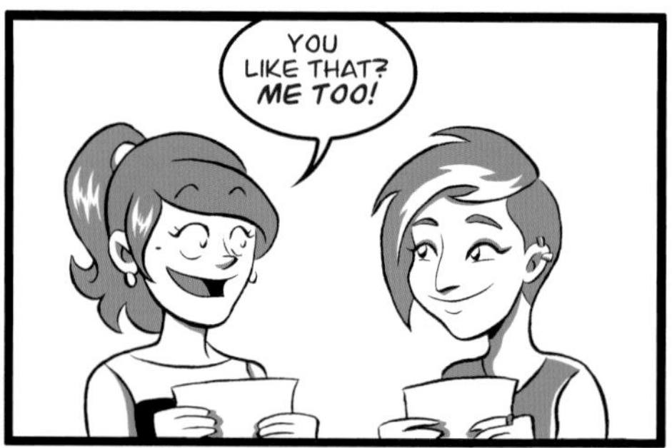
YOU LIKE THAT? ***ME TOO!***

THEN GET TO THE SEXY STUFF!

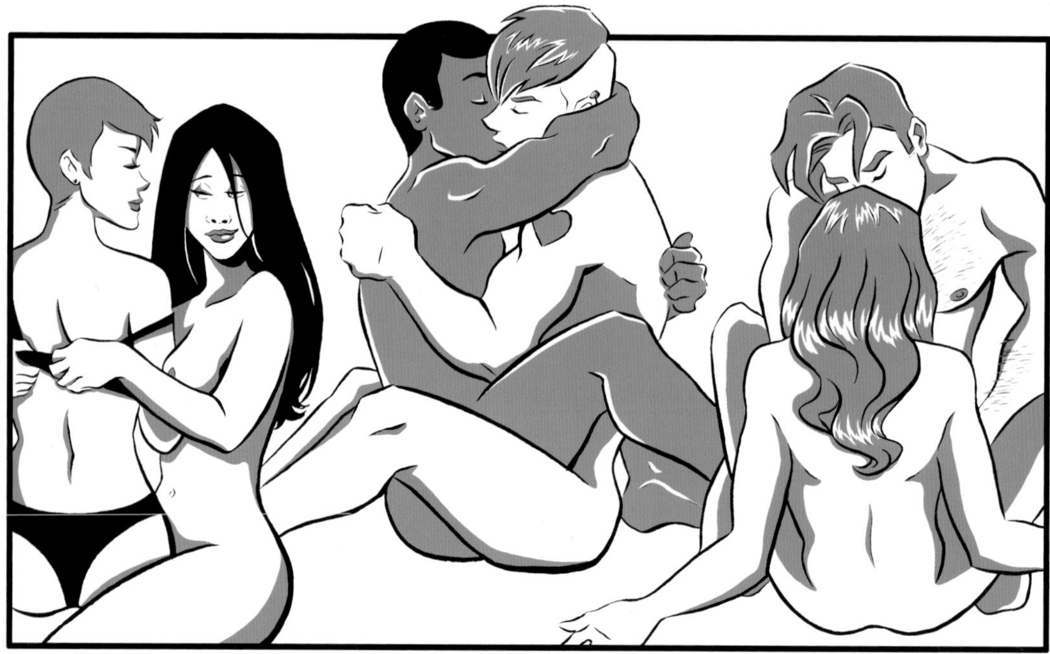

A LIST CAN HELP GET A ***CONVERSATION*** STARTED. HOPEFULLY, YOU'VE NOW GOT A WIDE ***VARIETY*** OF FUN THINGS TO TRY. YOU MIGHT FIND YOU CHECK A LOT ***OF "MAYBES." BE ADVENTUROUS BUT SAFE!*** YOU NEVER KNOW WHAT YOU MIGHT LIKE UNTIL YOU TRY IT.

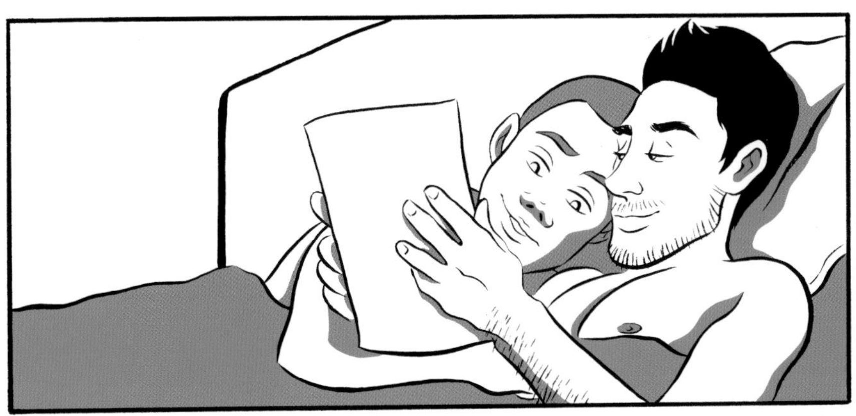

ALSO, IT CAN ***BUILD EXCITEMENT***, KNOWING THAT LATER ON, YOU'RE GOING TO BE DOING STUFF FROM YOUR LISTS.

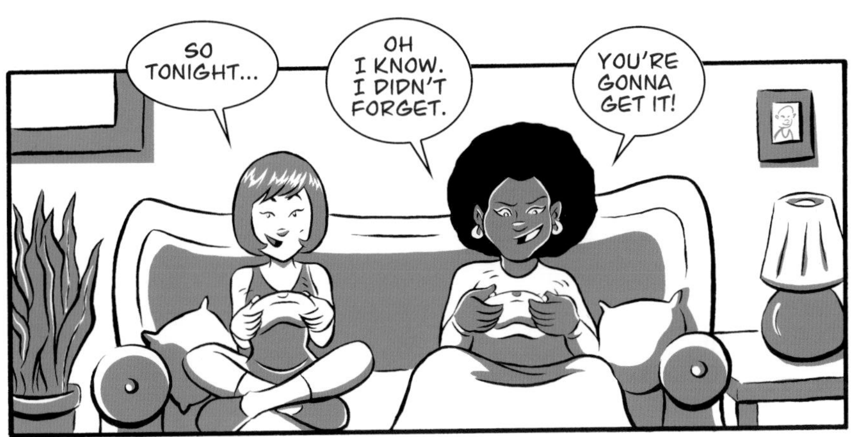
SO TONIGHT...
OH I KNOW. I DIDN'T FORGET.
YOU'RE GONNA GET IT!

BUT REMEMBER:

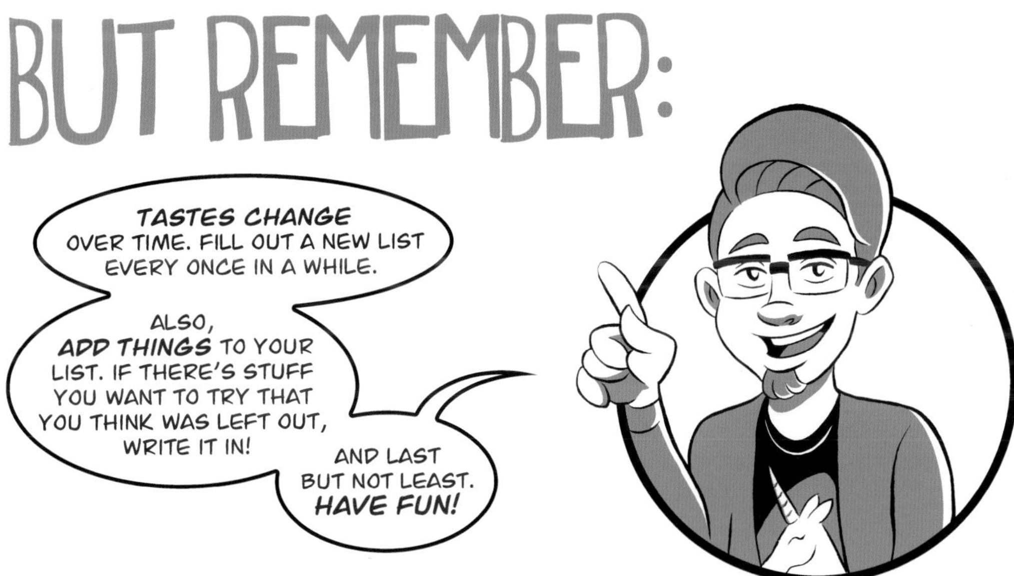
TASTES CHANGE OVER TIME. FILL OUT A NEW LIST EVERY ONCE IN A WHILE.
ALSO, ADD THINGS TO YOUR LIST. IF THERE'S STUFF YOU WANT TO TRY THAT YOU THINK WAS LEFT OUT, WRITE IT IN!
AND LAST BUT NOT LEAST. HAVE FUN!

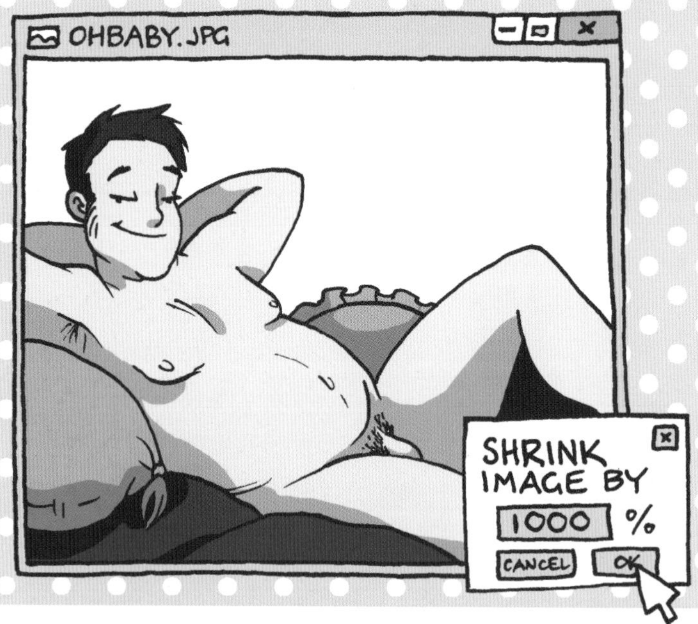

THREE GREATEST SFW FETISHES

by Ryan North & Trudy Cooper

qwantz.com & oglaf.com

unmasked BB font by blambot

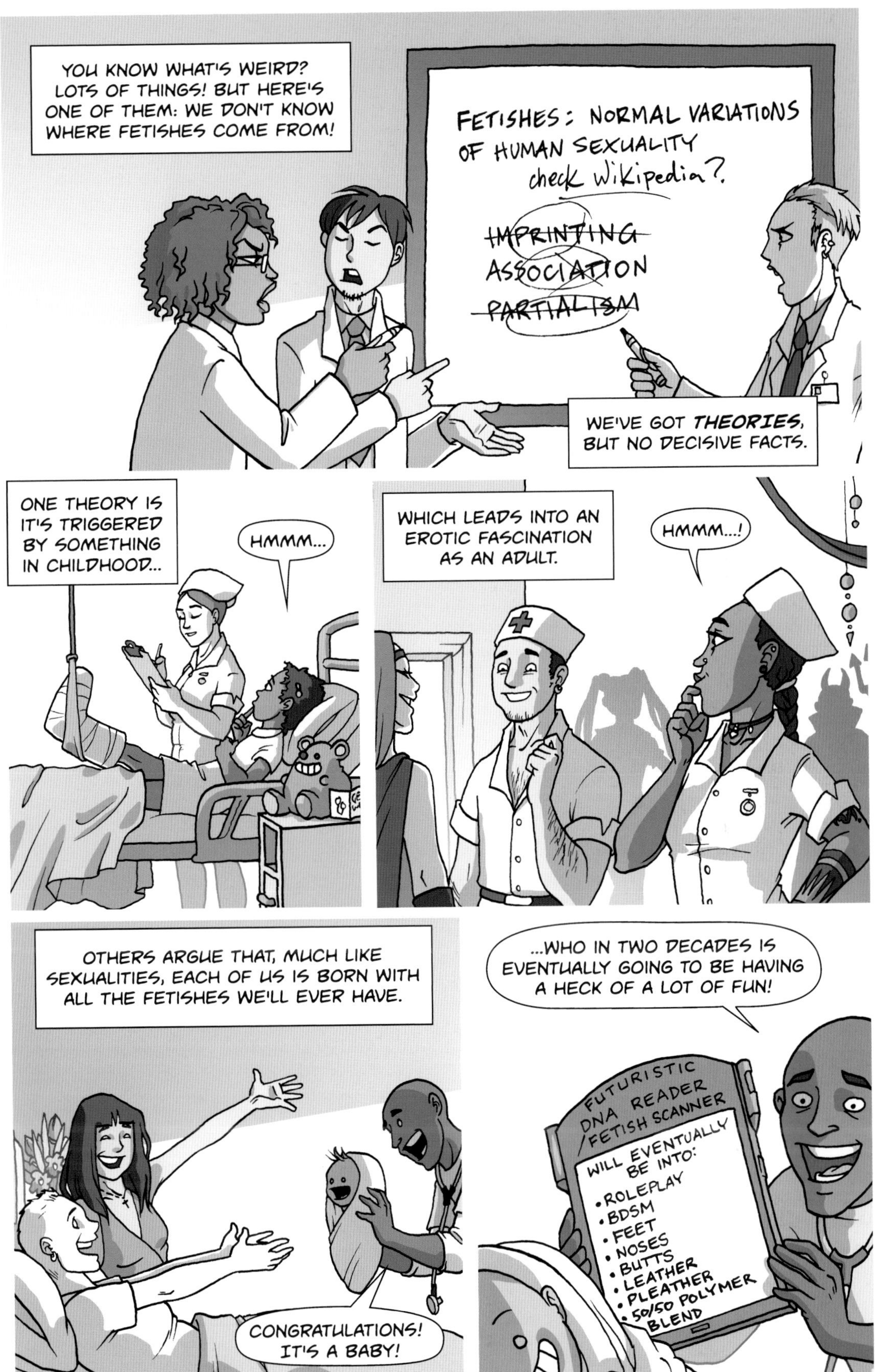
YOU KNOW WHAT'S WEIRD? LOTS OF THINGS! BUT HERE'S ONE OF THEM: WE DON'T KNOW WHERE FETISHES COME FROM!
FETISHES: NORMAL VARIATIONS OF HUMAN SEXUALITY
check Wikipedia?
IMPRINTING
ASSOCIATION
PARTIALISM
WE'VE GOT *THEORIES*, BUT NO DECISIVE FACTS.
ONE THEORY IS IT'S TRIGGERED BY SOMETHING IN CHILDHOOD...
HMMM...
WHICH LEADS INTO AN EROTIC FASCINATION AS AN ADULT.
HMMM...!
OTHERS ARGUE THAT, MUCH LIKE SEXUALITIES, EACH OF US IS BORN WITH ALL THE FETISHES WE'LL EVER HAVE.
CONGRATULATIONS! IT'S A BABY!
...WHO IN TWO DECADES IS EVENTUALLY GOING TO BE HAVING A HECK OF A LOT OF FUN!
FUTURISTIC DNA READER /FETISH SCANNER
WILL EVENTUALLY BE INTO:
• ROLEPLAY
• BDSM
• FEET
• NOSES
• BUTTS
• LEATHER
• PLEATHER
• 50/50 POLYMER BLEND

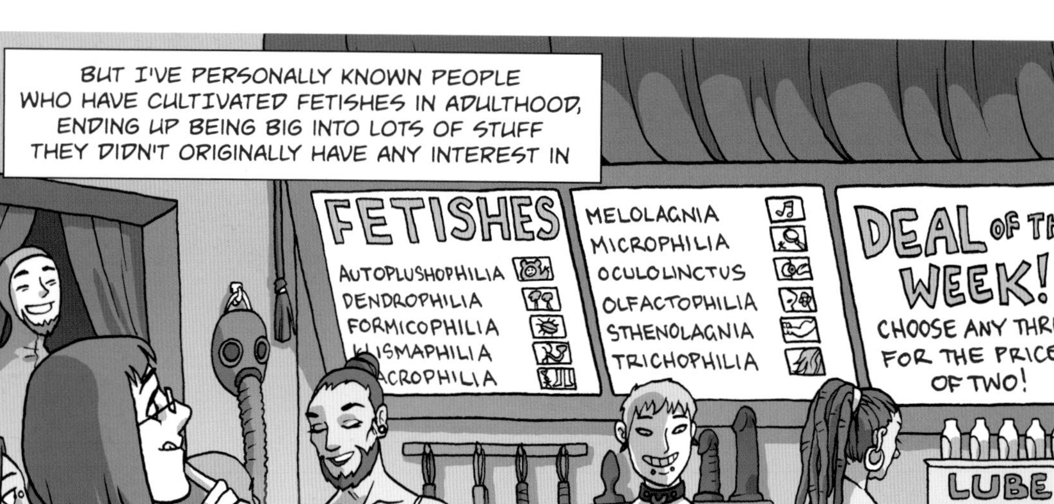
BUT I'VE PERSONALLY KNOWN PEOPLE WHO HAVE CULTIVATED FETISHES IN ADULTHOOD, ENDING UP BEING BIG INTO LOTS OF STUFF THEY DIDN'T ORIGINALLY HAVE ANY INTEREST IN
FETISHES
AUTOPLUSHOPHILIA
DENDROPHILIA
FORMICOPHILIA
MELOLAGNIA
MICROPHILIA
OCULOLINCTUS
OLFACTOPHILIA
STHENOLAGNIA
TRICHOPHILIA
DEAL OF TH
WEEK!
CHOOSE ANY THRE
FOR THE PRICE
OF TWO!
LUBE
USUALLY THIS WAS BECAUSE OF WANTING TO BE GIVING AND GAME WITH A PARTNER!

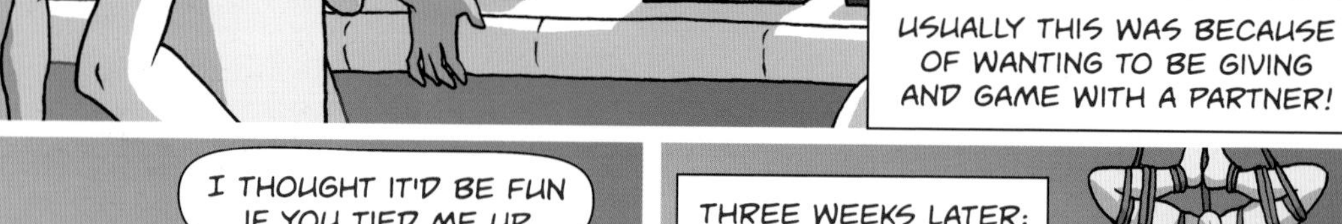

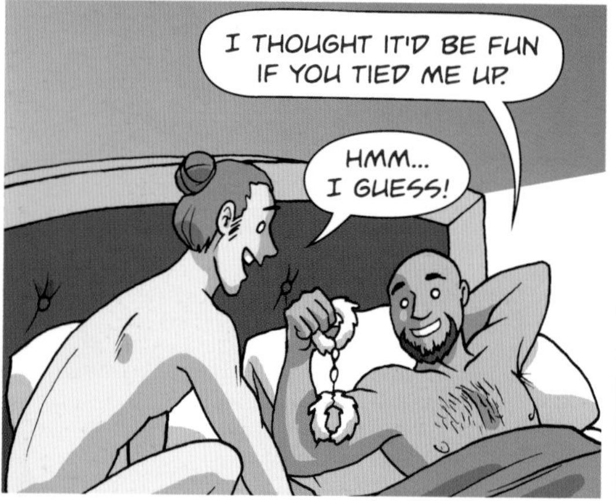

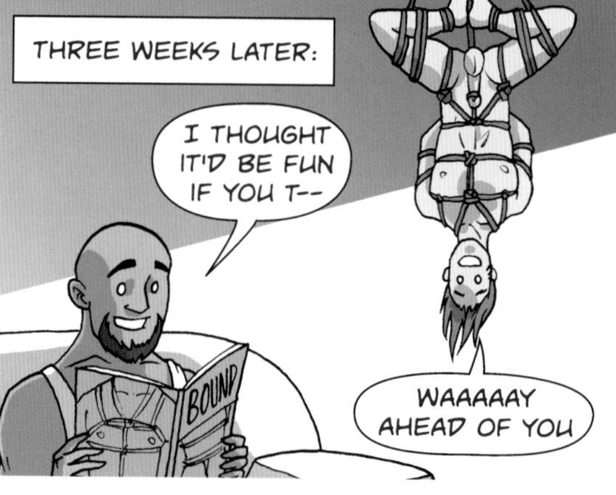
THREE WEEKS LATER:
I THOUGHT IT'D BE FUN IF YOU T--
WAAAAAY AHEAD OF YOU
BOUND

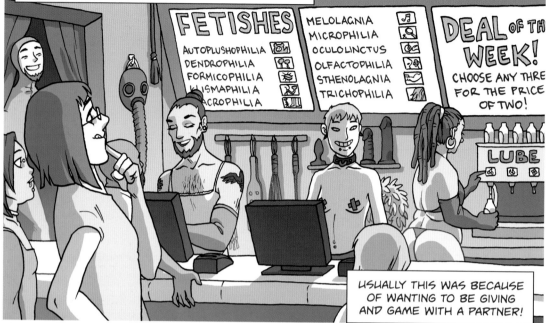

HOW DO YOU KNOW WHAT YOU'RE INTO UNLESS YOU'VE SEEN IT BEFORE, RIGHT? SO WHETHER YOU'RE LOOKING TO CULTIVATE A NEW FETISH, OR MERELY HOPING TO TRIP OVER ONE YOU NEVER EVEN KNOW YOU HAD, LET'S GO OVER...

THE THREE GREATEST

FETISHES

THAT I GUESS ARE SAFE FOR WORK, BECAUSE YOU CAN TOTALLY WATCH THEM ON YOUTUBE

FIRST UP:
BODY INFLATION

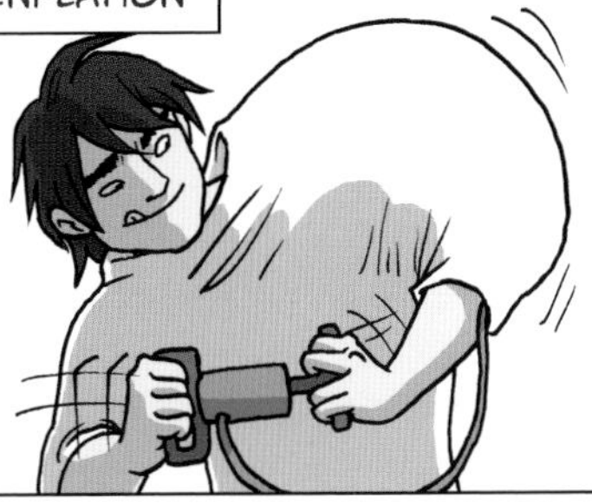

THIS IS WHERE YOU GET TURNED ON BY PEOPLE BEING INFLATED LIKE BALLOONS. THIS IS NOT POSSIBLE IN REAL LIFE (SURPRISE!), BUT YOU CAN SIMULATE IT WITH BALLOONS UNDER YOUR CLOTHES.

AND THERE'S NOTHING WRONG WITH A FETISH THAT CAN'T BE REALIZED IN REALITY! WHY SHOULD WE RESTRICT OUR IMAGINATIONS TO ONLY WHAT REALITY HAS TO OFFER, ANYWAY??

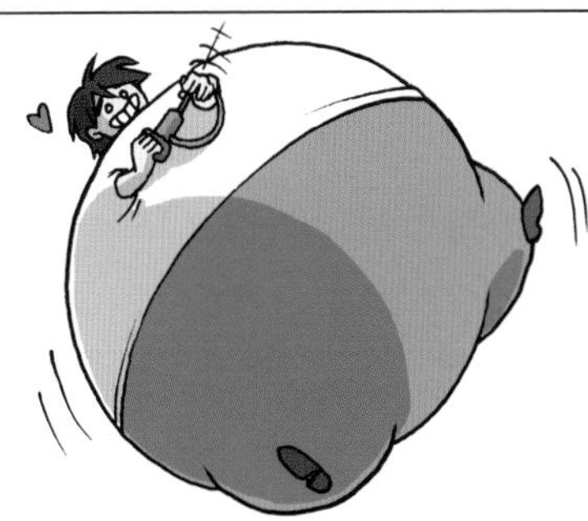

AMAZINGLY, AS LONG AS EVERYONE WHOSE BODY IS INFLATING KEEPS THEIR CLOTHES ON, THIS FLIES UNDER YOUTUBE'S RADAR.

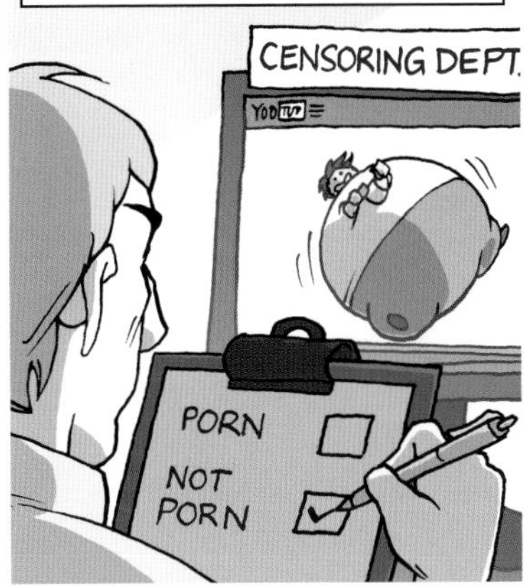

IT SEEMS THE YOUTUBE CENSORS ARE ALL...

WHY, THIS ISN'T SEX! THIS IS JUST CLOSE-UP EXPANSION SHOTS, ALL ANIMATED WITH THE SAME OBSESSIVE FOCUS ON THE MECHANICS OF SUCH AN ACT, MUCH LIKE YOU'D SEE IN THE PORN I'M FAMILIAR WITH!

MAYBE IT'S A DEMO REEL OR SOMETHING, I DUNNO

BUT IT'S *TOTALLY SEX*

THIS MEANS THERE'S TONS OF APPARENTLY SAFE-FOR-WORK BODY INFLATION VIDEOS AVAILABLE! CHECK THEM OUT: YOU MIGHT DISCOVER A NEW FETISH!

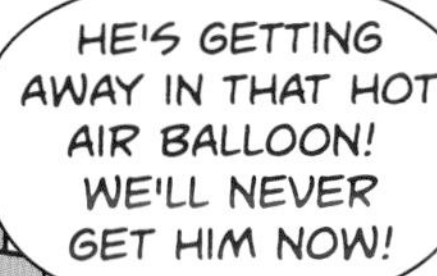

HE'S GETTING AWAY IN THAT HOT AIR BALLOON! WE'LL NEVER GET HIM NOW!

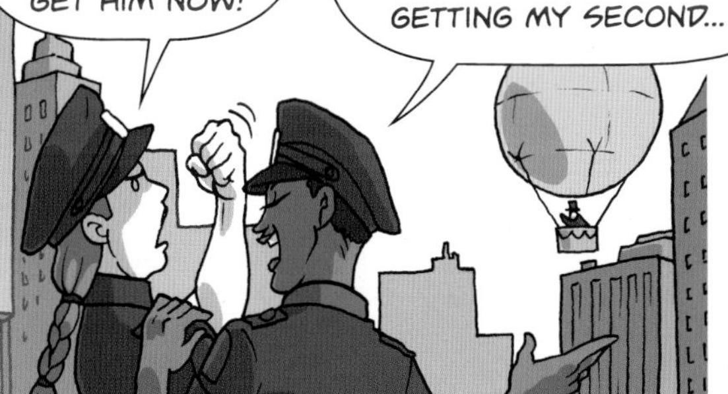

NEVER FEAR, PARTNER! WHAT THAT MALEVOLENT MISCREANT FAILS TO REALIZE IS THAT *I'M* JUST GETTING MY SECOND...

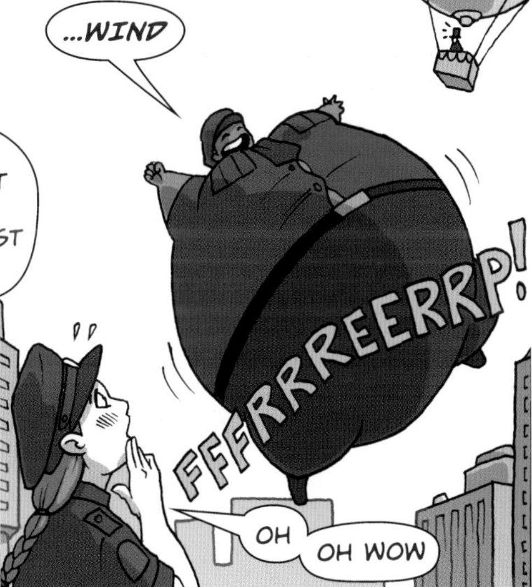

...WIND
FFFRRREERRP!
OH
OH WOW

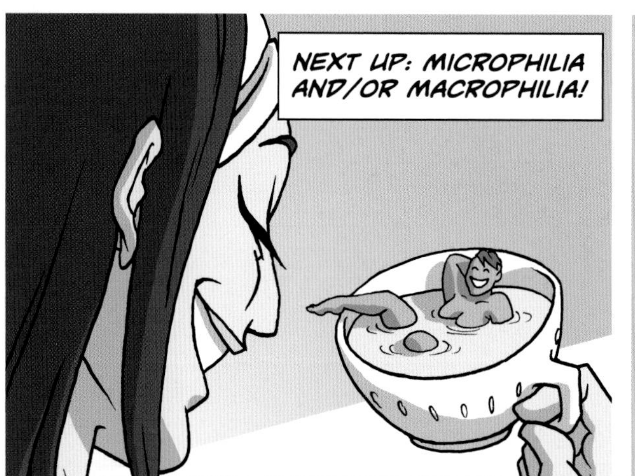
NEXT UP: MICROPHILIA AND/OR MACROPHILIA!
THIS IS WHERE YOU LOVE THE IDEA OF A TINY TINY PERSON OR A GIANT. AGAIN: TOTALLY IMPOSSIBLE, BUT ALSO TOTALLY EASY TO FAKE USING PHOTOSHOP, OR BY SETTING YOUR VIDEO CAMERA LOW TO THE GROUND TO FILM A TINY PERSON'S POV SHOTS AS "GIANTS" WALK AROUND!

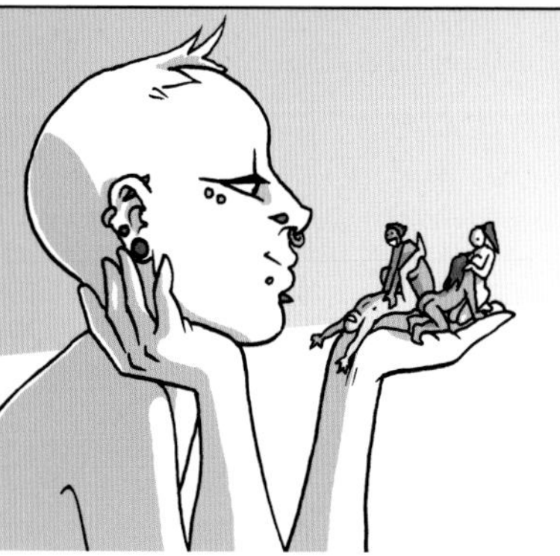
AGAIN, AS LONG AS EVERYONE KEEPS THEIR CLOTHES ON, YOUTUBE CENSORS WILL TOTALLY ASSUME THIS ISN'T PORN.BUT EVEN IF YOUTUBE IS BLOCKED, THE NICE THING ABOUT BEING INTO SHRINKING PEOPLE IS THAT YOU CAN MAKE YOUR OWN IMAGES REALLY EASILY!

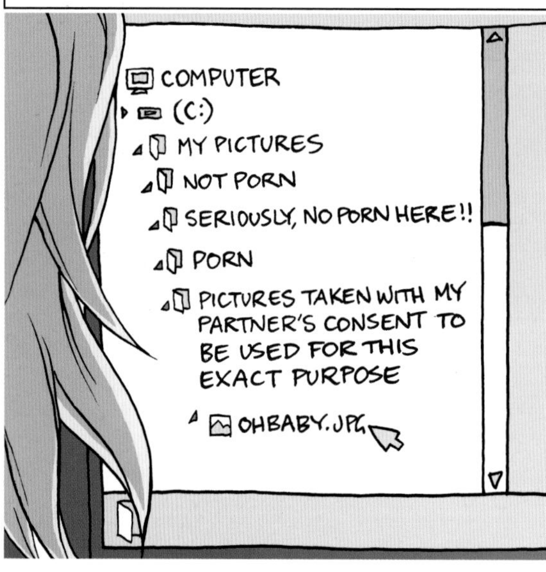
COMPUTER
(C:)
MY PICTURES
NOT PORN
SERIOUSLY, NO PORN HERE!!
PORN
PICTURES TAKEN WITH MY PARTNER'S CONSENT TO BE USED FOR THIS EXACT PURPOSE
OHBABY.JPG

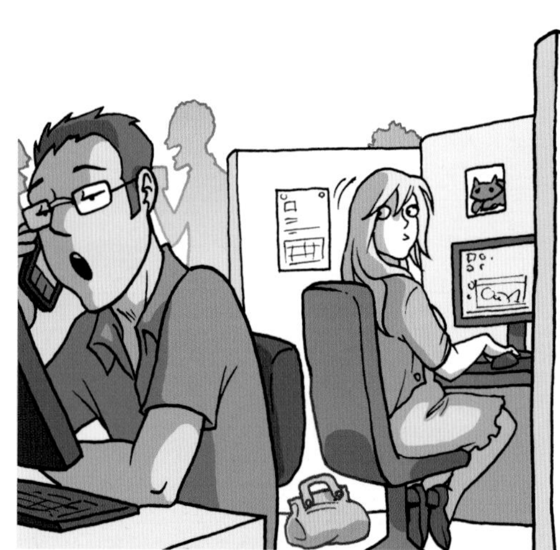

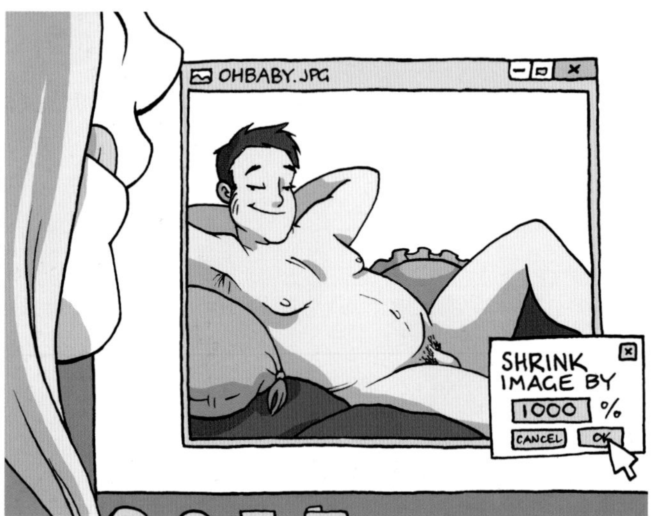
OHBABY.JPG
SHRINK IMAGE BY
1000 %
CANCEL
OK

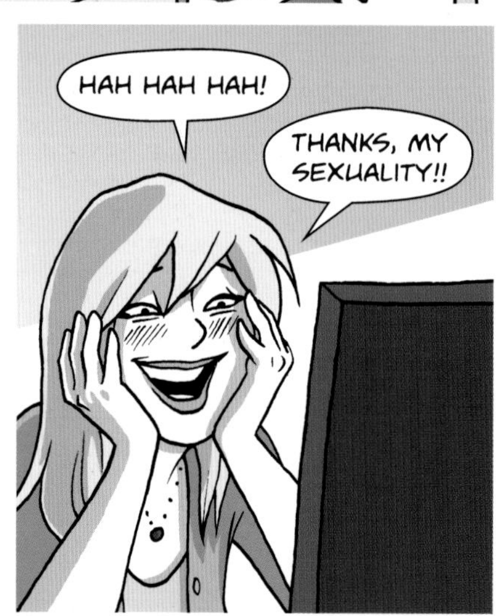
HAH HAH HAH!
THANKS, MY SEXUALITY!!

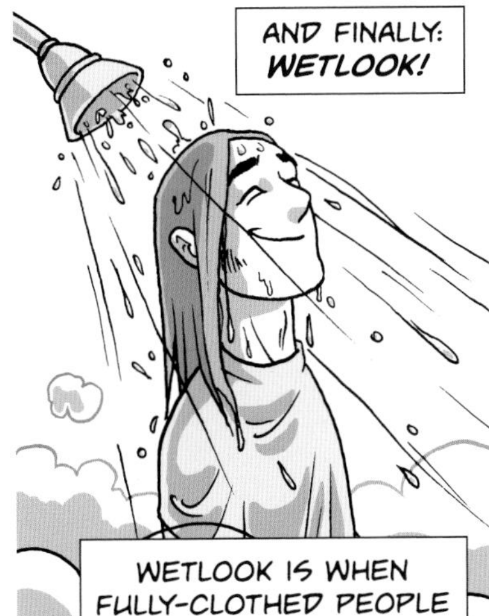
AND FINALLY:
WETLOOK!
WETLOOK IS WHEN FULLY-CLOTHED PEOPLE GET SOAKED.

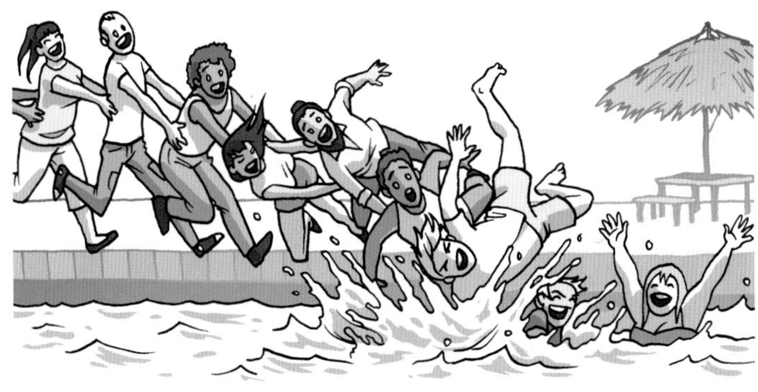
THANKS TO ITS FOCUS ON EVERYONE KEEPING THEIR CLOTHES ON, WETLOOK IS THE TRULY INVISIBLE FETISH. THAT MEGAMIX OF "CONGA LINE TUMBLES INTO THE POOL" MOVIE CLIPS? **TOTAL WETLOOK.**

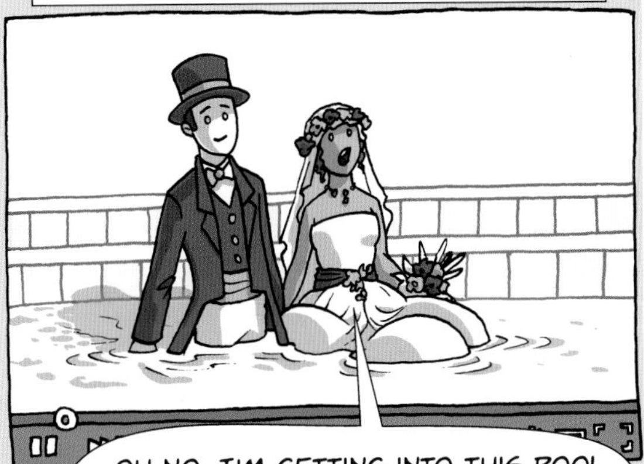
IF YOU DIDN'T KNOW ABOUT WETLOOK YOU MIGHT NOT EVEN REALIZE YOU'RE WATCHING PORN! IT'S JUST PEOPLE GETTING INTO WATER, RIGHT?
OH NO, I'M GETTING INTO THIS POOL FULLY CLOTHED, WHICH IS TECHNICALLY MORE ACCEPTABLE THAN A BATHING SUIT UNDER YOUTUBE'S ACCEPTABLE CONTENT POLICIES!

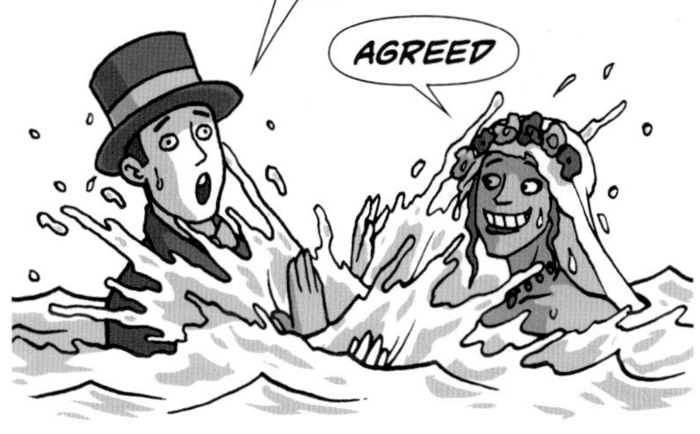
AND AS LONG AS THOSE POOR, SHELTERED CENSORS THINK SEX HAS TO INVOLVE PEOPLE GETTING NAKED, YOU'LL ALWAYS HAVE WETLOOK ON YOUTUBE!
OH NOOOO, NOW MY SUIT IS GETTING SOAKED TOO! WATER'S GETTING ALL OVER MY FULLY CLOTHED BODY! MY LOOK WILL BE SO WET WHEN THIS IS FILMED IN SLOW MOTION!
AGREED

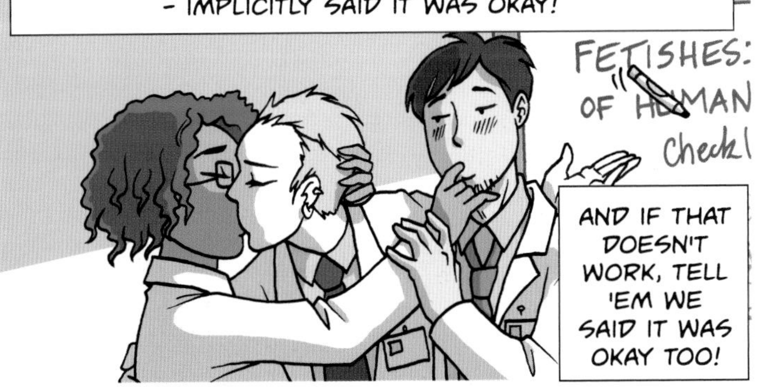
FEEL FREE TO LOOK UP ANY OF THESE FETISHES AT WORK! IF YOUR BOSS GETS MAD, TELL 'EM GOOGLE - A RESPECTED MULTINATIONAL CORPORATION WITH ACCESS TO MOST OF HUMANITY'S KNOWLEDGE - IMPLICITLY SAID IT WAS OKAY!
FETISHES:
OF HUMAN
Check!
AND IF THAT DOESN'T WORK, TELL 'EM WE SAID IT WAS OKAY TOO!

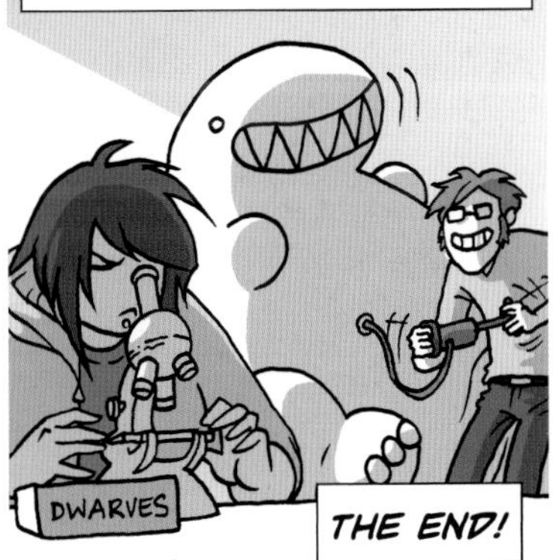
WE'RE INTERNET CARTOONISTS WITH NOTHING LEFT TO LOSE!
DWARVES
THE END!

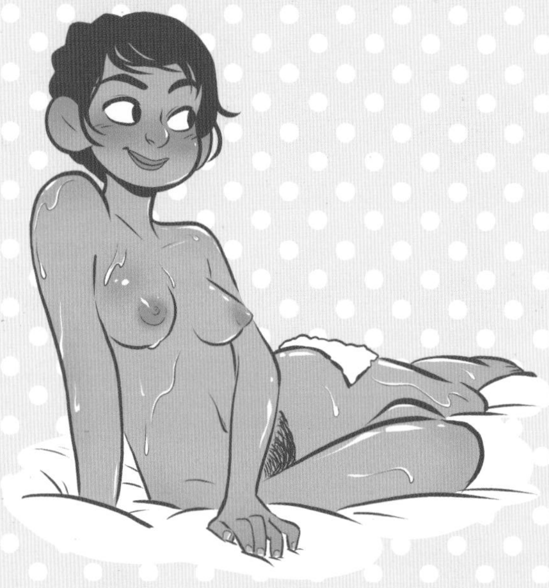

TOUCH THERAPY

by Tits McGee

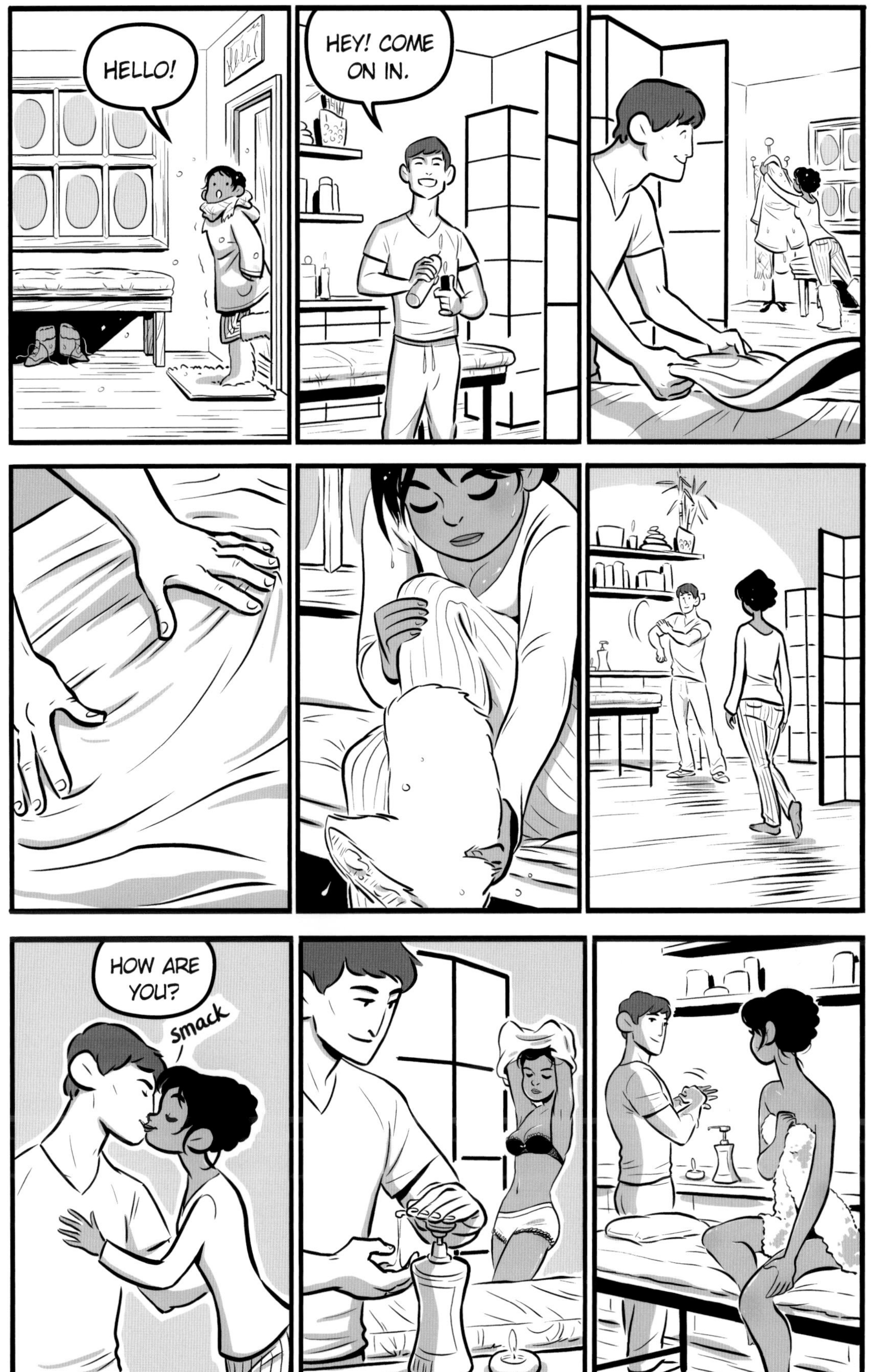
HELLO!
HEY! COME ON IN.
HOW ARE YOU?
smack

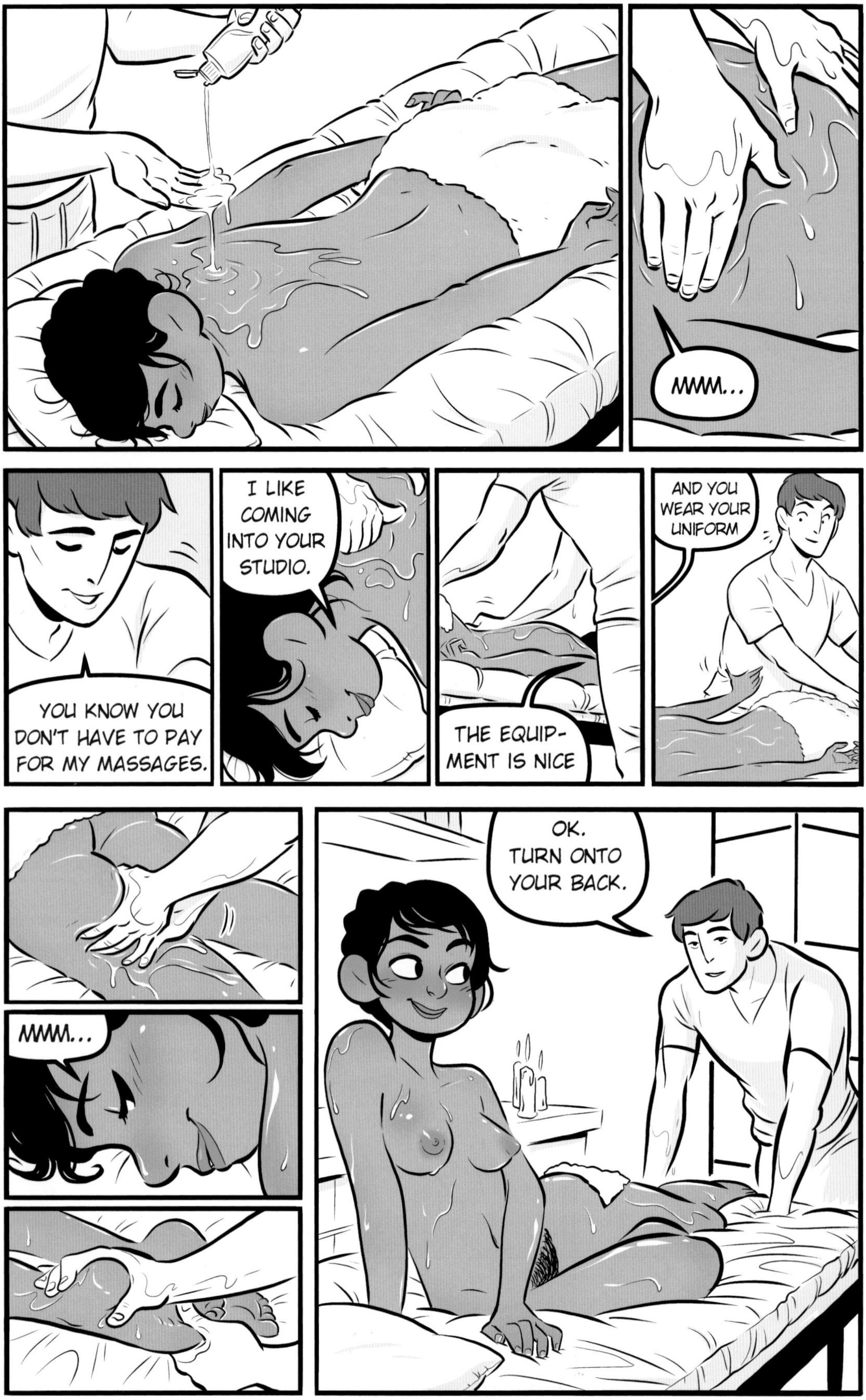

MMM...

YOU KNOW YOU DON'T HAVE TO PAY FOR MY MASSAGES.

I LIKE COMING INTO YOUR STUDIO.

THE EQUIP-MENT IS NICE

AND YOU WEAR YOUR UNIFORM

MMM...

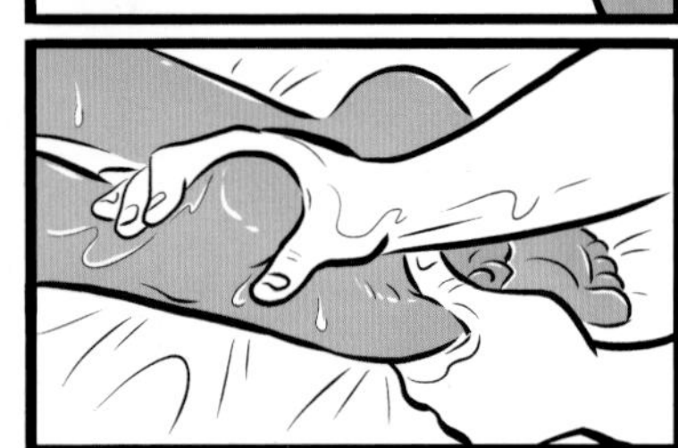

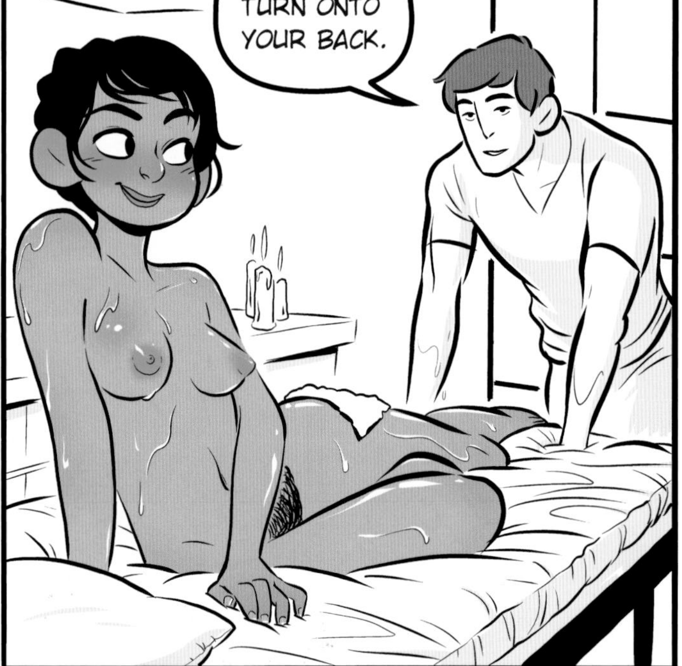

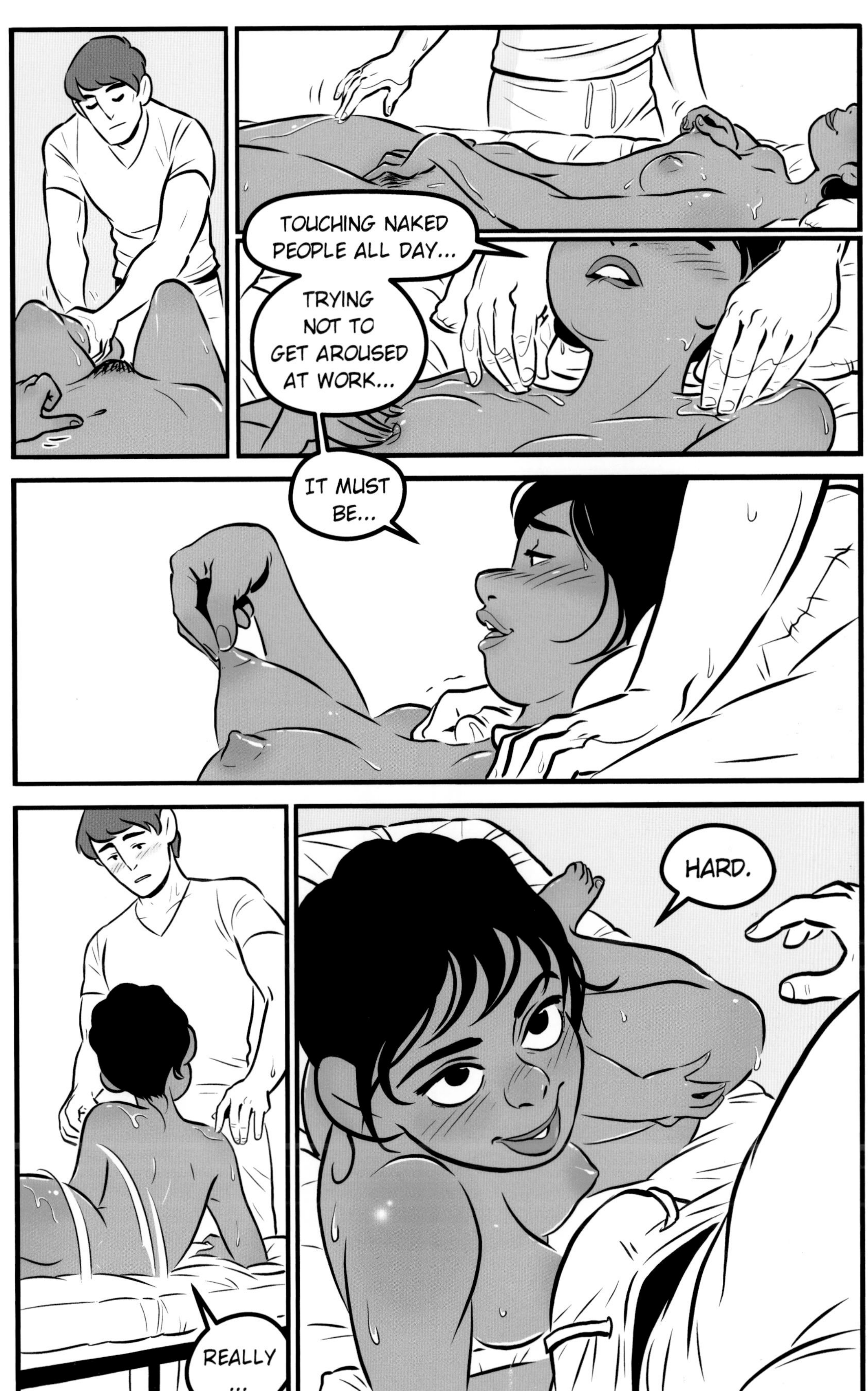
TOUCHING NAKED PEOPLE ALL DAY...
TRYING NOT TO GET AROUSED AT WORK...
IT MUST BE...
HARD.
REALLY ...

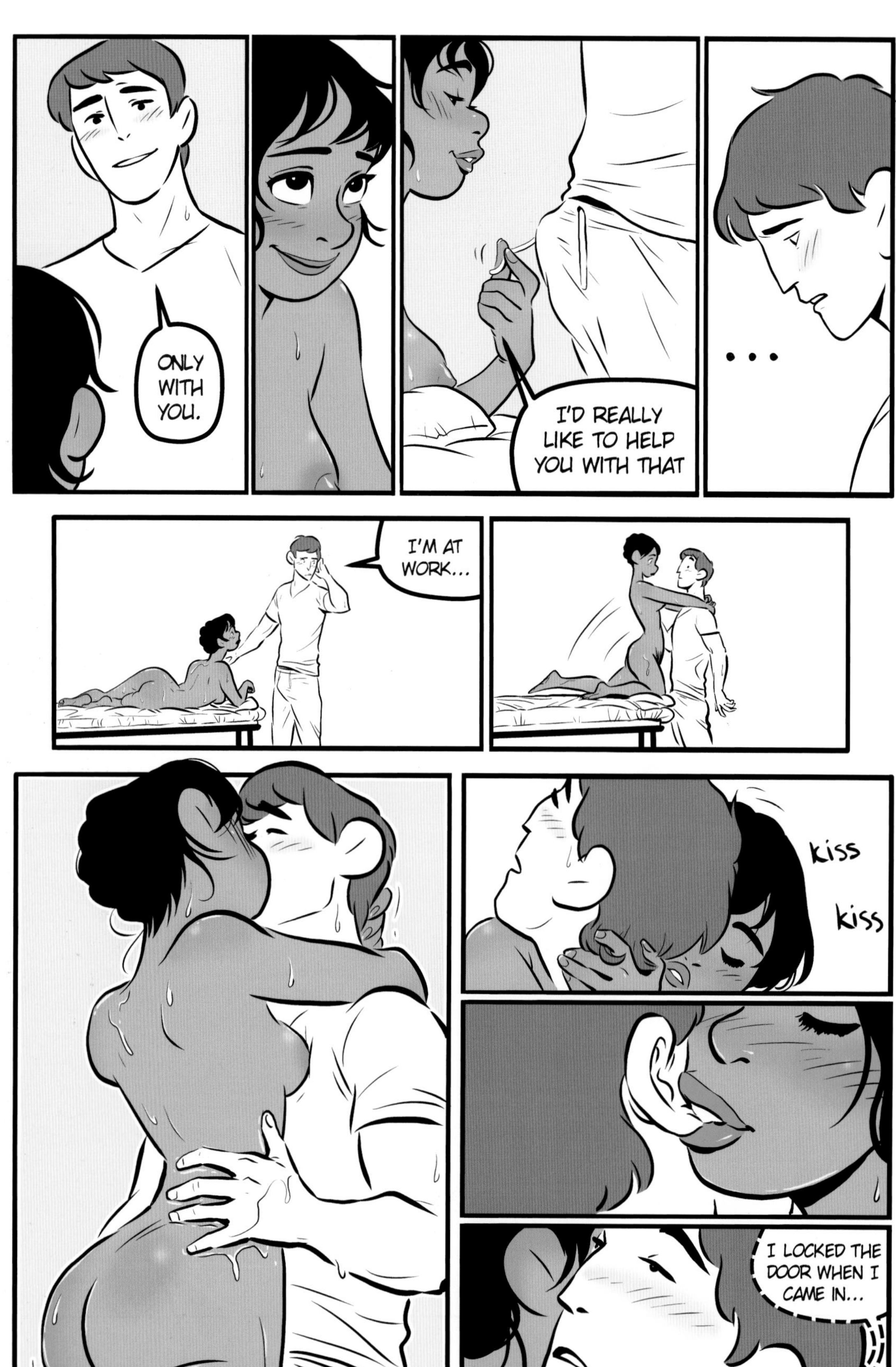
ONLY WITH YOU.
I'D REALLY LIKE TO HELP YOU WITH THAT
. . .
I'M AT WORK...
kiss
kiss
I LOCKED THE DOOR WHEN I CAME IN...

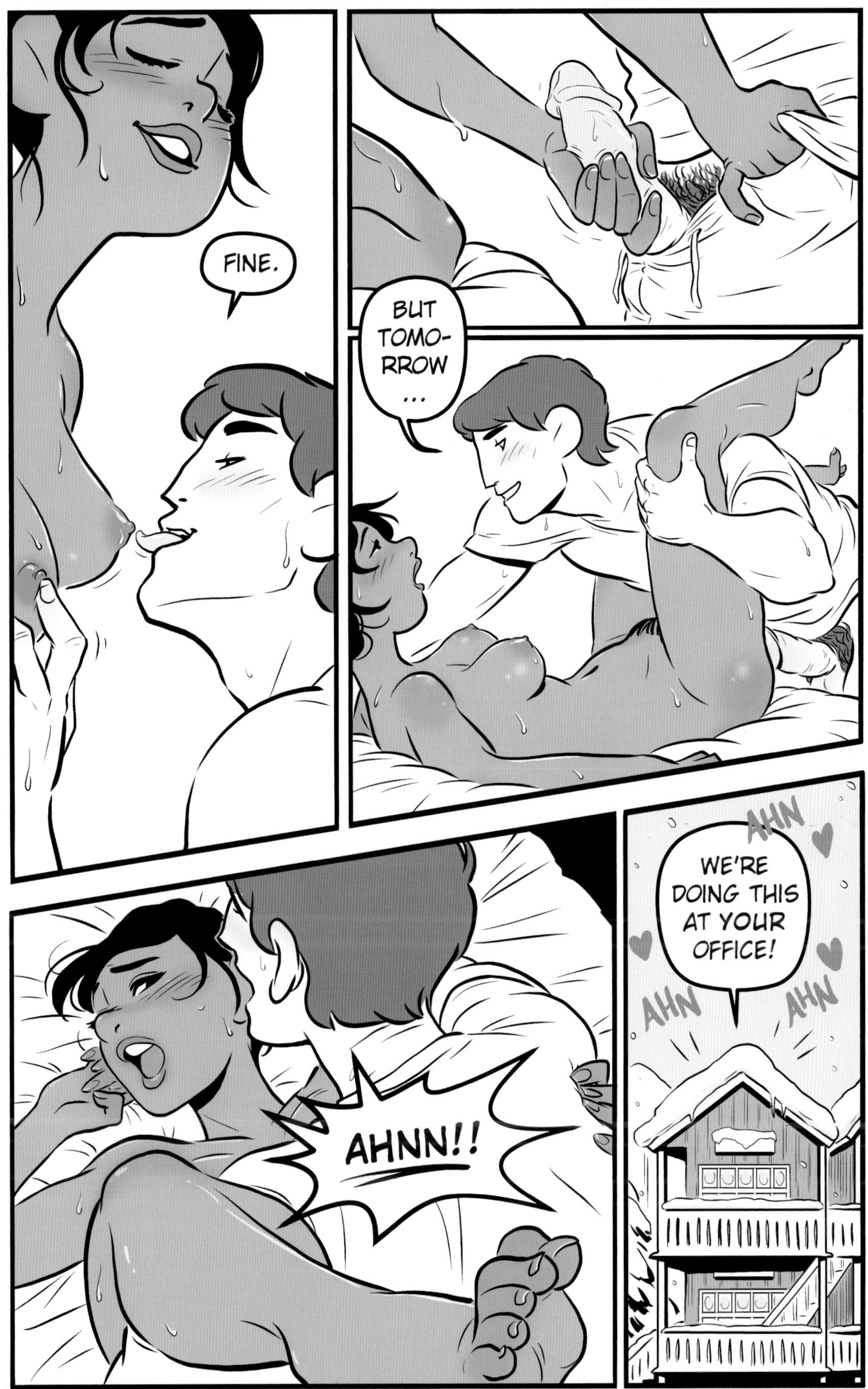
FINE.
BUT TOMO-RROW ...
AHNN!!
AHN
WE'RE DOING THIS AT YOUR OFFICE!
AHN
AHN

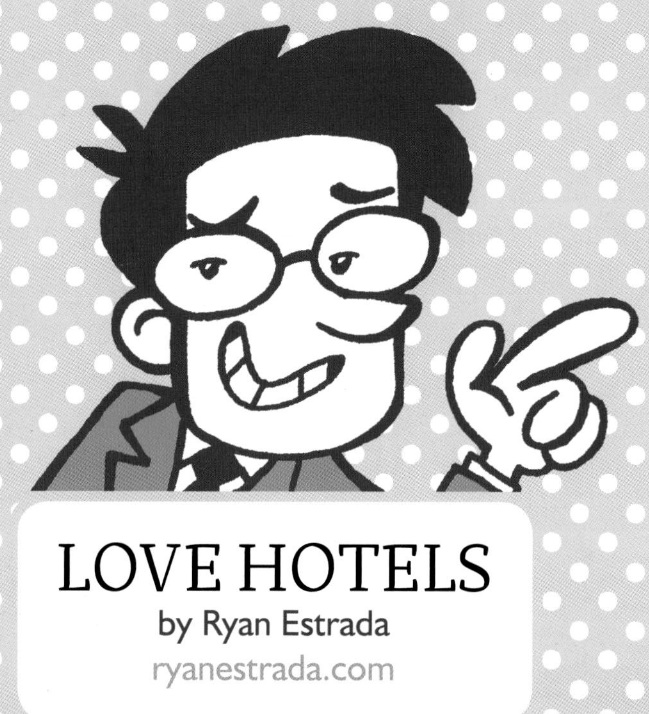

LOVE HOTELS

by Ryan Estrada

ryanestrada.com

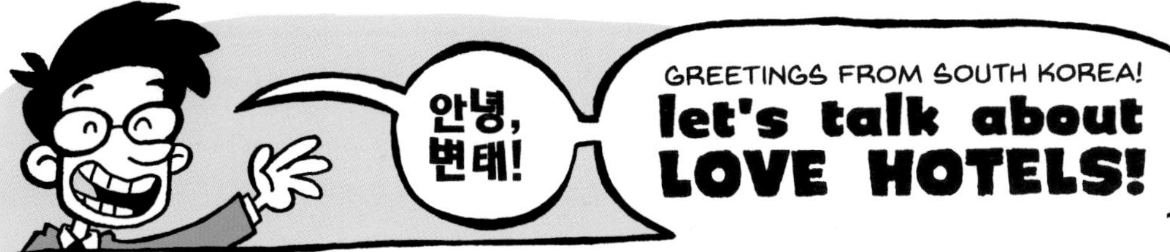

GREETINGS FROM SOUTH KOREA!

I KNOW THAT JUST TALKING ABOUT PAY-PER-HOUR NO-TELL MOTELS GIVES PEOPLE THE HEEBIE JEEBIES. I'M PRETTY SURE 70% OF THE WORLD'S USAGE OF THE WORD ***SEEDY*** IS SOLELY DEVOTED TO DESCRIBING THESE PLACES.

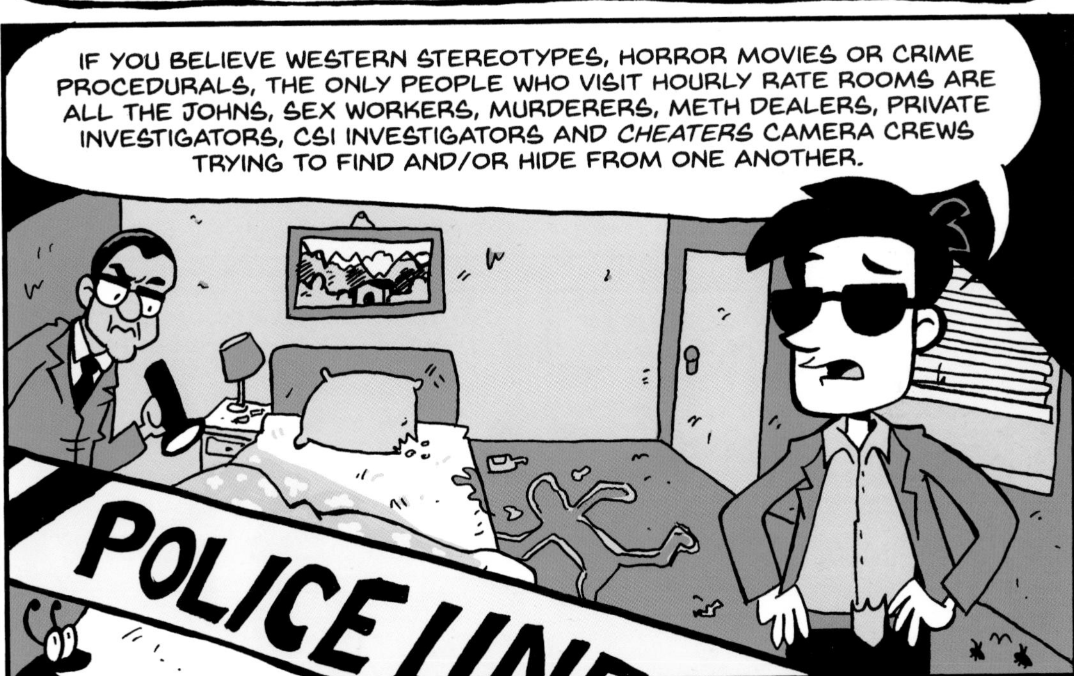

IF YOU BELIEVE WESTERN STEREOTYPES, HORROR MOVIES OR CRIME PROCEDURALS, THE ONLY PEOPLE WHO VISIT HOURLY RATE ROOMS ARE ALL THE JOHNS, SEX WORKERS, MURDERERS, METH DEALERS, PRIVATE INVESTIGATORS, CSI INVESTIGATORS AND *CHEATERS* CAMERA CREWS TRYING TO FIND AND/OR HIDE FROM ONE ANOTHER.
POLICE LINE

BUT IN ASIA, LOVE HOTELS ARE FOR EVERYONE.

MAYBE LIVING IN A SMALL APARTMENT WITH PAPER-THIN WALLS AND KIDS WHO ARE UP LATE STUDYING MAKES MARITAL ROMANCE AT HOME A DIFFICULT PROPOSITION.

MAYBE BECAUSE YOU'RE LIVING WITH YOUR EXTENDED FAMILY UNTIL YOU GET MARRIED, SO '*LET'S GO BACK TO MY PLACE*' ISN'T AN OPTION.

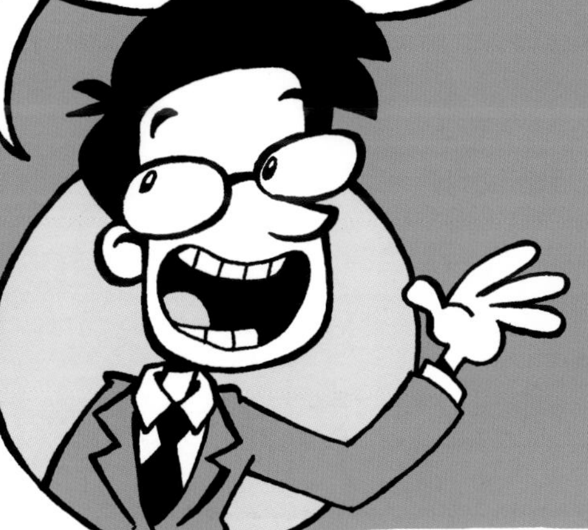

OR BECAUSE PUBLIC DISPLAYS OF AFFECTION ARE LOOKED DOWN UPON, AND YOU NEED A FRIENDLY, SEX-POSITIVE PLACE TO SMOOCH.

THERE ARE LOTS OF REASONS!

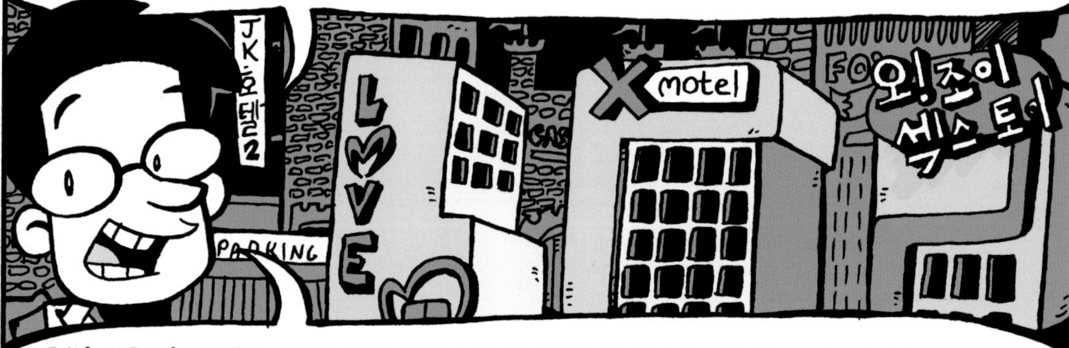

AN ENTIRE INDUSTRY HAS SPRUNG UP TO SATISFY ALL THESE REASONS. THERE ARE DOZENS IN EVERY NEIGHBORHOOD, AND THE NEWER THE LOVE HOTEL, THE MORE EFFORT THEY'VE PUT INTO OUTCLASSING THE COMPETITION.
JK 모텔2
LOVE

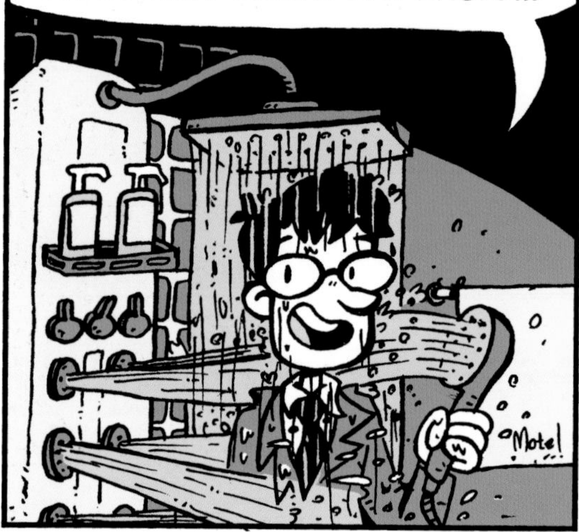

IF YOU WANNA GET SEXIED UP, YOU'LL FIND ONE OF THOSE HIGH-END SHOWERS WITH MASSAGE JETS FROM EVERY HEIGHT AND ANGLE...

WITH A WIDE SELECTION OF FANCY FRUIT-SCENTED SCRUBS, AND A SINGLE-SERVING SAMPLER PACK OF MOISTURIZERS, CREAMS, FACIAL MASKS, BUBBLE BATHS, BATH SALTS, AND LUBES.

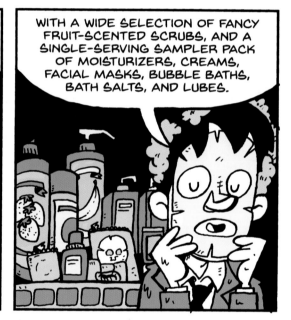

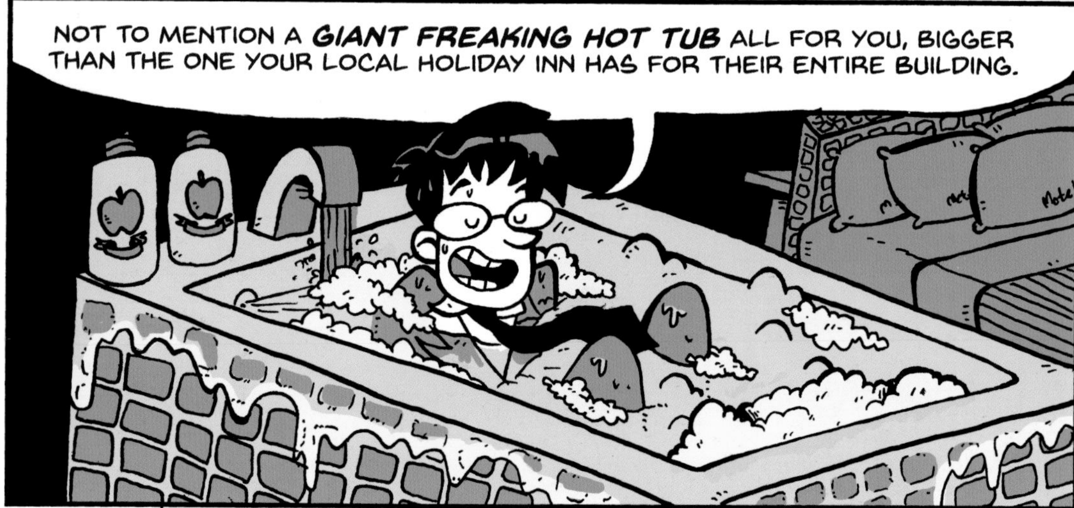

PARKING
THIS ARMS RACE OF ROMANCE MEANS THAT DEPENDING ON WHICH ONE YOU CHOOSE, FOR LIKE 30 BUCKS YOU CAN GET 3 HOURS IN A METICULOUSLY CLEAN ROOM WITH AN ***ENDLESS LIST OF THINGS TO DO:***

NOT TO MENTION A ***GIANT FREAKING HOT TUB*** ALL FOR YOU, BIGGER THAN THE ONE YOUR LOCAL HOLIDAY INN HAS FOR THEIR ENTIRE BUILDING.
Motel

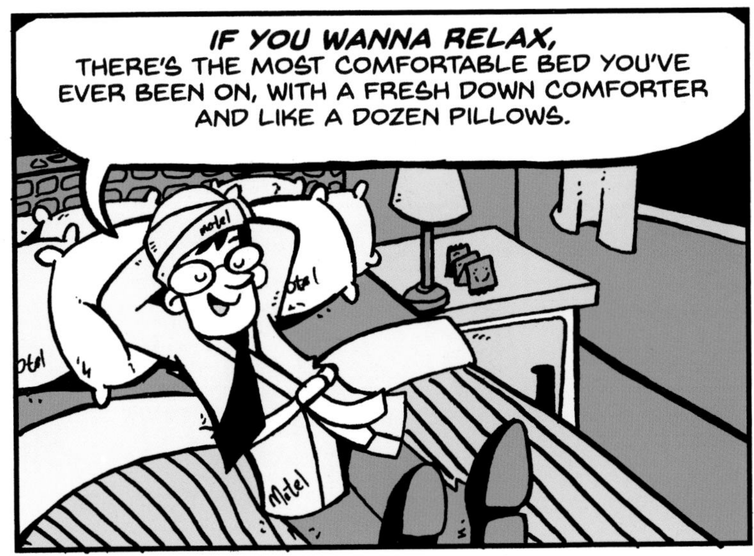
IF YOU WANNA RELAX, THERE'S THE MOST COMFORTABLE BED YOU'VE EVER BEEN ON, WITH A FRESH DOWN COMFORTER AND LIKE A DOZEN PILLOWS.
Motel

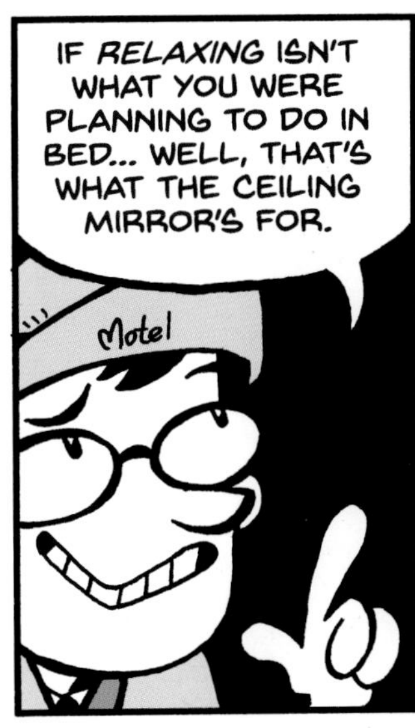
IF RELAXING ISN'T WHAT YOU WERE PLANNING TO DO IN BED... WELL, THAT'S WHAT THE CEILING MIRROR'S FOR.
Motel

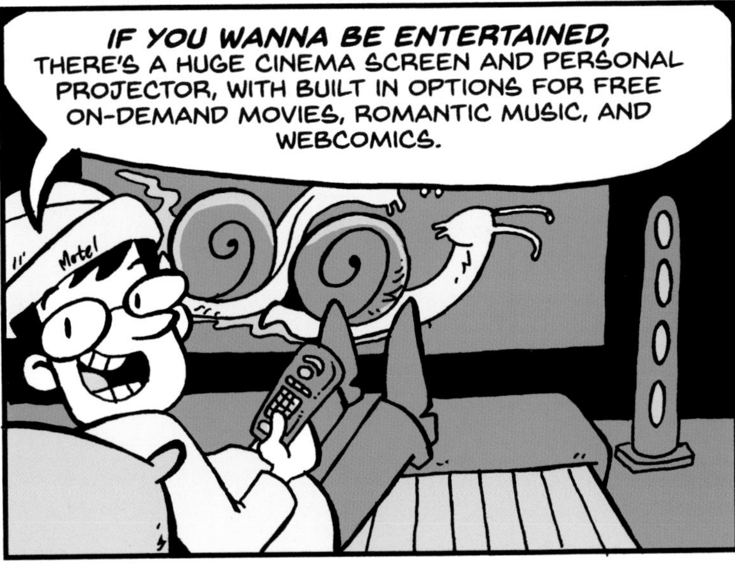
IF YOU WANNA BE ENTERTAINED, THERE'S A HUGE CINEMA SCREEN AND PERSONAL PROJECTOR, WITH BUILT IN OPTIONS FOR FREE ON-DEMAND MOVIES, ROMANTIC MUSIC, AND WEBCOMICS.
Motel

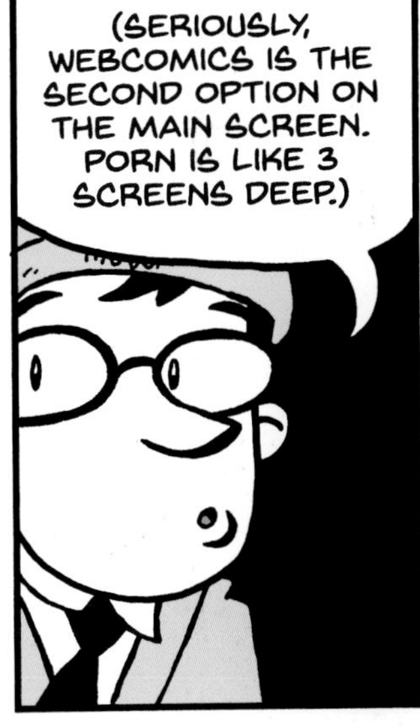
(SERIOUSLY, WEBCOMICS IS THE SECOND OPTION ON THE MAIN SCREEN. PORN IS LIKE 3 SCREENS DEEP.)

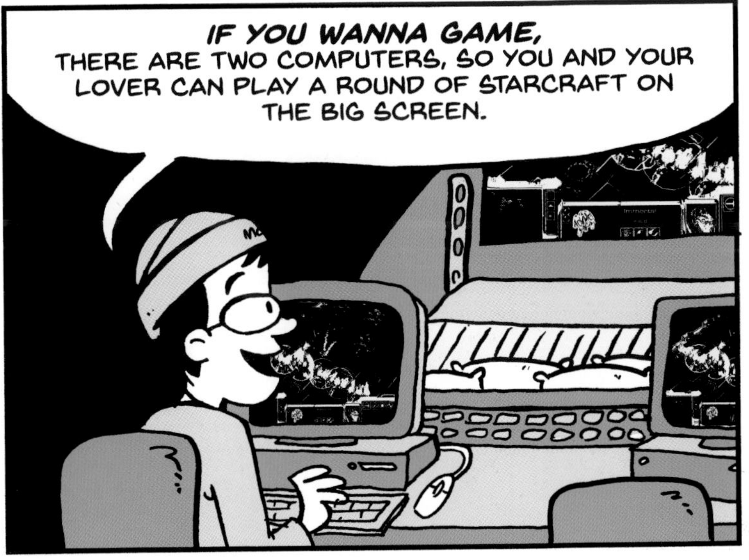
IF YOU WANNA GAME, THERE ARE TWO COMPUTERS, SO YOU AND YOUR LOVER CAN PLAY A ROUND OF STARCRAFT ON THE BIG SCREEN.

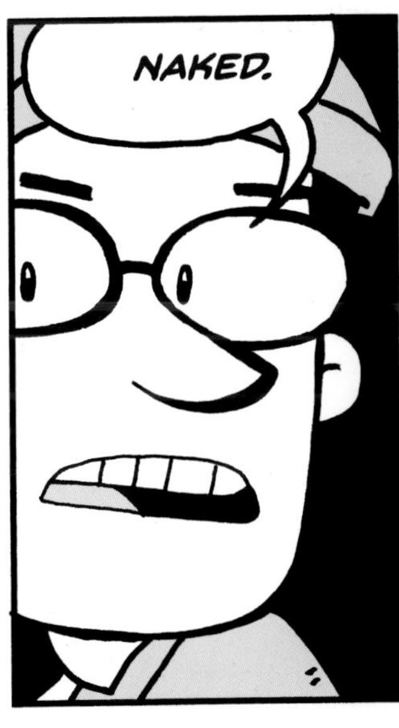
NAKED.

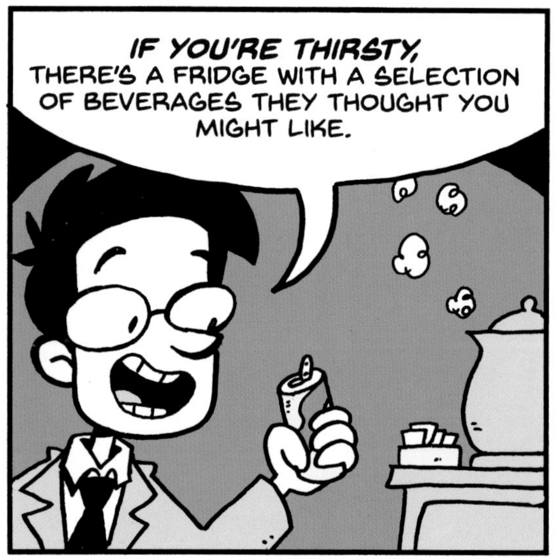
IF YOU'RE THIRSTY, THERE'S A FRIDGE WITH A SELECTION OF BEVERAGES THEY THOUGHT YOU MIGHT LIKE.

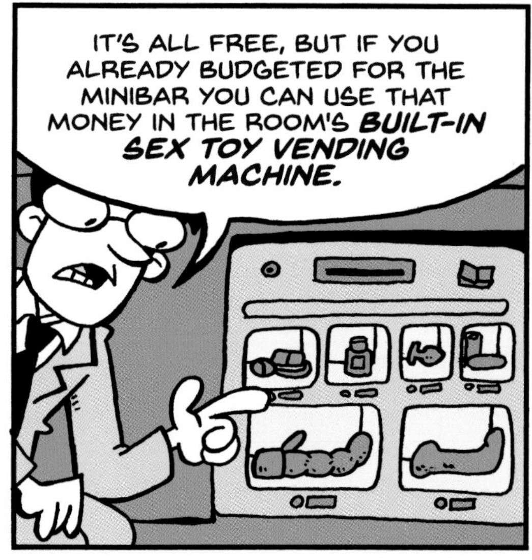
IT'S ALL FREE, BUT IF YOU ALREADY BUDGETED FOR THE MINIBAR YOU CAN USE THAT MONEY IN THE ROOM'S BUILT-IN SEX TOY VENDING MACHINE.

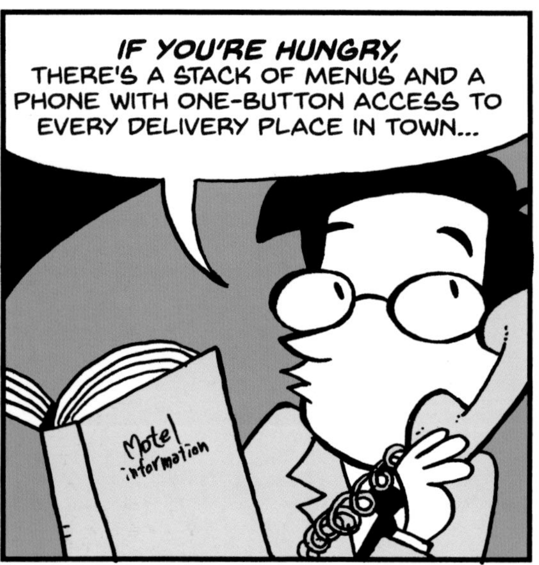
IF YOU'RE HUNGRY, THERE'S A STACK OF MENUS AND A PHONE WITH ONE-BUTTON ACCESS TO EVERY DELIVERY PLACE IN TOWN...
Motel information

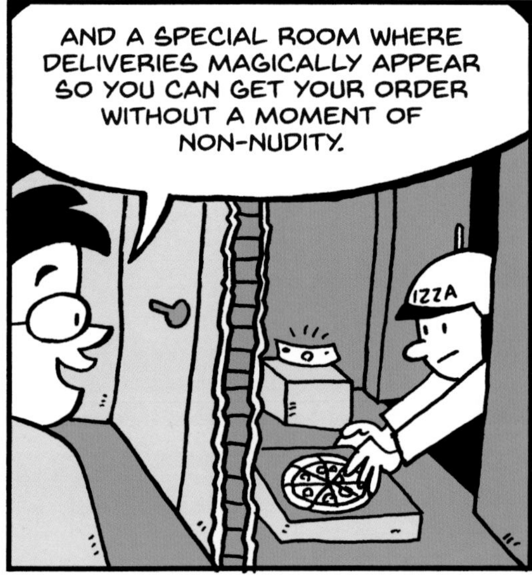
AND A SPECIAL ROOM WHERE DELIVERIES MAGICALLY APPEAR SO YOU CAN GET YOUR ORDER WITHOUT A MOMENT OF NON-NUDITY.
IZZA

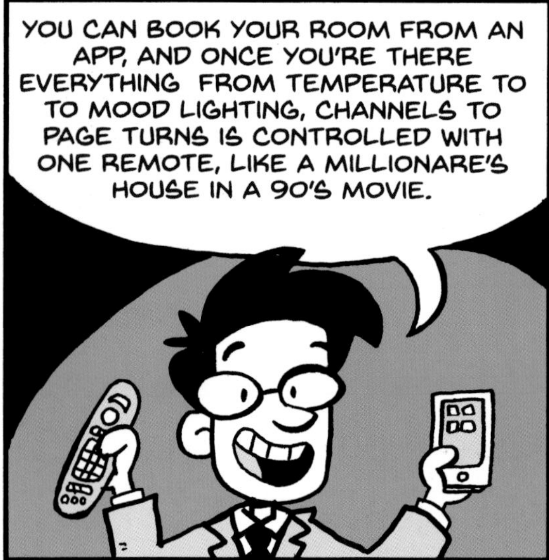
YOU CAN BOOK YOUR ROOM FROM AN APP, AND ONCE YOU'RE THERE EVERYTHING FROM TEMPERATURE TO TO MOOD LIGHTING, CHANNELS TO PAGE TURNS IS CONTROLLED WITH ONE REMOTE, LIKE A MILLIONARE'S HOUSE IN A 90'S MOVIE.

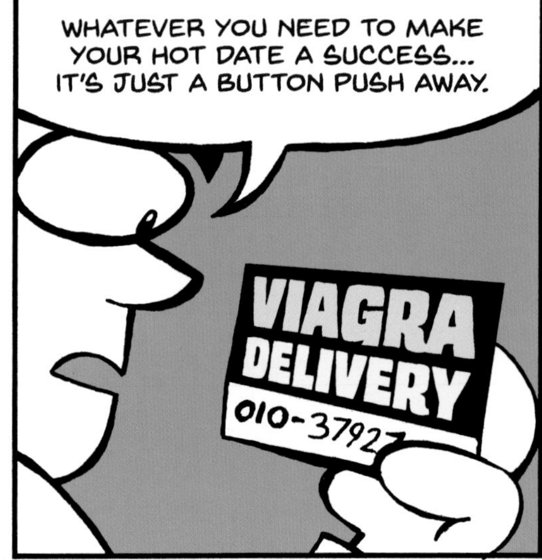
WHATEVER YOU NEED TO MAKE YOUR HOT DATE A SUCCESS... IT'S JUST A BUTTON PUSH AWAY.
VIAGRA DELIVERY
010-3792

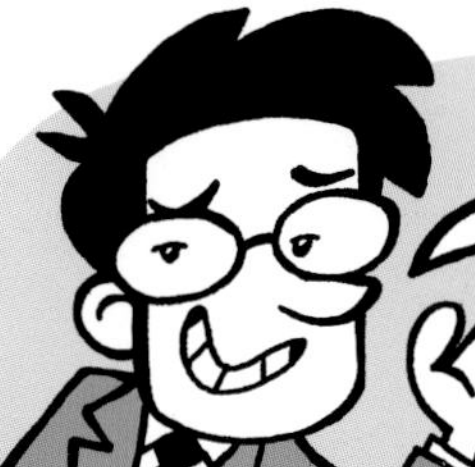
THERE'S ALWAYS SOME KIND OF FANCY DESIGN OR THEME, AND ***IF YOU'VE GOT A VERY PARTICULAR FETISH,*** YOU CAN FIND THE RIGHT THEME ROOM FOR YOU.

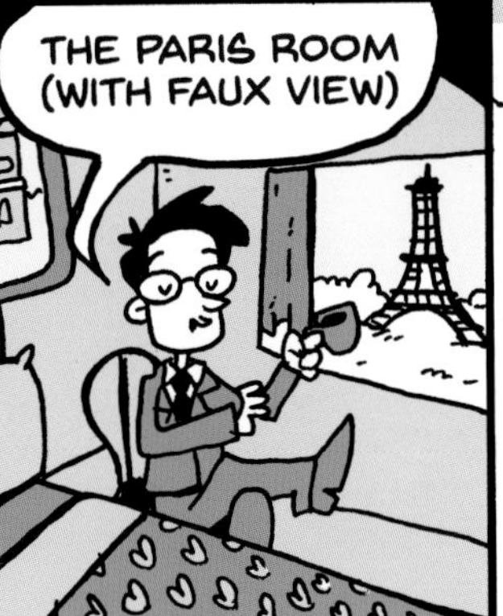
THE PARIS ROOM (WITH FAUX VIEW)

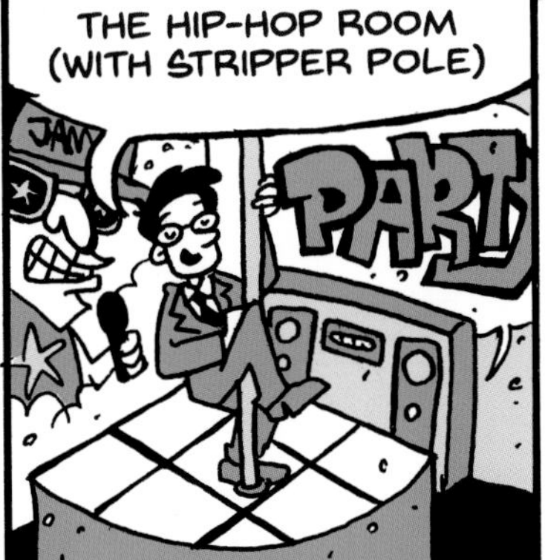
THE HIP-HOP ROOM (WITH STRIPPER POLE)
JAM
PART

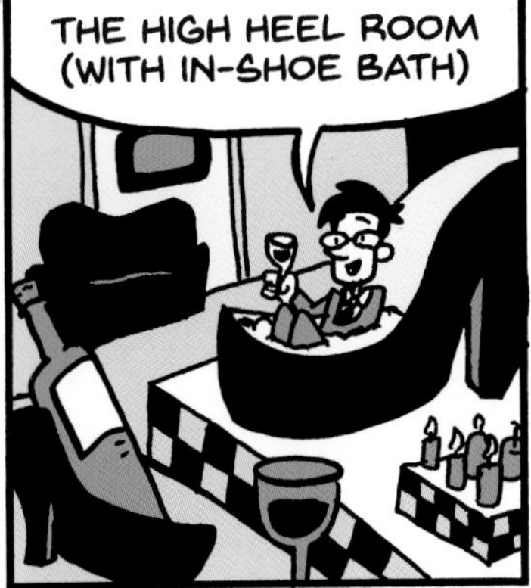
THE HIGH HEEL ROOM (WITH IN-SHOE BATH)

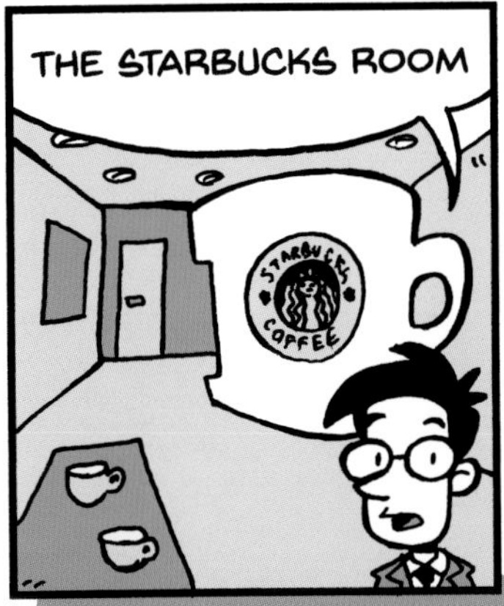
THE STARBUCKS ROOM
STARBUCKS COFFEE

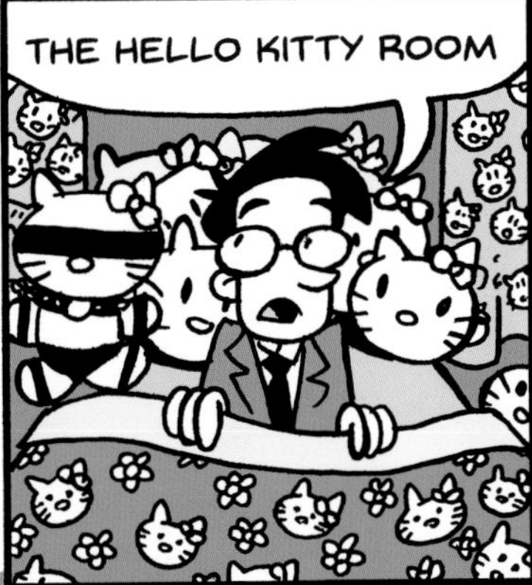
THE HELLO KITTY ROOM

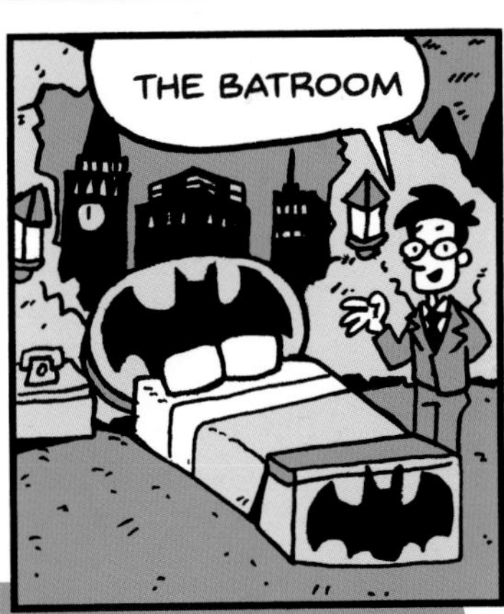
THE BATROOM

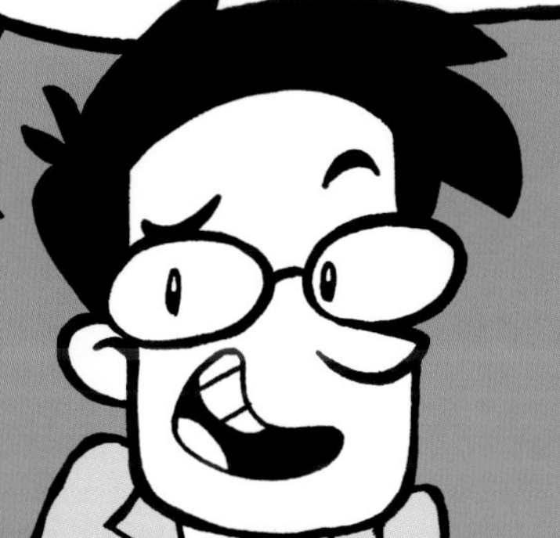
THERE ARE A MILLION KINDS OF LOVE HOTEL, A MILLION REASONS TO GO, AND A MILLION THINGS TO DO ONCE YOU GET THERE.
MANY TOURISTS STAY THERE EVEN WHEN THEY'RE TRAVELING ALONE... JUST BECAUSE IT'S USUALLY THE BEST, CHEAPEST OPTION IN TOWN. I KNOW I'D CHOOSE A *GLOW-IN-THE-DARK LOVE ROOM* OVER A BORING OLD *HILTON SUITE* ANY DAY OF THE WEEK.

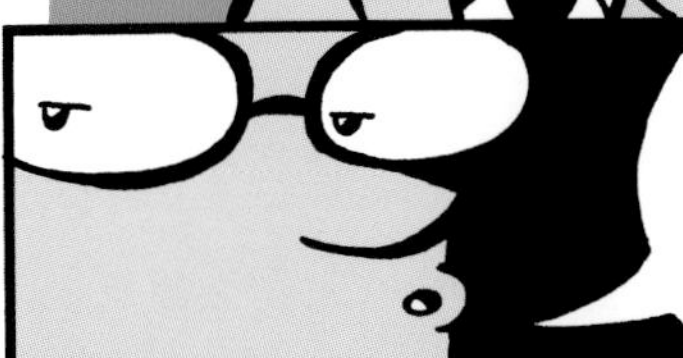
AND ***EVEN IF YOU ARE THERE*** FOR REASONS YOU MIGHT CONSIDER 'SEEDY,' YOU'LL BE PLEASED WITH THE HIDDEN PARKING LOT, PUSH-BUTTON CHECK-IN AND NINJA-LIKE STAFF THAT YOU KNOW EXIST ONLY BECAUSE OF HOW CLEAN EVERYTHING IS.

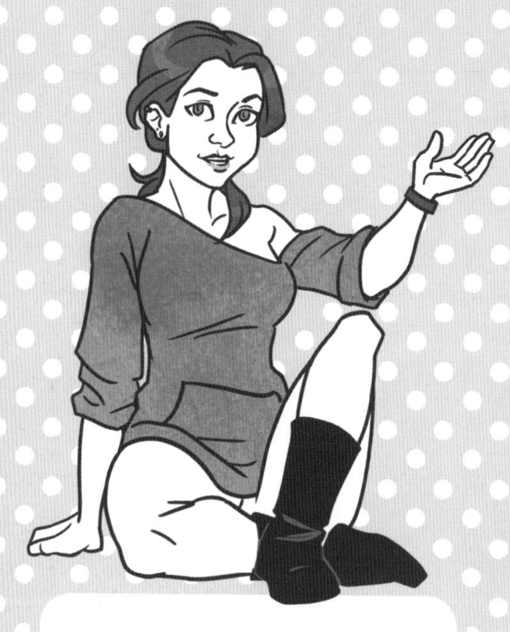

ASMR

by Grace Allison

gracifer.com

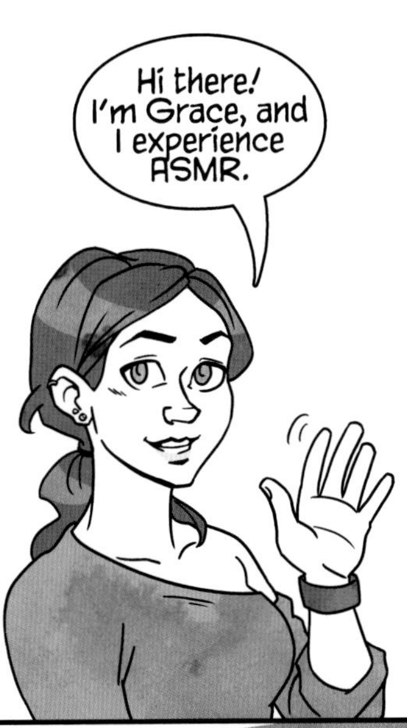
Hi there! I'm Grace, and I experience ASMR.

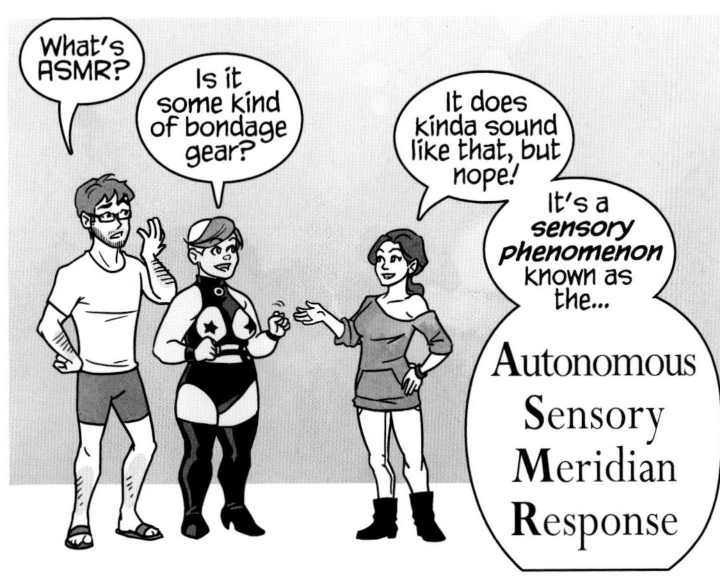
What's ASMR?
Is it some kind of bondage gear?
It does kinda sound like that, but nope!
It's a ***sensory phenomenon*** known as the...
Autonomous Sensory Meridian Response

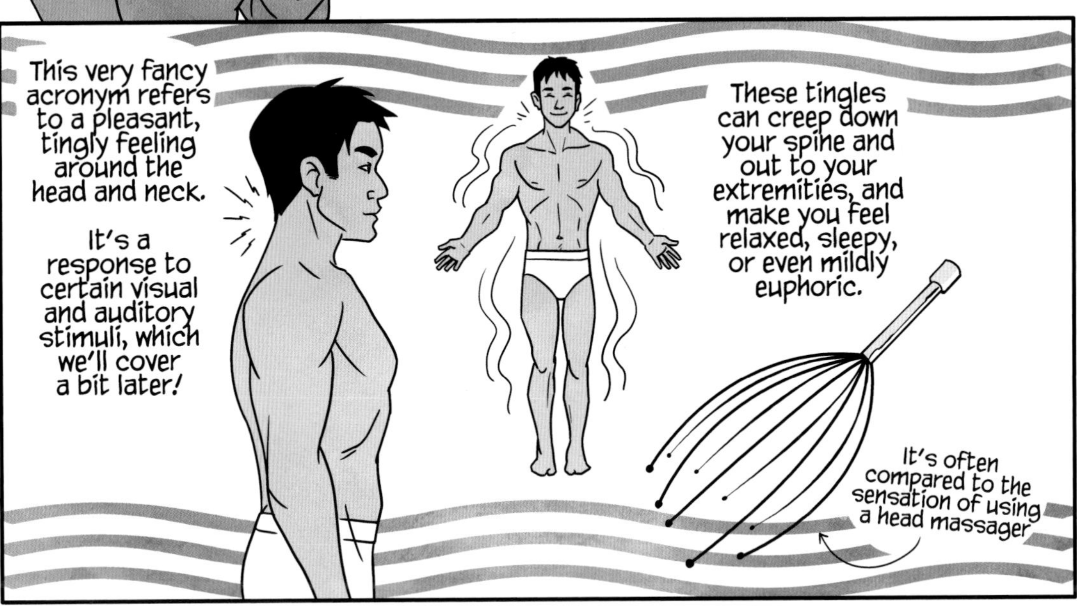
This very fancy acronym refers to a pleasant, tingly feeling around the head and neck.
It's a response to certain visual and auditory stimuli, which we'll cover a bit later!
These tingles can creep down your spine and out to your extremities, and make you feel relaxed, sleepy, or even mildly euphoric.
It's often compared to the sensation of using a head massager

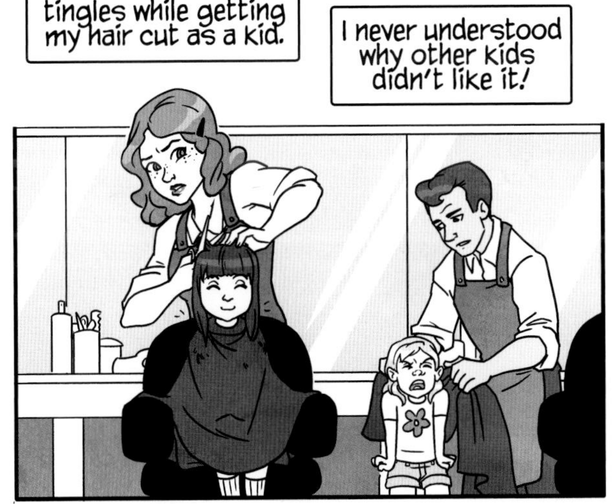
I first noticed ASMR tingles while getting my hair cut as a kid.
I never understood why other kids didn't like it!

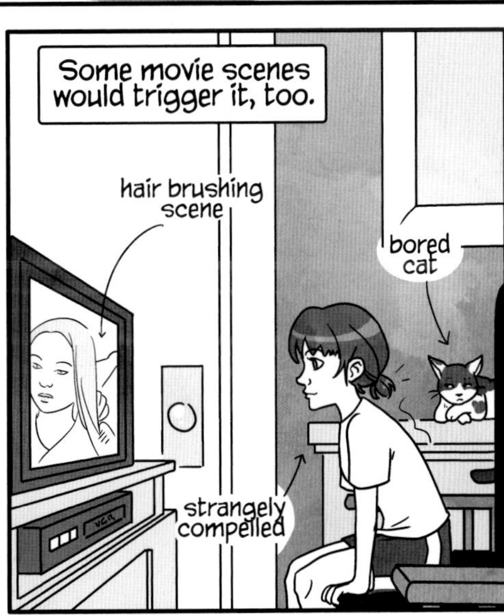
Some movie scenes would trigger it, too.
hair brushing scene
bored cat
strangely compelled
VCR

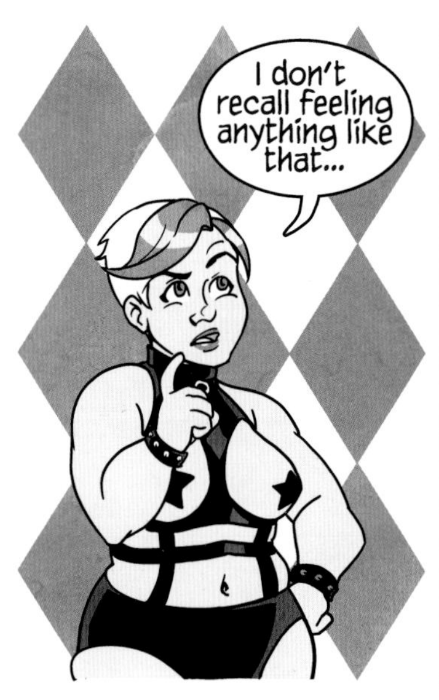
I don't recall feeling anything like that...

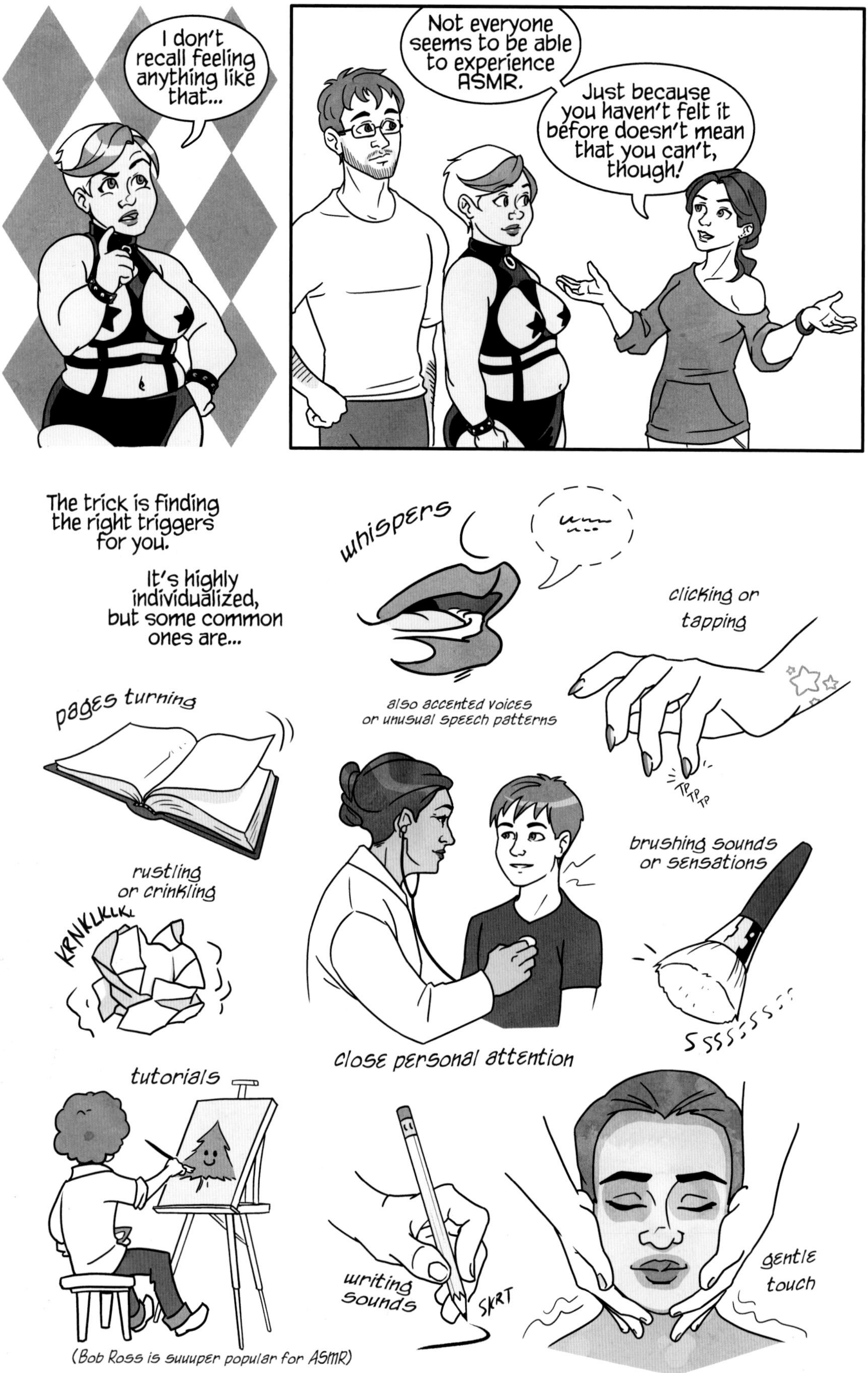

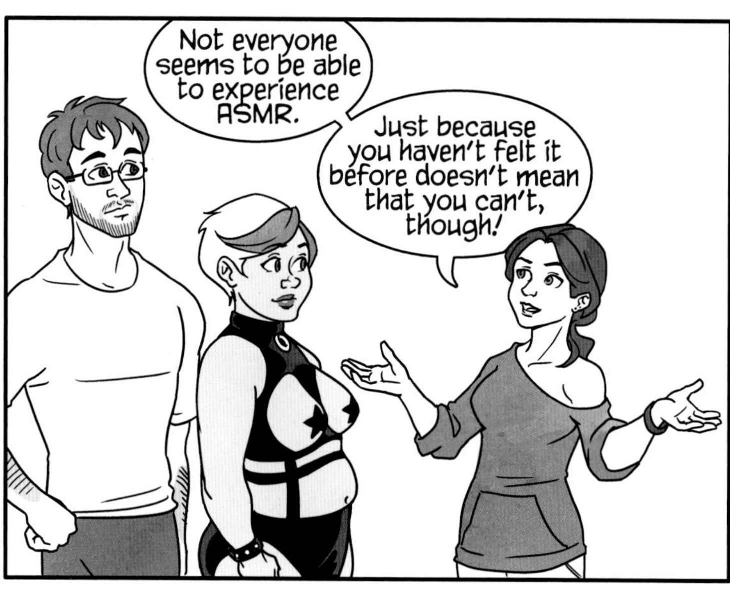
Not everyone seems to be able to experience ASMR.
Just because you haven't felt it before doesn't mean that you can't, though!

The trick is finding the right triggers for you.

It's highly individualized, but some common ones are...

whispers

also accented voices or unusual speech patterns

clicking or tapping

TP TP TP

pages turning

rustling or crinkling

KRNKLKLKL

brushing sounds or sensations

SSSSSSSS

close personal attention

tutorials

writing sounds

SKRT

gentle touch

(Bob Ross is suuuper popular for ASMR)

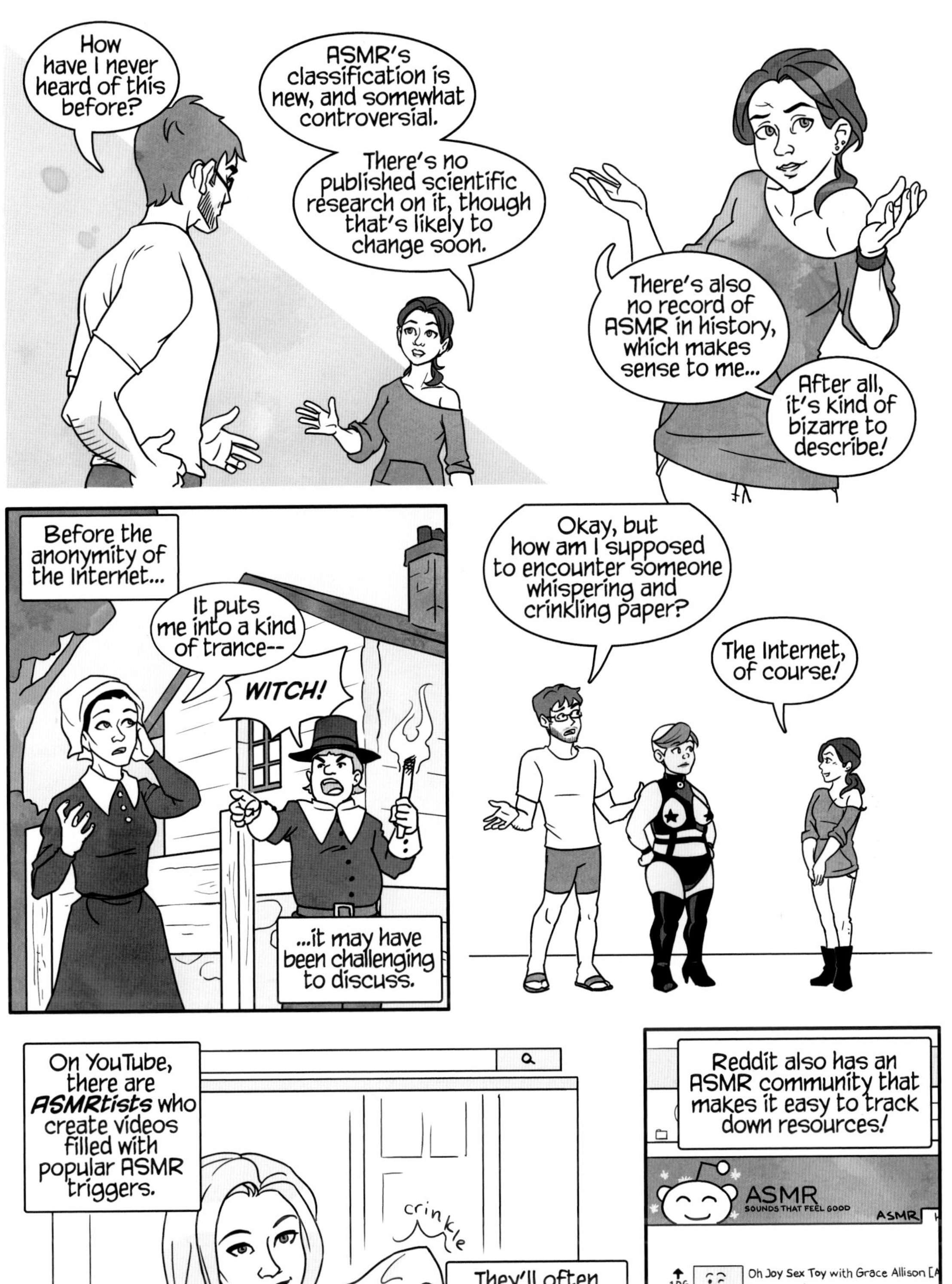
How have I never heard of this before?
ASMR's classification is new, and somewhat controversial.
There's no published scientific research on it, though that's likely to change soon.
There's also no record of ASMR in history, which makes sense to me...
After all, it's kind of bizarre to describe!
Before the anonymity of the Internet...
It puts me into a kind of trance--
WITCH!
...it may have been challenging to discuss.
Okay, but how am I supposed to encounter someone whispering and crinkling paper?
The Internet, of course!
On YouTube, there are ASMRtists who create videos filled with popular ASMR triggers.
crinkle
0:31 / 36:50
They'll often roleplay situations with close personal attention, and some use 3D (or binaural) microphones to make it more immersive.
Reddit also has an ASMR community that makes it easy to track down resources!
ASMR
SOUNDS THAT FEEL GOOD
Oh Joy Sex Toy with Grace Allison
(ohjoysextoy.com)
NSFW
ASMR Lotion Ear Massage [Ear to
Speaking][Massage][SoftlyRelax]
How to Drink Whisky with Richard
Accent] [Instructional] [Personal
Relaxing [Tapping] [Scratching]

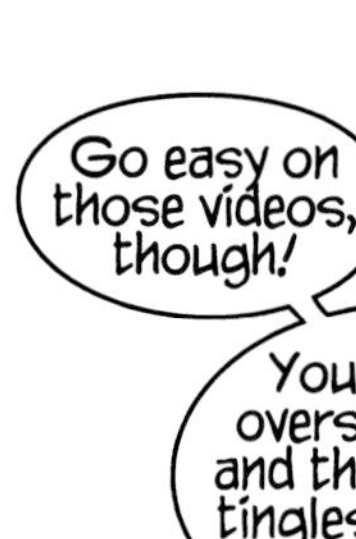

Go easy on those videos, though!

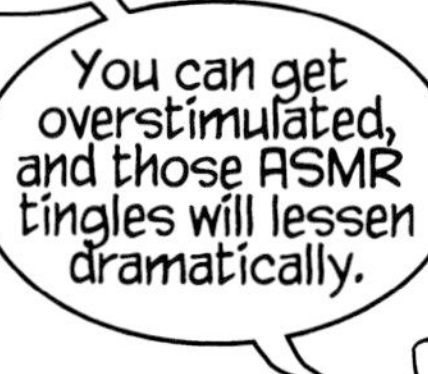

You can get overstimulated, and those ASMR tingles will lessen dramatically.

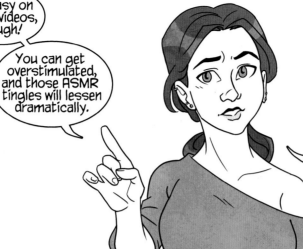

However, if you take a break for a few days, sensitivity will return.

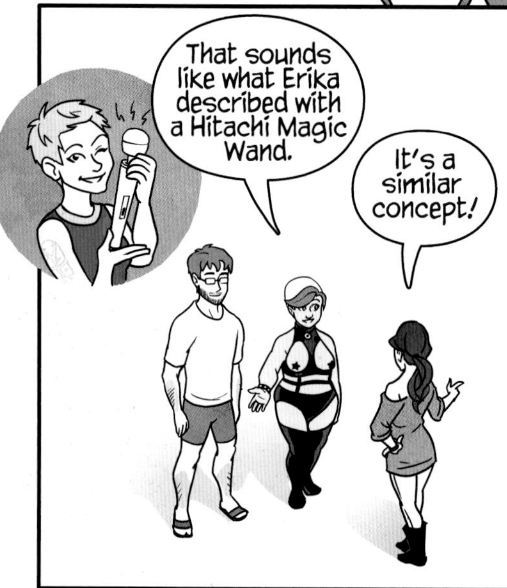

That sounds like what Erika described with a Hitachi Magic Wand.
It's a similar concept!

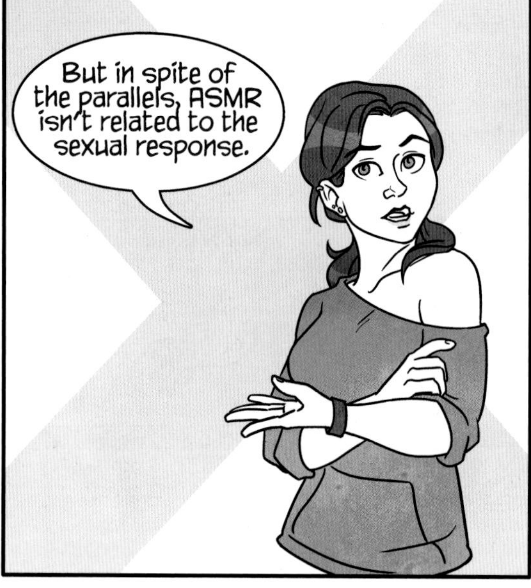

But in spite of the parallels, ASMR isn't related to the sexual response.

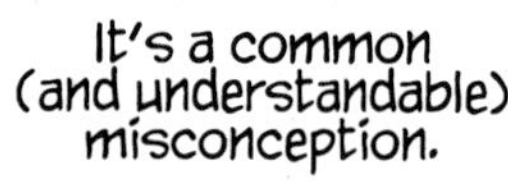

It's a common (and understandable) misconception.

ASMR is sensual experience, and the videos can seem very intimate. Plus, the sensation is often described as a ***braingasm.***

Still, for most ASMR-ers, sex takes them out of the right head space to enjoy those tingles!

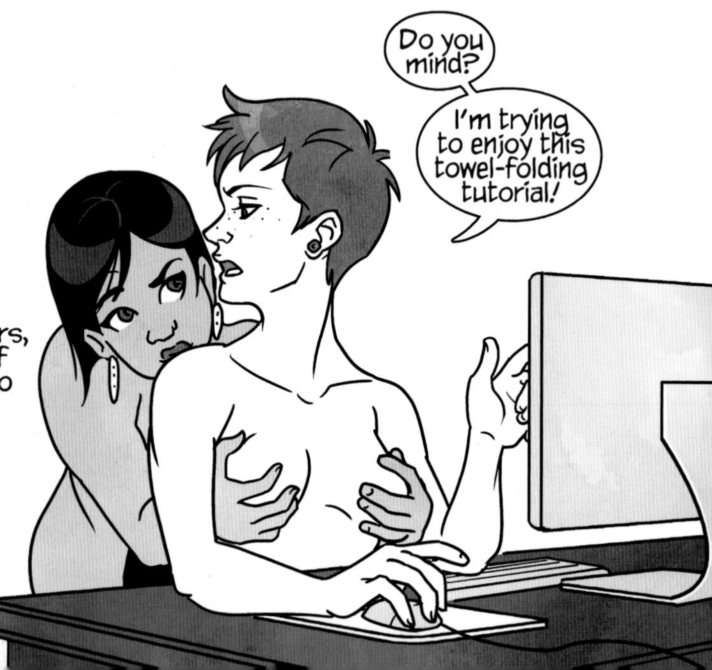

Do you mind?
I'm trying to enjoy this towel-folding tutorial!

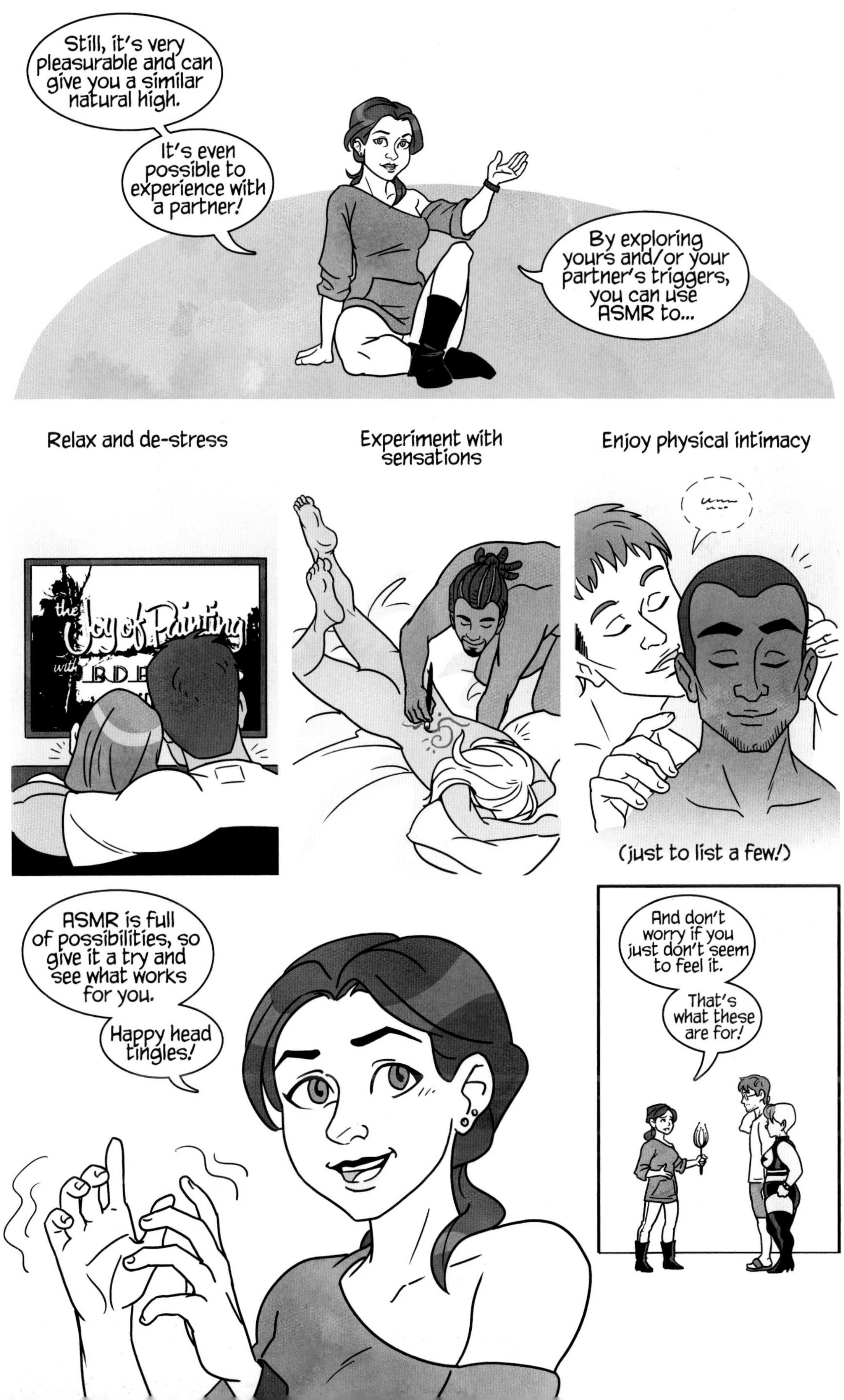

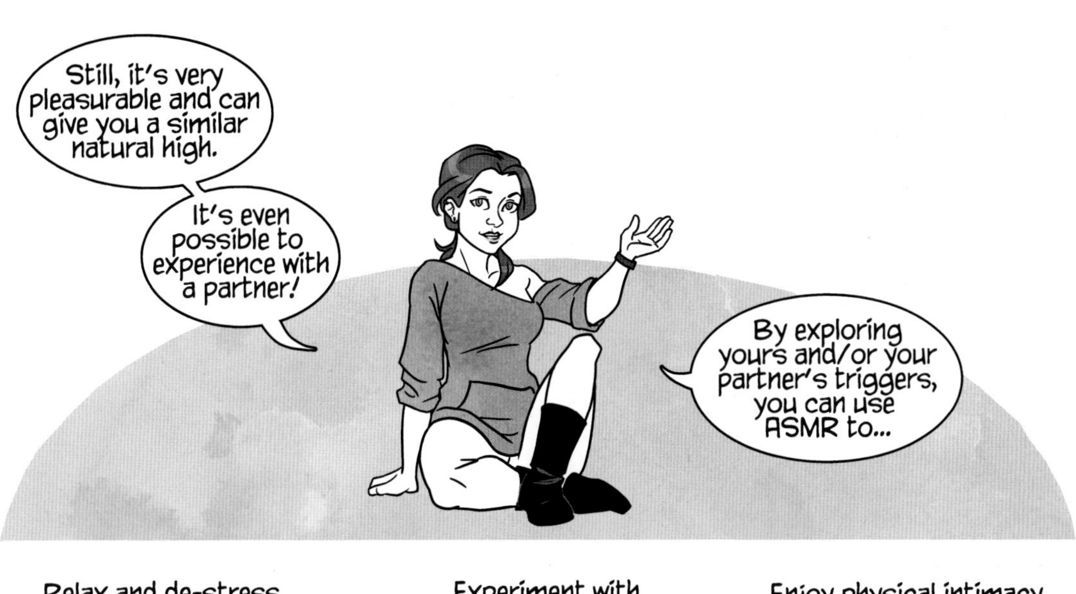
Still, it's very pleasurable and can give you a similar natural high.
It's even possible to experience with a partner!
By exploring yours and/or your partner's triggers, you can use ASMR to...

Relax and de-stress

Experiment with sensations

Enjoy physical intimacy

(just to list a few!)

ASMR is full of possibilities, so give it a try and see what works for you.

Happy head tingles!

And don't worry if you just don't seem to feel it.

That's what these are for!

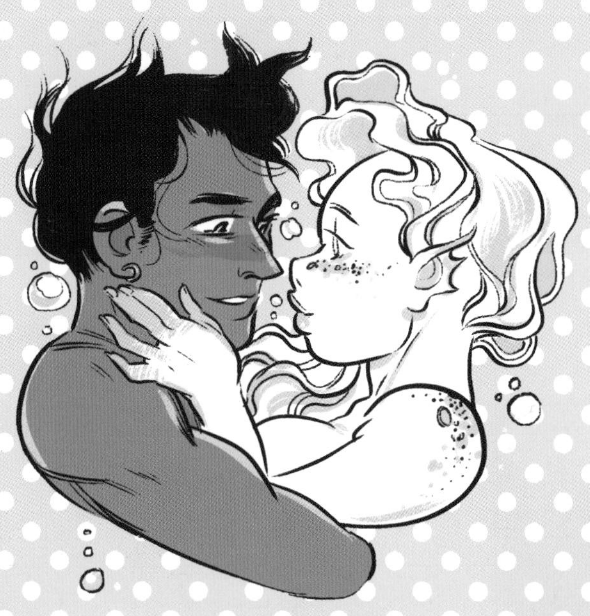

MERMAID

by Ghostgreen

ghostgreen.tumblr.com

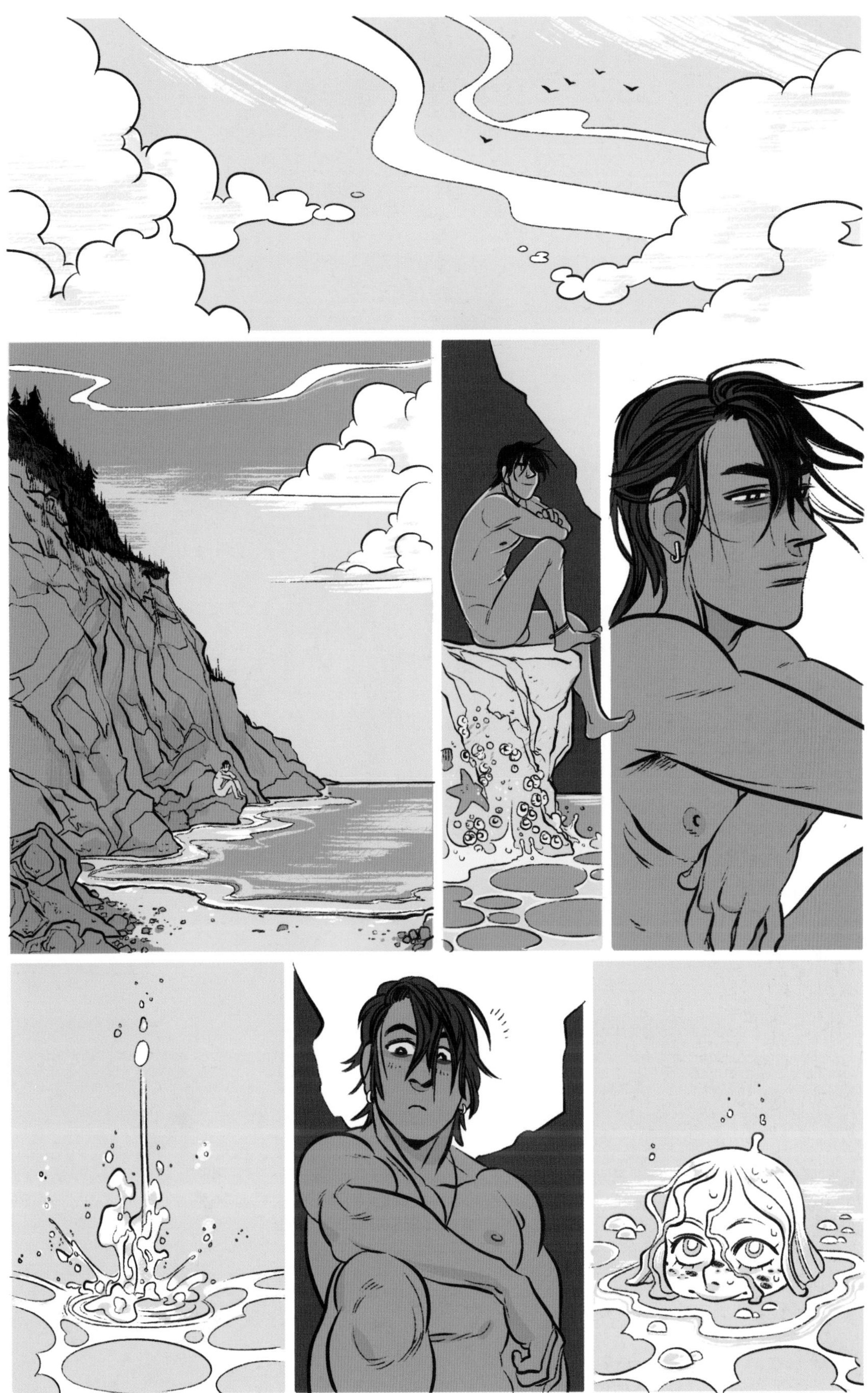

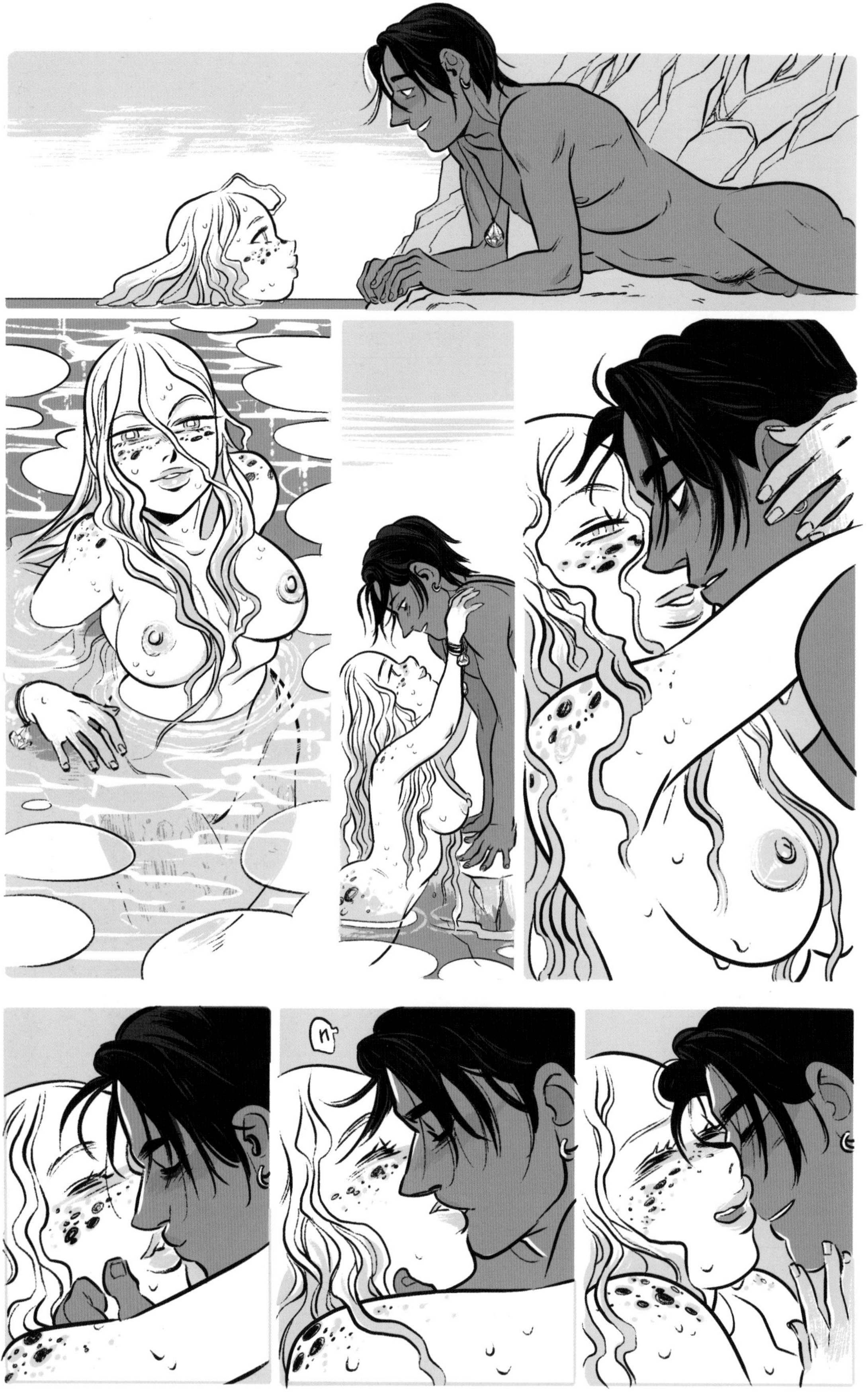
n

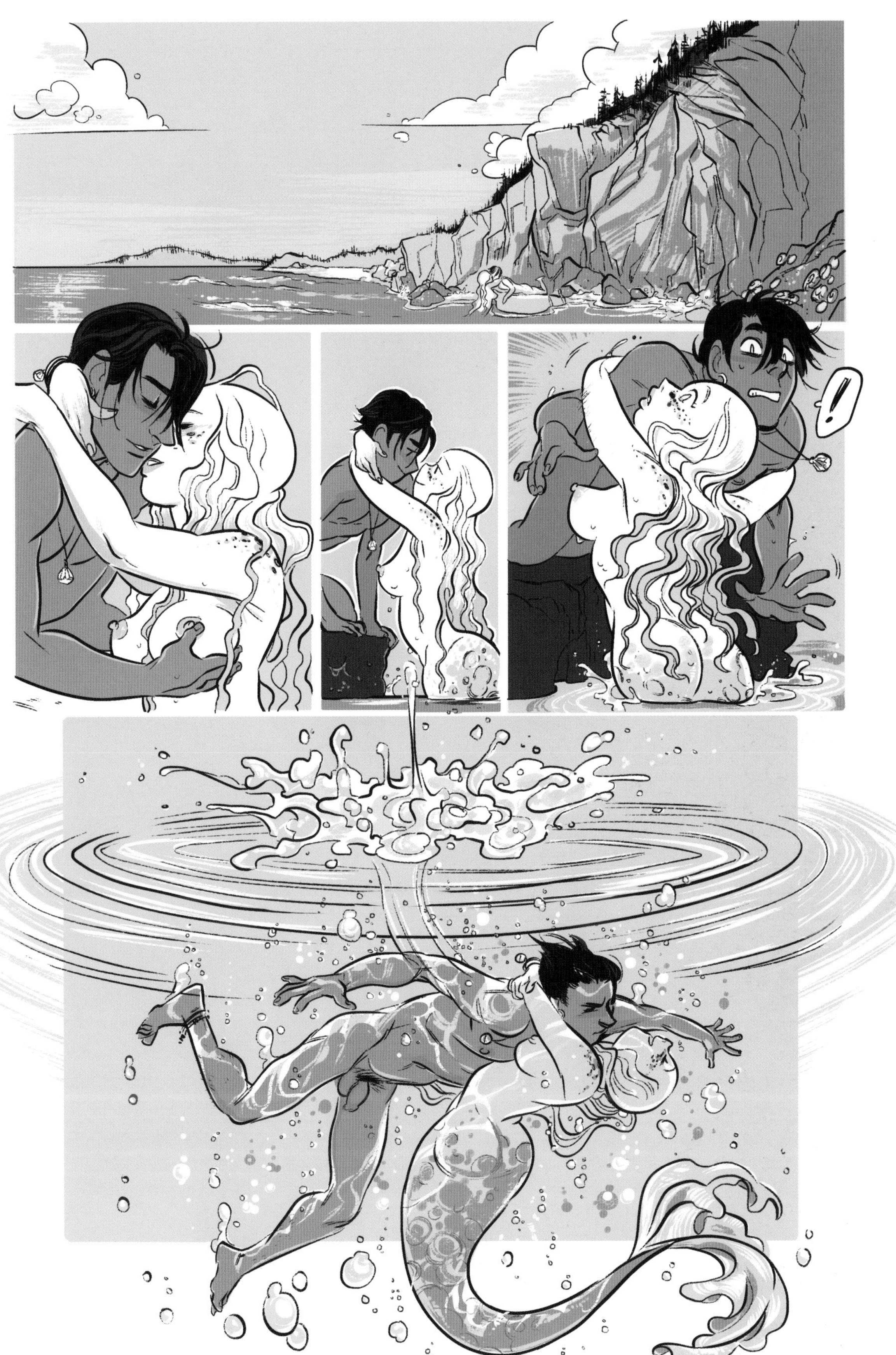

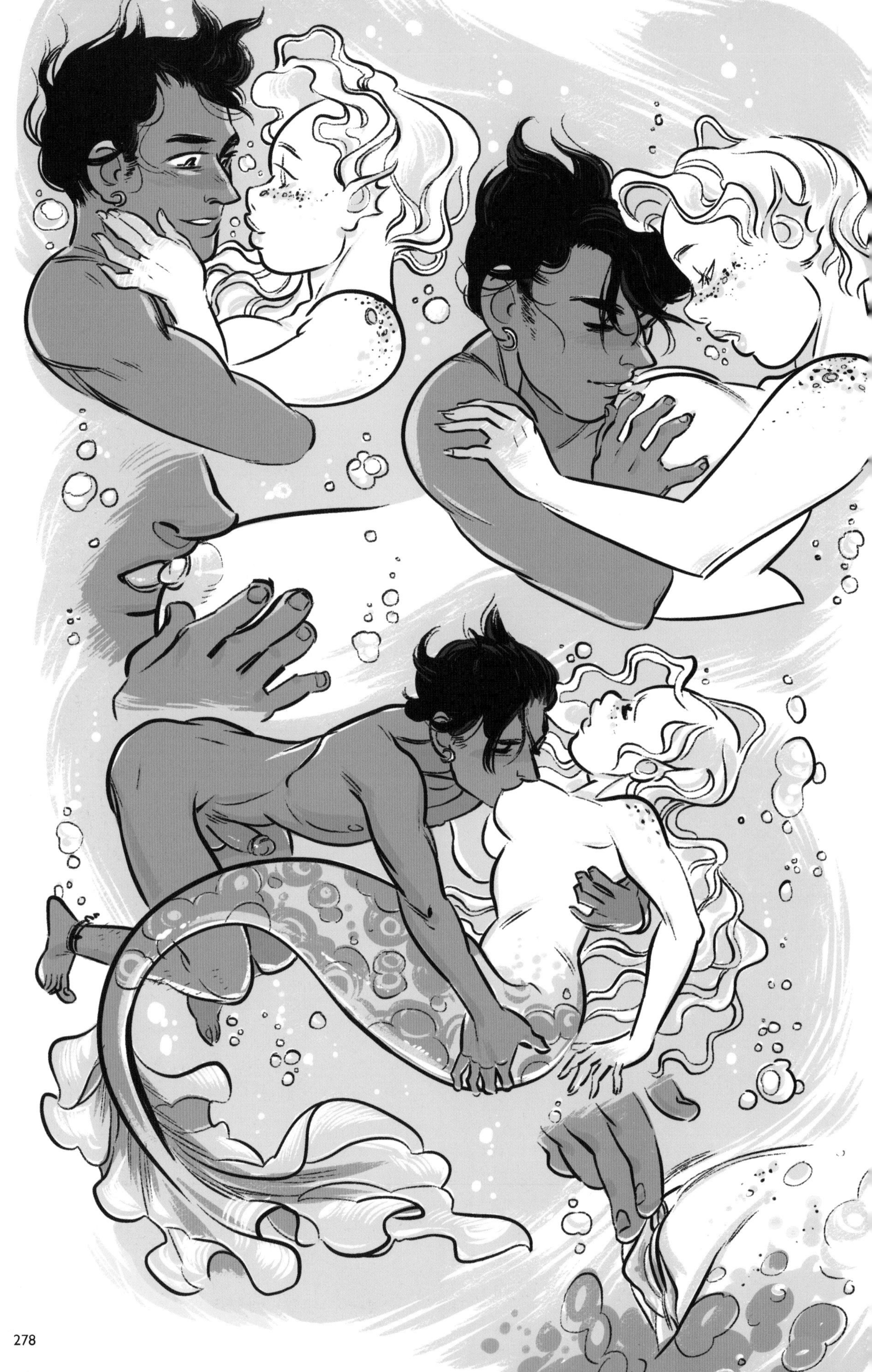

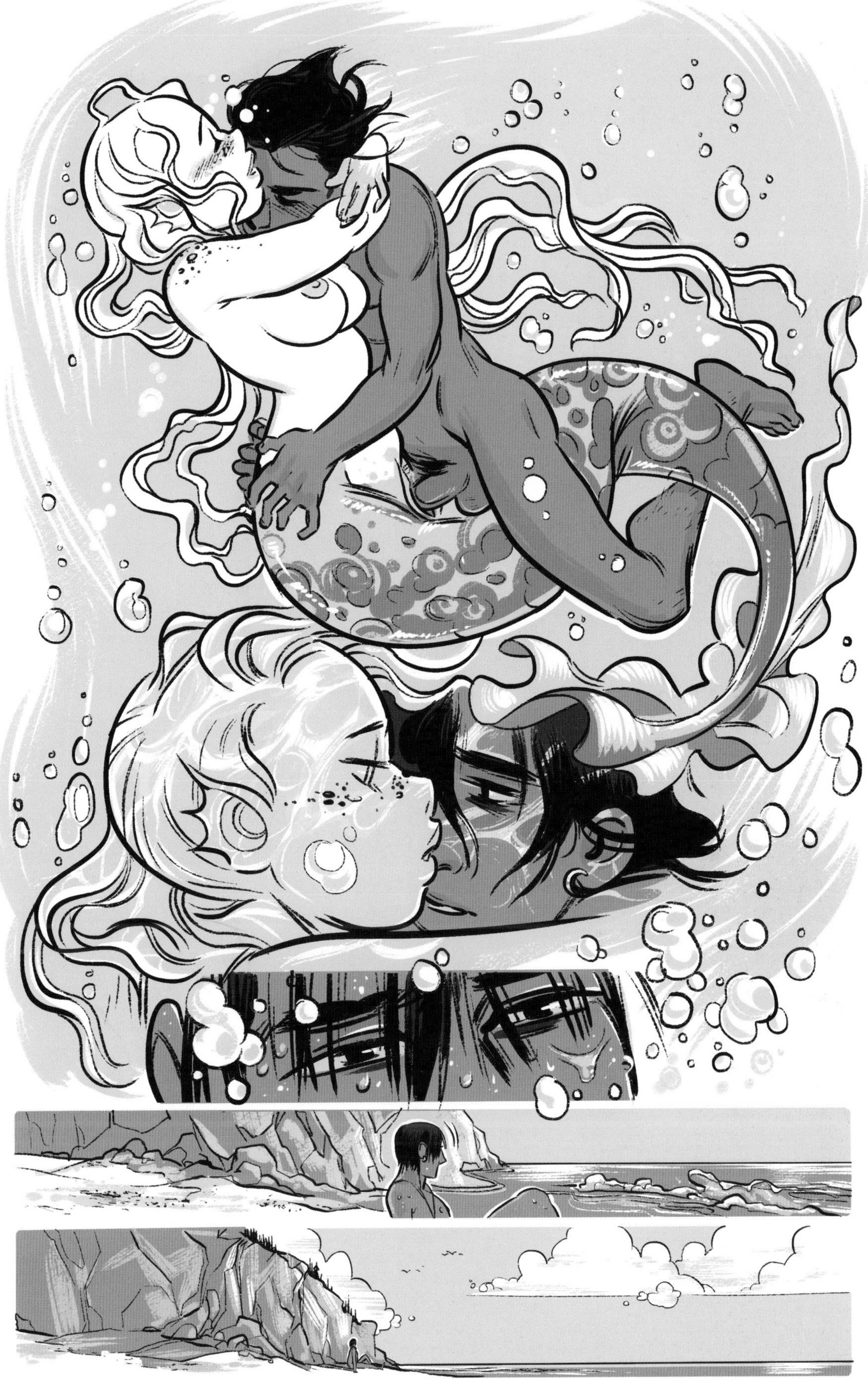

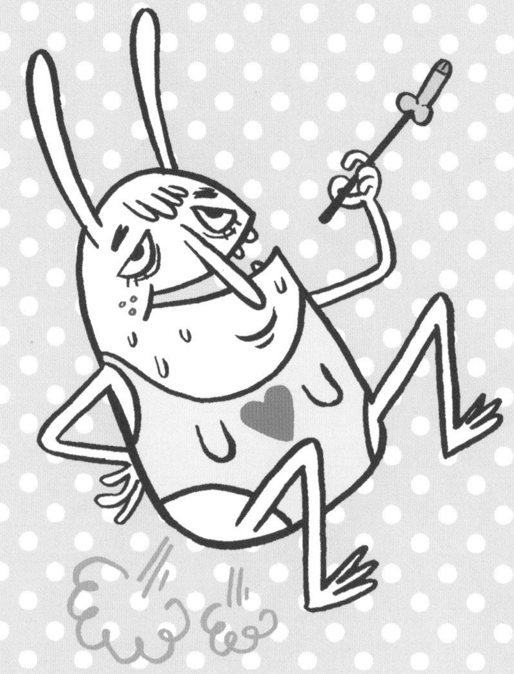

GENDERPLAY

by Mady G

madygcomics.tumblr.com

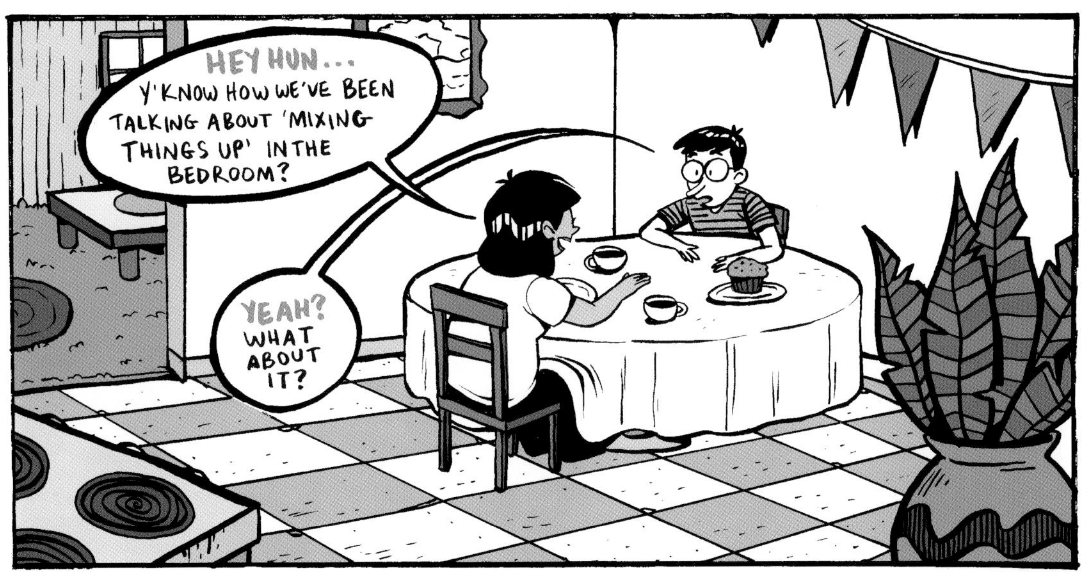
HEY HUN...
Y'KNOW HOW WE'VE BEEN TALKING ABOUT 'MIXING THINGS UP' IN THE BEDROOM?
YEAH? WHAT ABOUT IT?

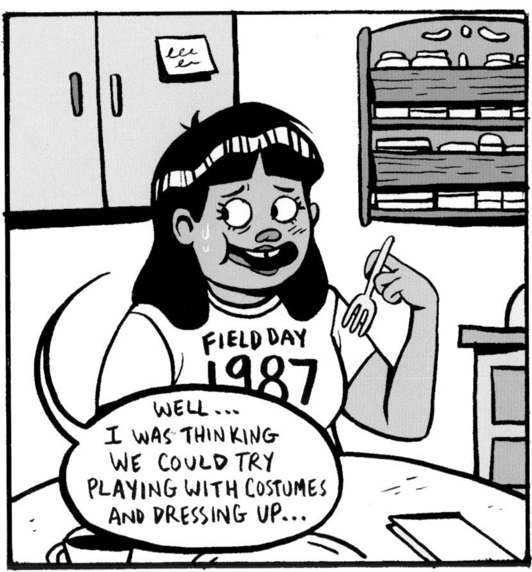
FIELD DAY 1987
WELL... I WAS THINKING WE COULD TRY PLAYING WITH COSTUMES AND DRESSING UP...

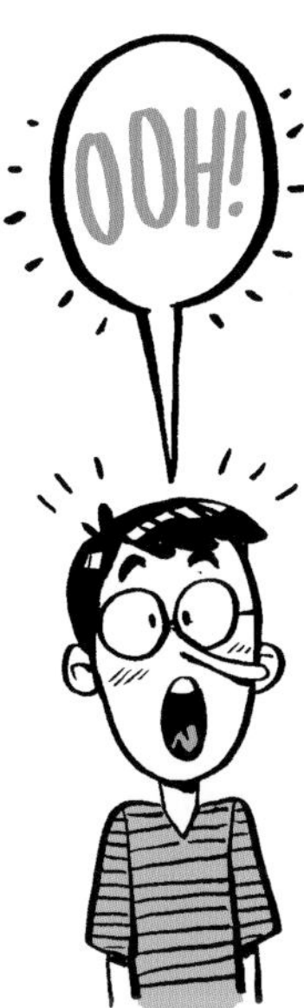
OOH!

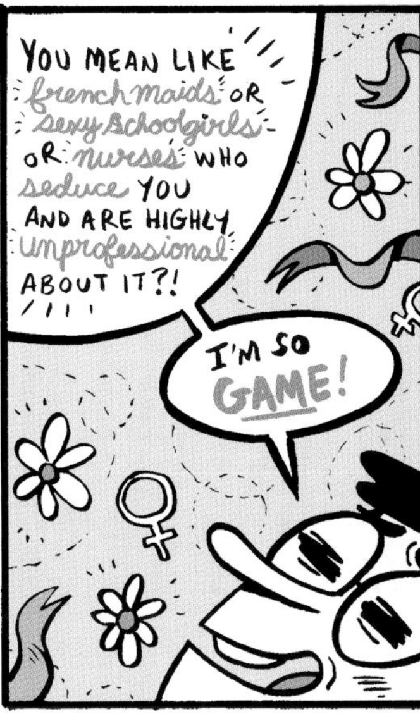
YOU MEAN LIKE french maids OR sexy schoolgirls OR nurses WHO seduce YOU AND ARE HIGHLY unprofessional ABOUT IT?!
I'M SO GAME!

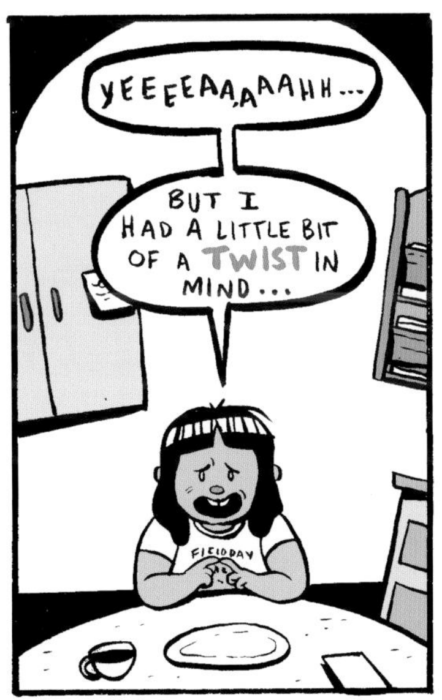
YEEEEAAAAAHH...
BUT I HAD A LITTLE BIT OF A TWIST IN MIND...

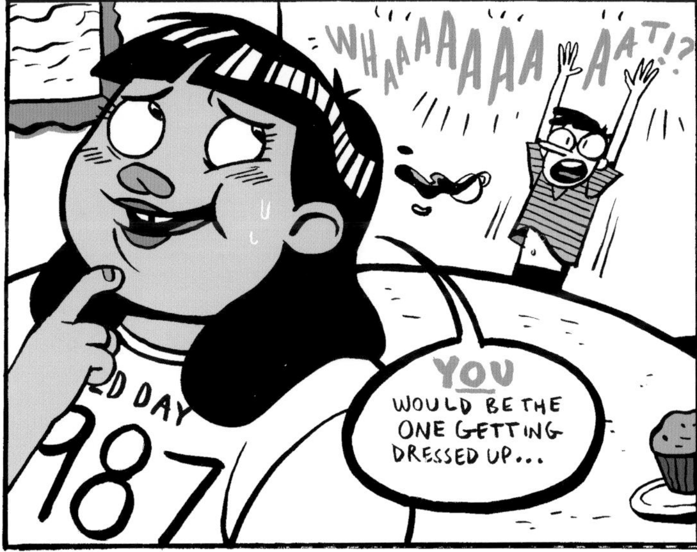
WHAAAAAAAAT!?
YOU WOULD BE THE ONE GETTING DRESSED UP...

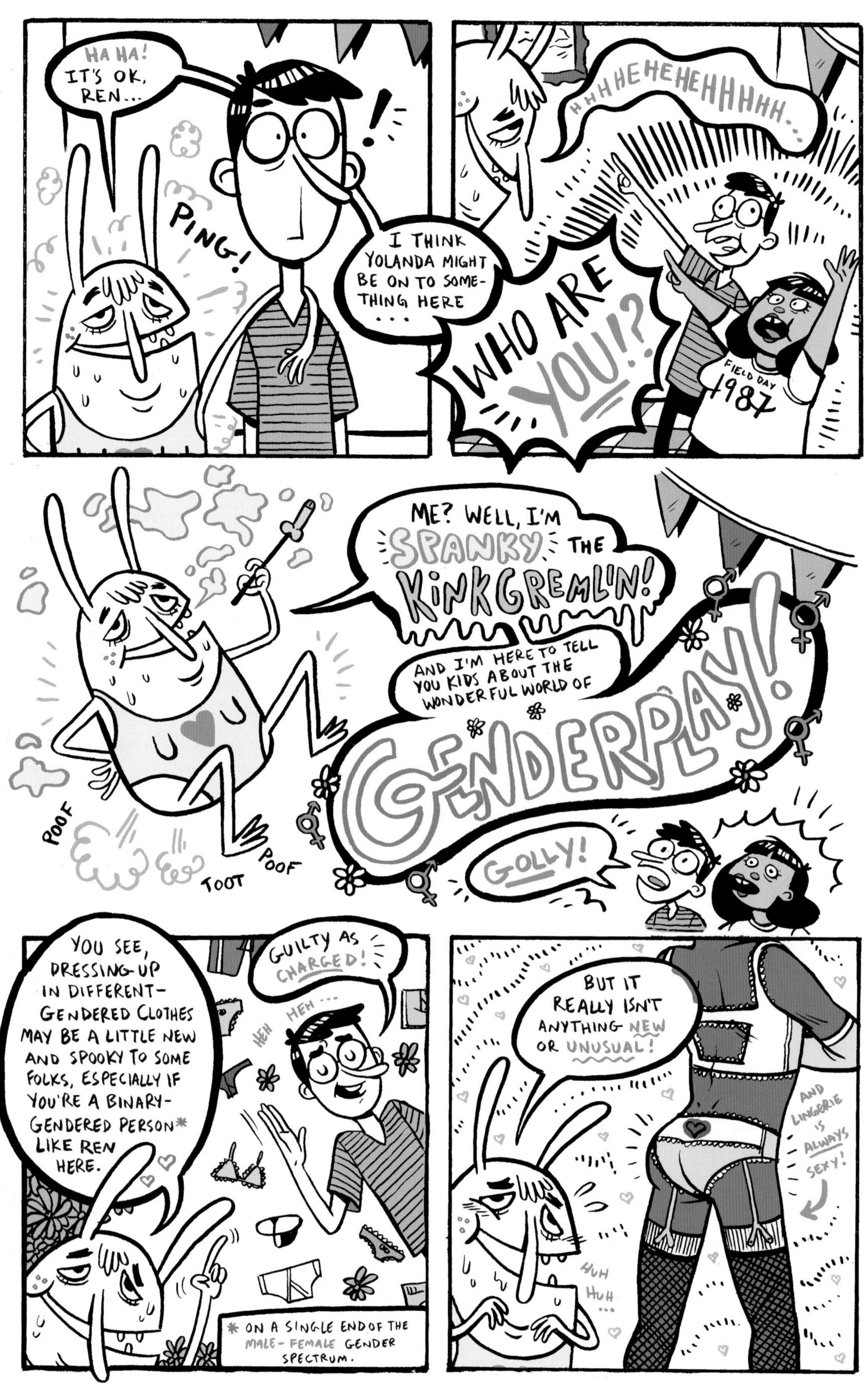
HA HA! IT'S OK, REN...
!
PING!
I THINK YOLANDA MIGHT BE ON TO SOMETHING HERE . . .
HHHHEHEHEHHHHHH...
WHO ARE YOU!?
FIELD DAY 1987
ME? WELL, I'M SPANKY THE KINKGREMLIN!
AND I'M HERE TO TELL YOU KIDS ABOUT THE WONDERFUL WORLD OF
GENDERPLAY!
POOF
TOOT
POOF
GOLLY!
YOU SEE, DRESSING-UP IN DIFFERENT-GENDERED CLOTHES MAY BE A LITTLE NEW AND SPOOKY TO SOME FOLKS, ESPECIALLY IF YOU'RE A BINARY-GENDERED PERSON* LIKE REN HERE.
GUILTY AS CHARGED!
HEH HEH...
* ON A SINGLE END OF THE MALE-FEMALE GENDER SPECTRUM.
BUT IT REALLY ISN'T ANYTHING NEW OR UNUSUAL!
AND LINGERIE IS ALWAYS SEXY!
HUH HUH...

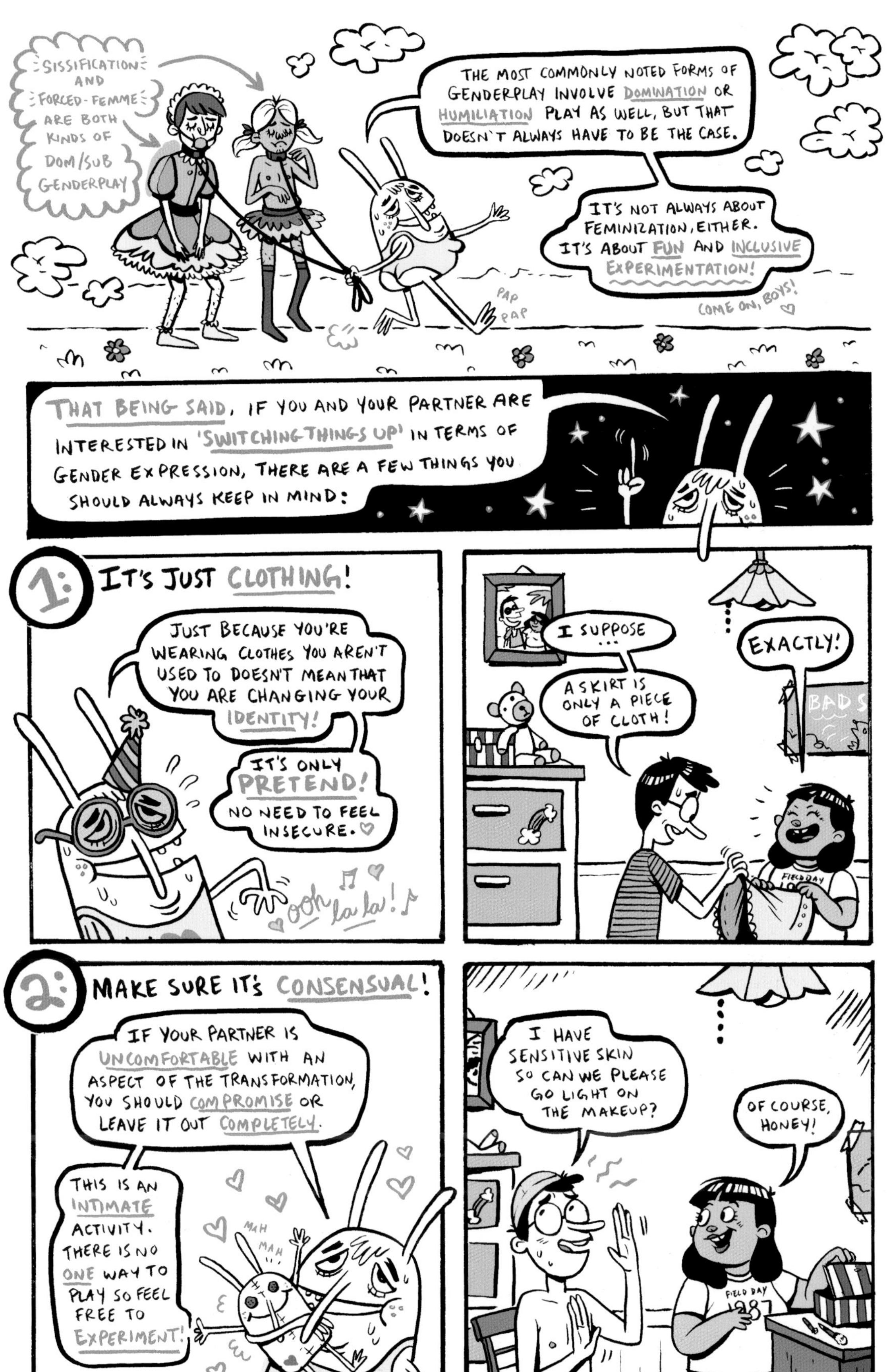
SISSIFICATION AND FORCED-FEMME ARE BOTH KINDS OF DOM/SUB GENDERPLAY
THE MOST COMMONLY NOTED FORMS OF GENDERPLAY INVOLVE DOMINATION OR HUMILIATION PLAY AS WELL, BUT THAT DOESN'T ALWAYS HAVE TO BE THE CASE.
IT'S NOT ALWAYS ABOUT FEMINIZATION, EITHER. IT'S ABOUT FUN AND INCLUSIVE EXPERIMENTATION!
PAP PAP
COME ON, BOYS!
THAT BEING SAID, IF YOU AND YOUR PARTNER ARE INTERESTED IN 'SWITCHING THINGS UP' IN TERMS OF GENDER EXPRESSION, THERE ARE A FEW THINGS YOU SHOULD ALWAYS KEEP IN MIND:
1: IT'S JUST CLOTHING!
JUST BECAUSE YOU'RE WEARING CLOTHES YOU AREN'T USED TO DOESN'T MEAN THAT YOU ARE CHANGING YOUR IDENTITY!
IT'S ONLY PRETEND! NO NEED TO FEEL INSECURE.
ooh la la!
I SUPPOSE...
A SKIRT IS ONLY A PIECE OF CLOTH!
EXACTLY!
FIELD DAY
2: MAKE SURE IT'S CONSENSUAL!
IF YOUR PARTNER IS UNCOMFORTABLE WITH AN ASPECT OF THE TRANSFORMATION, YOU SHOULD COMPROMISE OR LEAVE IT OUT COMPLETELY.
THIS IS AN INTIMATE ACTIVITY. THERE IS NO ONE WAY TO PLAY SO FEEL FREE TO EXPERIMENT!
MAH MAH
I HAVE SENSITIVE SKIN SO CAN WE PLEASE GO LIGHT ON THE MAKEUP?
OF COURSE, HONEY!
FIELD DAY 1987

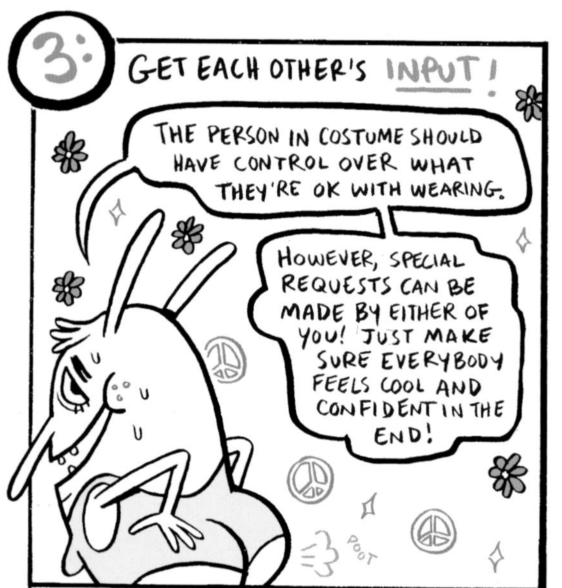
3:
GET EACH OTHER'S INPUT!
THE PERSON IN COSTUME SHOULD HAVE CONTROL OVER WHAT THEY'RE OK WITH WEARING.
HOWEVER, SPECIAL REQUESTS CAN BE MADE BY EITHER OF YOU! JUST MAKE SURE EVERYBODY FEELS COOL AND CONFIDENT IN THE END!
POOT

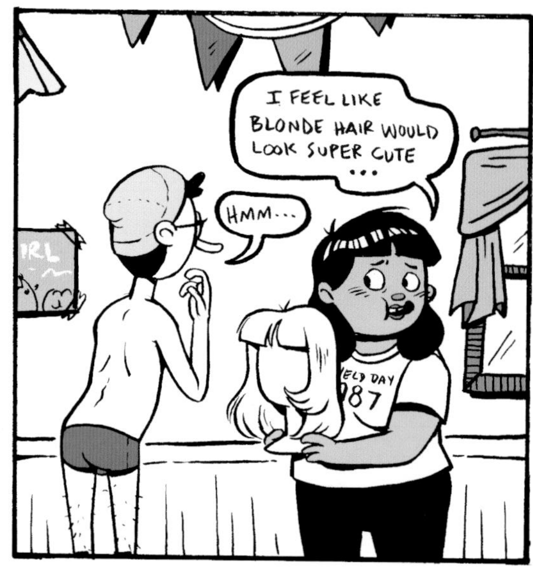
I FEEL LIKE BLONDE HAIR WOULD LOOK SUPER CUTE ...
HMM...

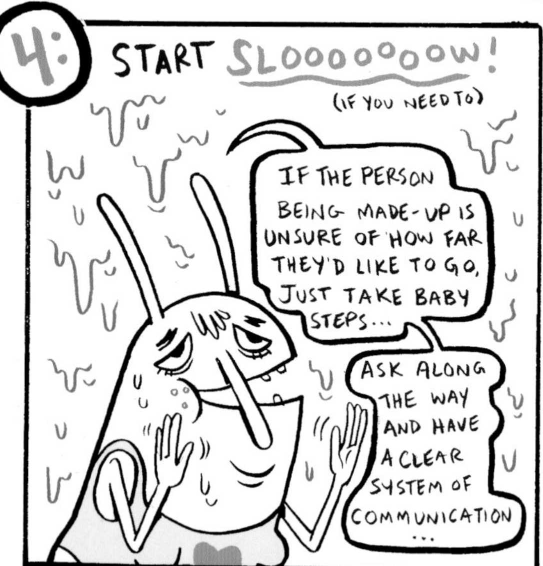
4:
START SLOOOOOOOW!
(IF YOU NEED TO)
IF THE PERSON BEING MADE-UP IS UNSURE OF HOW FAR THEY'D LIKE TO GO, JUST TAKE BABY STEPS...
ASK ALONG THE WAY AND HAVE A CLEAR SYSTEM OF COMMUNICATION ...

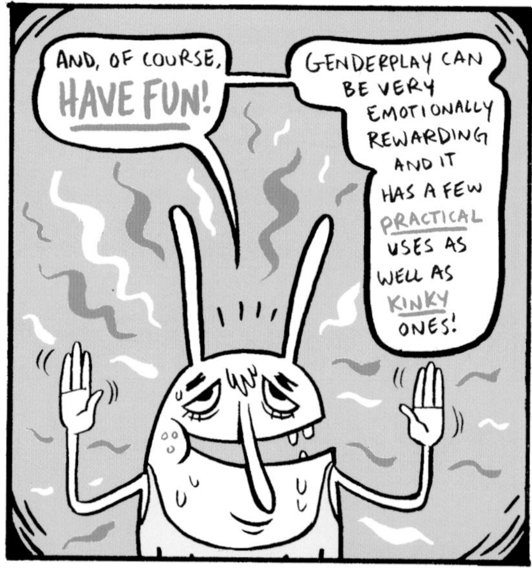
AND, OF COURSE, HAVE FUN!
GENDERPLAY CAN BE VERY EMOTIONALLY REWARDING AND IT HAS A FEW PRACTICAL USES AS WELL AS KINKY ONES!

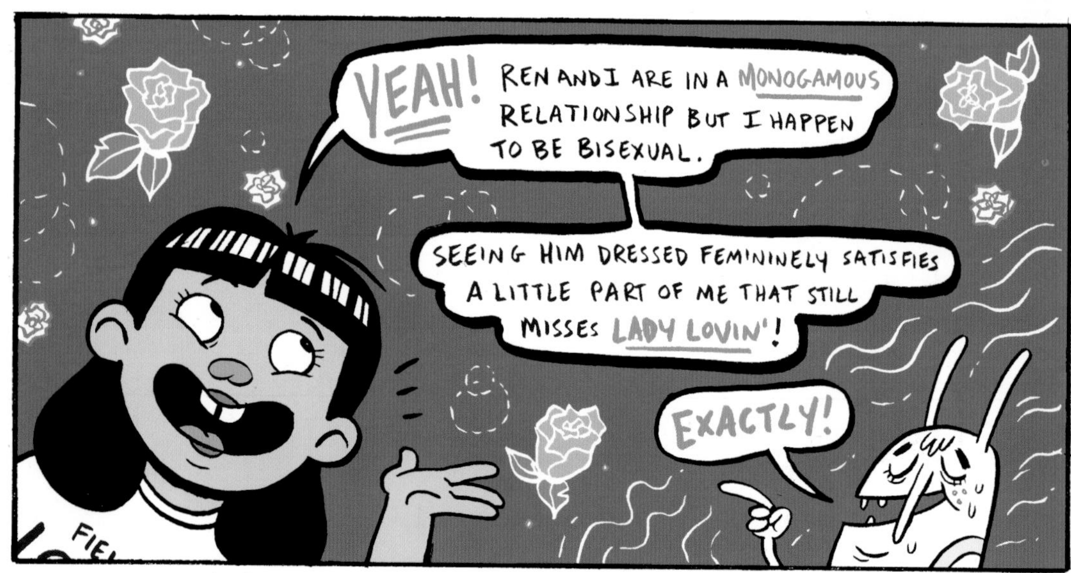
YEAH! REN AND I ARE IN A MONOGAMOUS RELATIONSHIP BUT I HAPPEN TO BE BISEXUAL.
SEEING HIM DRESSED FEMININELY SATISFIES A LITTLE PART OF ME THAT STILL MISSES LADY LOVIN'!
EXACTLY!

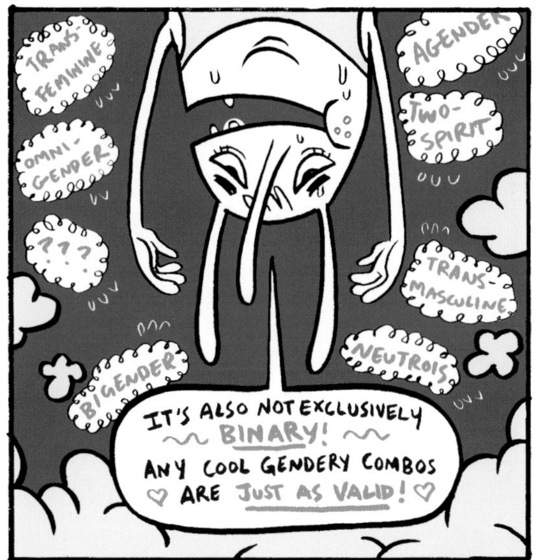
TRANS-FEMININE
AGENDER
TWO-SPIRIT
OMNI-GENDER
???
TRANS-MASCULINE
BIGENDER
NEUTROIS
IT'S ALSO NOT EXCLUSIVELY BINARY! ANY COOL GENDERY COMBOS ARE JUST AS VALID!

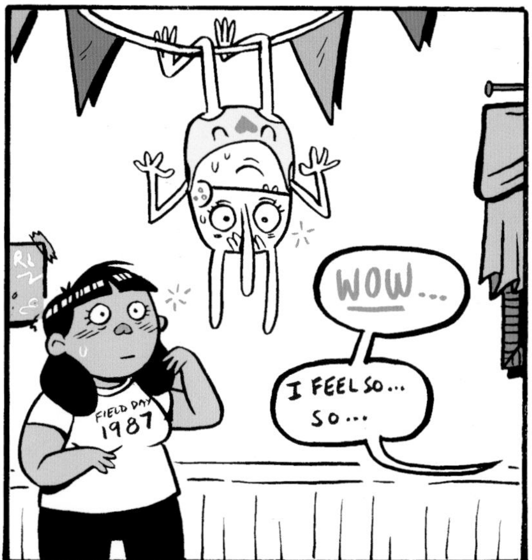
FIELD DAY 1987
WOW...
I FEEL SO... SO...

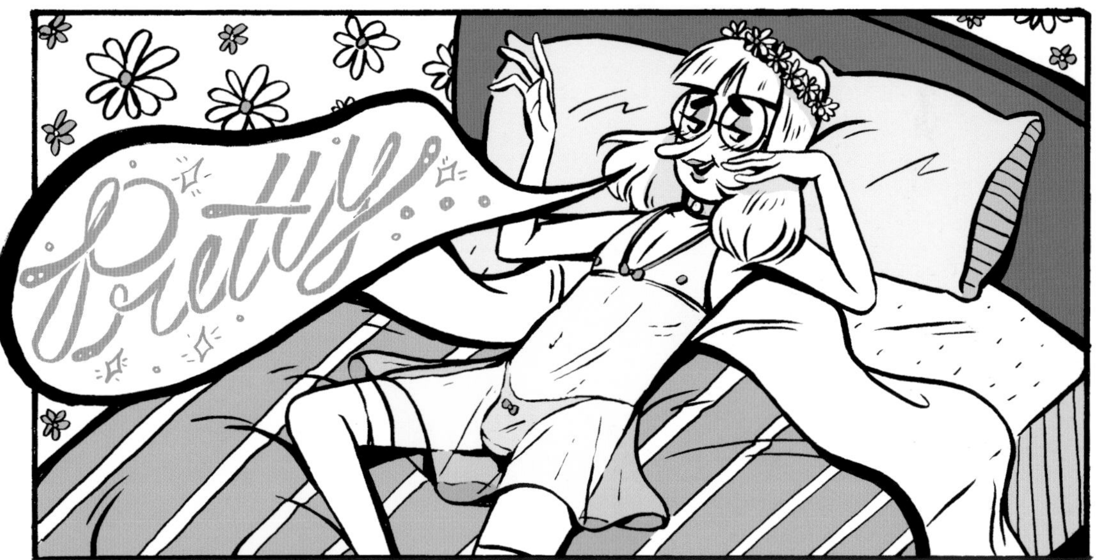
Pretty

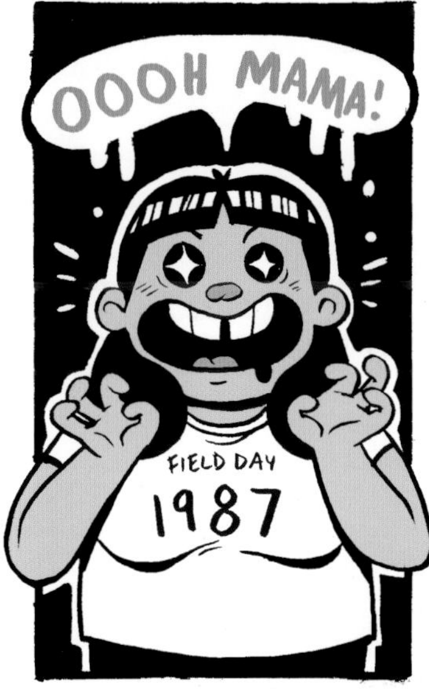
OOOH MAMA!
FIELD DAY 1987

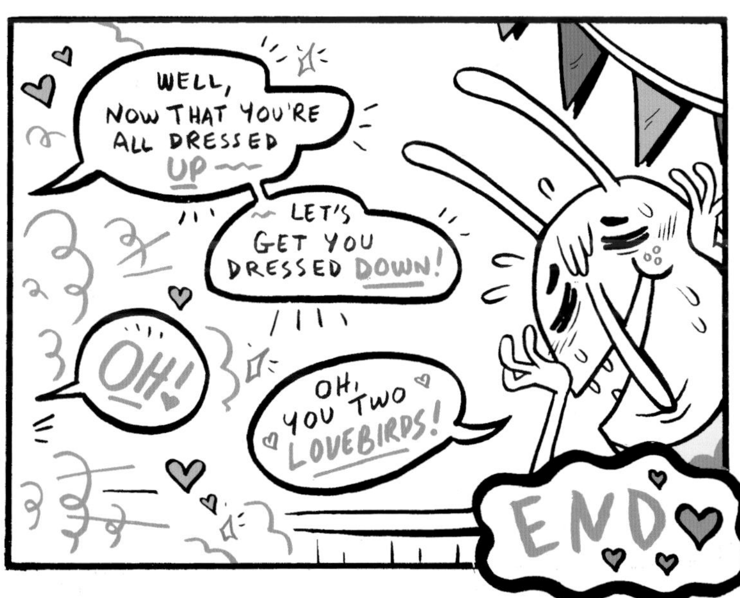
WELL, NOW THAT YOU'RE ALL DRESSED UP
LET'S GET YOU DRESSED DOWN!
OH!
OH, YOU TWO LOVEBIRDS!
END

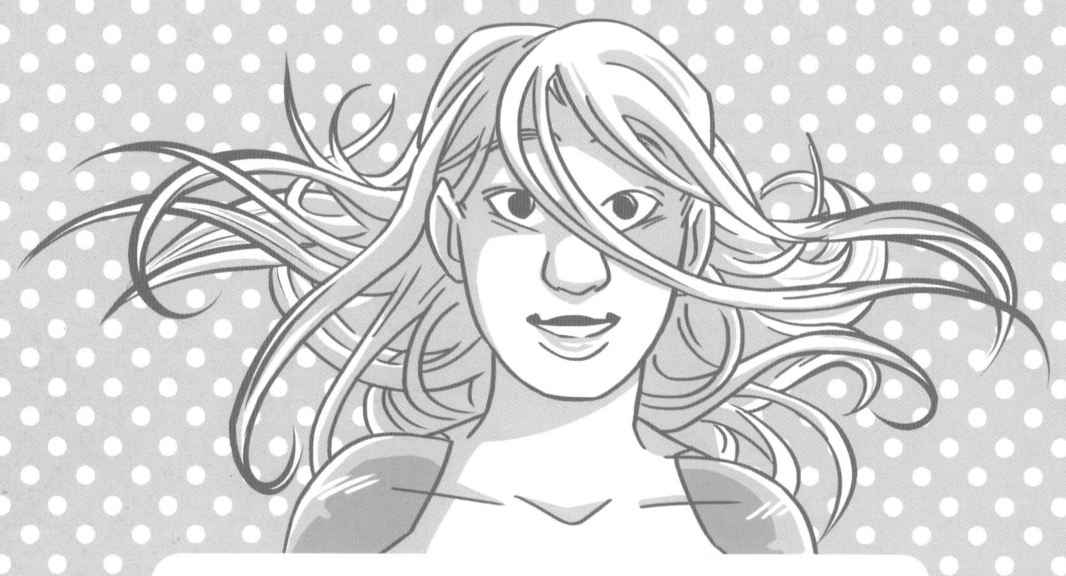

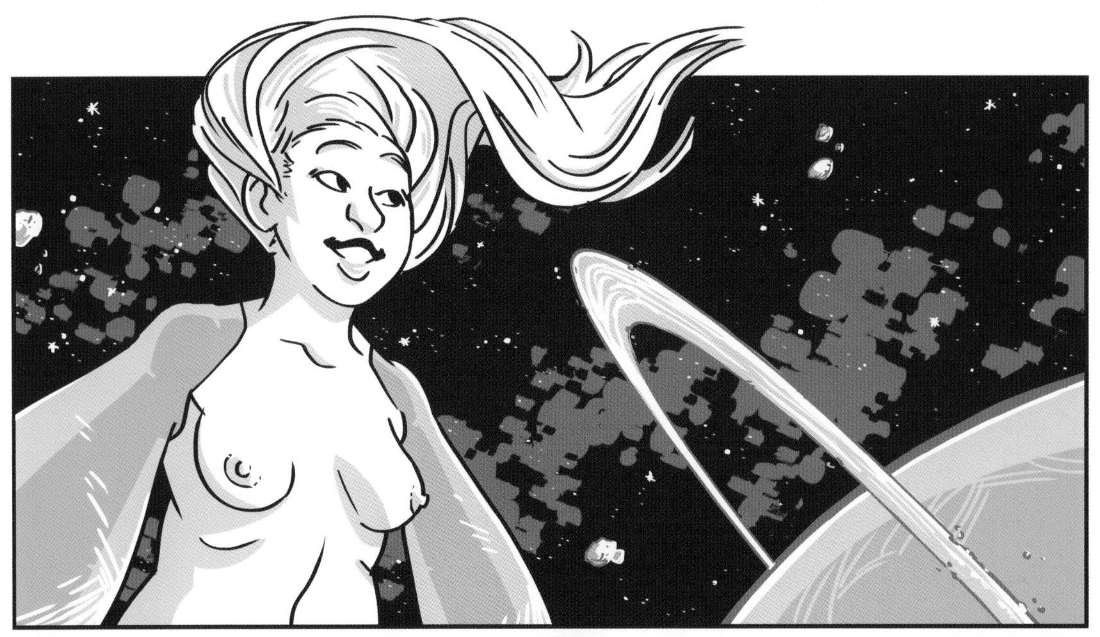
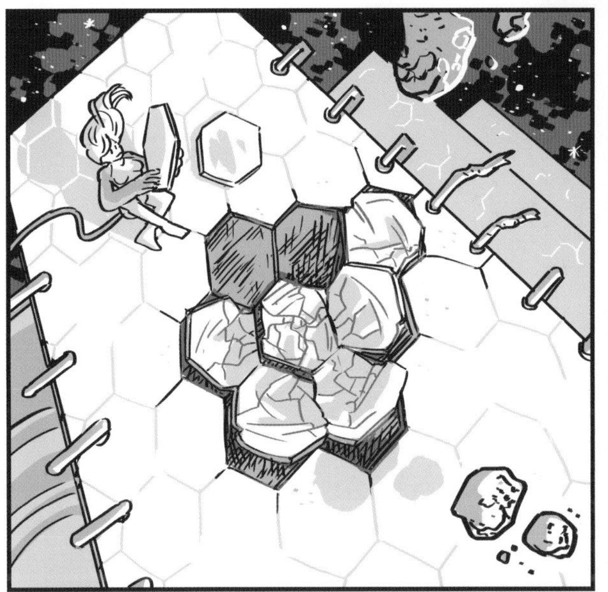
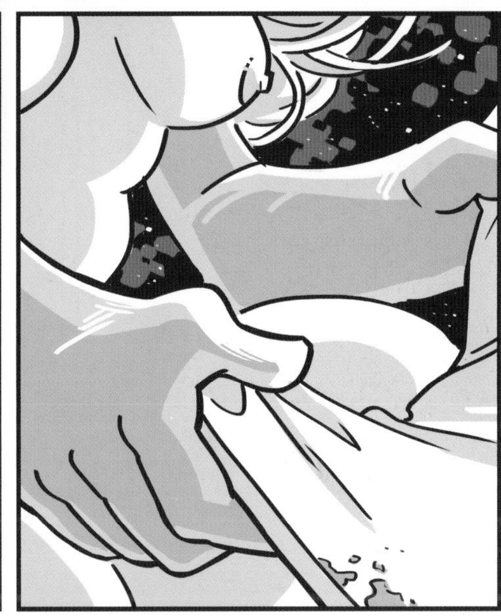
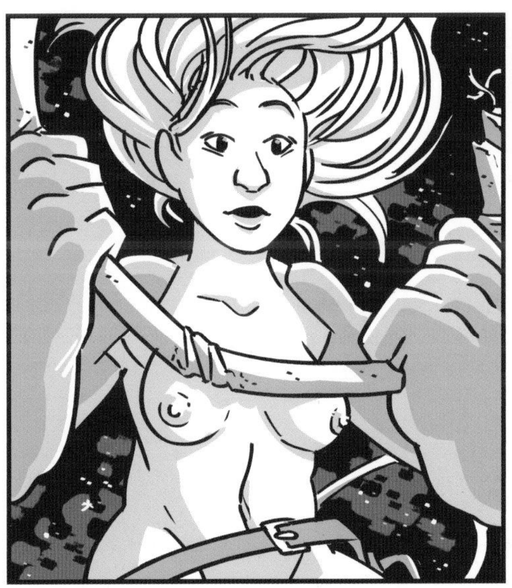
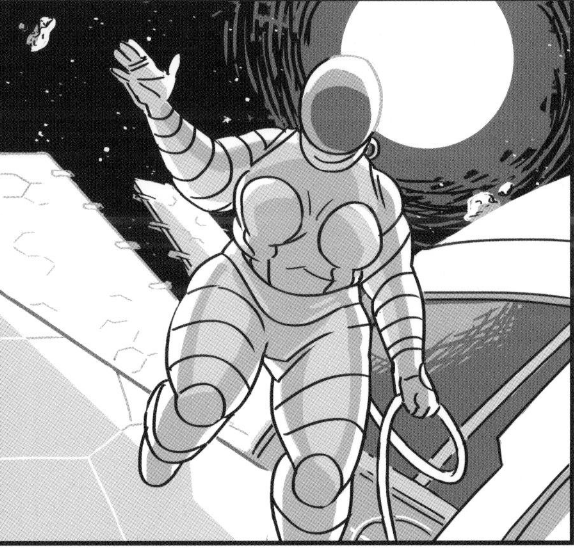

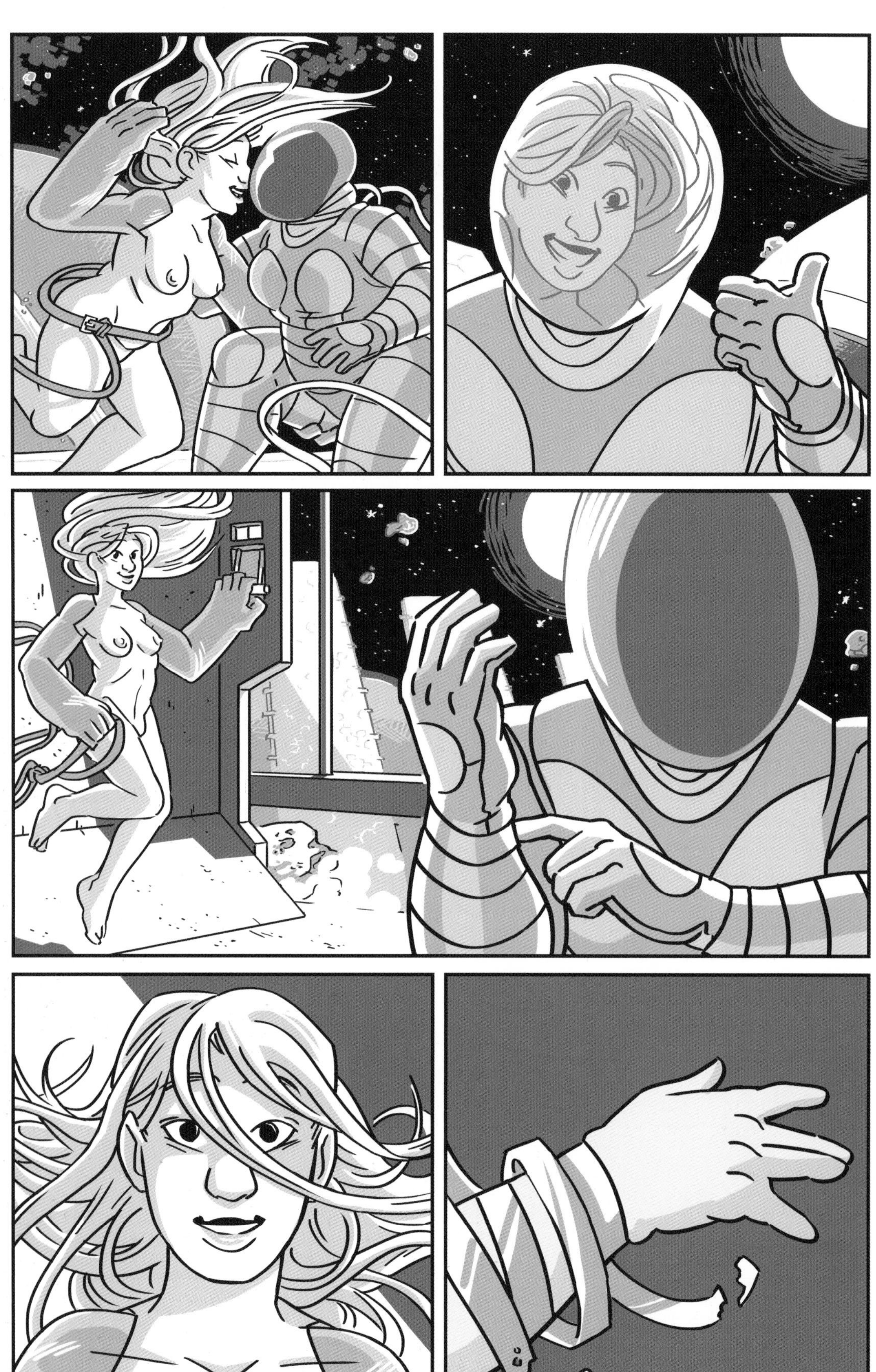

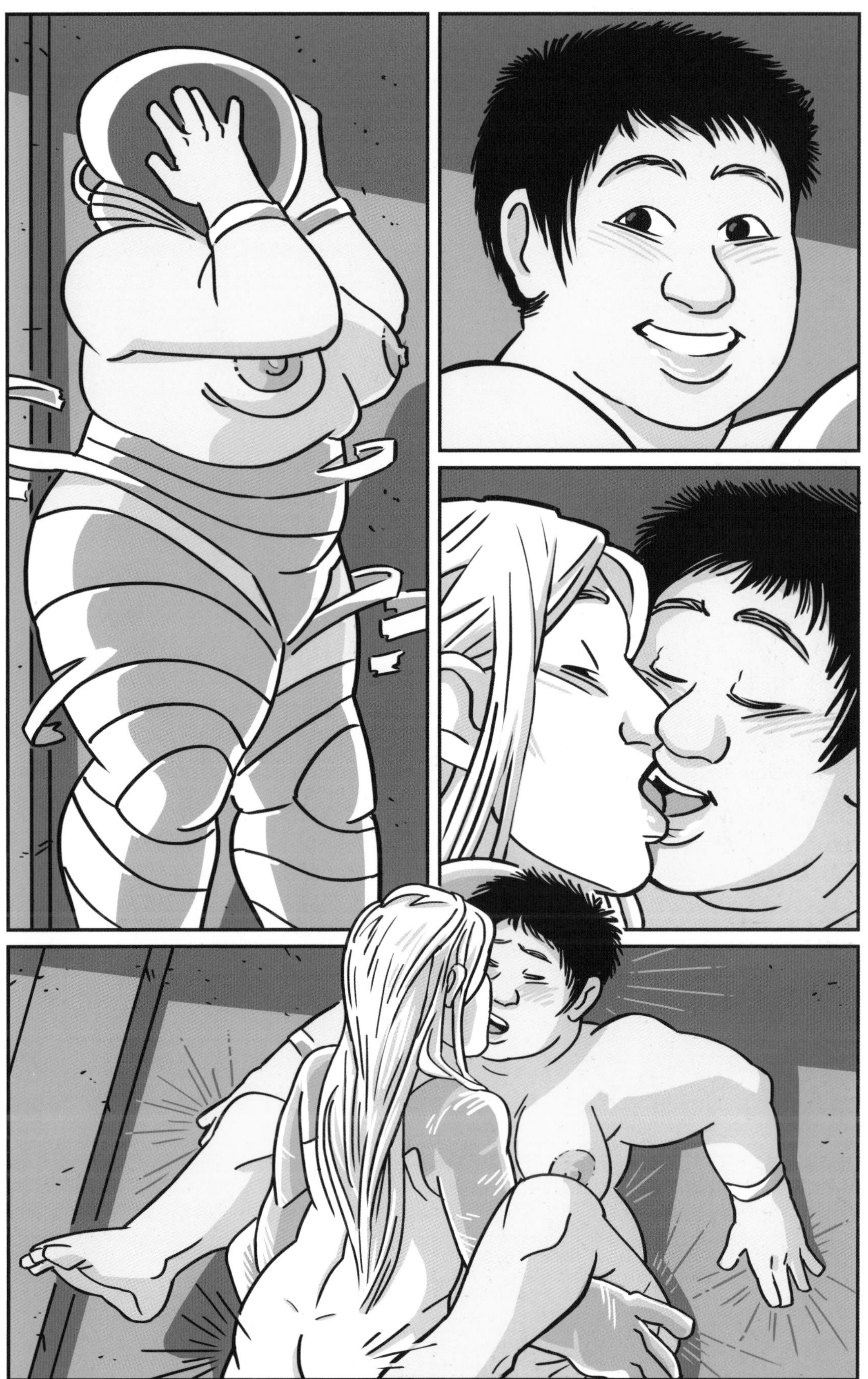

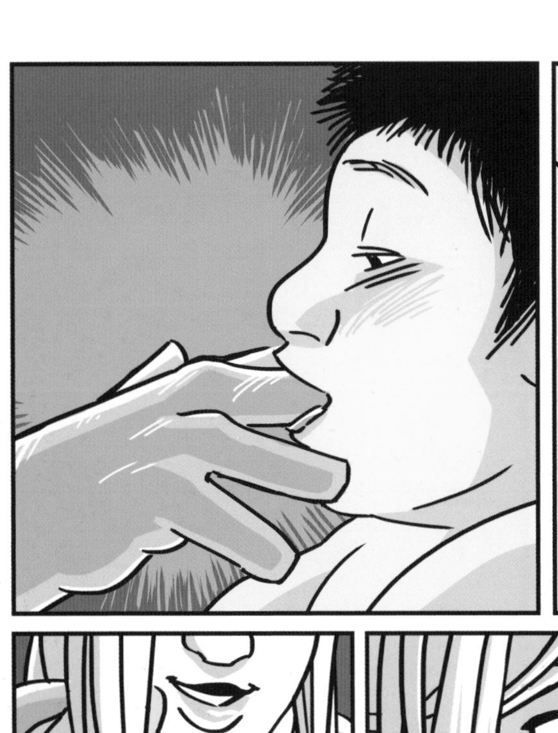
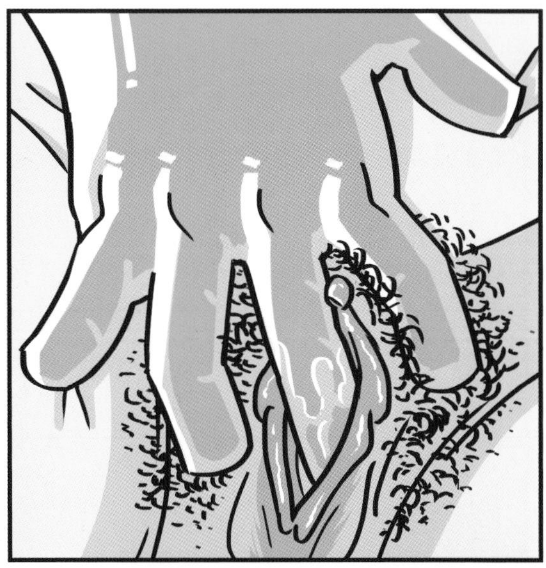
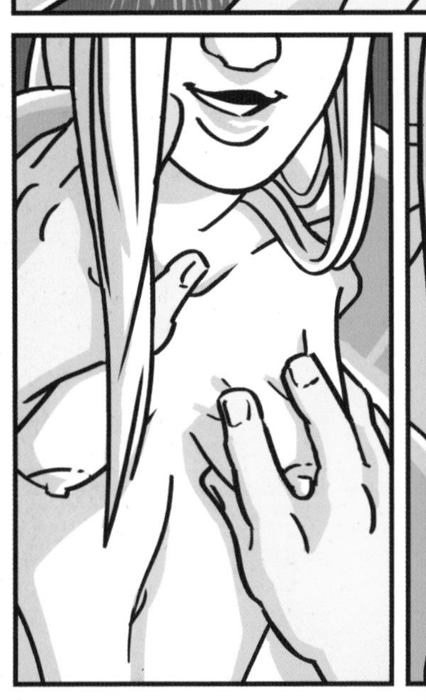
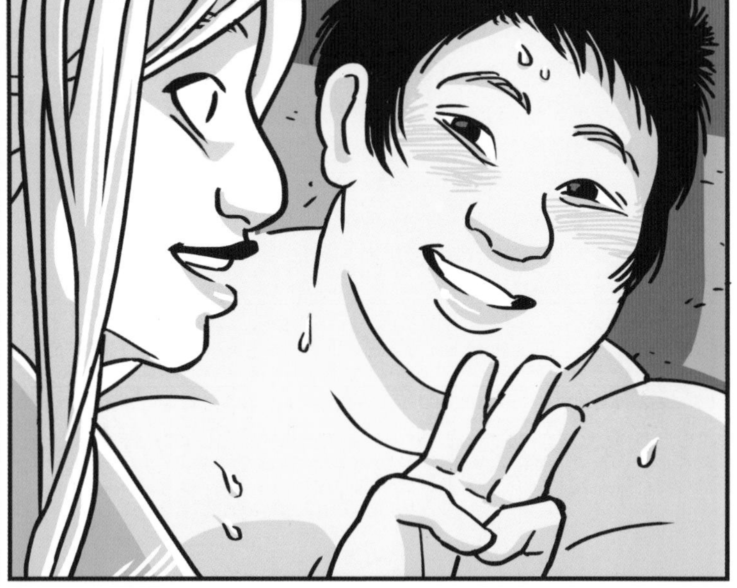
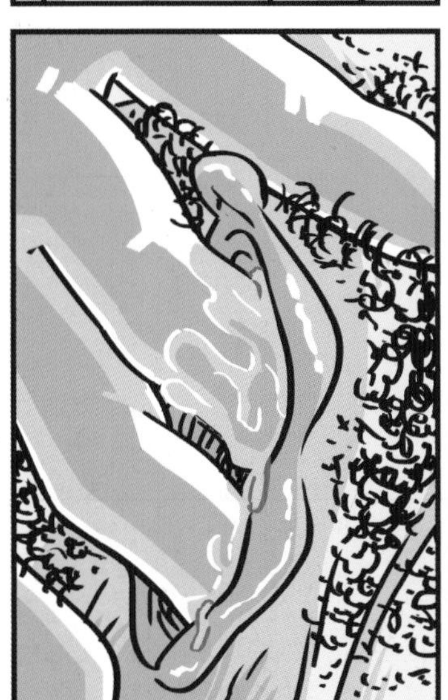
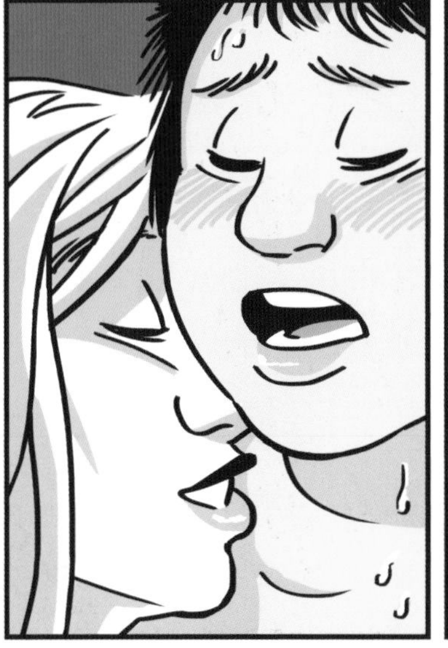
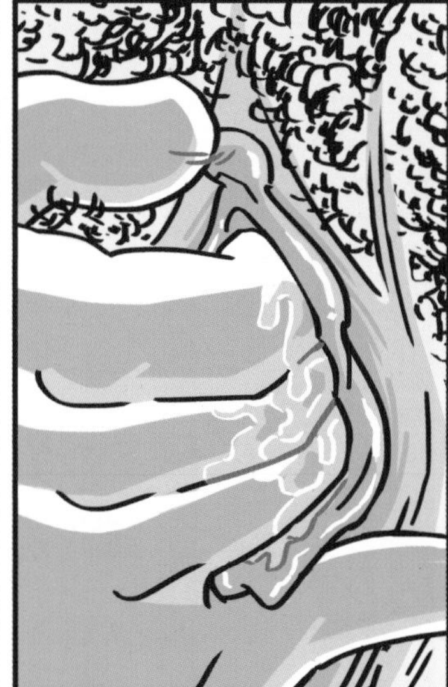

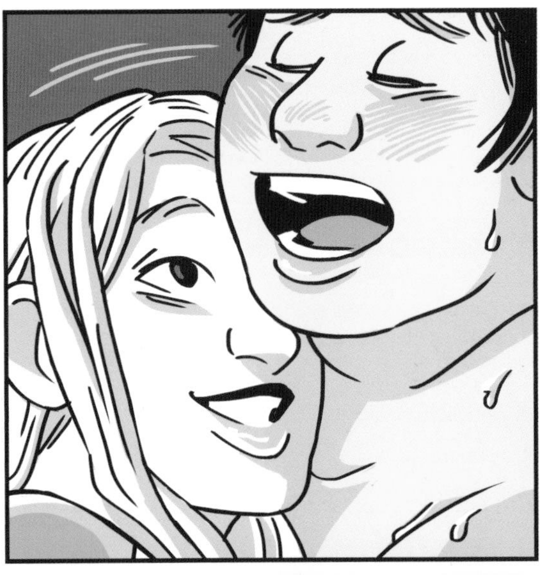
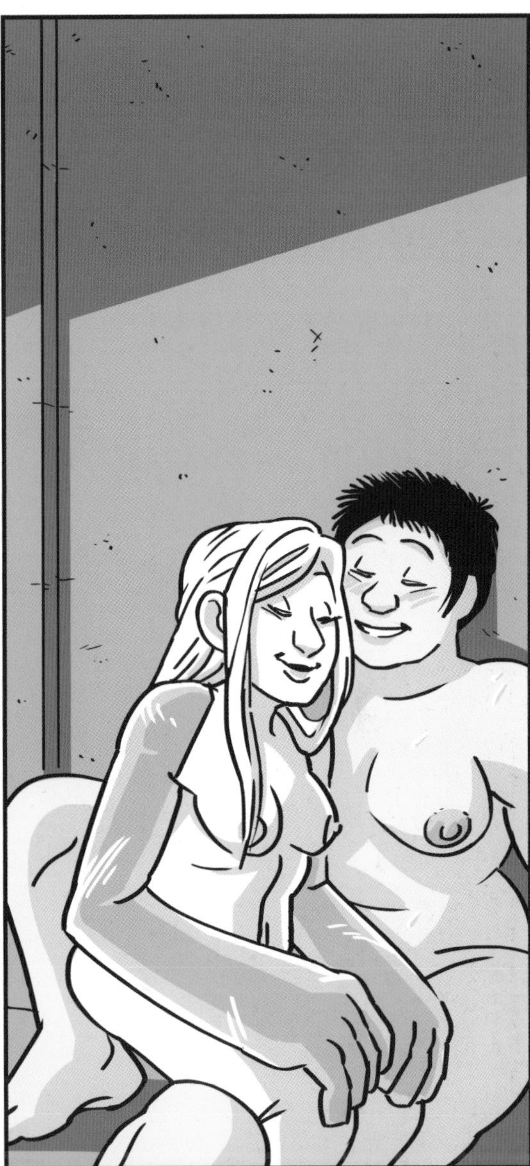
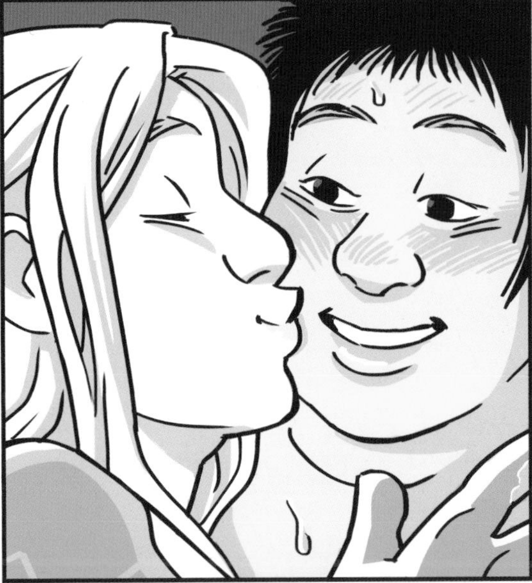
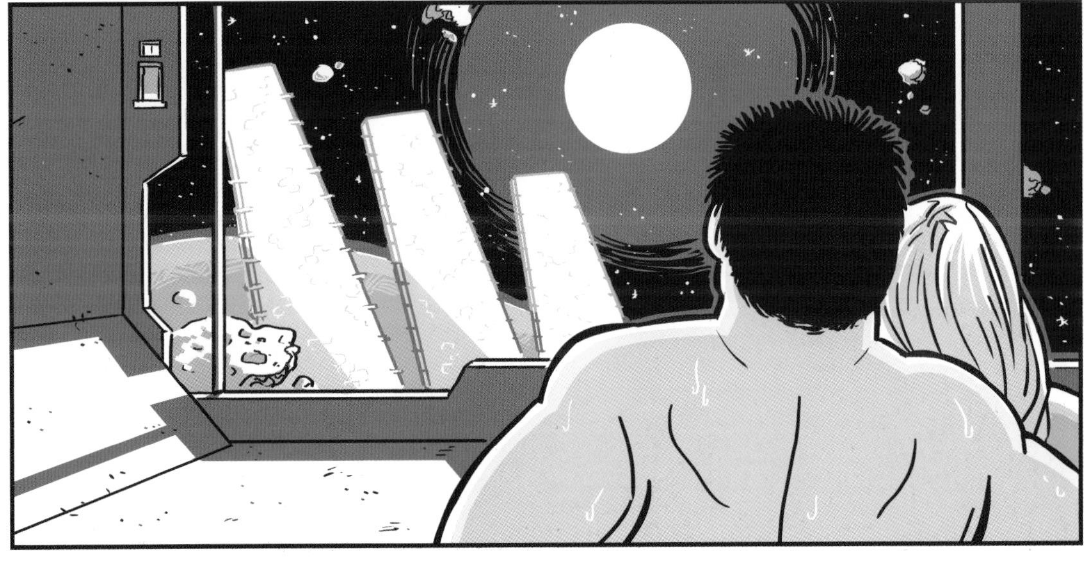

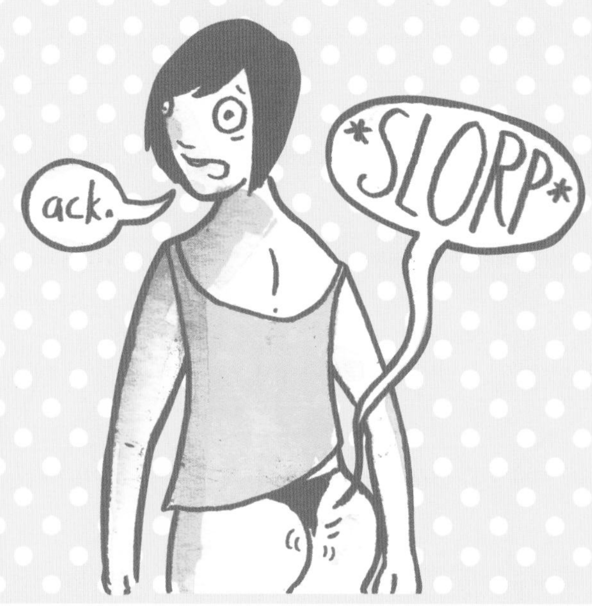

HORRIFIC SEX TOY MISTAKES

by Shing Yin Khor

sawdustbear.com

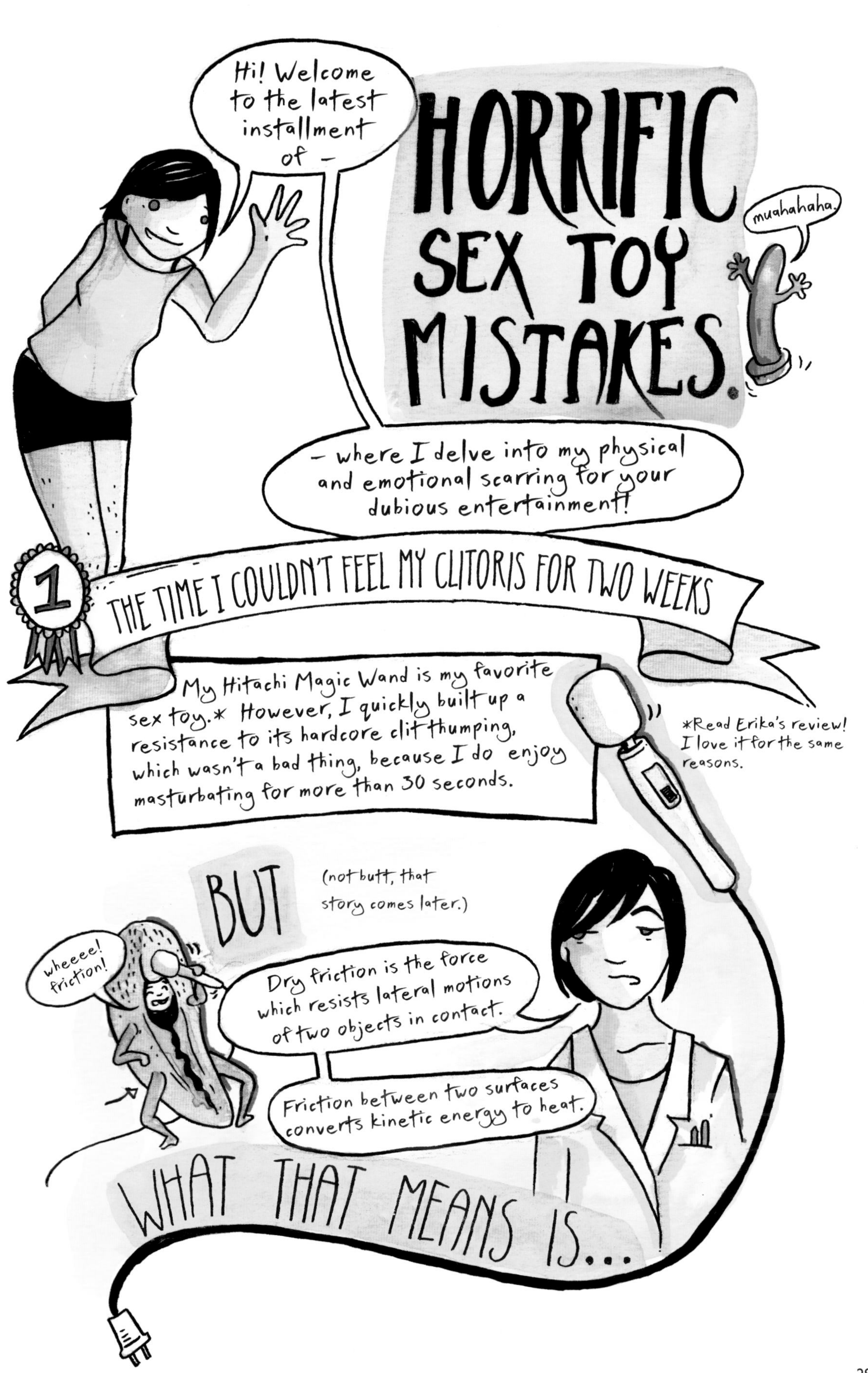
Hi! Welcome to the latest installment of –
HORRIFIC SEX TOY MISTAKES.
muahahaha.
– where I delve into my physical and emotional scarring for your dubious entertainment!
1
THE TIME I COULDN'T FEEL MY CLITORIS FOR TWO WEEKS
My Hitachi Magic Wand is my favorite sex toy.* However, I quickly built up a resistance to its hardcore clit thumping, which wasn't a bad thing, because I do enjoy masturbating for more than 30 seconds.
*Read Erika's review! I love it for the same reasons.
BUT
(not butt, that story comes later.)
wheeee! friction!
Dry friction is the force which resists lateral motions of two objects in contact.
Friction between two surfaces converts kinetic energy to heat.
WHAT THAT MEANS IS...

If you can get off in 5 minutes, things are just great!

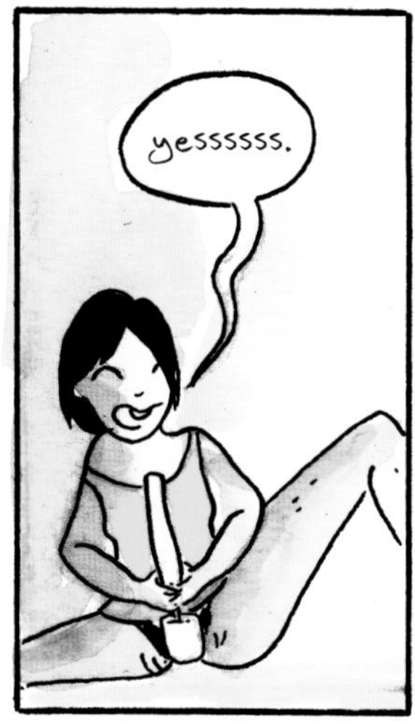
yessssss.

Fifteen minutes is pretty good too.

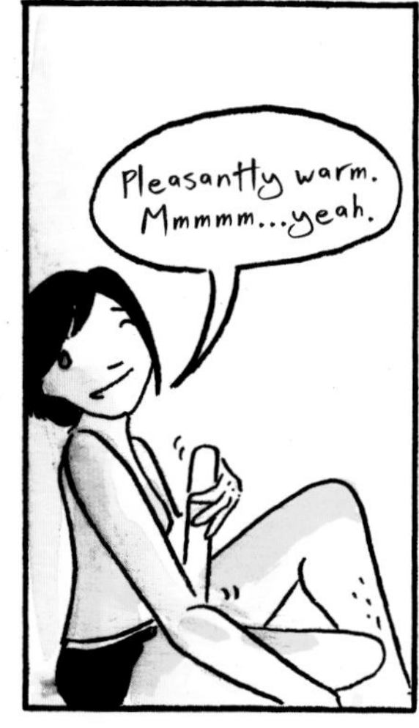
Pleasantly warm. Mmmmm...yeah.

But, if it maybe takes more than 25 minutes...

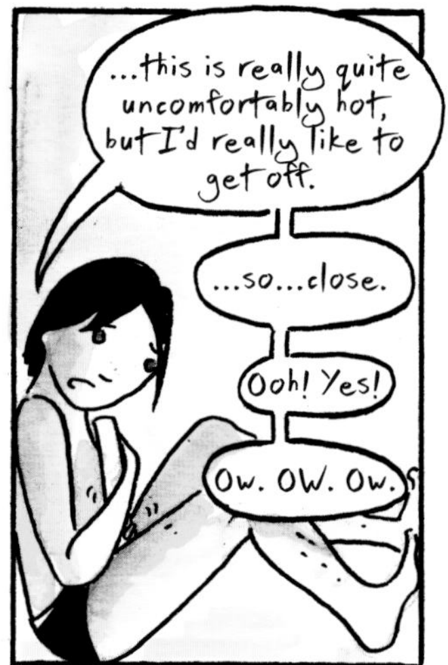
...this is really quite uncomfortably hot, but I'd really like to get off.
...so...close.
Ooh! Yes!
Ow. OW. Ow.

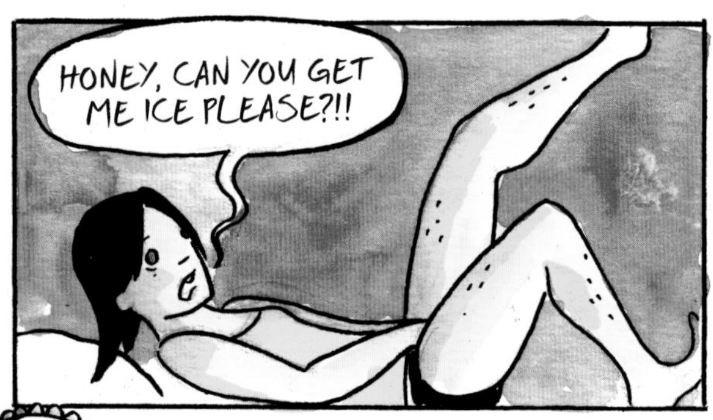
HONEY, CAN YOU GET ME ICE PLEASE?!!

AND THAT IS HOW I BURNT MY CLITORIS!

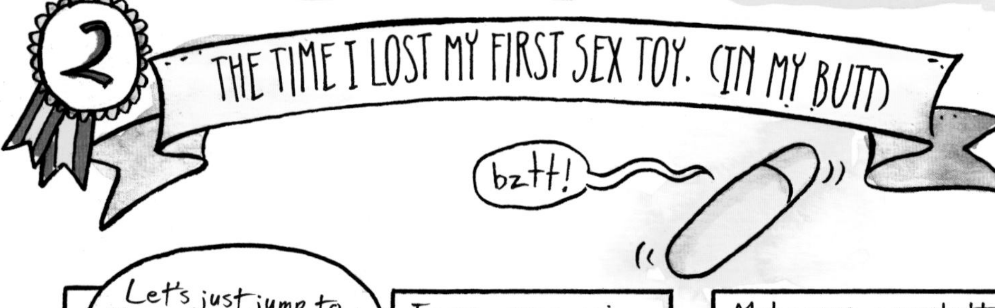
2
THE TIME I LOST MY FIRST SEX TOY. (IN MY BUTT)
bztt!

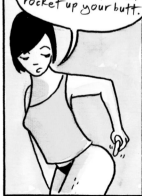

Let's just jump to the educational part. Don't stick a pocket rocket up your butt.

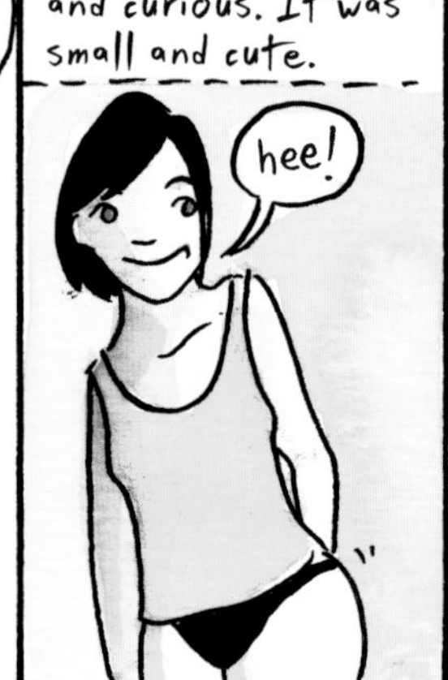
I was young, naive, and curious. It was small and cute.
hee!

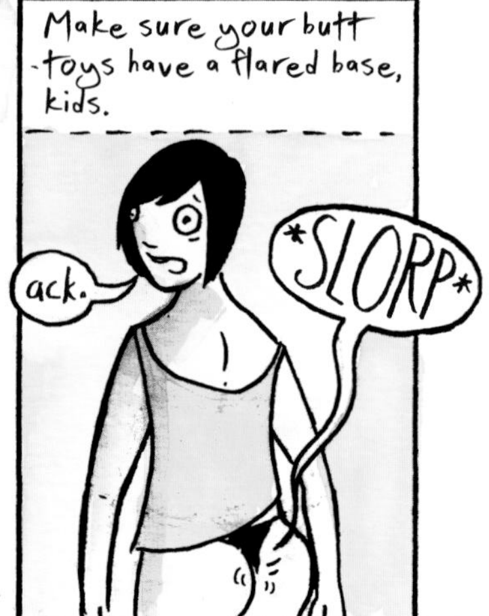
Make sure your butt-toys have a flared base, kids.
ack.
SLORP

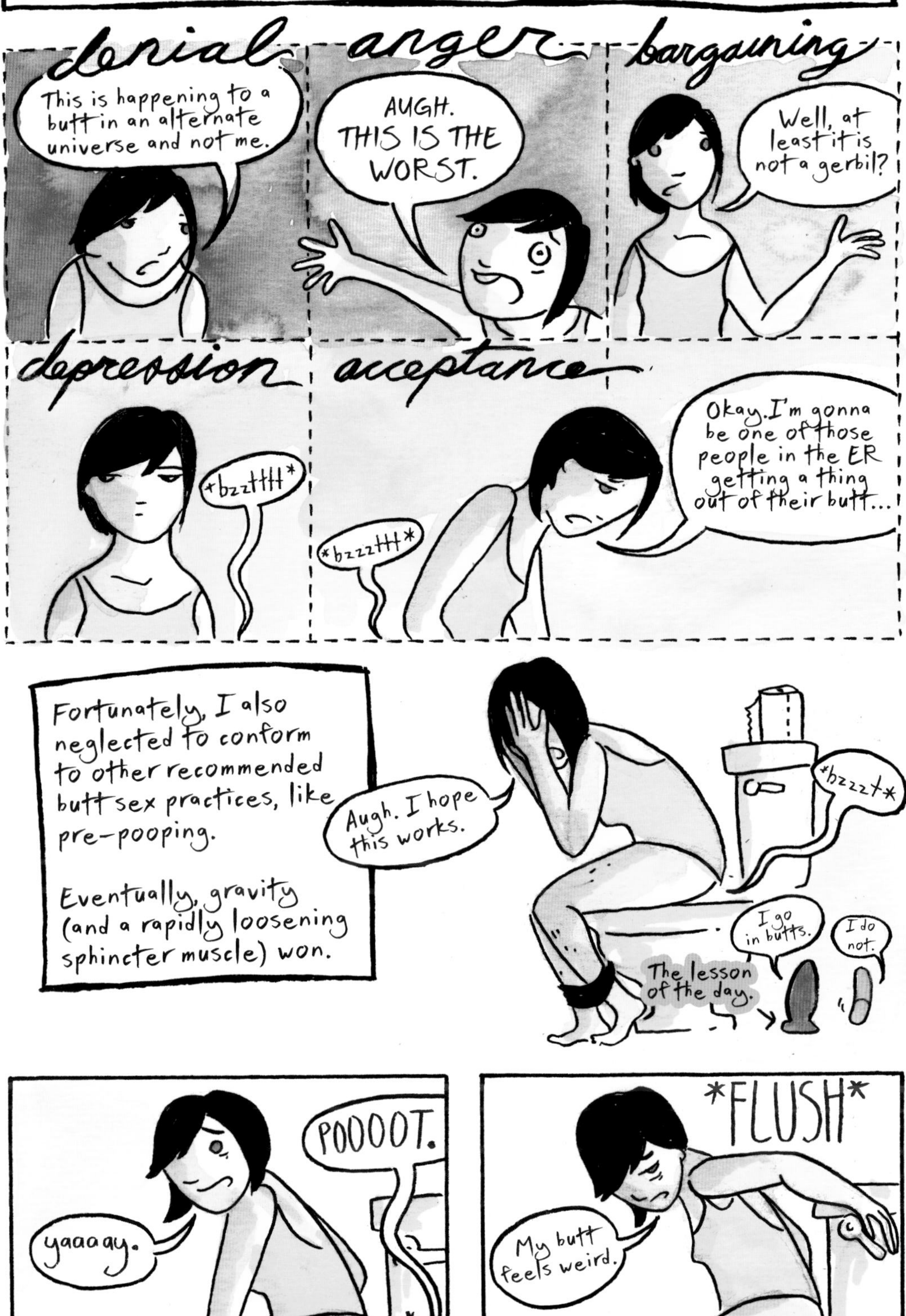
It turns out that the Kubler-Ross model can absolutely be applied to situations such as "Help, I have a vibrating bullet vibe up my ass and I don't know how to get it out."
denial
This is happening to a butt in an alternate universe and not me.
anger
AUGH. THIS IS THE WORST.
bargaining
Well, at least it is not a gerbil?
depression
bzztttt
acceptance
bzzzttt
Okay. I'm gonna be one of those people in the ER getting a thing out of their butt...
Fortunately, I also neglected to conform to other recommended butt sex practices, like pre-pooping.
Eventually, gravity (and a rapidly loosening sphincter muscle) won.
Augh. I hope this works.
bzzzt
I go in butts.
I do not.
The lesson of the day.
POOOOT.
yaaaay.
PLOP
FLUSH
My butt feels weird.

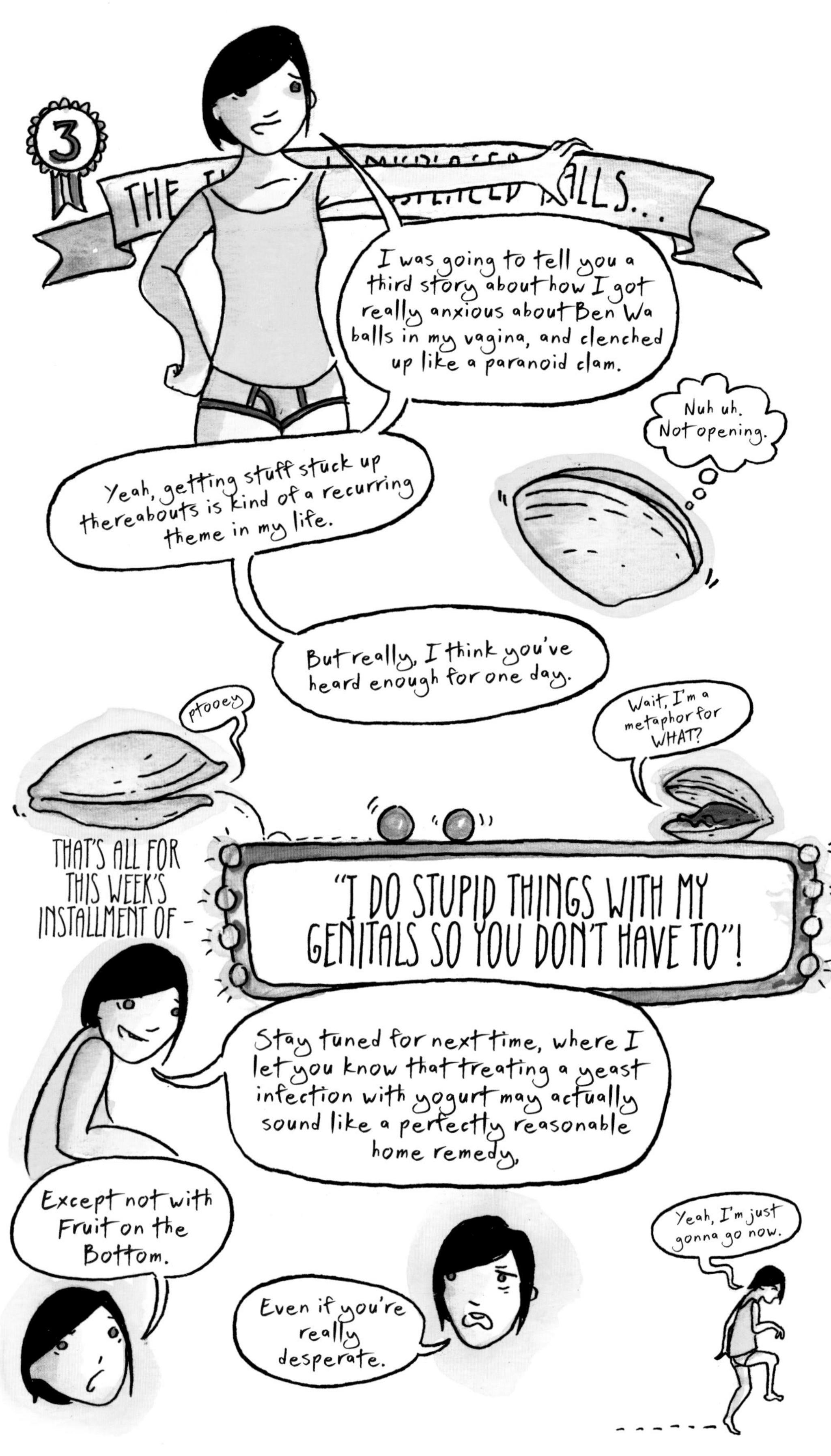
3
I was going to tell you a third story about how I got really anxious about Ben Wa balls in my vagina, and clenched up like a paranoid clam.
Yeah, getting stuff stuck up thereabouts is kind of a recurring theme in my life.
Nuh uh. Not opening.
But really, I think you've heard enough for one day.
ptooey
Wait, I'm a metaphor for WHAT?
THAT'S ALL FOR THIS WEEK'S INSTALLMENT OF –
"I DO STUPID THINGS WITH MY GENITALS SO YOU DON'T HAVE TO"!
Stay tuned for next time, where I let you know that treating a yeast infection with yogurt may actually sound like a perfectly reasonable home remedy,
Except not with Fruit on the Bottom.
Even if you're really desperate.
Yeah, I'm just gonna go now.

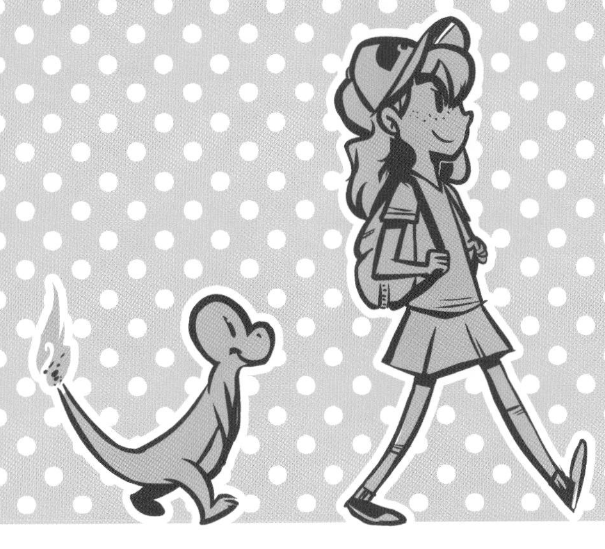

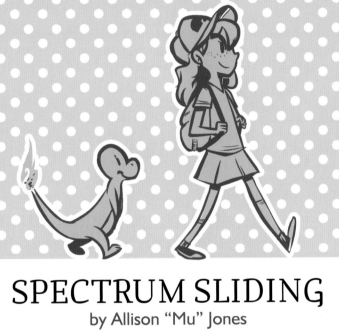

SPECTRUM SLIDING

by Allison “Mu” Jones

kismesister.tumblr.com

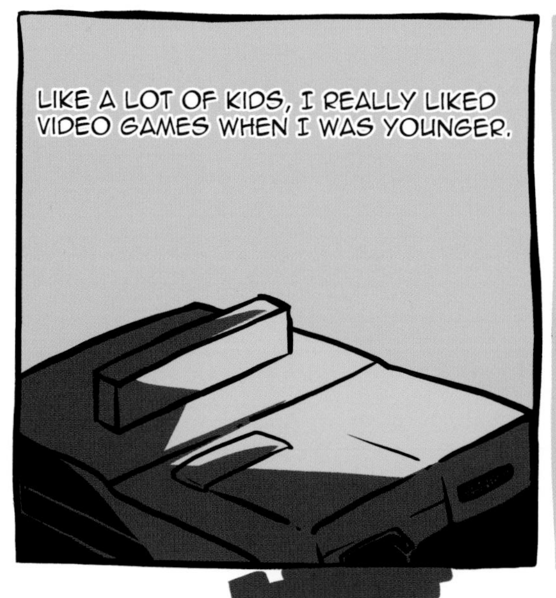

LIKE A LOT OF KIDS, I REALLY LIKED VIDEO GAMES WHEN I WAS YOUNGER.

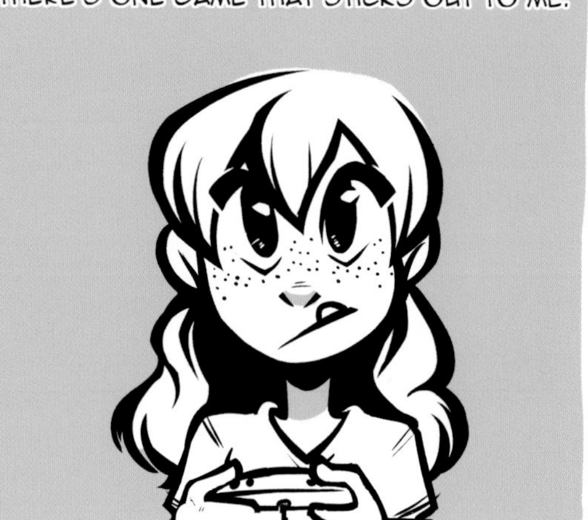

THERE'S ONE GAME THAT STICKS OUT TO ME.

SUPER MARIO BROS. 2

IT WAS THE ONLY GAME WE HAD WHERE YOU COULD ACTUALLY PLAY AS A *GIRL*.

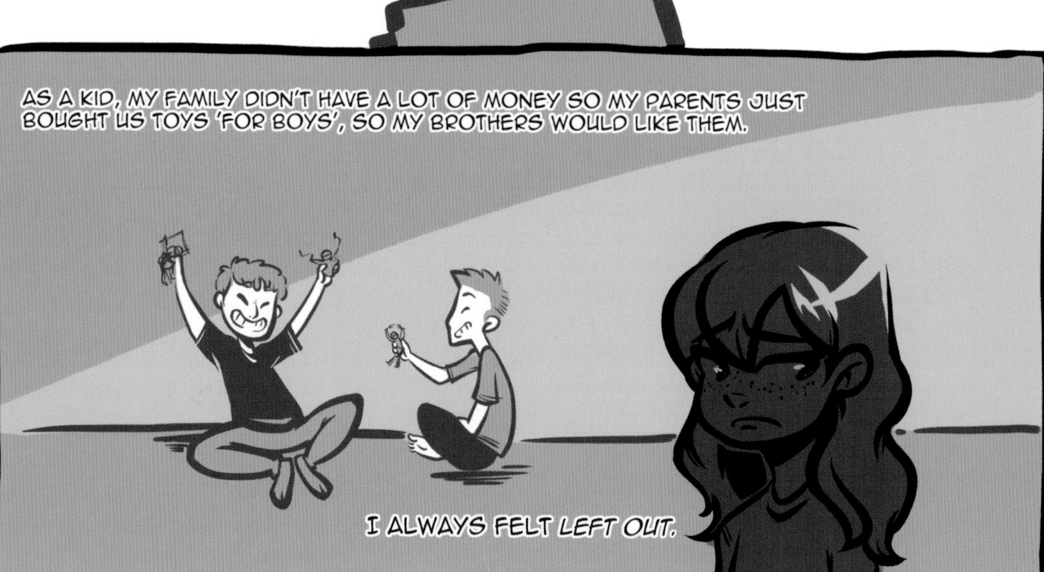

AS A KID, MY FAMILY DIDN'T HAVE A LOT OF MONEY SO MY PARENTS JUST BOUGHT US TOYS 'FOR BOYS', SO MY BROTHERS WOULD LIKE THEM.
I ALWAYS FELT *LEFT OUT.*

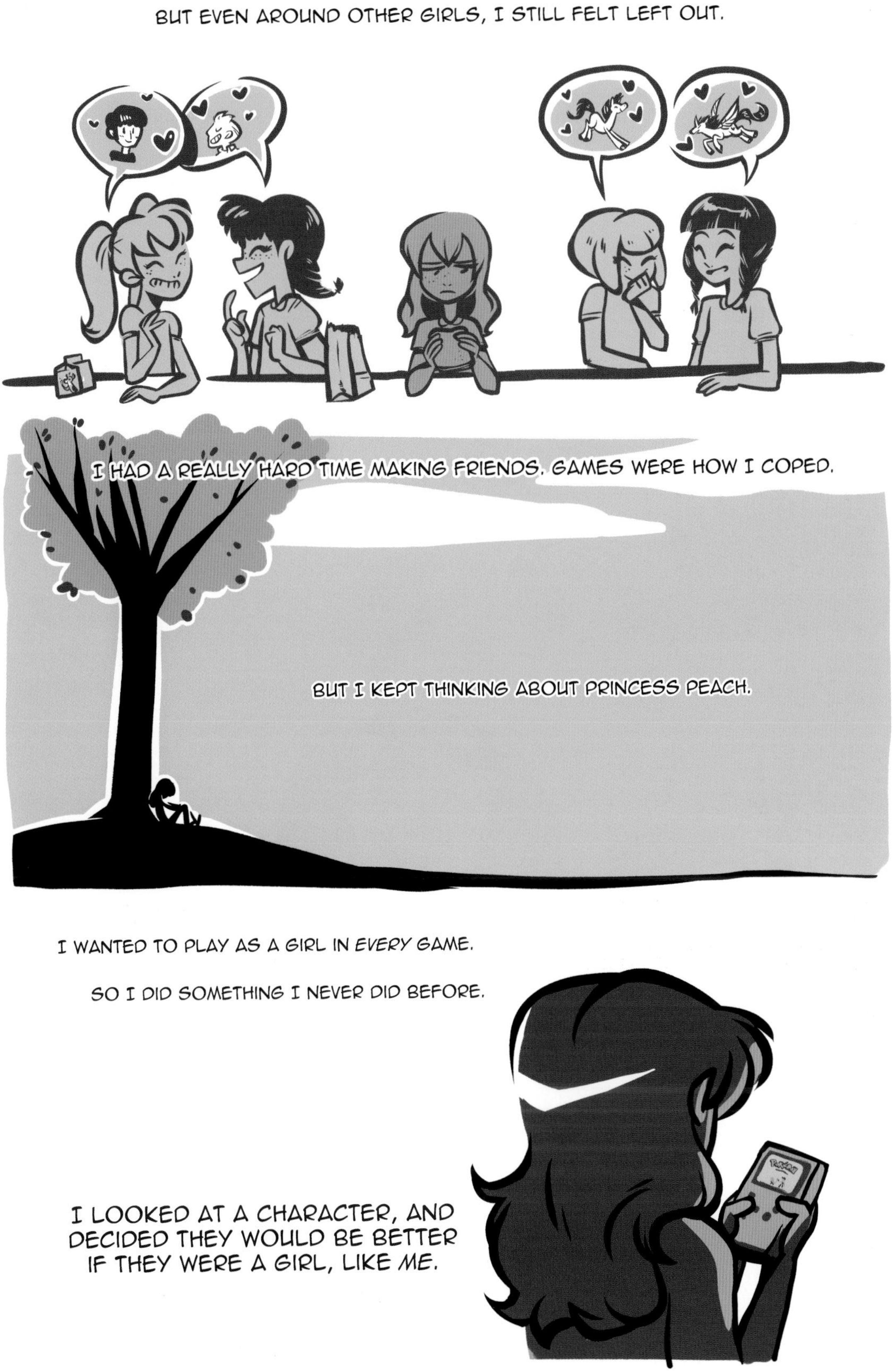

BUT EVEN AROUND OTHER GIRLS, I STILL FELT LEFT OUT.

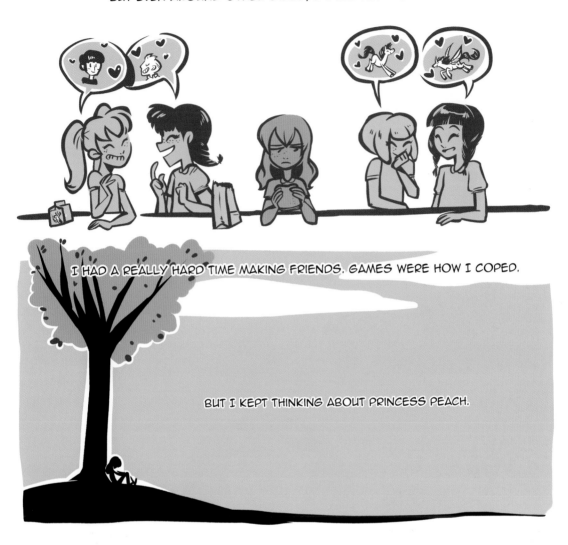

I HAD A REALLY HARD TIME MAKING FRIENDS. GAMES WERE HOW I COPED.

BUT I KEPT THINKING ABOUT PRINCESS PEACH.

I WANTED TO PLAY AS A GIRL IN *EVERY* GAME.

SO I DID SOMETHING I NEVER DID BEFORE.

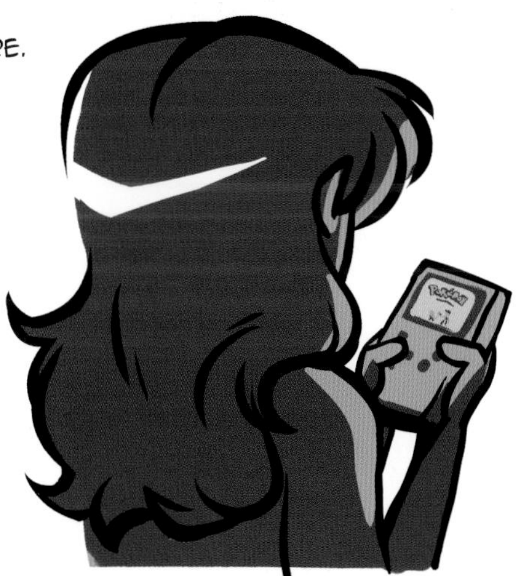

I LOOKED AT A CHARACTER, AND DECIDED THEY WOULD BE BETTER IF THEY WERE A GIRL, LIKE *ME*.

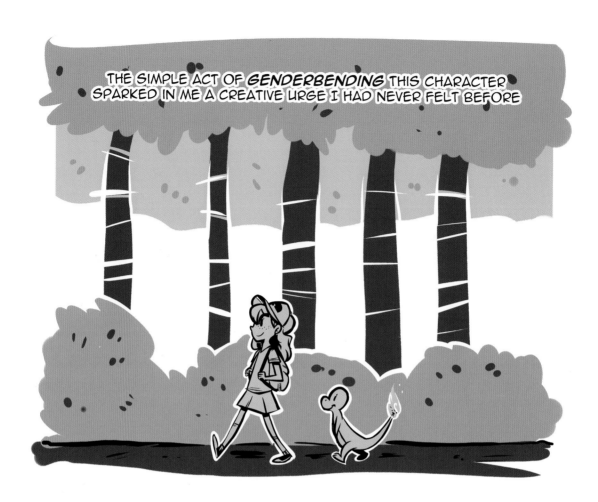

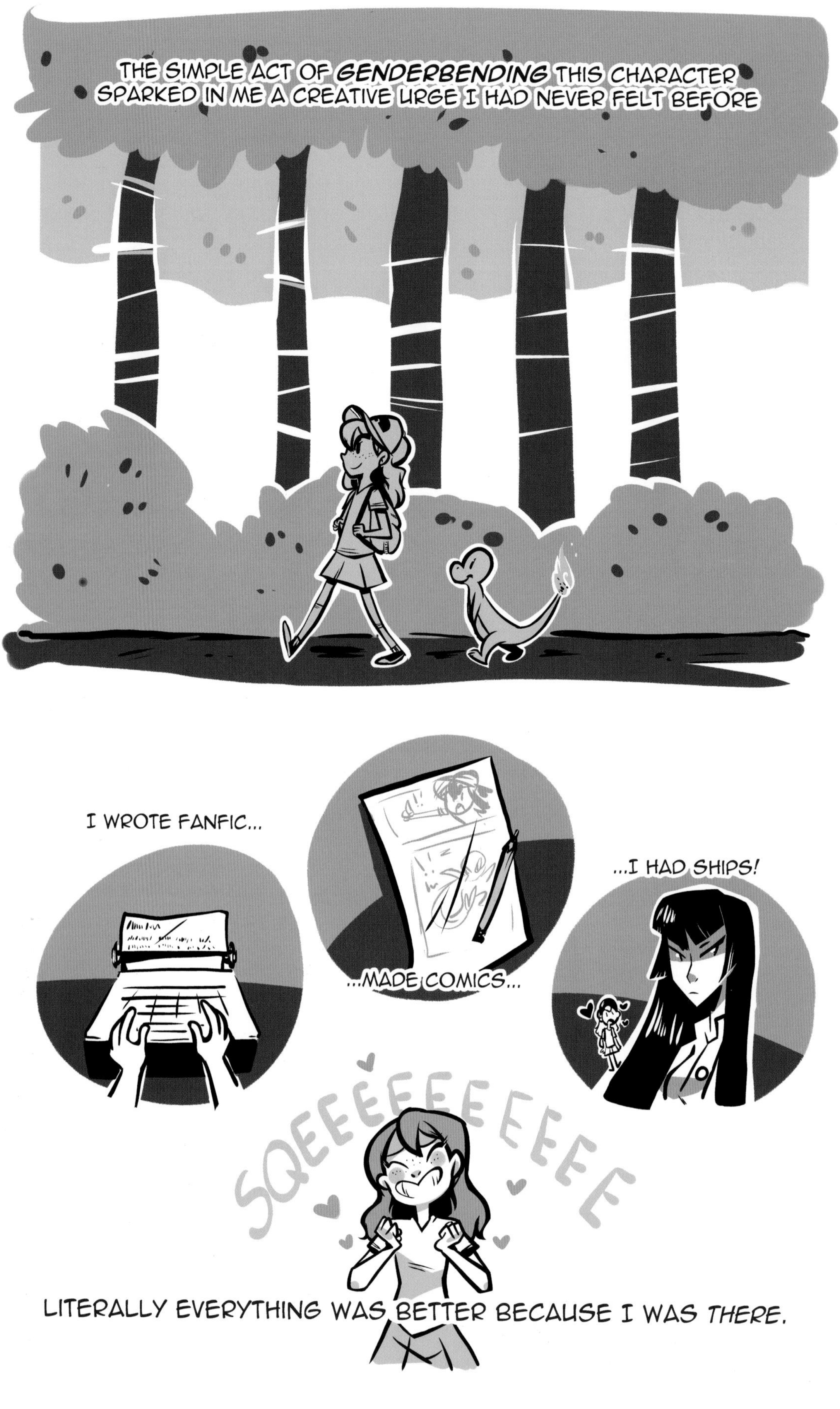

THE SIMPLE ACT OF ***GENDERBENDING*** THIS CHARACTER SPARKED IN ME A CREATIVE URGE I HAD NEVER FELT BEFORE

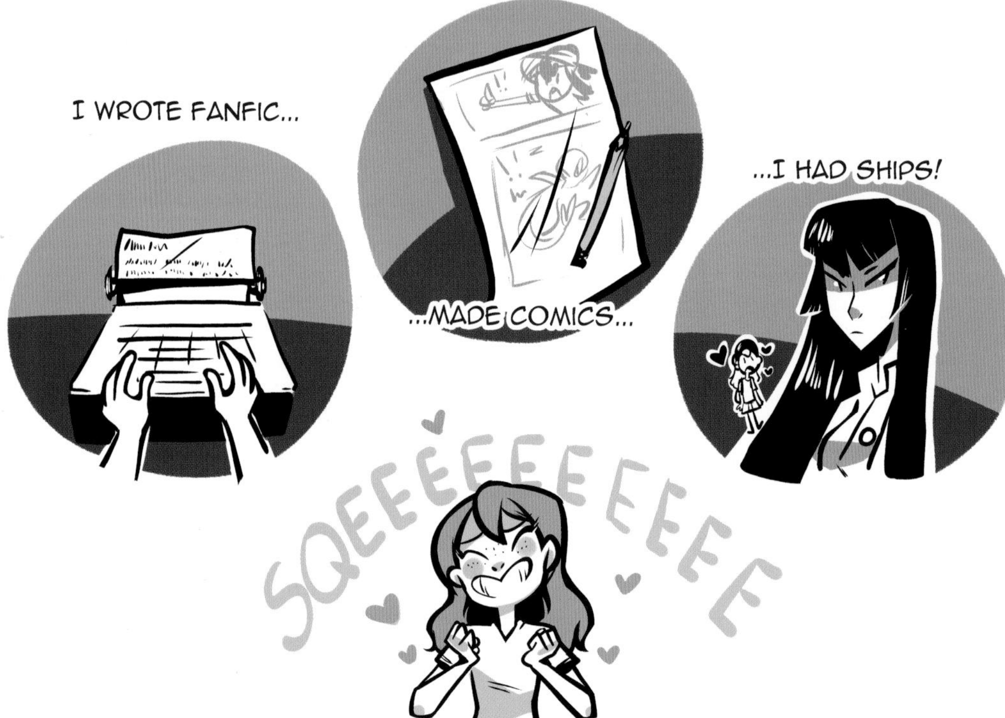

I WROTE FANFIC...
...MADE COMICS...
...I HAD SHIPS!
SQEEEEEEEEEE

LITERALLY EVERYTHING WAS BETTER BECAUSE I WAS *THERE.*

GENDERBENDING PROMPTED MY FIRST DIVE INTO FANDOM, AND I COULDN'T BE MORE GRATEFUL! BUT THE TERM ITSELF IS PRETTY LIMITED. I PICKED UP ***SPECTRUMSLIDE*** A FEW YEARS BACK, THOUGH!!

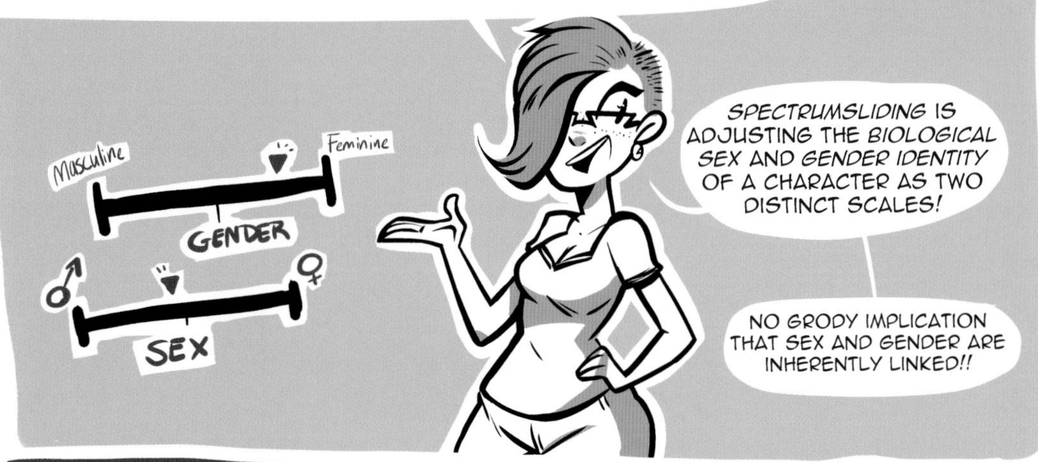

Masculine
Feminine
GENDER
SEX
SPECTRUMSLIDING IS ADJUSTING THE BIOLOGICAL SEX AND GENDER IDENTITY OF A CHARACTER AS TWO DISTINCT SCALES!
NO GRODY IMPLICATION THAT SEX AND GENDER ARE INHERENTLY LINKED!!

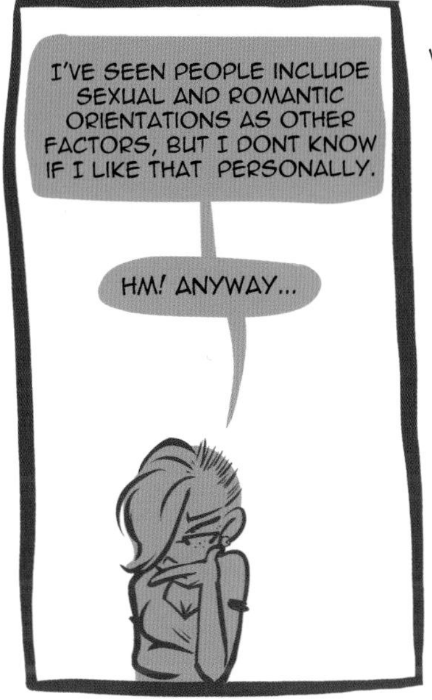

I'VE SEEN PEOPLE INCLUDE SEXUAL AND ROMANTIC ORIENTATIONS AS OTHER FACTORS, BUT I DONT KNOW IF I LIKE THAT PERSONALLY.
HM! ANYWAY...

I LOVE IT WHEN PEOPLE TAKE SOMETHING THEY LOVE AND RUN WITH IT IN A DIRECTION THAT'S CLEARLY VERY PERSONAL TO THEM, AND SPECTRUMSLIDE FANWORKS ARE FULL OF THAT!! THERE'S SEXY PINUPS, HEARTBREAKING HEADCANONS AND LITERALLY ***EVERYTHING*** IN BETWEEN.

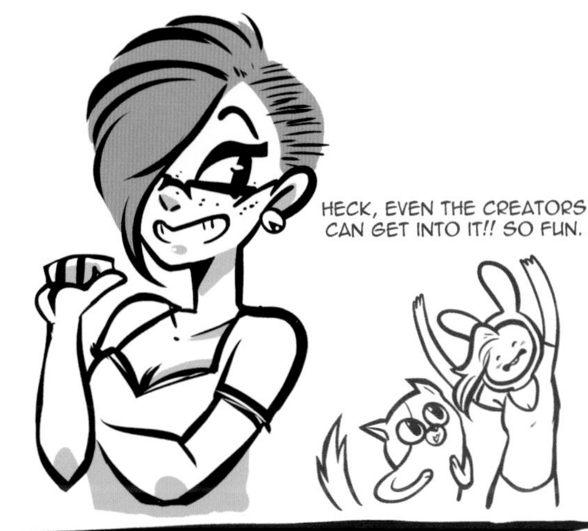

HECK, EVEN THE CREATORS CAN GET INTO IT!! SO FUN.

IT IS LITERALLY MY FAVORITE TROPE OF ALL TIME. IT ADDS SOME MUCH NEEDED DIVERSITY TO MEDIA I ALREADY LOVE!

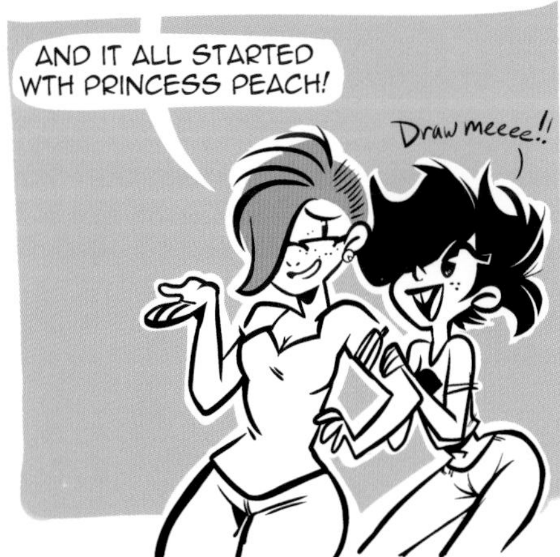

AND IT ALL STARTED WTH PRINCESS PEACH!
Draw meeee!!

MAYBE THAT SOUNDS SILLY, BUT FOR A LITTLE GIRL WHO FELT *INVISIBLE* ...

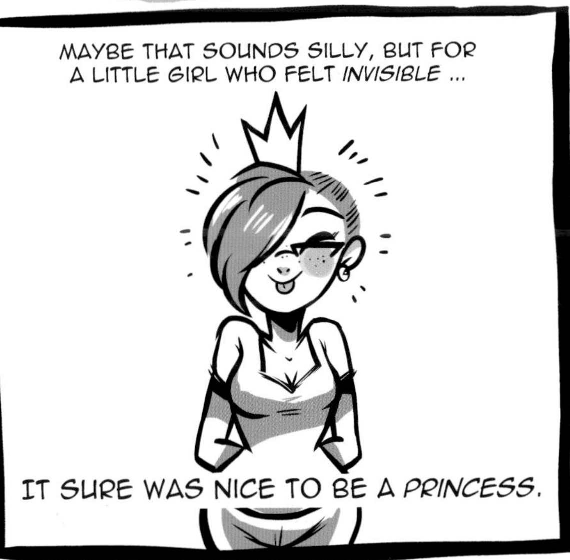

IT SURE WAS NICE TO BE A *PRINCESS.*

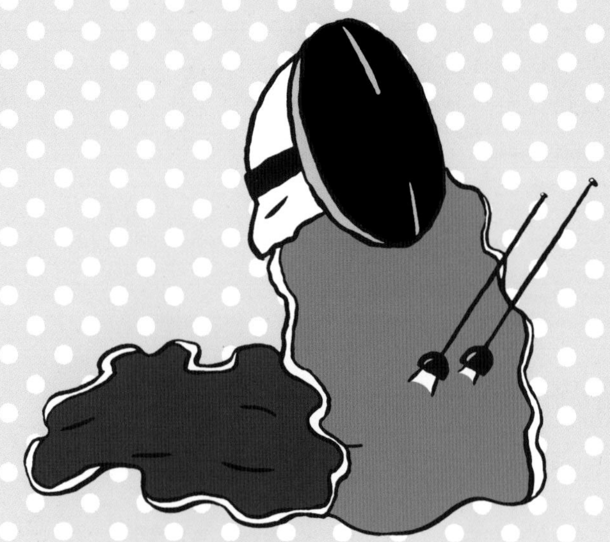

PENIS FENCING

by Jeannette Langmead

jimmyjanesays.com

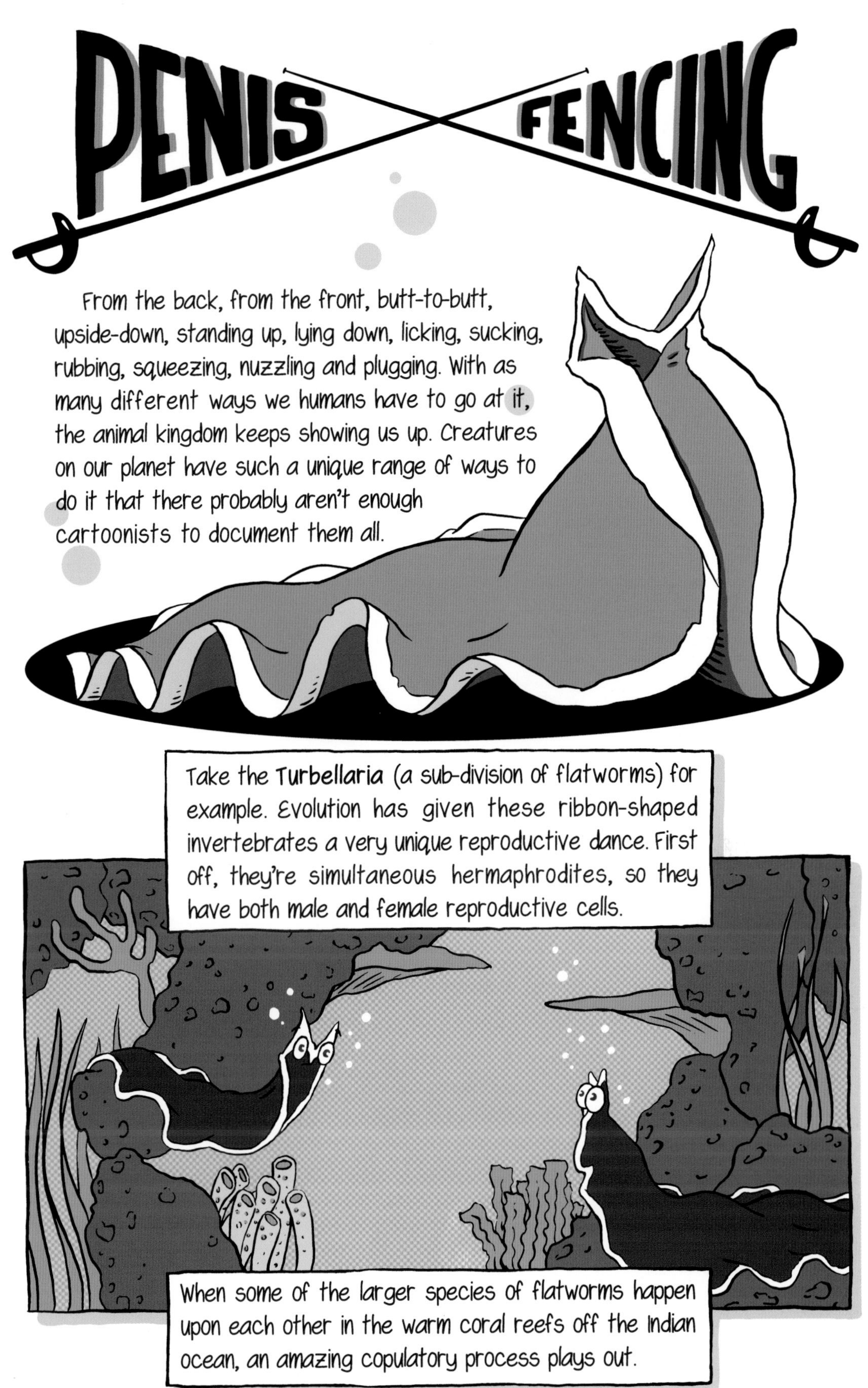
PENIS FENCING
From the back, from the front, butt-to-butt, upside-down, standing up, lying down, licking, sucking, rubbing, squeezing, nuzzling and plugging. With as many different ways we humans have to go at it, the animal kingdom keeps showing us up. Creatures on our planet have such a unique range of ways to do it that there probably aren't enough cartoonists to document them all.
Take the **Turbellaria** (a sub-division of flatworms) for example. Evolution has given these ribbon-shaped invertebrates a very unique reproductive dance. First off, they're simultaneous hermaphrodites, so they have both male and female reproductive cells.
When some of the larger species of flatworms happen upon each other in the warm coral reefs off the Indian ocean, an amazing copulatory process plays out.

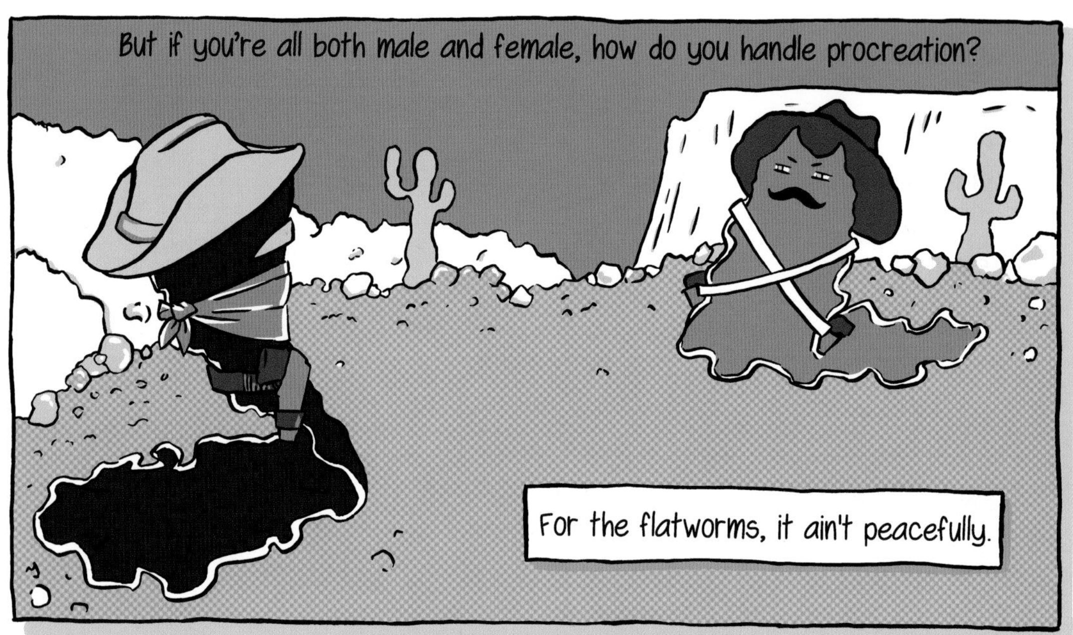

But if you're all both male and female, how do you handle procreation?
For the flatworms, it ain't peacefully.

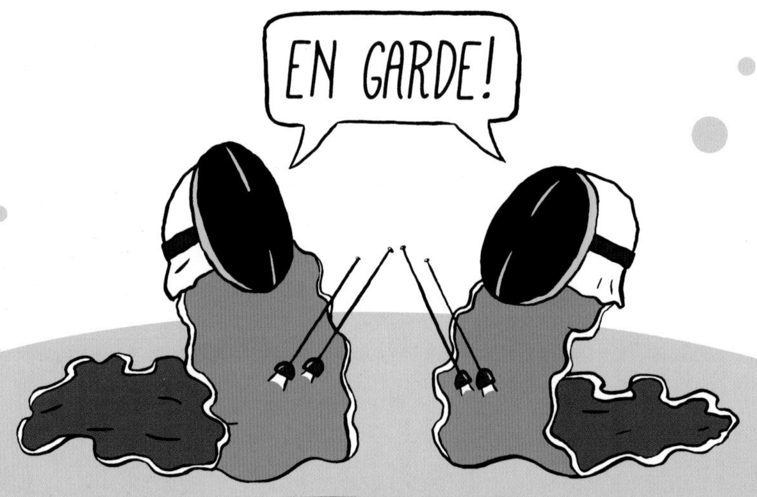

EN GARDE!
A violent battle begins where the flatworms use their dagger-like double penises to try and stab each other.

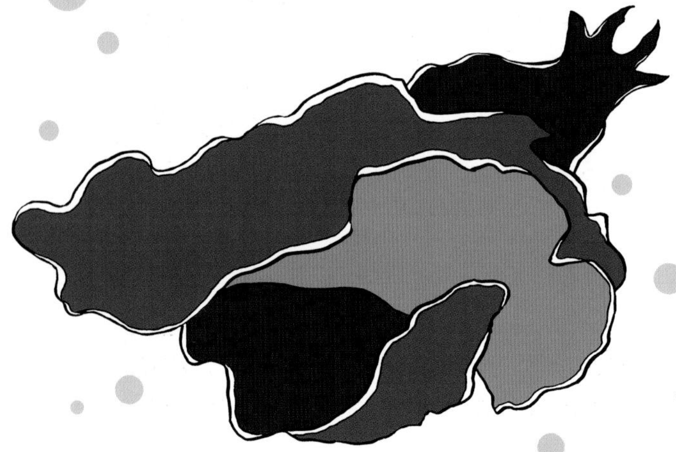

The fight is referred to as **'penis fencing'** by scientists.

Scientists do a really great job at naming things.

For the Turbellaria a penis fencing triumph is loading sperm into your dueling partner's skin. Once a successful stab is made the puncture creates a father out of the winner and a mother out of the defeated.

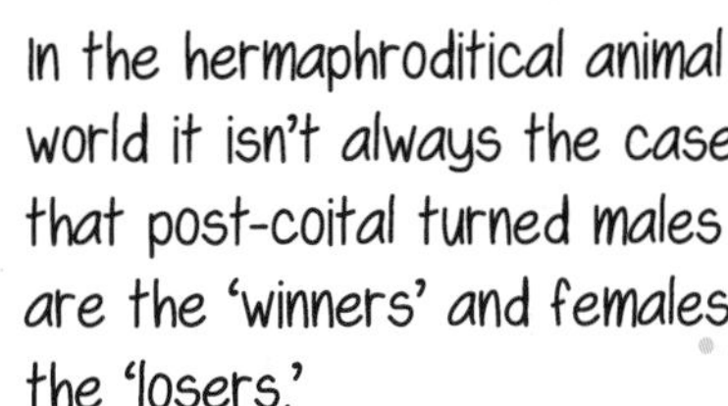

In the hermaphroditical animal world it isn't always the case that post-coital turned males are the 'winners' and females the 'losers.'

For flatworms it is though.

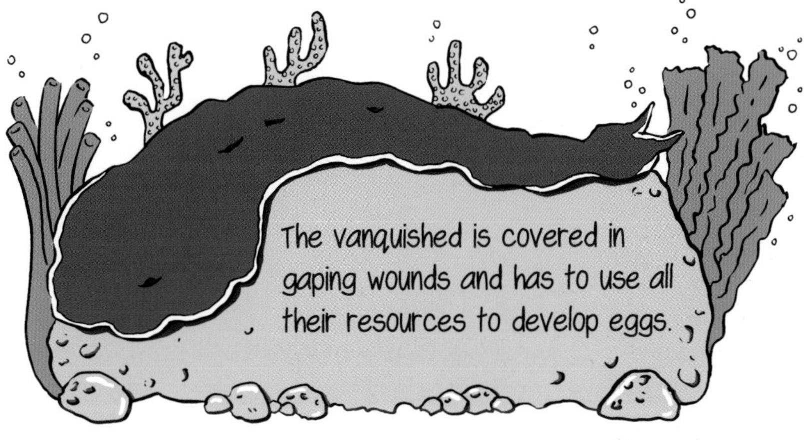

The vanquished is covered in gaping wounds and has to use all their resources to develop eggs.

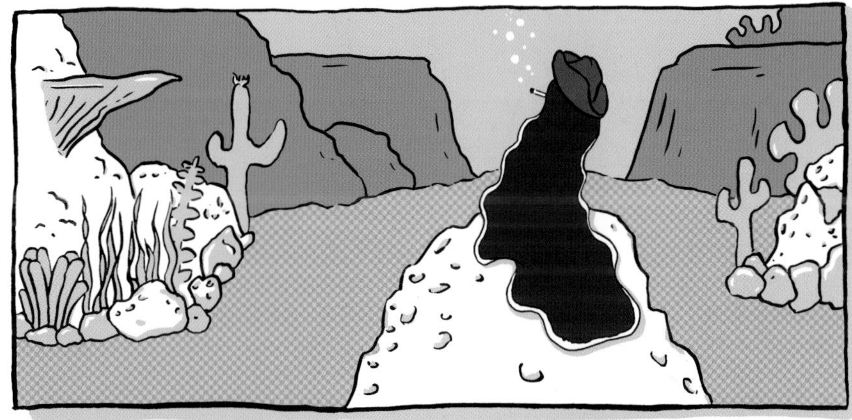

The victorious remain unencumbered by parenthood, free to seek out a new dueling partner and take another stab at penis fencing.

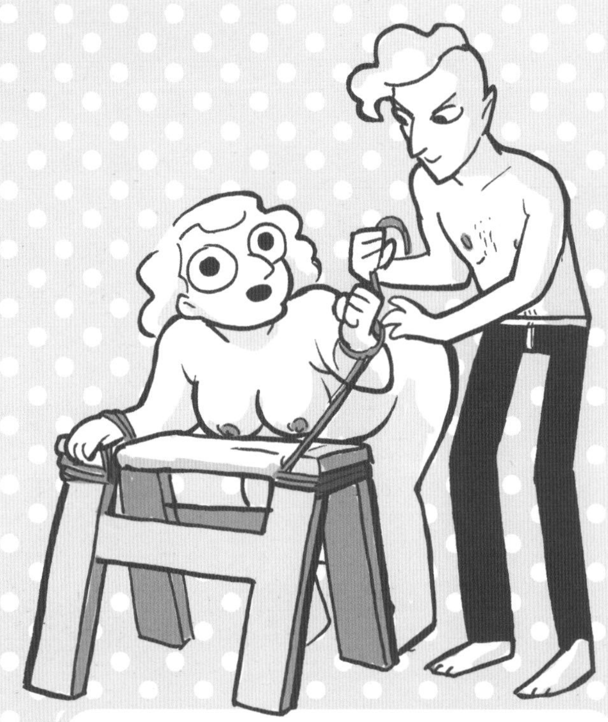

BDSM SAFETY

by Abby Howard

jspowerhour.com

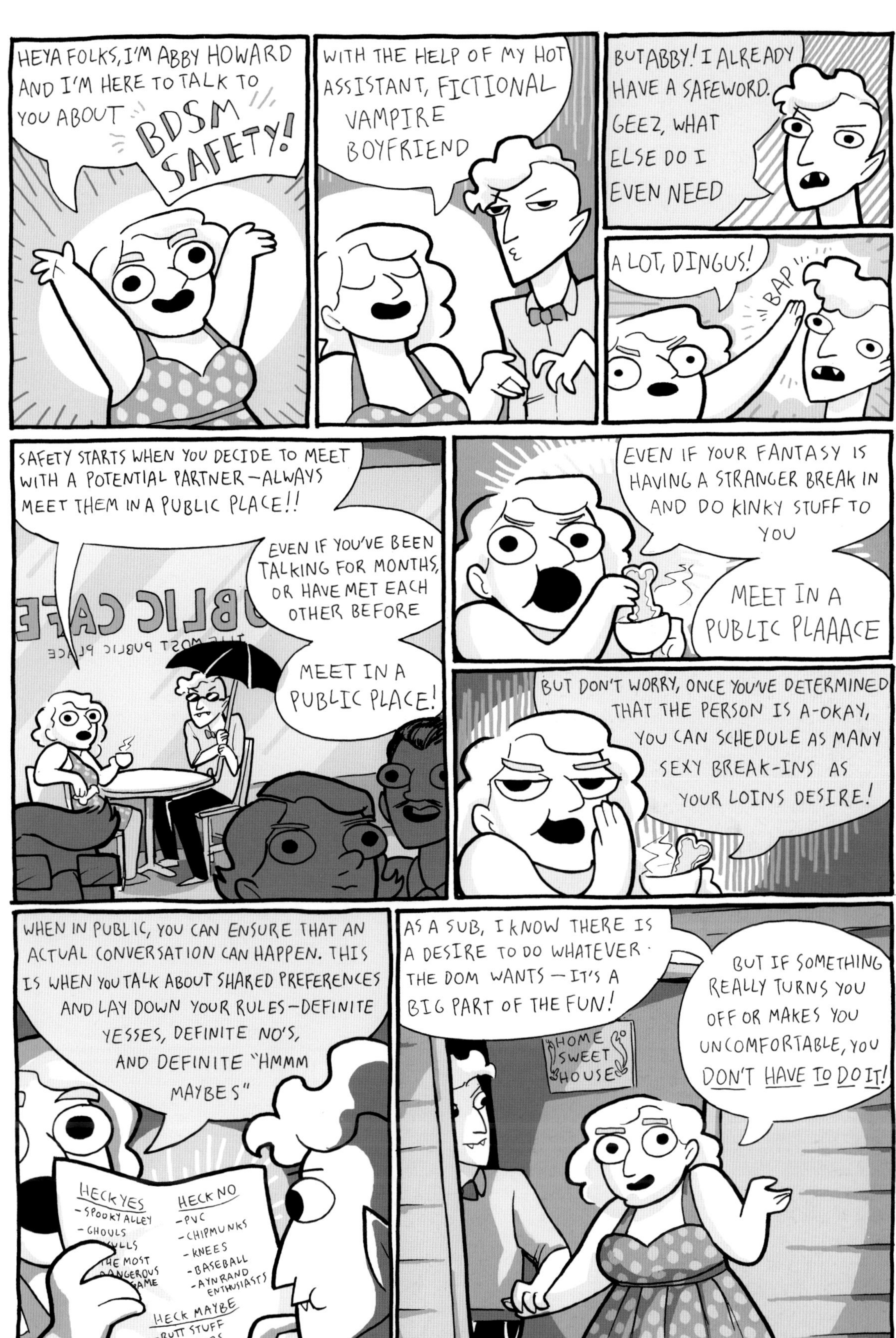
HEYA FOLKS, I'M ABBY HOWARD AND I'M HERE TO TALK TO YOU ABOUT BDSM SAFETY!
WITH THE HELP OF MY HOT ASSISTANT, FICTIONAL VAMPIRE BOYFRIEND
BUT ABBY! I ALREADY HAVE A SAFEWORD. GEEZ, WHAT ELSE DO I EVEN NEED
A LOT, DINGUS!
BAP
SAFETY STARTS WHEN YOU DECIDE TO MEET WITH A POTENTIAL PARTNER—ALWAYS MEET THEM IN A PUBLIC PLACE!!
EVEN IF YOU'VE BEEN TALKING FOR MONTHS, OR HAVE MET EACH OTHER BEFORE
MEET IN A PUBLIC PLACE!
EVEN IF YOUR FANTASY IS HAVING A STRANGER BREAK IN AND DO KINKY STUFF TO YOU
MEET IN A PUBLIC PLAAACE
BUT DON'T WORRY, ONCE YOU'VE DETERMINED THAT THE PERSON IS A-OKAY, YOU CAN SCHEDULE AS MANY SEXY BREAK-INS AS YOUR LOINS DESIRE!
WHEN IN PUBLIC, YOU CAN ENSURE THAT AN ACTUAL CONVERSATION CAN HAPPEN. THIS IS WHEN YOU TALK ABOUT SHARED PREFERENCES AND LAY DOWN YOUR RULES—DEFINITE YESSES, DEFINITE NO'S, AND DEFINITE "HMMM MAYBES"
HECK YES
-SPOOKY ALLEY
-GHOULS
HECK NO
-PVC
-CHIPMUNKS
-KNEES
-BASEBALL
-AYN RAND ENTHUSIASTS
HECK MAYBE
-BUTT STUFF
-ICE CHIPS
-DINOSAUR ROLEPLAY
AS A SUB, I KNOW THERE IS A DESIRE TO DO WHATEVER THE DOM WANTS—IT'S A BIG PART OF THE FUN!
HOME SWEET HOUSE
BUT IF SOMETHING REALLY TURNS YOU OFF OR MAKES YOU UNCOMFORTABLE, YOU DON'T HAVE TO DO IT!

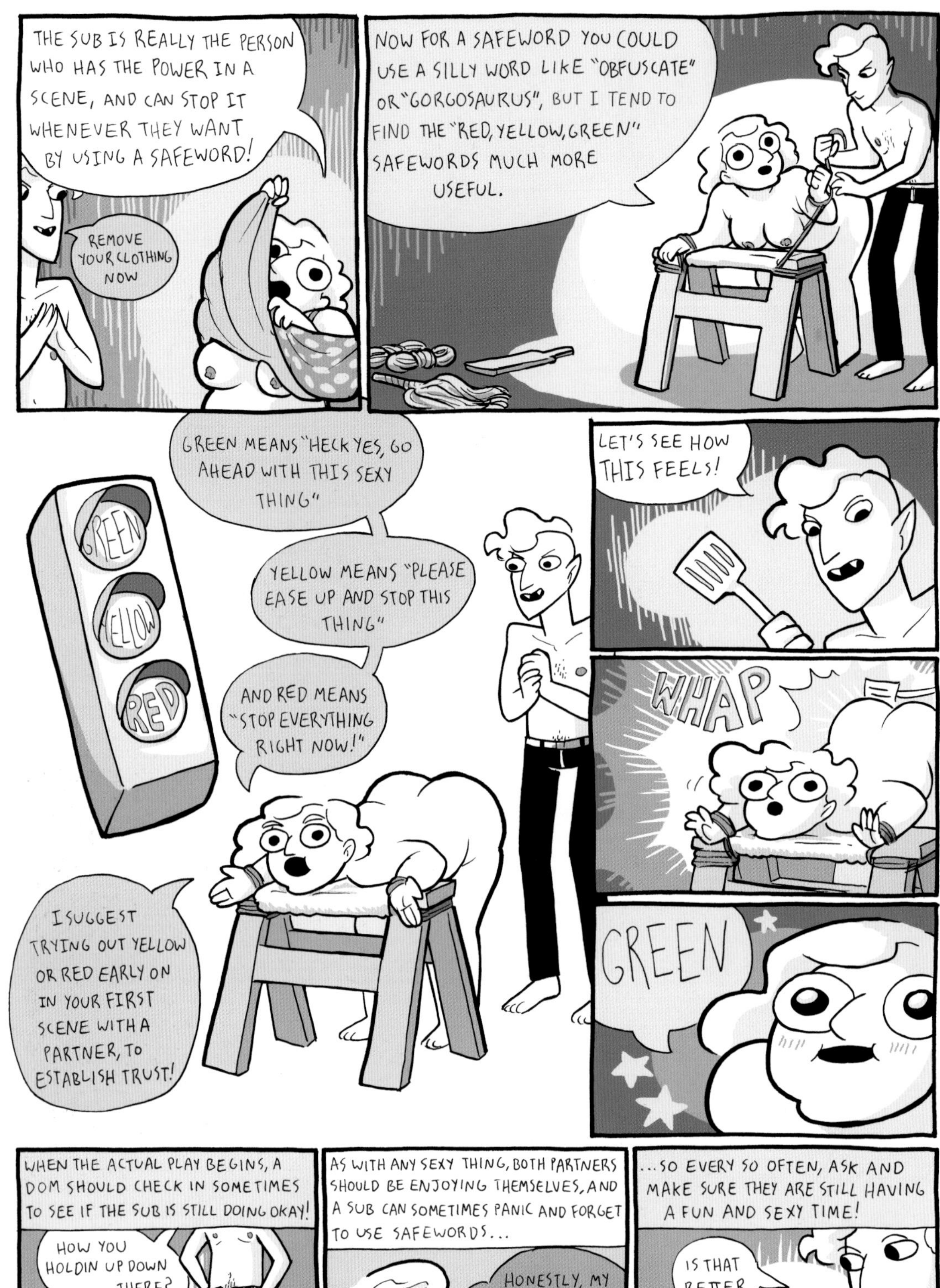
THE SUB IS REALLY THE PERSON WHO HAS THE POWER IN A SCENE, AND CAN STOP IT WHENEVER THEY WANT BY USING A SAFEWORD!
REMOVE YOUR CLOTHING NOW
NOW FOR A SAFEWORD YOU COULD USE A SILLY WORD LIKE "OBFUSCATE" OR "GORGOSAURUS", BUT I TEND TO FIND THE "RED, YELLOW, GREEN" SAFEWORDS MUCH MORE USEFUL.
GREEN MEANS "HECK YES, GO AHEAD WITH THIS SEXY THING"
YELLOW MEANS "PLEASE EASE UP AND STOP THIS THING"
AND RED MEANS "STOP EVERYTHING RIGHT NOW!"
GREEN
YELLOW
RED
I SUGGEST TRYING OUT YELLOW OR RED EARLY ON IN YOUR FIRST SCENE WITH A PARTNER, TO ESTABLISH TRUST!
LET'S SEE HOW THIS FEELS!
WHAP
GREEN
WHEN THE ACTUAL PLAY BEGINS, A DOM SHOULD CHECK IN SOMETIMES TO SEE IF THE SUB IS STILL DOING OKAY!
HOW YOU HOLDIN UP DOWN THERE?
AS WITH ANY SEXY THING, BOTH PARTNERS SHOULD BE ENJOYING THEMSELVES, AND A SUB CAN SOMETIMES PANIC AND FORGET TO USE SAFEWORDS...
HONESTLY, MY NIPS ARE 'BOUT TO FALL OFF. I'M CALLIN' YELLOW!
...SO EVERY SO OFTEN, ASK AND MAKE SURE THEY ARE STILL HAVING A FUN AND SEXY TIME!
IS THAT BETTER
YES, MY NIPS WILL LIVE ANOTHER DAY

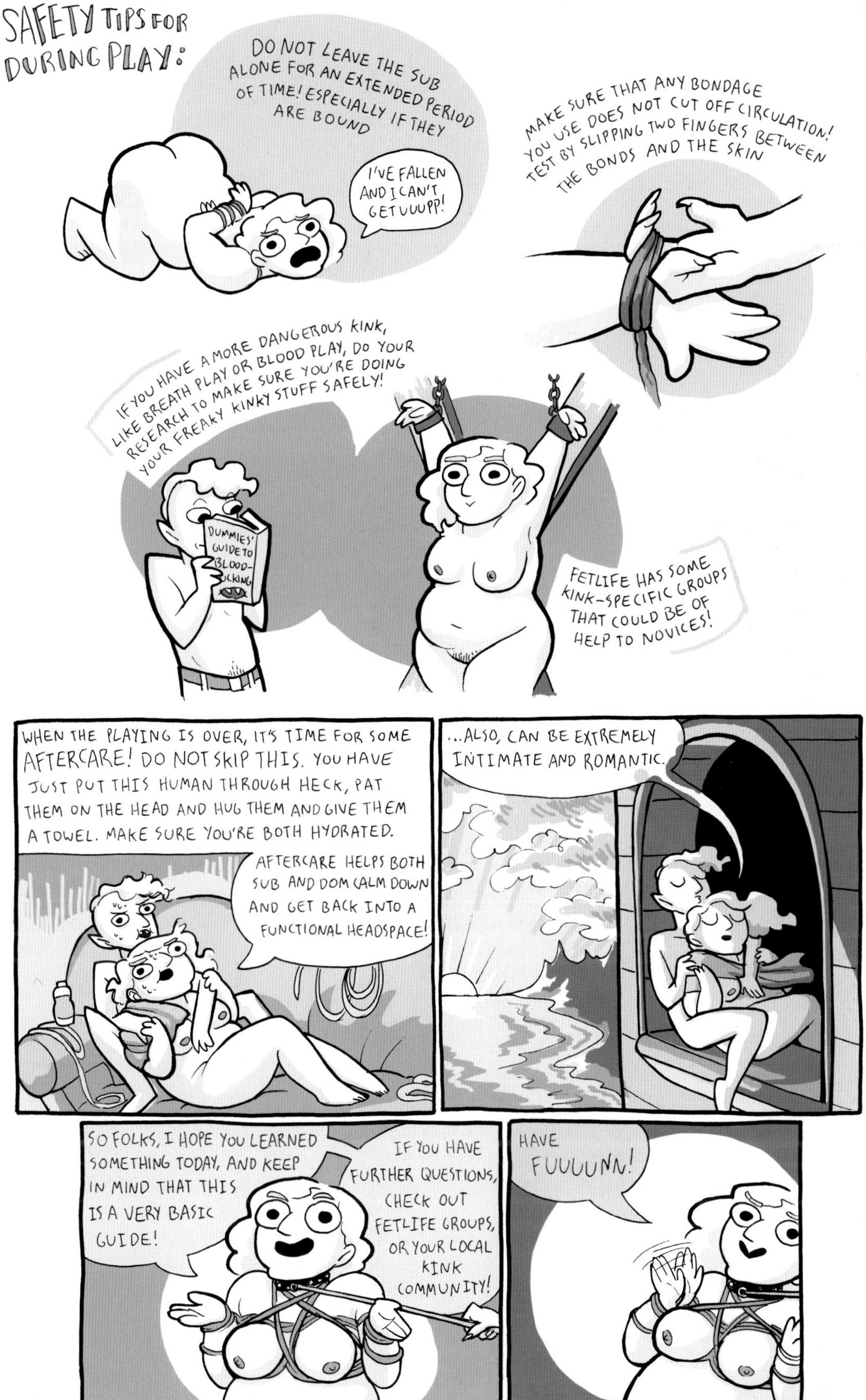

SAFETY TIPS FOR DURING PLAY:

DO NOT LEAVE THE SUB ALONE FOR AN EXTENDED PERIOD OF TIME! ESPECIALLY IF THEY ARE BOUND

I'VE FALLEN AND I CAN'T GET UUUPP!

MAKE SURE THAT ANY BONDAGE YOU USE DOES NOT CUT OFF CIRCULATION! TEST BY SLIPPING TWO FINGERS BETWEEN THE BONDS AND THE SKIN

IF YOU HAVE A MORE DANGEROUS KINK, LIKE BREATH PLAY OR BLOOD PLAY, DO YOUR RESEARCH TO MAKE SURE YOU'RE DOING YOUR FREAKY KINKY STUFF SAFELY!

DUMMIES' GUIDE TO BLOOD-SUCKING

FETLIFE HAS SOME KINK-SPECIFIC GROUPS THAT COULD BE OF HELP TO NOVICES!

WHEN THE PLAYING IS OVER, IT'S TIME FOR SOME AFTERCARE! DO NOT SKIP THIS. YOU HAVE JUST PUT THIS HUMAN THROUGH HECK, PAT THEM ON THE HEAD AND HUG THEM AND GIVE THEM A TOWEL. MAKE SURE YOU'RE BOTH HYDRATED.

AFTERCARE HELPS BOTH SUB AND DOM CALM DOWN AND GET BACK INTO A FUNCTIONAL HEADSPACE!

...ALSO, CAN BE EXTREMELY INTIMATE AND ROMANTIC.

SO FOLKS, I HOPE YOU LEARNED SOMETHING TODAY, AND KEEP IN MIND THAT THIS IS A VERY BASIC GUIDE!

IF YOU HAVE FURTHER QUESTIONS, CHECK OUT FETLIFE GROUPS, OR YOUR LOCAL KINK COMMUNITY!

HAVE FUUUUNN!

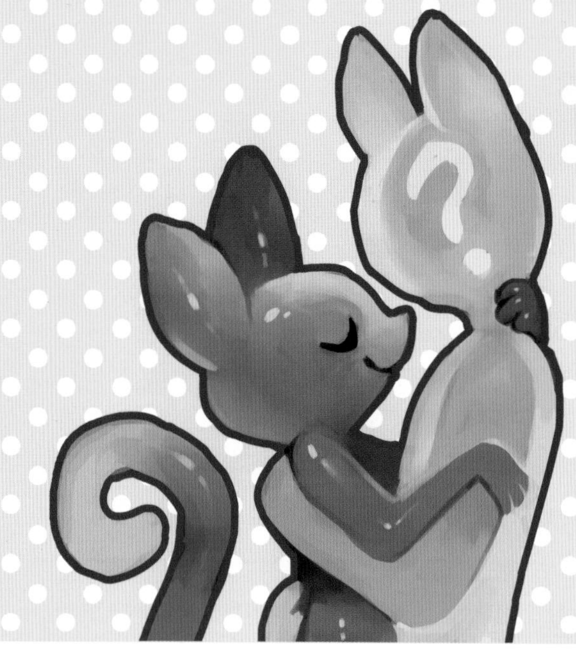

OPEN TO CHANGE

by Purple Kecleon

patreon.com/forbiddenflora

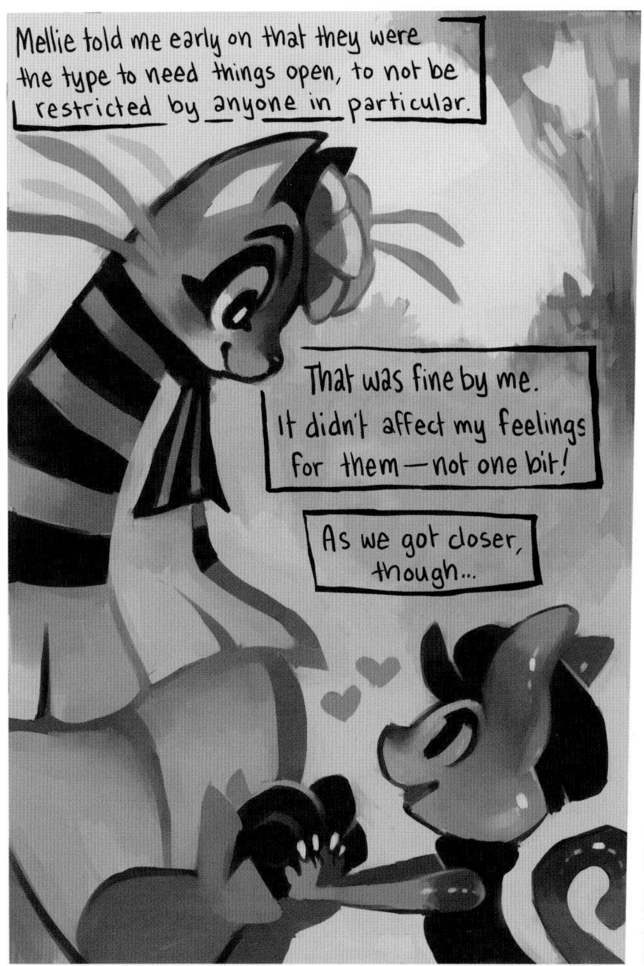
Mellie told me early on that they were the type to need things open, to not be restricted by anyone in particular.
That was fine by me. It didn't affect my feelings for them—not one bit!
As we got closer, though...

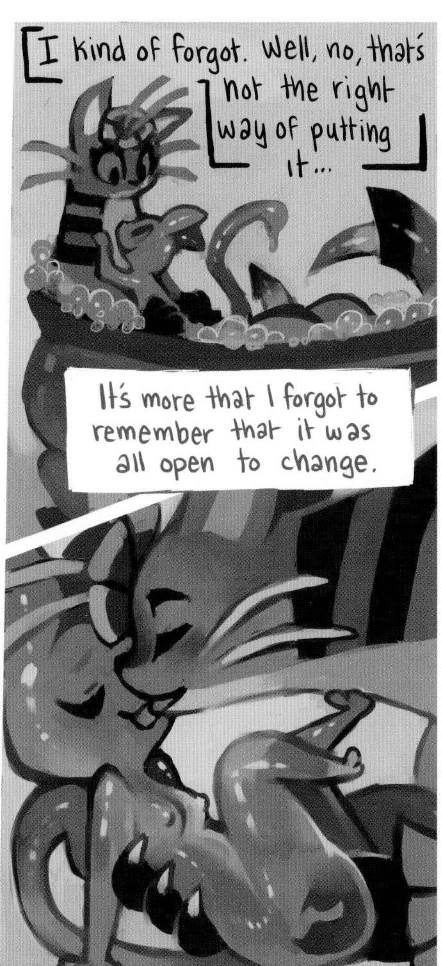
I kind of forgot. Well, no, that's not the right way of putting it...
It's more that I forgot to remember that it was all open to change.

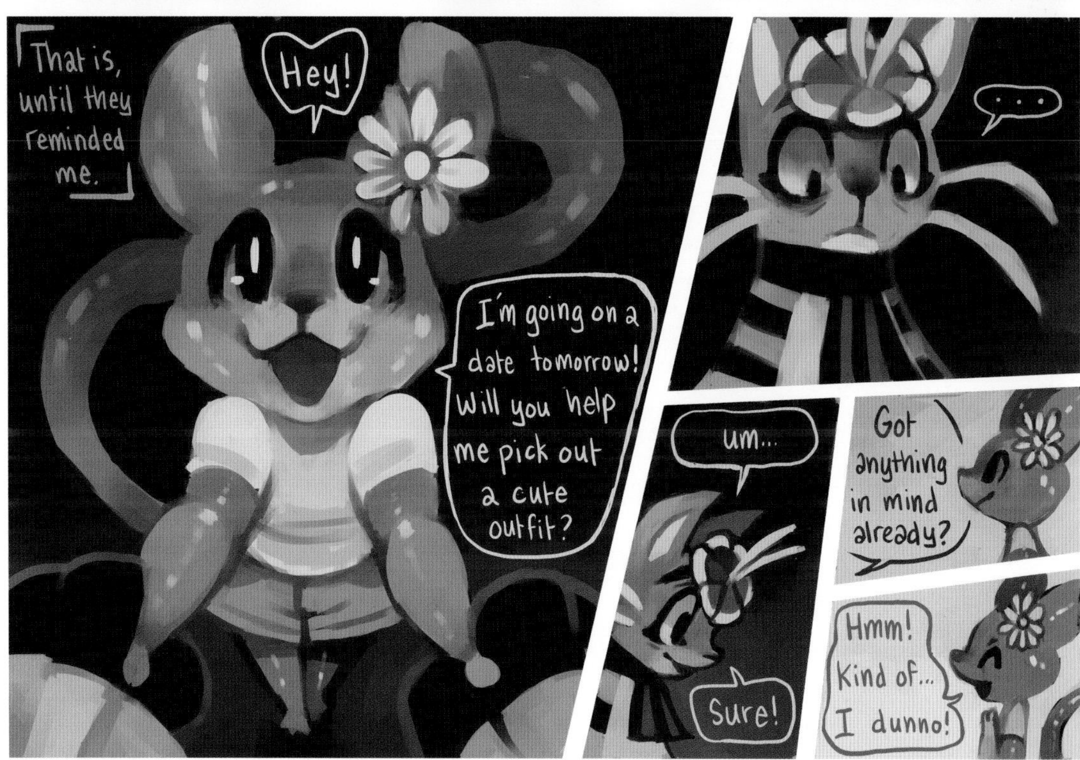
That is, until they reminded me.
Hey!
I'm going on a date tomorrow! Will you help me pick out a cute outfit?
...
um...
Sure!
Got anything in mind already?
Hmm! Kind of... I dunno!

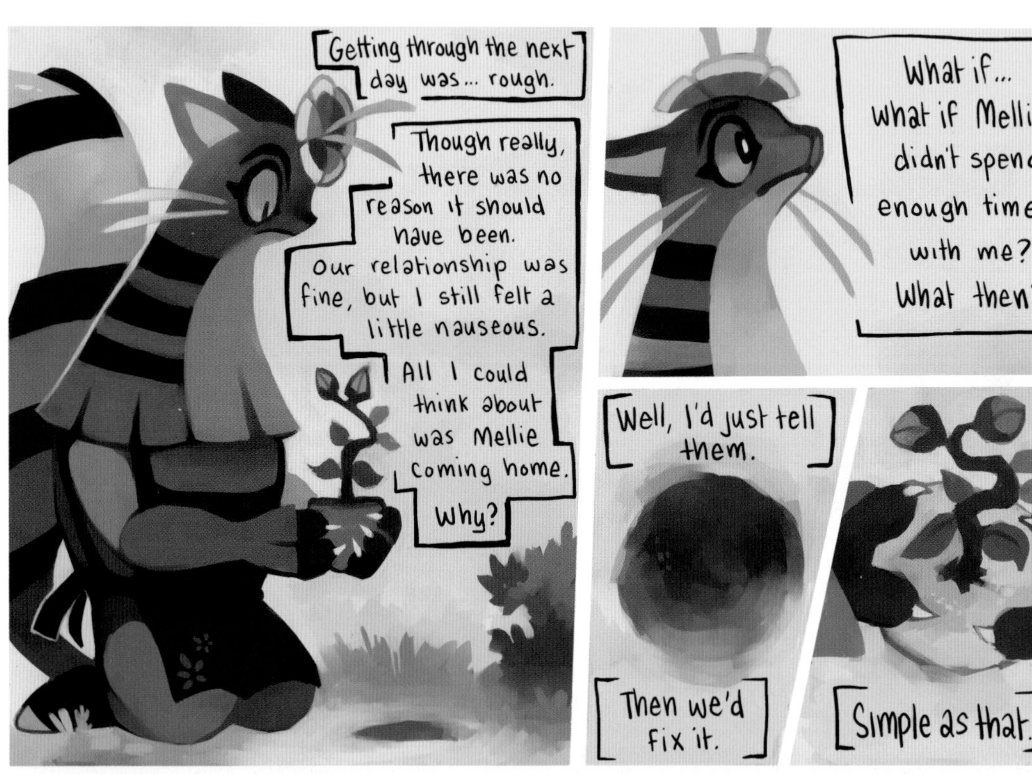
Getting through the next day was... rough.
Though really, there was no reason it should have been.
Our relationship was fine, but I still felt a little nauseous.
All I could think about was Mellie coming home.
Why?
What if... what if Mellie didn't spend enough time with me? What then?
Well, I'd just tell them.
Then we'd fix it.
Simple as that.

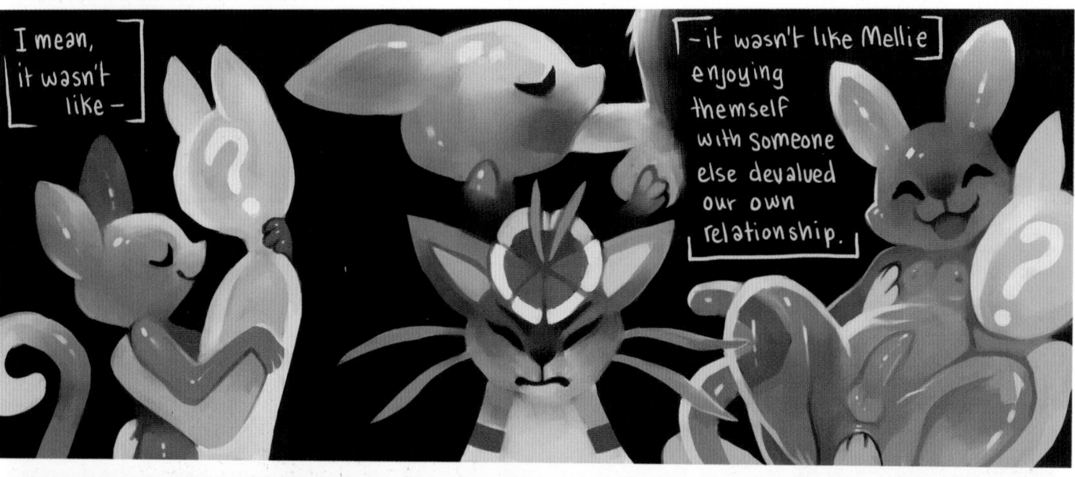
I mean, it wasn't like -
-it wasn't like Mellie enjoying themself with someone else devalued our own relationship.

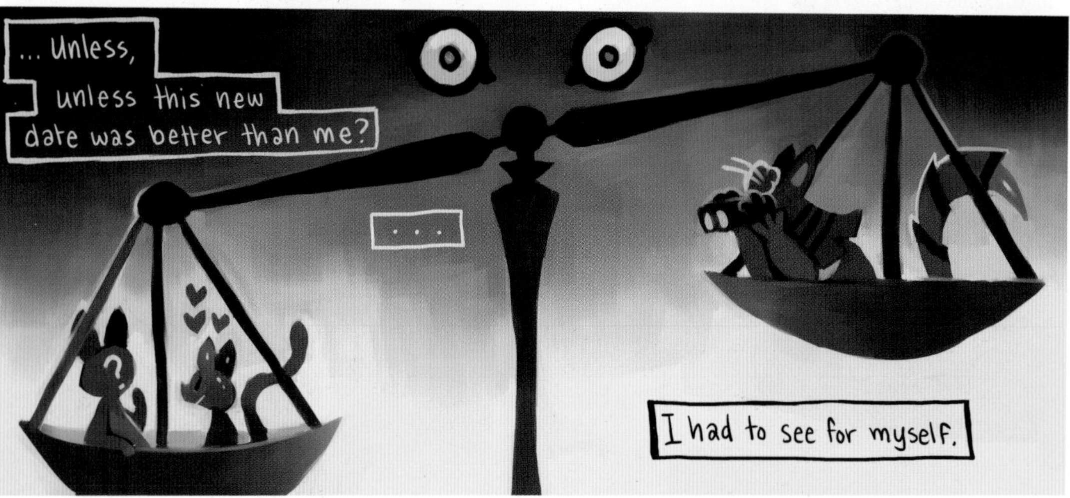
... Unless, unless this new date was better than me?
...
I had to see for myself.

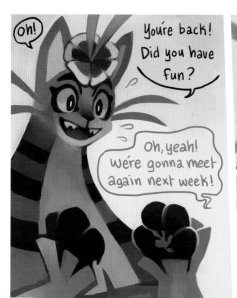
Oh!
You're back! Did you have fun?
Oh, yeah! We're gonna meet again next week!

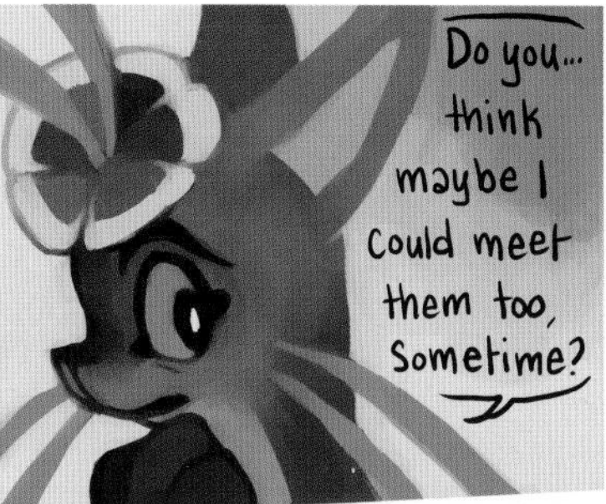
Do you... think maybe I could meet them too, Sometime?

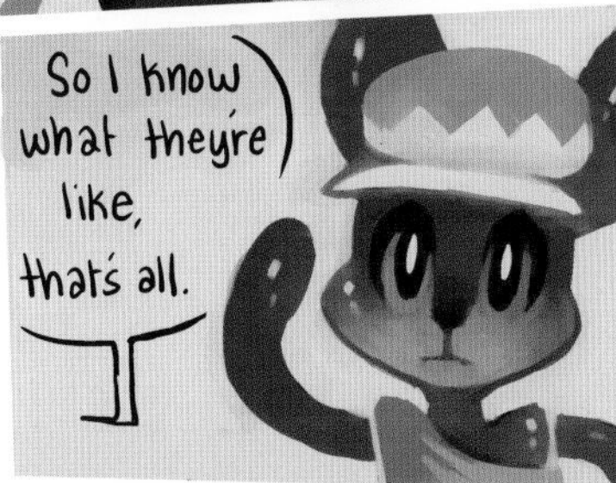
So I know what they're like, that's all.

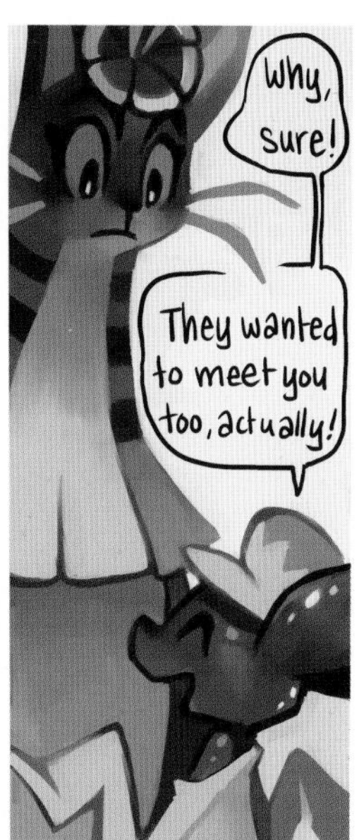
Why, sure!
They wanted to meet you too, actually!

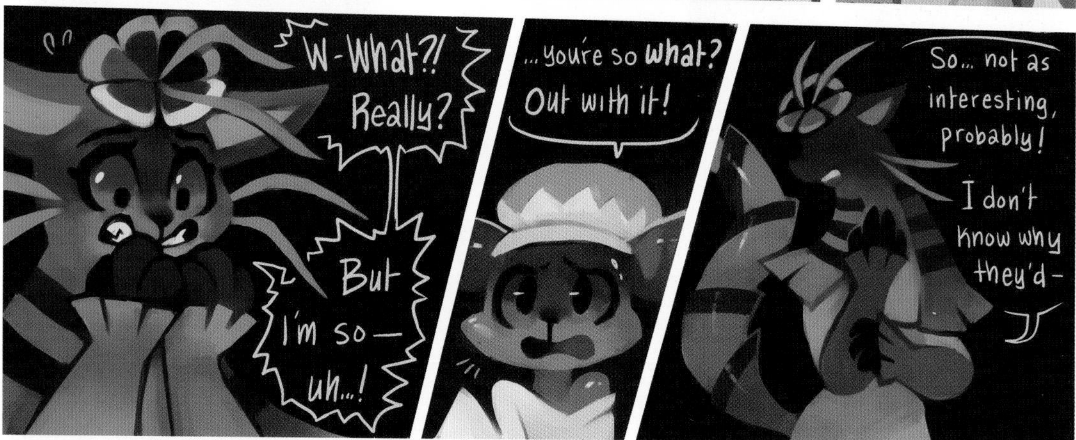
W-What?! Really?
But I'm so— uh...!
...you're so what? Out with it!
So... not as interesting, probably!
I don't know why they'd-

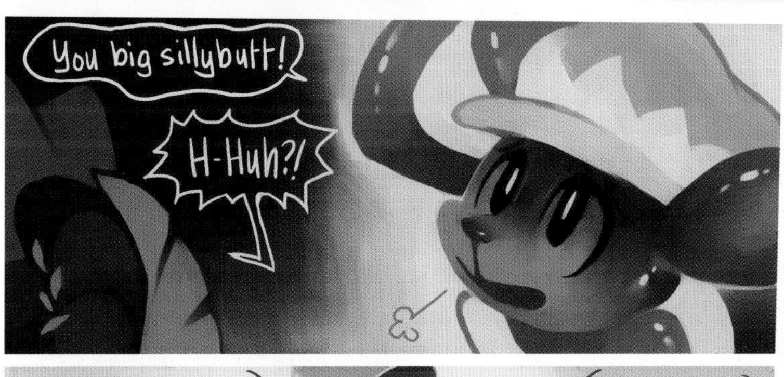
You big sillybutt!
H-Huh?!

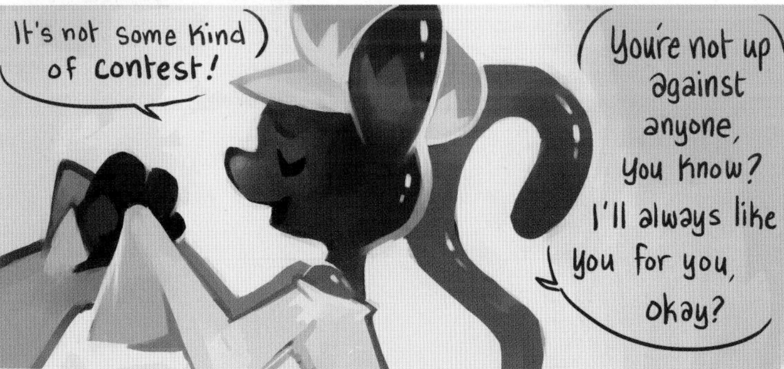
It's not some kind of contest!
You're not up against anyone, you know? I'll always like you for you, okay?

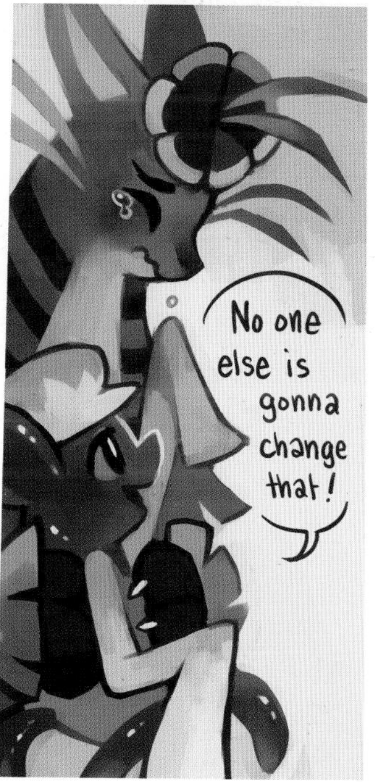
No one else is gonna change that!

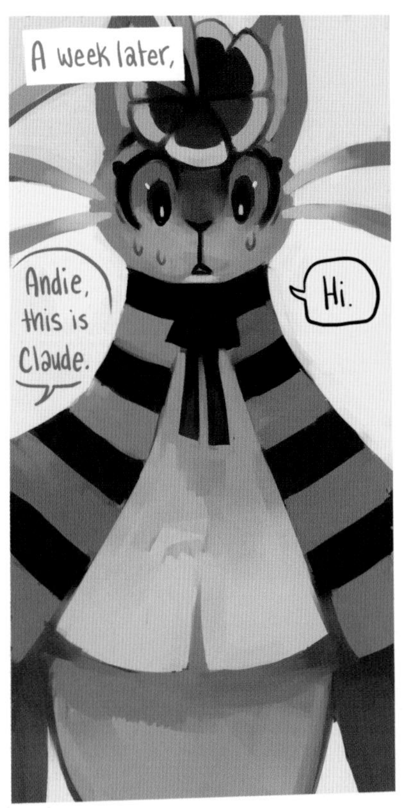
A week later,
Andie, this is Claude.
Hi.

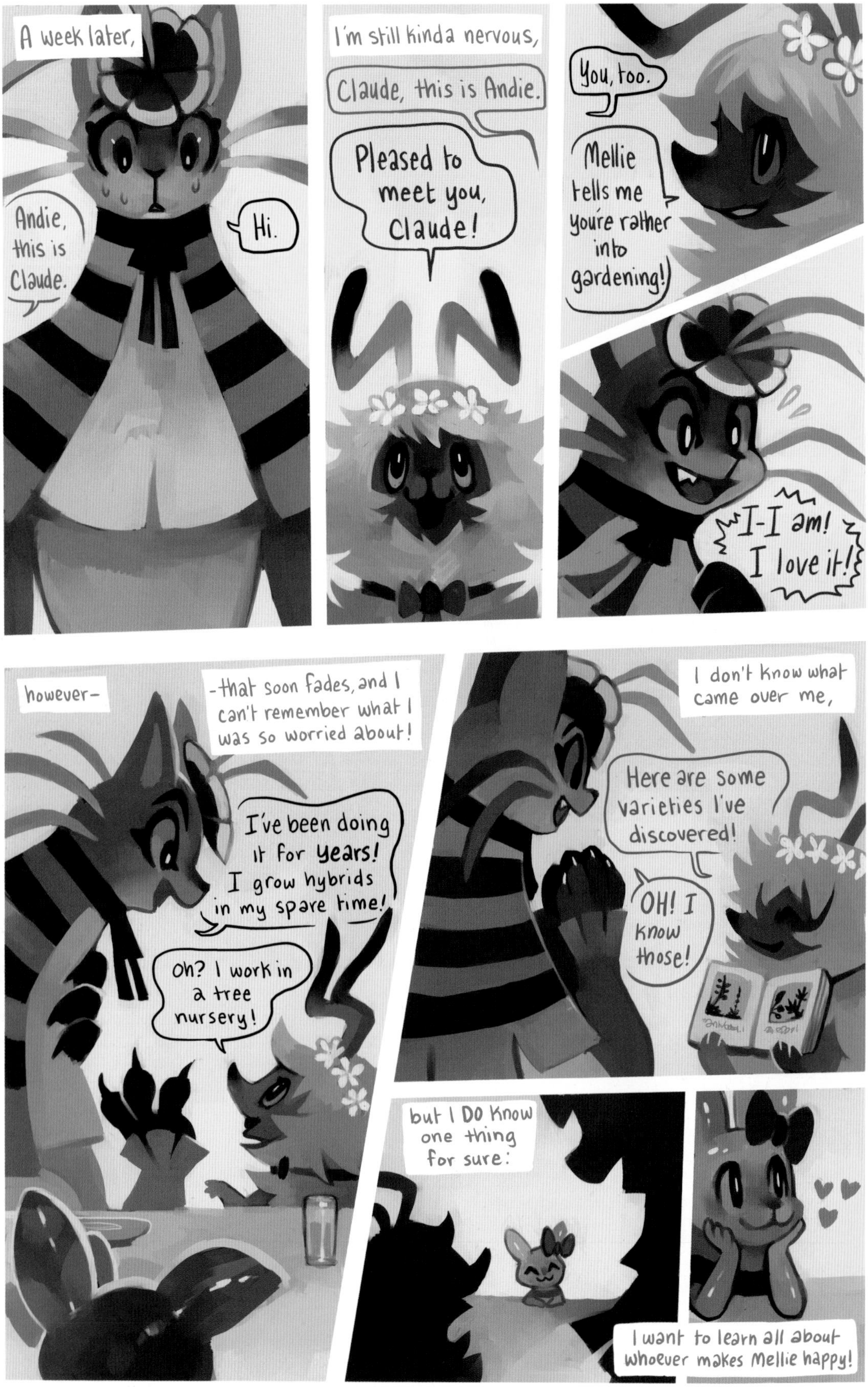

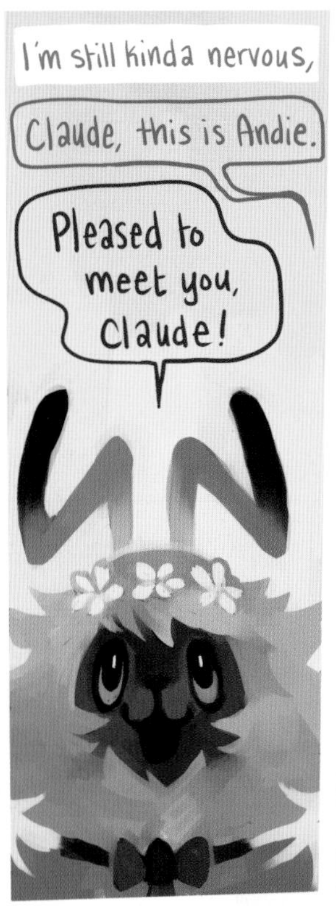
I'm still kinda nervous,
Claude, this is Andie.
Pleased to meet you, Claude!

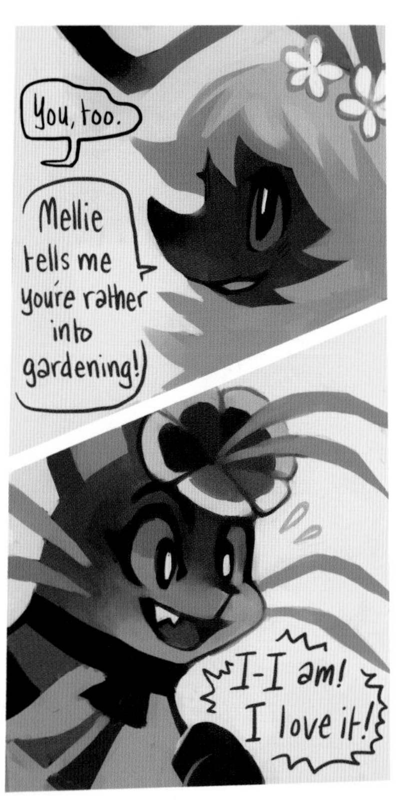
You, too.
Mellie tells me you're rather into gardening!
I-I am! I love it!

however-
-that soon fades, and I can't remember what I was so worried about!
I've been doing it for **years!** I grow hybrids in my spare time!
Oh? I work in a tree nursery!

I don't know what came over me,
Here are some varieties I've discovered!
OH! I know those!

but I DO know one thing for sure:

I want to learn all about whoever makes Mellie happy!

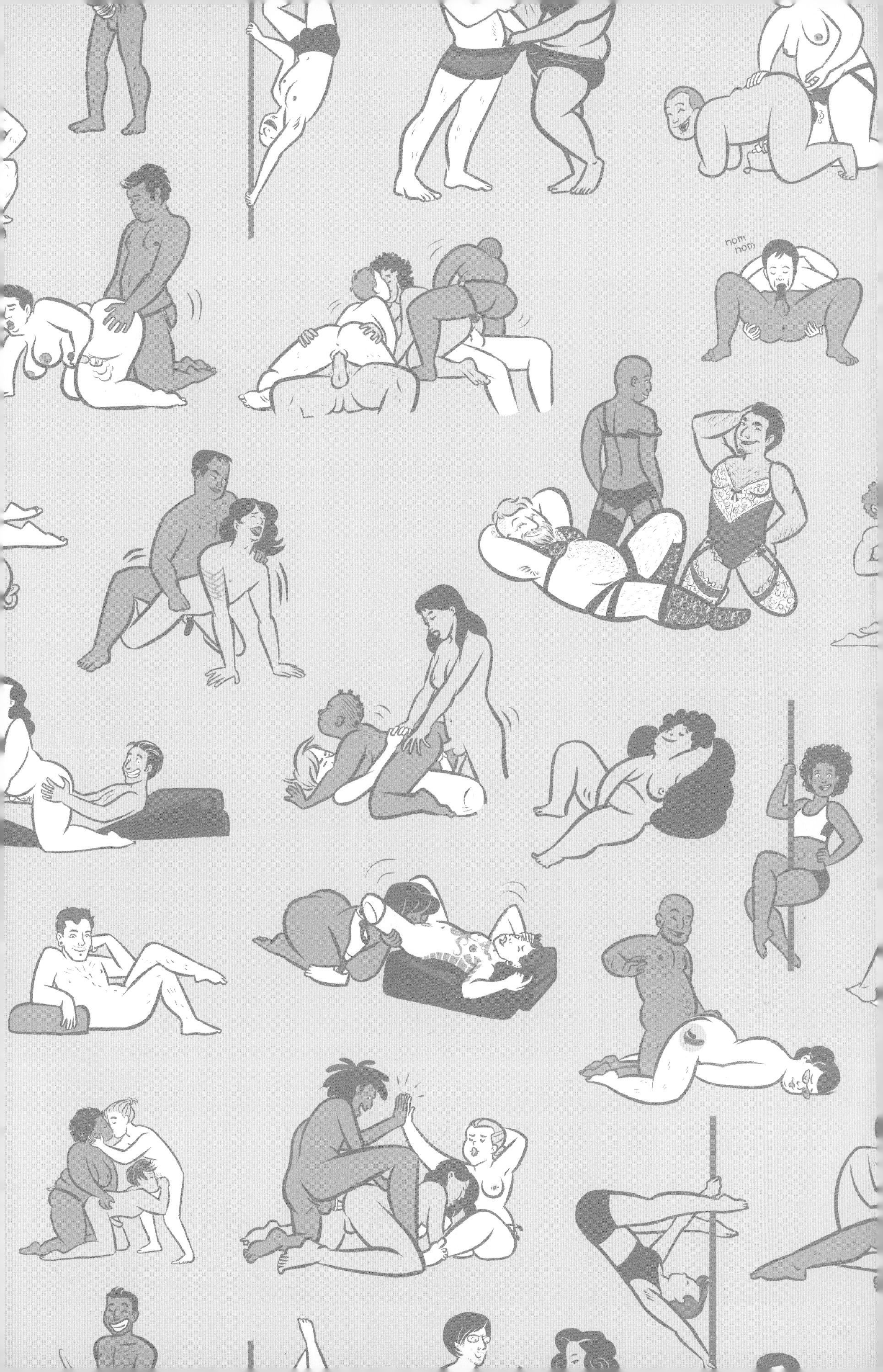
nom
nom

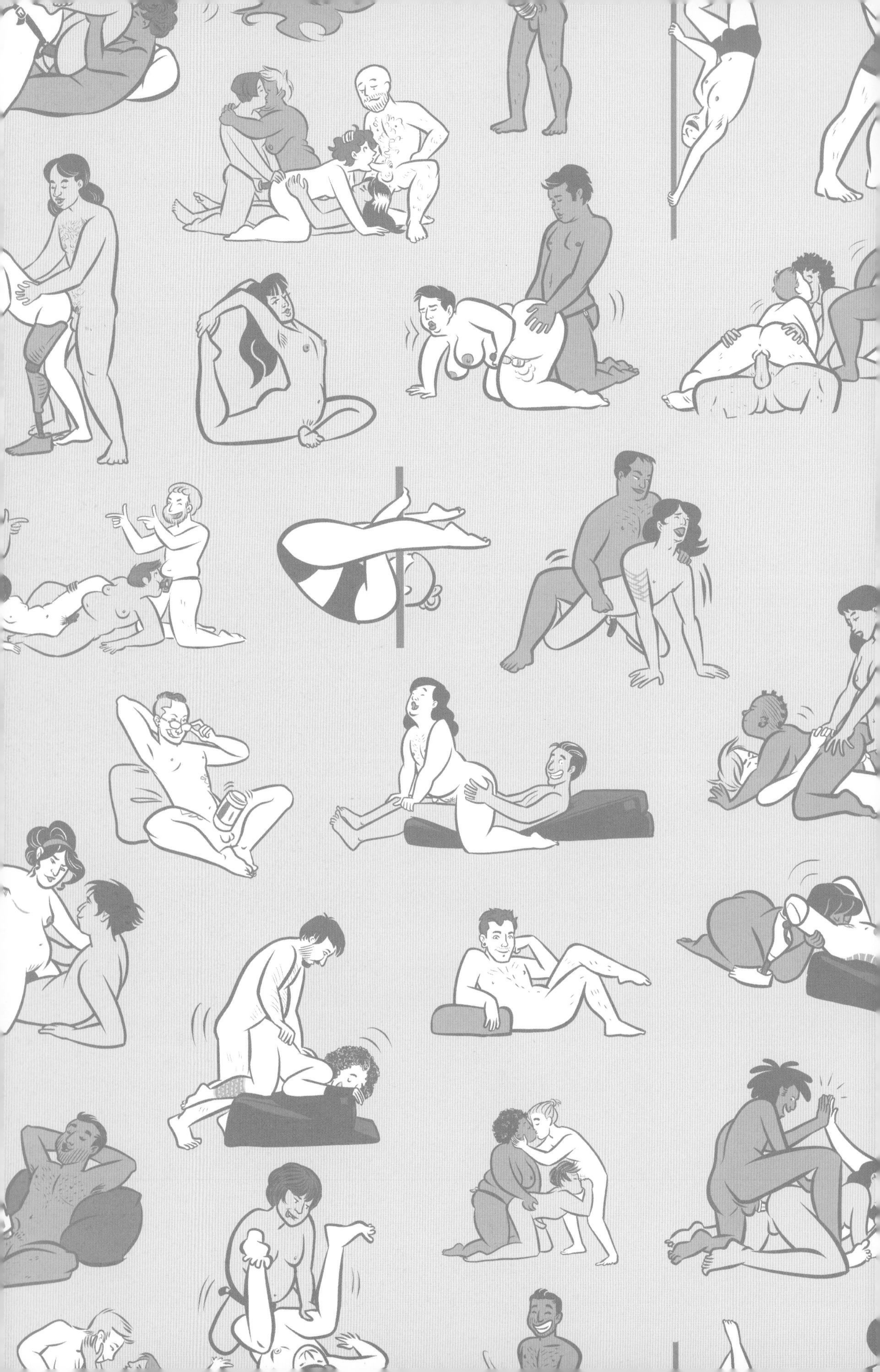

Bonus Material

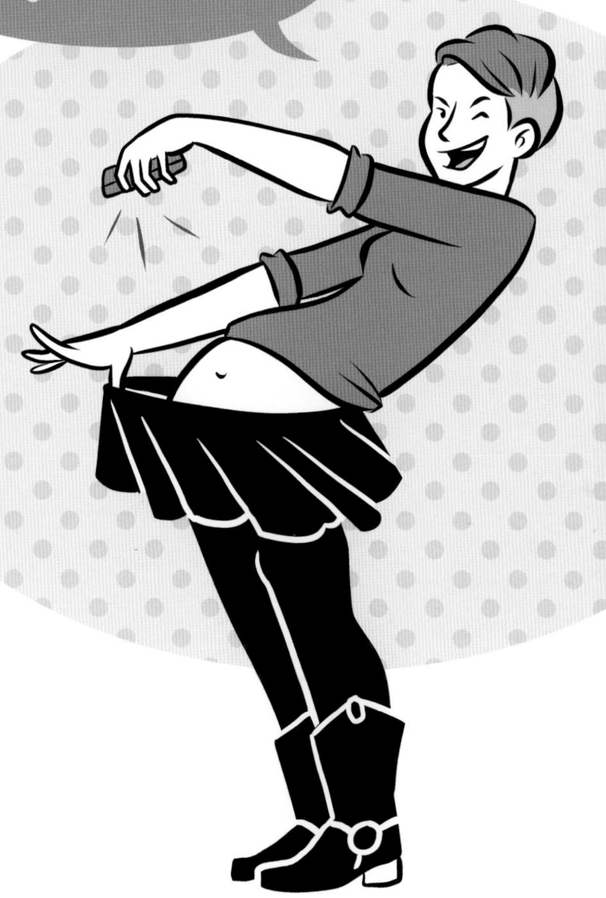

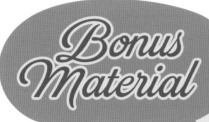

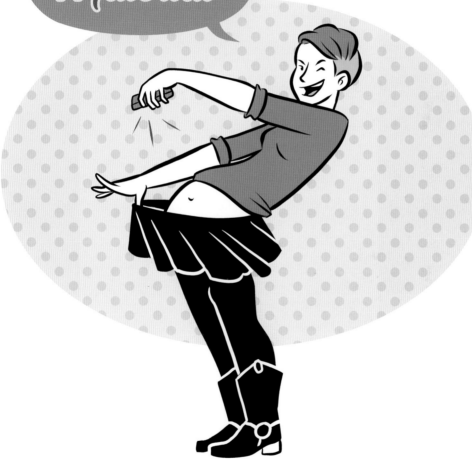

Business Stuff

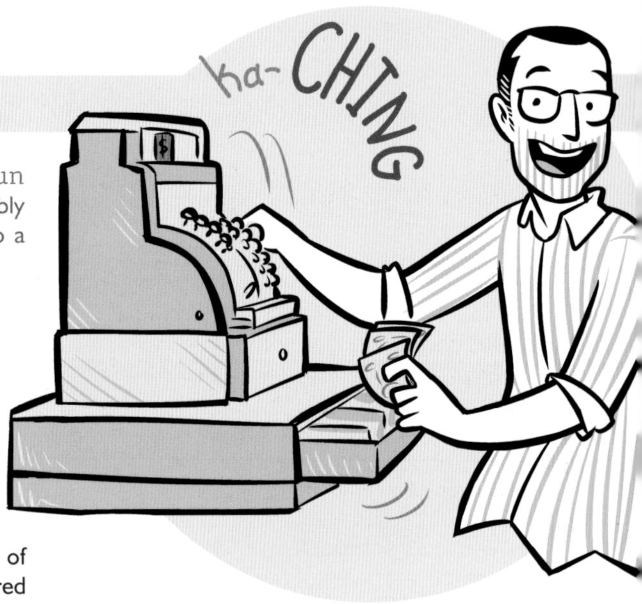

We get a lot of emails asking about how we run Oh Joy Sex Toy as a business and how we could possibly be working on it full time, so I thought I would do a write up on the business side of things!

Oh Joy Sex Toy is a small business that we run out of our home and Erika's space at Periscope Studio. We review sex toys, make education comics and showcase and hire guests artists.

WHERE DO YOU MAKE YOUR MONEY?

I see a lot of people take note of just one or two of our revenue steams and then make assumptions. The reality is we make our living from a BUNCH of different avenues, our business succeeds on a hundred small checks each month instead of any one big check. So where does the money come from?

Affiliate Sales! We're signed up under 21 different affiliate programs. Almost every link on our site is affiliated, so when a purchase is made somewhere we get our tiny cut. From each sale we earn: Amazon 7-8%, sex toy company/shop sales 15-20%, pornography subscriptions 50%.

Licensing! We actively sell licenses for our comics to other websites for a small fee. This fluctuates a bunch month to month.

Merchandising! Books, t-shirts, e-books, all great stuff that adds to our income.

Wholesaling Books! While we don't make much on a per-book basis this way, turning our stock into dollars helps keep the inventory flowing out and our PR with stores/product-reach good.

Patreon! Fans pledge to pay a certain amount for every comic that gets posted each month. This is the lion's share of our monthly income and the reason I can work on this full time! patreon.com/erikamoen

Kickstarter! A different form of income. By pushing pre-sales and pre-orders for our books on this platform we can accumulate wealth to spend on future guest artists (meaning we don't have to spend our own money on them) and not-yet sold book inventory.

Adverts! Maintained by our Hiveworks friend, we run two paid ads on our site!

Each one of these things contribute to the business as a whole and are all fed by the comic's fans. Each thing takes major time and work to maintain, and that does not even including making the comics!

WHAT DO YOU EACH DO?

Both Erika and I are overworked, even after I quit my day job! This is our current weekly setup.

Matt's core responsibilities:

- Chasing up all those affiliate programs
- Doing business emails (3-4 hours a day)
- Doing book design on OJST Vol. 2 and a compilation book of Erika's other comics
- Editing the script (Monday/Tuesday) or writing the script if it's a Matt-toy
- Coloring the comic once the inked pages are done (Thursday-Sunday)
- Recruiting and nagging guest artists to sign contracts & turn in pages
- Organizing and taking point on Kickstarter pre-work, during and post.
- Designing & organizing merch when possible
- Coordinating & planning with our fulfillment company
- Planning, scheduling, number crunching and forecasting.
- Website stuff
- Being pessimistic

Erika's core responsibilities:

- Business account management (includes tax stuff & invoices)
- Responding to business emails (1-2 hours a day)
- Script writing or editing Matt's script (Mondays)
- Comic Layout (Monday-Wednesday)
- Comic Pencils (Tuesdays-Wednesdays)
- Comic Inking (Thursday-Sunday)
- Additional art for the next books (Fridays if we're ahead)
- Sending licensed comics to syndicators
- Delivering wholesale books to local vendors on her bike
- Writing patron-only reports & essays on Patreon
- Correcting the dyslexic spelling of Matt's blog posts
- Being optimistic

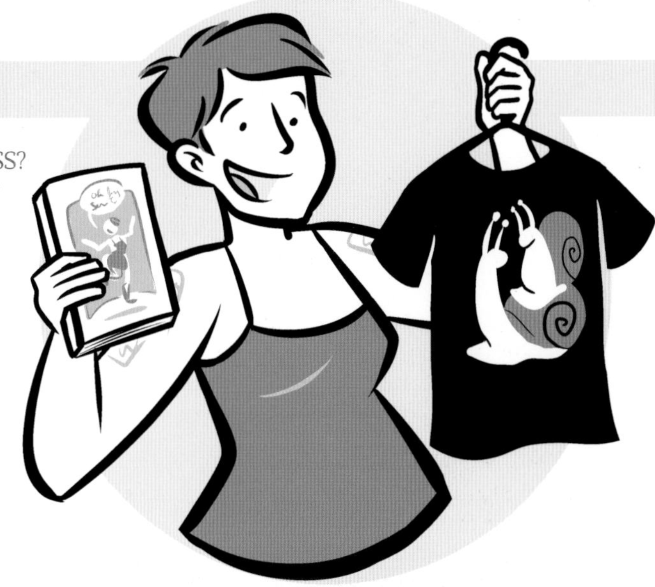

HOW DO YOU EXPECT TO GROW AS A BUSINESS?
Well this is actually a hard question! We've already grown a lot this past year and don't NEED to grow larger than we are. We're not chasing bigger bucks, we're not making a business we can hand down to our grandcats. Our aim is healthy sustainability. We're looking for the best way to keep going without experiencing burnout and enjoying our lives. A lot of small companies that experience early success put a huge emphasis on growth and expansion. There is a real danger of everything folding in and imploding when you rapidly expand, as people forget/never see their limits! We're more than aware of ours and are happy at the level we're at, so we have no plans for expansion.

If we DID want to grow larger, what would we do? Well probably hire a second cartoonist so we could update twice a week, but this would involve a lot of money and organization. There's also the idea of expanding Oh Joy into a brand of review webcomics with a fleet of different awesome talent reviewing non-sex products. But that sort of thing would need 3-4 people on board full time and a truck of cash.

In the short term: a compilation book of Erika's earlier autobio comics and OJST Mobile website are low-priority growth projects.

WHAT'S MY TAKE AWAY HERE?
Well, there's not much to learn here! I suppose you can walk away feeling like you know a little bit more about us as a company, about how we feed ourselves, and how we would want to grow if we weren't happy with the current level of pressure we already have =)
I suppose if you're a webcomicker and are looking for the insider scoop, I would tell you to go make an Amazon associates account right this second. And from today onward if you ever link to anything, make sure it's affiliate-linked up correctly. Those small %s on individual sales really DO add up. I would also tell you to get a no-additional-work, no-tiered-expansion Patreon set up. If you have fans, or are about to accumulate some, giving them an easy option to support your work is awesome. You don't need to bribe them with additional content, if people want to support you because of your comic, that is reason enough for them to back you.

Some handy links!

These may be comics-focused, but the advice in them applies to most people seeking a self-employed career on the internet.

WORK MADE FOR HIRE
workmadeforhire.net
An amazing freelancers/small-business resource.

LETS KICKSTART A COMIC PDF
ironcircus.com/shop
Spike's great comic resource for fresh Kickstarters.

HOW TO MAKE WEBCOMICS BOOK
Webcomic how-to GOLD.

THE WEBCOMICS HANDBOOK
Another how-to gem that we love.

WEBCOMICS.COM
A good informative site with a community of experts you can quiz.

THIS IS EVERYTHING I KNOW
spikedrewthis.tumblr.com
Spike's personal guide on how to "make it" in comics. (Search for this title to find it)

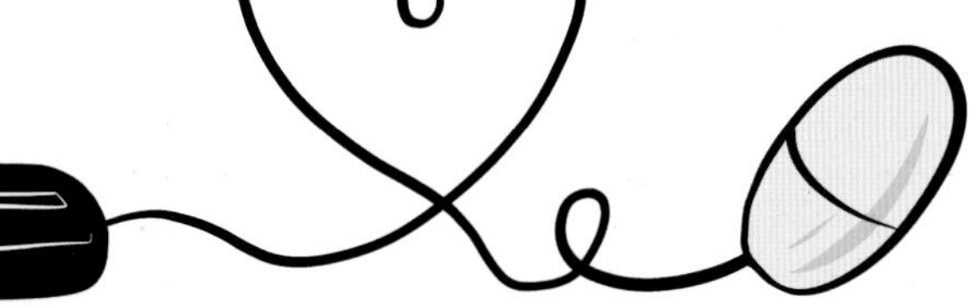

Using Reference

I USE A LOT OF PHOTO REFERENCE FOR OH JOY SEX TOY!

Drawing from photos allows an artist to study a figure thoroughly and pick up on the slight nuances of a posture or expression that they may otherwise not think of if they were drawing purely from their imagination. Or sometimes it's necessary to draw a pose from an extreme angle or an unusual position and a photo is required just to figure out where everything is supposed to go in the first place!

The human body sure can be a real pickle to draw.

Artists creating their own photo reference has a long, rich history. It's easy to find articles online that post a famous artist's reference photo next to their completed, well-know piece— just search for "Reference Photos" along with the names Alphonse Mucha, Norman Rockwell, or Toulouse Lautrec, just to name a few. You can even find videos of costumed actors performing on sets made for Disney artists to animate in classic films like Sleeping Beauty, Peter Pan, and so many more!

Two dozen other cartoonists and I all work in our shared office space at Periscope Studio in Portland, Oregon. At least once a day there's a mini photo shoot of artists posing for other artists so they can get exactly the right pose to draw for whatever comic or illustration they're working on. My studiomates and I are secretly in a ton of mainstream superhero comics! You just... wouldn't recognize us.

Personally, I love love LOVE to see other artist's photo reference. With that in mind, I thought you might enjoy seeing some of mine!

Love, Erika

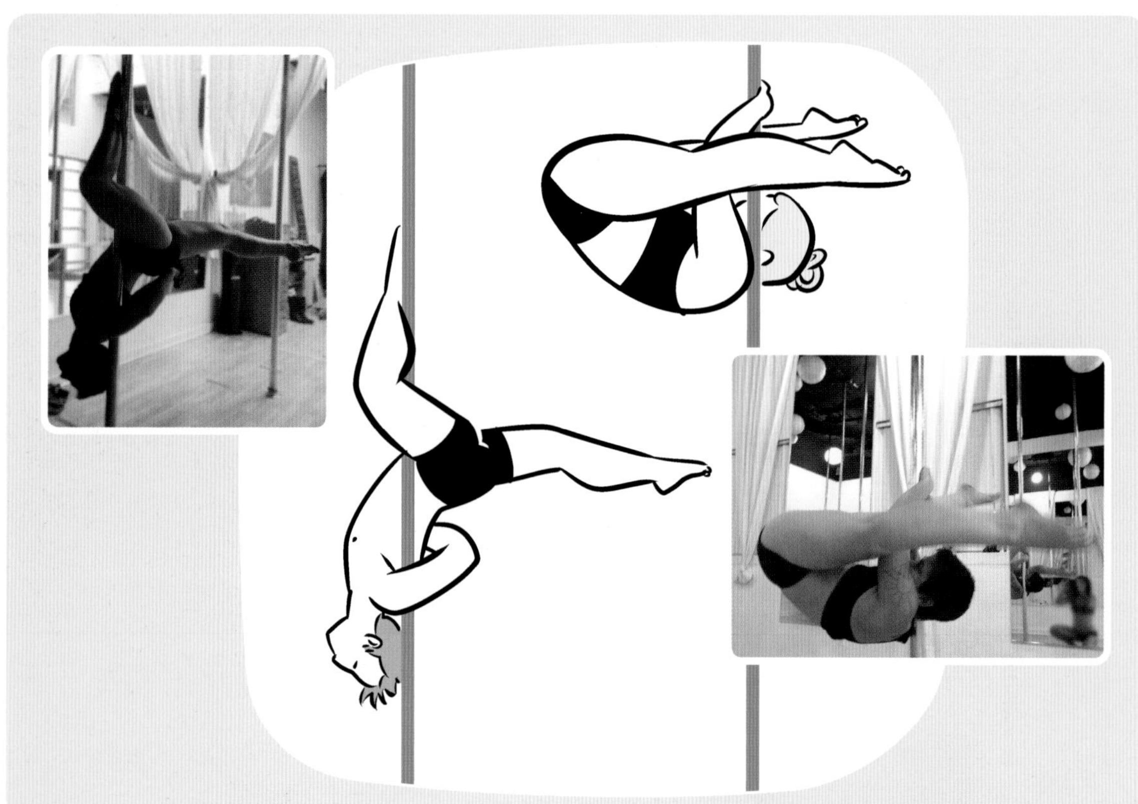

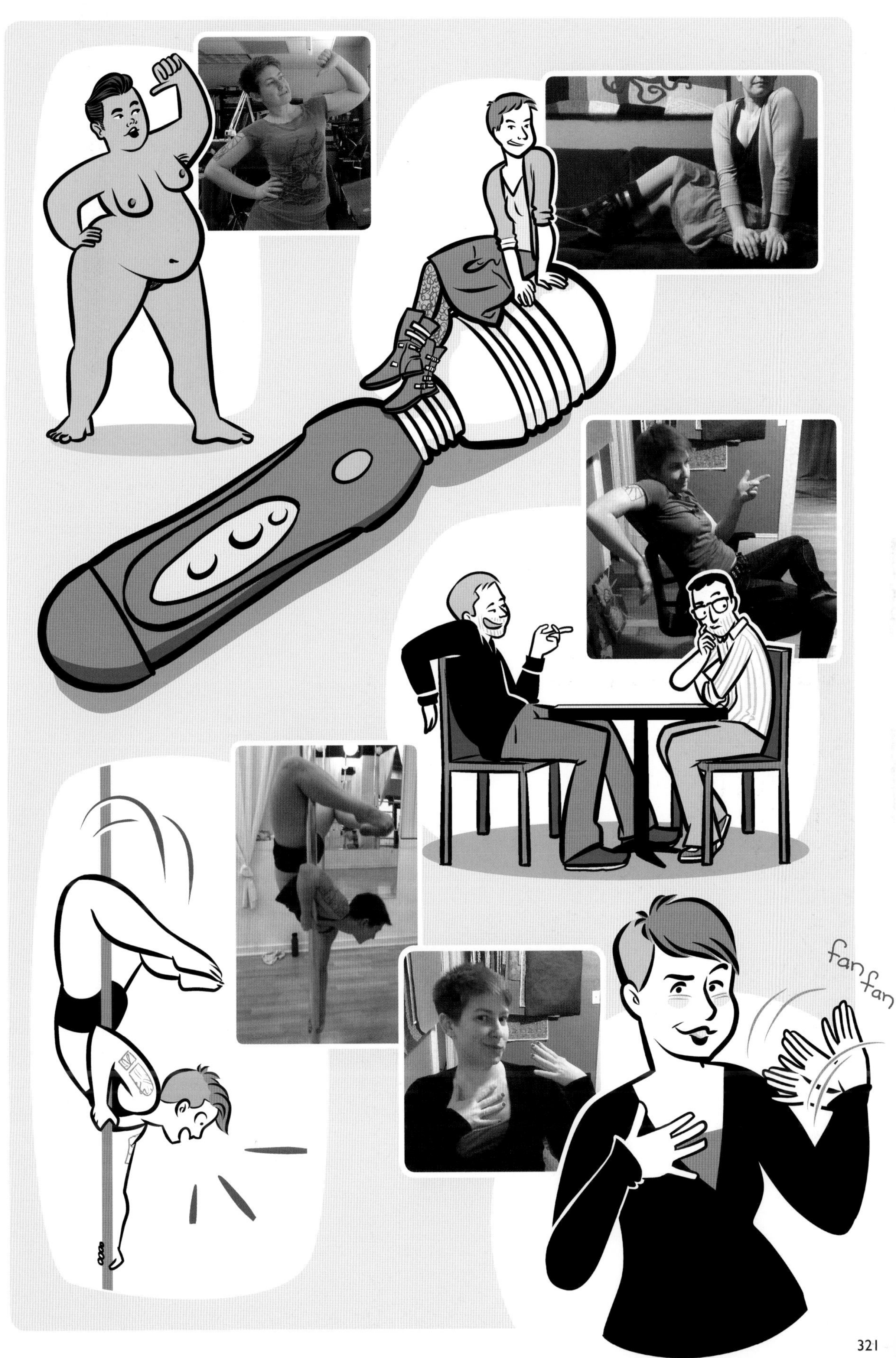
fan fan

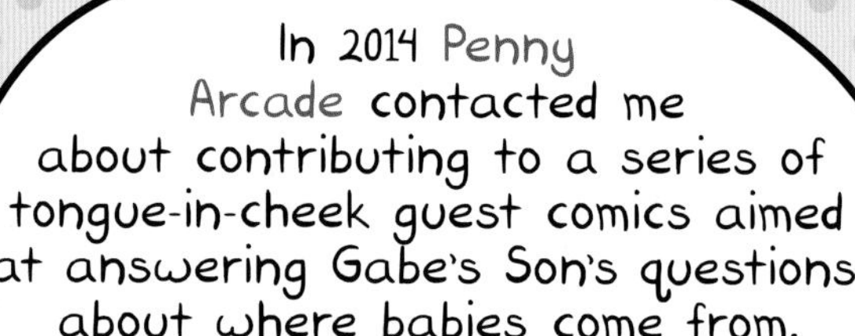
In 2014 Penny Arcade contacted me about contributing to a series of tongue-in-cheek guest comics aimed at answering Gabe's Son's questions about where babies come from.
Here is my answer!

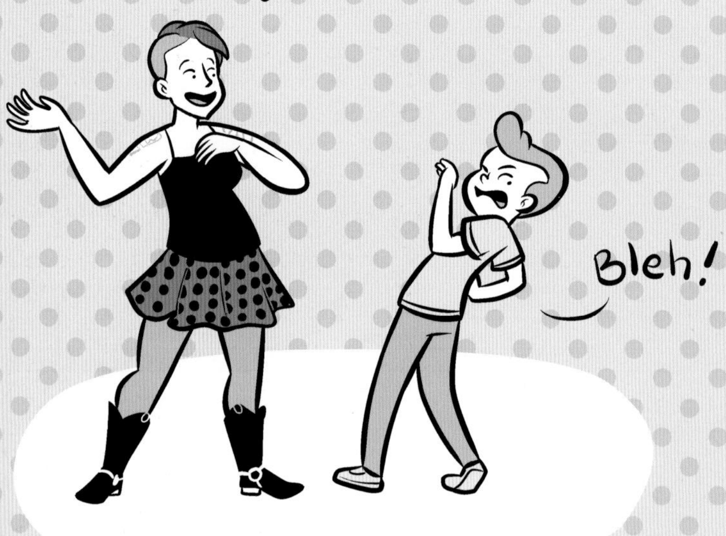
Bleh!

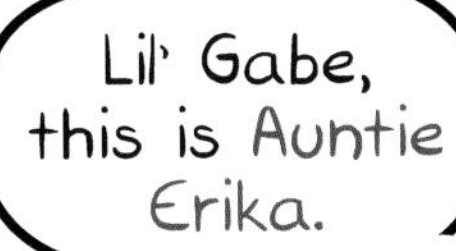

Lil' Gabe, this is Auntie Erika.

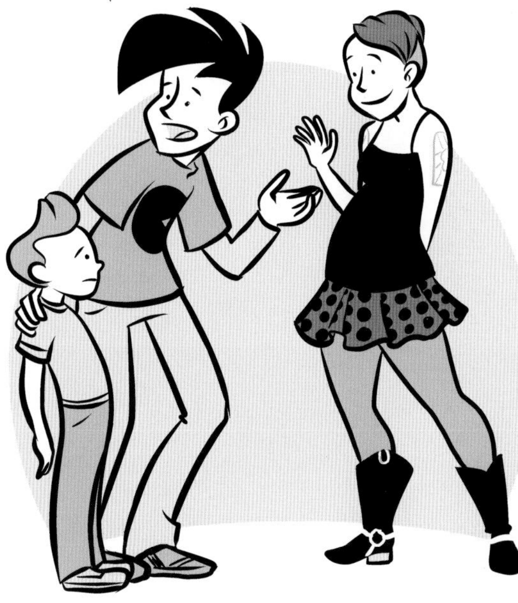

She's a full-time sex toy reviewer and sex education cartoonist, so despite my better judgement I'm going to entrust your malleable young mind in her hands.

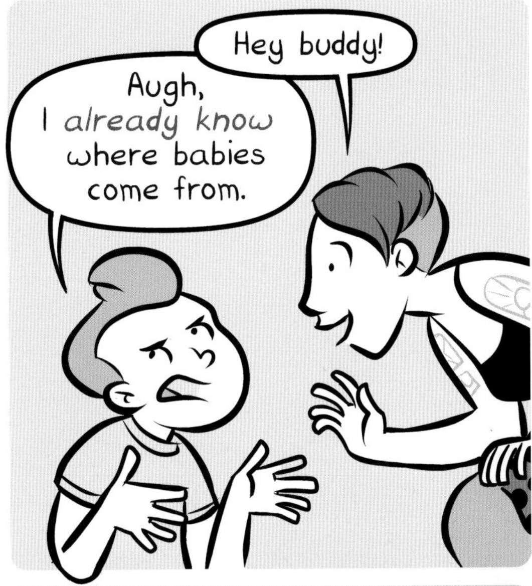

Hey buddy!
Augh, I *already know* where babies come from.

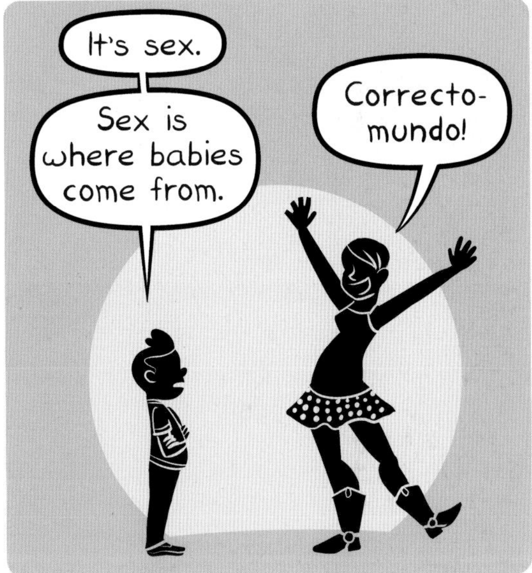

It's sex.
Sex is where babies come from.
Correcto-mundo!

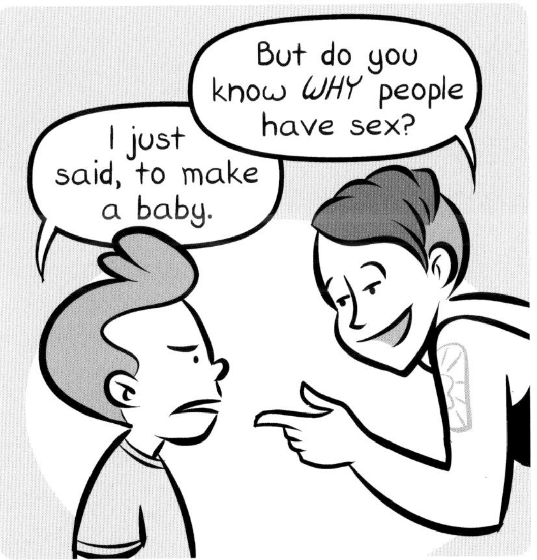

But do you know *WHY* people have sex?
I just said, to make a baby.

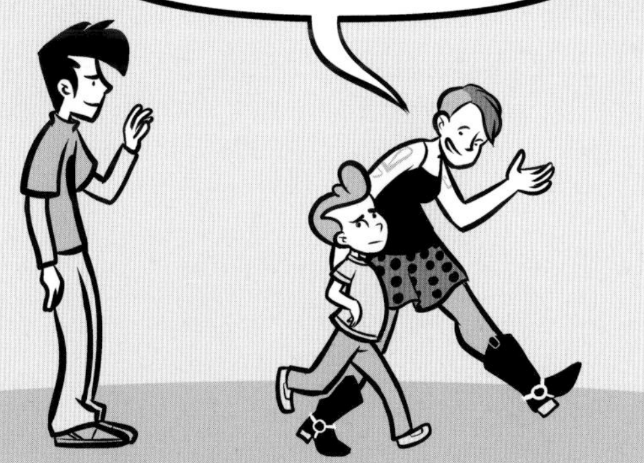

That's definitely why **some** people have sex **some** of the time, but sex actually serves a much bigger role than that.

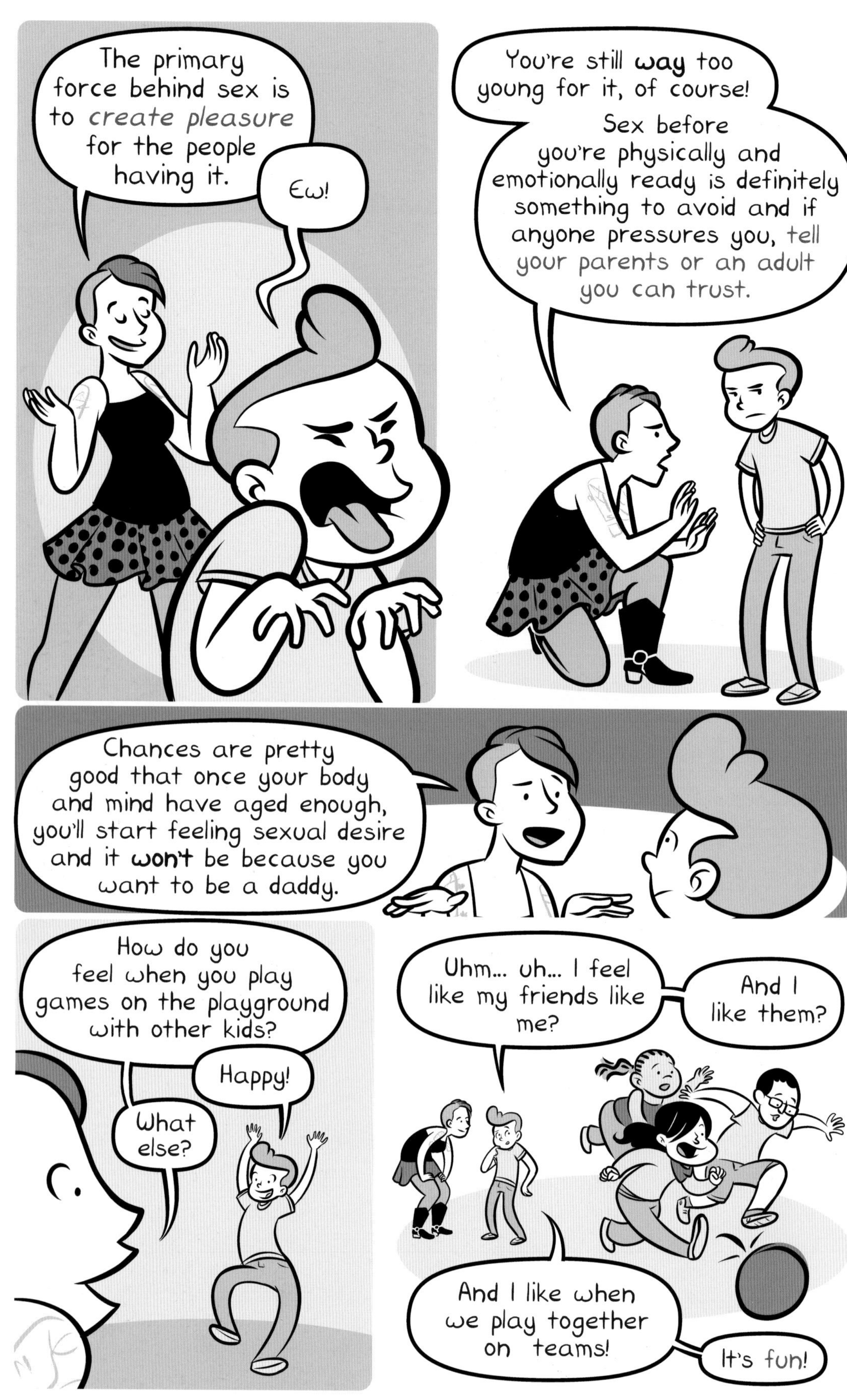
The primary force behind sex is to create pleasure for the people having it.
Ew!
You're still way too young for it, of course!
Sex before you're physically and emotionally ready is definitely something to avoid and if anyone pressures you, tell your parents or an adult you can trust.
Chances are pretty good that once your body and mind have aged enough, you'll start feeling sexual desire and it won't be because you want to be a daddy.
How do you feel when you play games on the playground with other kids?
Happy!
What else?
Uhm... uh... I feel like my friends like me?
And I like them?
And I like when we play together on teams!
It's fun!

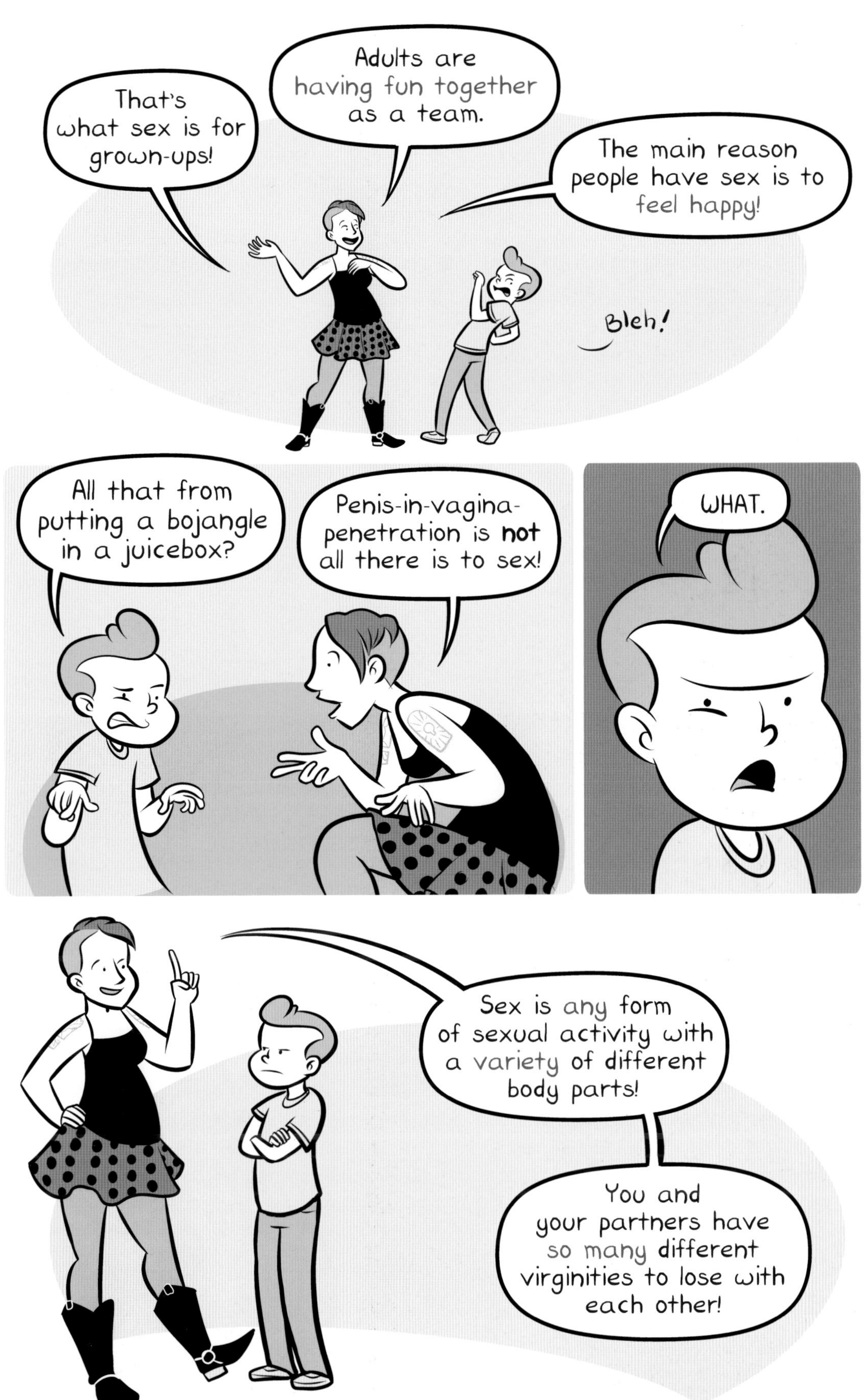
That's what sex is for grown-ups!
Adults are having fun together as a team.
The main reason people have sex is to feel happy!
Bleh!
All that from putting a bojangle in a juicebox?
Penis-in-vagina-penetration is **not** all there is to sex!
WHAT.
Sex is any form of sexual activity with a variety of different body parts!
You and your partners have so many different virginities to lose with each other!

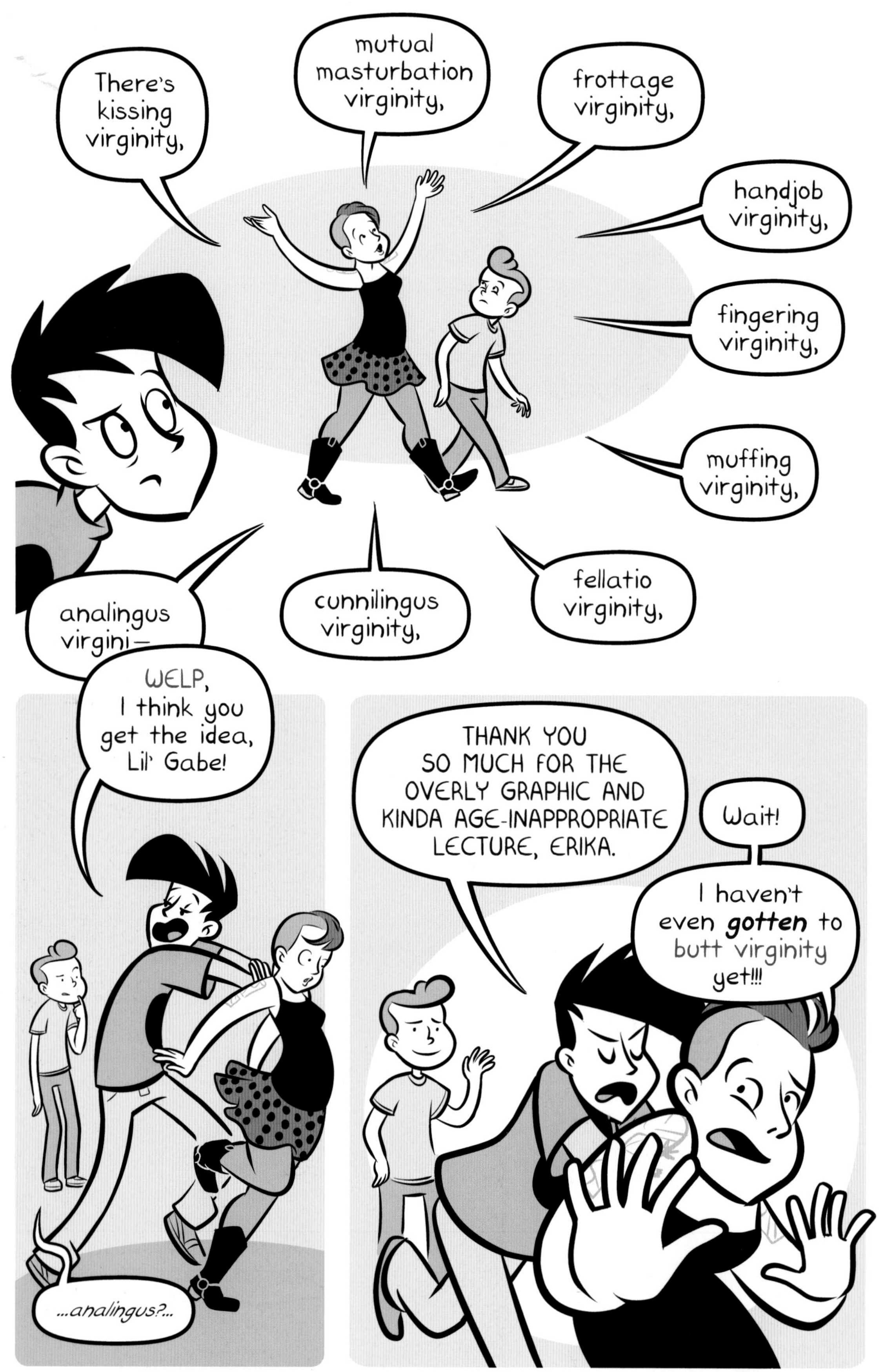
There's kissing virginity,
mutual masturbation virginity,
frottage virginity,
handjob virginity,
fingering virginity,
muffing virginity,
fellatio virginity,
cunnilingus virginity,
analingus virgini—
WELP, I think you get the idea, Lil' Gabe!
...analingus?...
THANK YOU SO MUCH FOR THE OVERLY GRAPHIC AND KINDA AGE-INAPPROPRIATE LECTURE, ERIKA.
Wait!
I haven't even **gotten** to butt virginity yet!!!

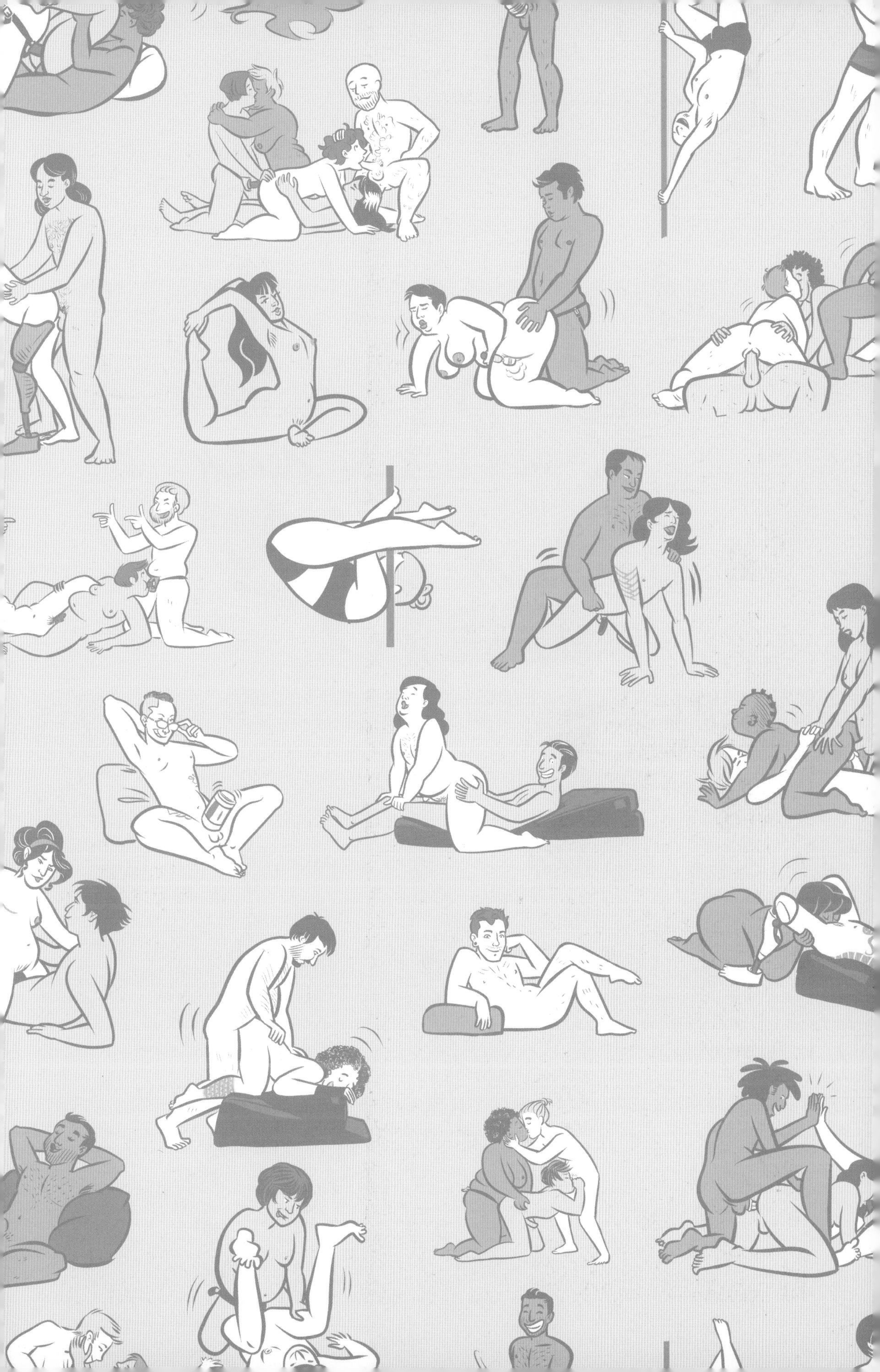

Oh Joy Sex Toy